HEALTH PROMOTION PLANNING

An Educational and Ecological Approach

HEALTH PROMOTION PLANNING

An Educational and Ecological Approach

THIRD EDITION

With a new chapter on technical applications of the Precede-Proceed model by Robert S. Gold of the University of Maryland and Nancy L. Atkinson of Macro International Inc.

Lawrence W. Green
Institute of Health Promotion Research
University of British Columbia

Marshall W. Kreuter
National Center for Chronic Disease Prevention and Health Promotion
Centers for Disease Control and Prevention

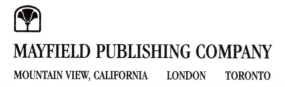

MAYFIELD PUBLISHING COMPANY

MOUNTAIN VIEW, CALIFORNIA   LONDON   TORONTO

Library of Congress Cataloging-in-Publication Data
Green, Lawrence W.
  Health promotion planning : an educational and ecological approach /
Lawrence W. Green, Marshall W. Kreuter. — 3rd ed.
      p.   cm.
  2nd ed. published with subtitle: An educational and environmental approach.
  ISBN 0-7674-0524-2
  1. Health promotion—United States. 2. Health education—United States—
Planning.   I. Kreuter, Marshall W.   II. Title.
RA427.8.G74   1999
613'.0973—dc21   98-52211
                                                                              CIP

Manufactured in the United States of America
10   9   8   7   6   5   4   3

Mayfield Publishing Company
1280 Villa Street
Mountain View, California 94041

Sponsoring editor, Michele Sordi; production, Greg Hubit Bookworks; manuscript editor, Molly Roth; design manager, Jean Mailander; text designer, Diane Beasley; cover designer, Jean Mailander; illustrations, Lotus Art; manufacturing manager, Randy Hurst. The text was set in 10/12 Times Roman by TBH Typecast and printed on 45# Highland Plus by R. R. Donnelley & Sons.

This book was printed on acid-free, recycled paper.

Dedicated, in memoriam, to William Griffiths, Ruby Isom, and Hod Ogden, three mentors and colleagues who helped shape 20th century health education and health promotion as we know them at the millennium.

Brief Contents

Contents

3   Epidemiological Assessment   83

4   Behavioral and Environmental Assessment   111

5   Educational and Ecological Assessment of Factors Affecting Health-Related Behavior and Environments   152

---

6   Administrative and Policy Assessment:
     Turning the Corner from PRECEDE to PROCEED   188

---

7   Evaluation and the Accountable Practitioner   218

Preface

A self-imposed pressure for another edition of this book began soon after the second edition appeared in print in 1991. The movement of the field of health promotion since then has been breathtaking in its pace and exhilarating in the development of its scientific and policy footings. Indeed, even as it was being published, the second edition seemed hopelessly dated by the quickened pace of change. The only solace was that the model retained its place in the toolkits of practitioners and policy makers around the world, even if the book's description of it could not keep pace with the changing circumstances. Users of the model presented in this book continued to apply it to the increasing range of population health, community health, school health, workplace health, and patient health issues. The book was translated in whole or in part into Chinese, Japanese, and French, with versions published in Shanghai, Tokyo, and Montreal. Some 700 applications of the model had been published as articles in the professional and scientific literature when the publisher prevailed on us to get busy with the third edition.

THE ECOLOGICAL APPROACH

With each new edition, we have needed to revise the subtitle to capture the essence of the field's accelerated drift from its health education roots (reflected in our first edition) toward a more comprehensive environmental approach (our second edition), and finally a more multisectoral and multilevel "ecological" approach. Before 1980, the field of action represented by health education and health promotion lacked a clear articulation of its boundaries, of its methods and procedures, and of the distinctions within the field between health education and health promotion. The philosophy, intellectual roots, and systematic descriptions of health education subspecialties were well represented in textbooks, and the research foundation of what was coming to be called health promotion was growing in every direction, including health education.

The contribution we sought to make with the first edition was a conceptual synthesis of these roots and foundations. Based on our academic syntheses of research from the 1970s, we presented a single framework on which disparate new research findings could be hung, a heuristic for theorists and planners, and a practical teaching and learning tool for practitioners, professors, and students trying to make sense of the field. That framework came to be called PRECEDE in the first edition (referring to predisposing, reinforcing, and enabling constructs in educational diagnosis and evaluation). It was further tested during the 1980s by many other academics and practitioners in field applications at local, state, provincial, and national levels, as well as in our own experiences as state, federal, and foundation officers. We collaborated in national efforts in support of disease prevention and health promotion objectives, in community health initiatives including CDC's PATCH program, in the Kaiser Family Foundation's "social reconnaissance" method of community health promotion grant making, and in developing a coalition of organizations in support of a national media-based nutrition campaign. These collaborative and individual experiences led us to question some of the limitations of PRECEDE and to formulate the additional policy, regulatory, and organizational constructs for educational and environmental development, which we called PROCEED. The second edition was thus born in 1991 with the new subtitle, "An Educational and Environmental Approach."

Since then, each of us has pursued yet different courses in our careers, one returning to academia in Canada, one embarking on a private-sector effort to support health planning, implementation, and evaluation. The field has rushed on and we have rushed to keep up with it, or to catch up with it, in bringing the experience of the 1990s to bear on this third edition. These experiences have confirmed our assumption in the second edition that what we characterized then as a combination of educational and environmental approach to health promotion was essentially an ecological approach.

What had been a growing interest in the social environmental dimensions of health in the 1980s became a revival of the ecological perspective on population health in the 1990s. This perspective demanded more than merely taking forces outside the person into account in planning programs. It demanded an intersectoral, interdisciplinary, and interorganizational strategy for integrating the forces operating at several levels and in various spheres to support people in their efforts to gain greater control over the determinants of their health.

OTHER EMERGENT EMPHASES OF THE 1990S

Besides the ecological renaissance in health promotion, the field responded to other challenges in the 1990s. Population health demanded a shift toward placing greater emphasis on the distal determinants of health, such as social conditions and policies—beyond the immediate risk factors that had preoccupied health promotion in the 1980s. Health promotion also concerned itself increasingly with coalition formation, capacity building, and sustainability as dimensions of community organization and development. In the United States, it centered increasingly on decentralized community organizations and managed care; in Canada on devolution from federal to provincial health care renewal. Participatory planning and the self-care movement converged on a growing interest in participatory research to arm citizens and consumers of health care with a greater capacity to control their own health and to develop the knowledge to do so. Participatory research for the planning and for the evaluation or monitoring of programs was emphasized in the second edition, as were capacity building and decentralized planning, but they take on new meaning in the third edition with the emerging language and the new fiscal implications of these thrusts in policy.

One consequence of participatory and decentralized planning has been a shift in focus from exclusively biomedical outcomes to increasingly holistic aspects of health, which people consider more important today than health professionals did in the past. The shift to quality of life in evaluation of medical care and to social impact in population health policy assessment has been entirely consistent with the previous editions of this book. Quality of life and social impact assessment have been the starting point in the PRECEDE planning process from its beginnings in cost-benefit analysis and its roots in community development approaches to public health planning. We have merely aligned the language in the third edition more squarely with the 1990s terminology and research on these aspects of health promotion.

NEW TECHNOLOGIES AND PARTICIPATORY APPROACHES

Knowledge development was once a matter mostly of search or research. With the explosion of new information and communication technologies in the 1990s, the search for existing knowledge became a task of sifting and managing the glut of information now seemingly all too accessible. As John Naisbitt (1982) said in *Megatrends,* "We are drowning in information and starved for knowledge" (p. 24). If accelerating and expanding the dissemination and diffusion of information were health promotion issues of the past decades, one needs to replace, at least, acceleration with organizing and applying information more strategically. Practitioners increasingly turned to PRECEDE-PROCEED to help them match, and sometimes reconcile, the "best practices" knowledge from research conducted afar with the information and knowledge generated locally on the problem, population, and circumstances at hand. The indigenous knowledge of a community did not always align with the evidence-based guidelines coming from research conducted elsewhere, with different people, at a different time.

The opportunity to work with Robert Gold in developing applications of PRECEDE-PROCEED with new technologies came to us in the early 1990s. A grant to Macro International from the National Cancer Institute in the United States and one to the University of British Columbia from the National Cancer Institute of Canada made possible a collaboration reflected in the new final chapter of this edition. We are indebted to Bob Gold, Nancy Meyer Atkinson, and Maria Fernandez for their contributions to the invention and development of the software we gave yet another acronym, EMPOWER (Enabling Methods of Planning and Organizing Within Everyone's Reach). Mike Chiasson, a postdoctoral fellow, along with Chris Lovato, Dawne Milligan, Louise Potvin, and other colleagues at UBC's Institute of Health Promotion Research, helped in the further development, internationalization, and field testing of the software. Mike has carried us onward in the development of our web integration of PRECEDE-PROCEED with a more generic application of the concepts, methods, and research evidence into NETPOWER. We have also developed a web site to support the users of this book on an ongoing basis.

OTHER CHANGES

Besides the change in our subtitle, reflecting the main theoretical reorientation of the field in the 1990s, and the addition of a new chapter on technological applications, reflecting the main methodological advances in this decade, this edition brings a few more changes. One of the most notable is the change in labels for phases in the model from "diagnosis" to "assessment." This change was not merely a concession to those who resented the medical bias they saw in the word *diagnosis* and the apparent contradiction they found therefore in the terms *social diagnosis* and *educational diagnosis,* among others. We could have ridden that storm out on the argument that medicine does not own the word *diagnosis.* We substitute *assessment* because of another compelling nuance of the nineties. Communities have risen up against the tendency of politicians, professionals, and official agencies to start with their problems, to ignore their inherent strengths and assets, and to "diagnose" their needs. We owe debts of gratitude to John McKnight and Peter Benson for their superb efforts to illuminate that very point. We incorporate McKnight's "asset mapping" approach in Chapter 2 and Benson's concept of "development assets" in Chapter 10.

Within this expanded scope, we continue to emphasize an educational approach to health promotion as the essential starting point, even when the ultimate interventions must be more coercive, regulatory, or economic. Indeed, the public support and acceptance of new legislation and regulation depends on adequate preparation of the electorate through education. Many good legislative bills that would have improved the public's health have failed to pass or have been repealed because their sponsors failed to build an educated constituency for them. The continuing commitment to an educational approach to health, even within the political context of health promotion, is reflected in the subtitle of this edition.

Our continuing attempt to address the essentially political dimension of health promotion has brought a further departure from our more strictly scientific and technological approach to health education in the first edition. At that time, we tried to avoid ideological traps by taking a value-free stance with respect to methods, except for one overriding principle or philosophy: that behavior change should be voluntary. We remain committed to that educational philosophy in this edition, and it remains the basis for the development of an educational approach as an extension to a more purely ecological approach. At the same time, we recognize that the social policy targets of health promotion sometimes call for aggressive and even coercive measures to regulate the behavior of those individuals, corporations, and government officials whose actions influence the health of others. The essential rule of thumb we suggest for justifying more coercive means of changing behavior or lifestyle is when the behavior in question threatens the health or well-being of others, such as drunk driving or the promotion of unhealthful products to children. This rule runs into gray areas, of course, when the alleged threat to the well-being of others is something more remote, such as the long-term economic cost to society incurred by people who smoke or engage in other high-risk behavior today that *might* result in chronic illness or disability later. It also runs into value conflicts with constitutional protections such as the right to free speech, which protects advertising as well as the press and the individual.

As we come to grips with more and more of these value-laden choices in health promotion, we must develop and sharpen the political understanding and skill of those who plan health promotion programs. We have put this burden particularly on Chapter 2, which focuses on the quality-of-life assessment or "social diagnosis." There we emphasize methods of assuring the active involvement of people in assessing their own needs and evaluating their own progress and programs. This is especially relevant at the local level, where values can be weighed within the context of the social culture and economy. Again, the educational perspective prevails, with the emphasis on participation and enabling people to take greater control of the decisions influencing their quality of life, but we have tried to reflect more of the political realities in carrying out this frequently neglected phase of the assessment process.

ACKNOWLEDGMENTS

The frameworks for planning and evaluation presented in this text grew out of our combined and cumulative experience in practice, research, teaching, consultation, and government service, all guided and enriched by significant teachers, colleagues and students. PRECEDE included an amalgamation of Ronald Andersen's Behavioral Model of Families' Use of Health Services; Albert Bandura's social learning theory; Hochbaum, Rosenstock, and Becker's Health Belief Model; J. Mayone Stycos' decision model on couples' adoption of family planning methods; Kurt Lewin's force-field analysis; and Edward E. Bartlett's Methods and Strategies in Health Education. These models influenced our ways of thinking about health and planning. Equally influential was our collaboration at Johns Hopkins University in the late 1970s with Joshua Adeniyi, Edward Bartlett, Robert Bertera, Lee Bone, Judith Chwalow, Wendy Cuneo, Lawren Daltroy, Sigrid Deeds, Sharon Dorfman, Michael Eriksen, Donald Fedder, Marion Field-Fass, Jack Finlay, Susan Fischman, Andrew Fisher, Brian Flynn, Stuart Fors, Pearl German, Andrea Gielen, Josephine Gimble, Myron Hatcher, Elizabeth Howze, Haille Kahssay, Howard Kalmer, David Levine, Carol Lewis, Frances Marcus Lewis, Virginia Li, Donald Morisky, Patricia Dolan Mullen, Kay Partridge, Barbara Rimer, Debra Roter, Rima Rudd, Julliette Sayegh, Makhdoom Shah, Nasra Shah, William Ward, Richard Windsor, and others.

PROCEED was a product of the Health Field Concept of Laframboise and the Lalonde Report for Canada and ecological concepts revived in epidemiology during the 1970s. It was influenced centrally by our experience in the U.S. federal initiative in disease prevention and health promotion with Julius Richmond, James O. Mason, Michael McGinnis, Martha Katz, Hod Ogden, Dennis Tolsma, Henry Montes, Donald Iverson, Lloyd Kolbe, Patricia Mullen, and others. This era included the opportunity to participate in the development of the first round of national objectives in disease prevention and health promotion, the Model Standards for Community Preventive Health Services, and participation in similar processes with several state and local health agencies. Our increased emphasis on implementation issues was influenced by work with Judith Ottoson, Bruce and Denise Simons-Morton, and Susan Brink. Our increased emphasis on participatory research methods was influenced by work on the Background Paper for the 1983 World Health Assembly, work at CDC in developing the PATCH program, and work at the Kaiser Family Foundation in developing the social reconnaissance approach to community health grant making. More recently, opportunities to prepare reports—on participatory research in health promotion for the Royal Society of Canada, on the issue of measuring social capital in public health programs for CDC, on both drug abuse prevention and linking research and practice for the National Academy of Science, on Health Impact Assessment for Health Canada, and on coalitions for the Health Services Administration—have influenced this edition.

For sabbatical opportunities to work on the book and the software supporting it and for chances to observe overseas applications, we are indebted also to Gerjo Kok, Patricia Van Assema, Evelyne deLeeuw, and Hein de Vries at the University of Maastricht in the Netherlands, and to Rob Sanson-Fisher at Newcastle University in Australia. We also thank colleagues in the World Bank, the World Health

Organization, the HealthWays Foundation and Victoria Health Promotion Foundation in Australia, the Kansas Health Foundation, the National Cancer Institute of Canada, and the National Health Research Development Program.

Besides the students, fellows, and colleagues we acknowledged in the first and second editions, we are indebted to the following, among others, for additional insights, helpful suggestions and feedback from their experience with PRECEDE-PROCEED: John Allegrante, Kay Bartholomew, Charles Basch, Allan Best, Bob Cadman, Margaret Cargo, Treena Chomik, Mark Daniel, Nicole Dedobbeleer, Willy de Haes, David DeJoy, Shafik Dharamsi, Margo Dijkstra, Mark Dignan, Ron Dovell, Suzanne Duke, Garry Eggar, Jack Farquhar, Stephen Fawcett, Edwin Fisher, Jerold Floyd, Vincent Francisco, C. James Frankish, Anne George, Dean Gerstein, Gary Gilmore, Gaston Godin, Robert Goodman, Nell Gottlieb, Carol Herbert, Harry Hubball, Bonnie Jeffery, Joy Johnson, Jack Jones, Laura Kann, Lloyd Kolbe, Fred Kroger, Dick Levinson, Chris Lovato, Marjorie MacDonald, Karen Mann, Patrick McGowan, Heather McLeod Williams, Ken McLeroy, Susan Mills, Charles Nelson, Gary Nelson, Michele O'Neill, Elan Paluck, Guy Parcel, Louise Potvin, John Raeburn, Pamela Ratner, Marilyn Rice, Lucie Richard, Irving Rootman, Jean Shoveller, Bruce and Denise Simons-Morton, David Sleet, Joan Wharf Higgins, Sally Willis Stewart, Abraham Wandersman, and Lynne Young.

We also thank the following people for their helpful reviews of the third edition: Patti Herring, Loma Linda University; Michael Peterson, University of Delaware; and Janet S. Reis, University of Illinois.

The final compilation of revisions and development of a workbook and web site to go with this edition were facilitated by Mike Chiasson, Jim Frankish, Wendy Klein, Glen Moulton, Pam Ratner, and Mary Sun at UBC and Sonja Greene, Nicole Lezin, and Laura Young at Health 2000. Michele Sordi took over from Serina Beauparlant as our editor at Mayfield. She and her assistant, Bessie Weiss, provided patient encouragement and support throughout the revision process. April Wells-Hayes and Greg Hubit handled production arrangements for Mayfield. We are also grateful for our outstanding copy editor, Molly Roth, who helped make this edition more readable than the last.

Lawrence W. Green, Vancouver
Marshall W. Kreuter, Atlanta

Chapter 1

Health Promotion and a Framework for Planning

We shall begin this chapter by reviewing some of the historic, economic, ecological, and epidemiological reasons for health promotion's emergence as the best hope of long-range improvements in quality of life and population health.[1] This chapter also introduces the two components of the health-planning framework. The first is an assessment phase referred to as **PRECEDE**[2] (for *pre*disposing, *re*inforcing, and *e*nabling *c*onstructs in *e*ducational/*e*cological *d*iagnosis and *e*valuation). The second is a developmental stage of planning that follows the assessment and initiates the implementation and evaluation process. This second component is called, conveniently, **PROCEED** for *p*olicy, *r*egulatory, and *o*rganizational *c*onstructs in *e*ducational and *e*nvironmental *d*evelopment.

HEALTH PROMOTION'S EMERGENCE OUT OF HEALTH SCIENCES, POLICY, AND ORGANIZATION

Most scholars, policy makers, and practitioners in this field would pick 1974 as the point in history that marks the beginning of the health promotion era. In that year, Canada published its landmark policy statement, *A New Perspective on the Health of Canadians.*[3] In the United States, Congress passed Public Law 94-317, the Health Information and Health Promotion Act, which created the Office of Health Information and Health Promotion, later renamed the Office of Disease Prevention and Health Promotion. This set in motion the effort now known as *Healthy People 2000,* a decidedly objective, evidence-based setting of goals and targets for health promotion and disease prevention.

1

Historical roots of health promotion

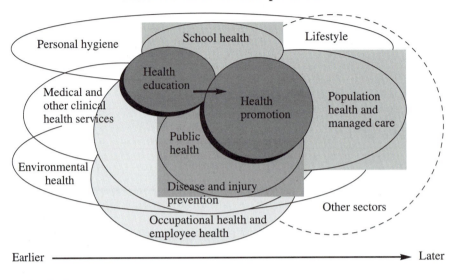

FIGURE 1-1

A relatively new sphere of policy, programs, and practice, the emergence of health promotion is a product of several historical movements and applied sciences in health.

Figure 1-1 locates health education and promotion in relation to their historical roots. Each of the earliest spheres of policy, programs, and practice remains viable and active in its own right. The evolution and interaction of each has produced new conditions with the emergence of new fields of policy and practice bearing on health.

Health promotion draws on those health sciences, programs, practices, and policies that relate to the health of human populations. We must move beyond the tidy boundaries of health institutions, for much of what relates to the health of human populations happens in other sectors, such as schools, industry, social services, and welfare. Other sectors of growing importance to health include recreation and transportation, building and waste management, taxation and regulation, and commercial services and trade. The questions we have struggled with increasingly in recent years are whether the expanded scope of health **policy**, **programs**, and practice, along with the other determinants of health, makes greater precision of measurement and intervention less relevant to the health of populations. Precision has been the hallmark of studies that make individuals the unit of analysis and that use medical or other institutions for maximum experimental control. As one moves outward from patient education and classroom health education to the community level where other practitioners have the opportunity to make a difference, the unit of analysis becomes whole clinics, schools, workplaces, and other organizational levels of analysis. This has called for a return to some **ecological** foundations of the health sciences.[4]

The ability to measure health and to evaluate efforts in developing, protecting, and restoring health has developed to the point of diminishing returns on greater precision in some areas.[5] The more precisely health professionals have tried to measure health itself, for example, the more they have seemed to lose sight of the larger whole of health. Reducing ill health to submolecular levels has improved the ability of medicine to intervene with increasing precision and effectiveness regarding specific illnesses. Yet, the intense focus on that level has caused a neglect of the whole person, the family, and the larger social influences on health. The more precise and controlled health practitioners have tried to be in evaluating health promotion programs, the more they seem to have lost the essential elements of participation and relevance. This is most problematic when the loss of participation or relevance occurs among those responsible for action, including those personally affected by the problems or issues.[6] This has caused a return to some educational foundations of health programs, policies, professions, and technologies.[7]

In the drift of medicine to high technology and specialization, some countries have neglected their development of primary care, though most people could benefit from simpler services most of the time.[8] Even nations that have made primary care central to their medical care systems have stacked the incentives for the practitioners in favor of technical rather than social, cultural, and behavioral aspects of care.[9] Disease prevention and health promotion services in clinical settings have suffered accordingly.[10] Outreach to populations from hospital settings seem to have been motivated by public relations rather than sincere attempts to transform the way health services relate to the social, cultural, and behavioral aspects of health.

Within the flow of science, the drift of medicine toward measuring and explaining disease and health in submolecular units has also swept epidemiology toward the same reductionist tendencies, emphasizing individual risk factors over social determinants of health.[11] Swimming upstream against these tendencies have been efforts to put technological resources more at the disposal of people seeking greater control over their own lives, with less dependency on professionals, technicians, and large, impersonal institutions.[12] In this postmodern time, when philosophy, the arts, and the social sciences are giving greater recognition to experiential knowledge and diversity while calling into question the certainty or universality of positivist scientific truth, the personalization and decentralization of the generation and application of knowledge finds a receptive audience.[13] Also swimming upstream against the technological, economic, and globalization imperatives of our time is a growing concern over how the unbridled application of such imperatives affects the environment.[14] These responses to the mixed blessings of our era have resulted in calls for more participatory, socially responsive, environmentally friendly approaches to epidemiology and other scientific and professional practices in health. This book seeks to pick up these strands and show how one might apply them.

THE ERA OF RESOURCE-BASED PLANNING AND EVALUATION

From 1945 to the 1970s, this drift of medical care toward high technology, and the hospital-based resources needed to support that technology, dragged the focus of health **planning** from outcomes to the cost of resources. Measurement and evaluation had to help justify, defend, and eventually contain the costs of the new technologies and resources. Because of this, measurement and evaluation changed its focus from the health outcomes in populations to the appropriate uses and applications of the resources. With that shift came the broader tendency in regional and community health planning toward a resource-based rather than a population-based planning and development cycle. The hospitals, personnel, and technology became ends in themselves. As such, they became the objects of measurement and evaluation in most health planning and development.

As shown in Figure 1-2, this change diverted attention away from the health needs of populations and toward their use or consumption of the resources and services offered.[15] Government health agencies sponsored social and behavioral science research in the 1950s and 1960s that focused mostly on increasing people's use of new technologies, services, and facilities. For instance, in the late 1950s, the Health Belief Model emerged initially to explain the results of studies on why people used or failed to use mobile chest X-ray services to screen for tuberculosis.[16] This influential model evolved in the 1960s to assess why people did not make greater use of immunization services[17] and eventually came to address the more generic question of why people use or fail to use health services.[18]

Similarly, the Precede-Proceed model[19] for health promotion planning and evaluation was first published as a **cost-benefit** evaluation model applied to patient education as a means of decreasing the use of emergency room services by asthmatic adults.[20] It was built initially on Andersen's model of families' use of health services[21] and original work on use of family-planning services.[22] PRECEDE and other models in patient education were further developed and tested in the 1970s to understand patient "compliance" with prescribed medical regimens, another rapidly developing medical technology or resource. In each instance, the starting point for measurement and evaluation in health education, patient counseling, and many other areas of applied social and behavioral sciences in health was a technology, facility, service, or other resource.

During the 1960s, even the significant work on community participation was framed in the context of the role of local residents in supporting the planning and development of health services and resources.[23] This role was often called *consumer* participation, where the commodity was the expanding services of the medical resources; research centered on the role of consumers participating in

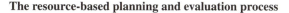

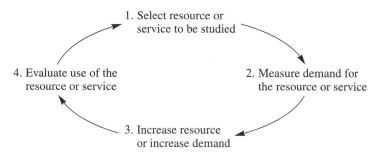

The resource-based planning and evaluation process

FIGURE 1-2

The resource-based planning cycle: This process has dominated most of the development and financing of health care systems in the United States since World War II. It produces a spiral of increased resources and increased demand for resources that drive the costs of health services upward even though a population's medical needs might be declining with improved health and living conditions.

"health systems agencies."[24] Most retrospective commentaries on this era view the "maximum feasible participation" mandate of federal laws to have failed in their purpose of reforming the system and containing costs. Moynihan refers to this indictment and the distortion of the legislative intent in the use of citizen participants in local health boards as "maximum feasible misunderstanding."[25]

In another reflection on the consequence of this experience, Morone concludes that the view of citizen participation having failed because it did not succeed in controlling costs misses its most important contribution—reigning in the monopoly and monolith of medicine:

> For in those late-night disputes the medical profession lost its trusteeship over American medicine. In every community, groups of lay people were making judgements on proposals submitted by medical professionals. In so doing they were transforming the way Americans think about health care policy. . . . A 4-to-3 vote may have been won . . . but in the process of having to vote and appeal at all, they [the medical profession] lost their hegemony over medical policy.[26]

Consequences. The resource-based planning and evaluation cycle resulted in locking the development process into a spiral of justifying existing and emerging resources, services, and technologies as ends in themselves. These resources were becoming more numerous and more expensive. The cost of health care was escalating. After two decades of seeking to increase the use of services, health education's new order of business in the 1970s became the reduction of "overutilization" and unnecessary use of medical care services. The President's Committee on Health Education in 1973,[27] the Health Information and Health

Promotion Act (PL 94-317) in 1974,[28] and the Health Maintenance Organization Act of 1973[29] all sought to *reduce* the public's use of health services. They sought to do so, in part, by developing educational strategies and incentives that would help the public to become more self-sufficient in health, to prevent diseases and injuries, to promote health, and to become better informed "consumers" of health care services.

In the agencies and foundations funding health services research, this gave rise to an interest in the self-care movement.[30] This movement grew out of the 1960s from a convergence of the women's movement; the do-it-yourself, self-help, and self-improvement movements; and the emergence of self-help and mutual aid groups.[31] Some of these fed on growing antiprofessionalism or at least some disenchantment with experts controlling one's life or pocketbook.[32]

The resource-based planning and evaluation cycle had another effect on health and behavioral researchers: It caused them to reason by analogy from medical successes that their scientific quest should be to find the best intervention to achieve a specific type of health-related behavior change. Practitioners and the agencies funding health services and public health research eagerly embraced this search for magic bullet solutions to the behavioral change problems presented by medical care and public health.[33] A generation of highly controlled, randomized trials and fine-grained behavioral research ensued.[34] By trial and error, these tested specific ways to improve patient compliance.[35] They included ways to reduce broken appointments, to educate mothers not to bring a child in for each earache or sore throat, to improve smoking cessation, and to modify a range of specific consumer and self-care behaviors. The targets of such "interventions" were as much those behaviors thought to account for some of the "unnecessary" and "inappropriate" use of health services as those accounting for leading causes of death or disability.[36]

The Magic Bullet Approach. The magic bullet approach to behavioral research in health was nowhere more evident than in smoking-cessation studies, which dominated the funded behavioral research in the 1970s and early 1980s. During this time, social and behavioral researchers conducted hundreds of studies on each of several focused techniques for stopping smoking.[37] Smoking-cessation research gained prominence with the growing recognition of tobacco as the leading cause of preventable deaths in Western countries and from the concomitantly growing public demand for ways to quit smoking. Its foothold in biomedical-research funding agencies, such as the U.S. National Institutes of Health (NIH), also came about because it lent itself to the kind of research NIH reviewers were most comfortable approving. Most important was the possibility of conducting highly controlled, randomized trials. Of nearly equal attraction, however, was specificity of measurement (quit versus relapsed, number of cigarettes smoked daily). The potential to verify verbal reports of behavior by measuring traces of tobacco in saliva, urine, or blood samples further enhanced the acceptability of smoking-cessation research among biomedical researchers. The further possibility of pin-pointing the relative **cost-effectiveness** of alternative smoking cessation methods made this work of interest to those trying to rationalize and finance preventive services within the evolving medical care system.[38] These precise measurement possibilities gave this line of research a status among the biomedical sciences that was difficult to match by other social, behavioral, and educational research initiatives in the health fields.[39]

Measurement conveniences were not the only fuel for tobacco research. Theory also motivated funders to support both the cessation and the prevention aspects of smoking research. Behavioral scientists found relatively generous grant support for their theory-testing ideas and found smoking a good testing ground for theories of behavioral disposition and change. This tradition of testing social psychological theories while building better interventions for health education and health promotion has been carried forward in Europe as well as North America.[40]

Only the research on patient compliance with prescribed medical regimens could compete in those funding agencies. Their advantage centered on those areas of medication that had a similar set of biomedical markers to serve as "objective" measures of drug error behavior to verify verbal reports. A meta-analysis of the cumulative clinical trial literature on this subject for the Pharmaceutical Manufacturers' Association in the mid-1980s concluded, however, that there was no magic bullet. Although the more than 100 studies demonstrated average effect sizes that amounted to a solid record of substantial reductions in drug errors and improvements in physiological outcomes from patient education, analysts could find little evidence of one method having superiority over others across different population groups. The analysts concluded that the patient education interventions were effective because of the planning that went into the strategic selection of methods that matched the learning and behavioral needs of the patients.[41] This observation, consistent with the principles on which the Precede-Proceed model is based, has caused some to question the wisdom of importing the idea of "evidence-based practice" to health promotion from the medical field.[42] Human biology is relatively uniform across the human species; however, human behavior, culture, and social change processes are not uniform enough to permit a single set of "best practices" to suffice the way medical best practices might.

Besides supporting smoking cessation and patient compliance research, funding agencies concerned with cost-containment issues in health care supported most of the applied social and behavioral research in health of that era. Those studies were pursued vigorously during the 1970s and early 1980s. The health resource imperative and the need to contain the cost of resources drove the research priorities. Emergency room visits, for example, provided a focal point for behavioral and social science research in health because many of the costs in this center could not be fully recovered from patients, insurance, or welfare systems. Cost savings or efficiencies from averting unnecessary visits to emergency rooms (ERs) or accomplishing other functions in the ER lent themselves to a precision of measurement of behavioral outcomes that seldom had to deal with long-term, complicated issues of health outcomes and quality-of-life or social outcomes.[43] The motivation for funding such research, once again, had more to do with rationalizing the use of the medical facilities or resources than with solving the health problem of a population. That unholy alliance—between precise control methodologies and funders' emphasis on the needs of health care systems rather than the primary health needs of populations—has given a reductionist texture to the current body of knowledge in health education.

A Call for Change. Recent examples of the conflict of precision and relevance inherent in resource-based planning and evaluation reveal the growing skepticism surrounding some programs. School health-education curricula, the mass media, and focused community-level programs in health promotion have come under increased scrutiny. Those that have shown the greatest difficulty accounting for their impact on lifestyle changes are substance abuse prevention,[44] alcohol-impaired driving,[45] tobacco use by adolescents,[46] and HIV/AIDS and cardiovascular disease prevention.[47] The disenchantment centers not on the settings and communication technologies themselves as appropriate channels for addressing these problems,[48] but rather on their limited ability to influence complex lifestyles and social trends without engaging wider social forces. School curricula alone increasingly gave way to comprehensive school-community approaches to the adolescent substance abuse and tobacco control issues,[49] teenage pregnancy prevention,[50] and injury prevention.[51] Mass media have outgrown their role as mere transmitters of information. Now they encompass more interactive features of the local environment,[52] as well as "media advocacy" as a means of mobilizing social and political support for policy and regulatory changes in alcohol, tobacco, HIV, and cardiovascular disease control.[53]

These expansions of the necessary scope of programs to effect complex lifestyle and social trends in behavior or health call for new methods of research and evaluation. Researchers have begun to revive and reinstate methods that have languished. The dominant emphasis has shifted from psychological and behavioral factors, which lend themselves to precise measure, to more difficult to measure and control factors, such as social, cultural, and political ones.[54]

The resource-based planning and evaluation cycle manifested itself also in the education sector as new, sometimes expensive, educational technologies emerged in the 1970s. These refocused school health educators and researchers for a time away from **comprehensive school health** onto methods and techniques of classroom teaching.[55] Disillusionment with the search for technological fixes and universal interventions has driven theory, measurement, and evaluation to new challenges in health, education, and other sectors.

This disillusionment has other sources as well. Consumers and the public show increasing discontent with the institutional systems of health, social, and educational services. Social and behavioral scientists express a growing discomfort with the biomedical imperatives driving their health research. Further, researchers and the philosophers of science exhibit ever more disdain for the positivist traditions of science dictating the rules of evidence and the methods of generating knowledge. Add to this ferment the growing impatience and even hostility of the public with their passive role as subjects (objects) of research who feel exploited as individuals and sometimes compromised and maligned as groups. This is especially problematic for minority groups and disadvantaged communities, as well as practitioners working under adverse circumstances, when the results paint them in an unfavorable light.

THE SHIFT FROM RESOURCE-BASED TO POPULATION-BASED PLANNING AND EVALUATION

The alternative to the resource-based planning and evaluation cycle is the population-based planning and evaluation cycle, shown in Figure 1-3. This process was implicit in the early epidemiological approaches to public health planning that prevailed when planners emphasized communicable disease control in Western countries in the 19th and early 20th centuries. This cycle continues in many developing countries, although they too have been caught up in the resource-based planning spiral as they seek to replicate the technological features of Western medicine.

The population-based approach to planning and evaluation starts with the identification of a specific human population (see Figure 1-3). This could be, for

Prototype of population-based planning and evaluation approaches

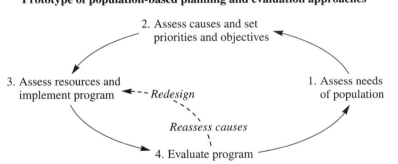

FIGURE 1-3

The population-based planning cycle: Breaking the resource-based planning habit has called for greater attention to population needs and outcomes as the starting and ending points in the planning and evaluation cycle.

example, a population of patients using a clinical service or the population of students in a classroom; in any case, the population-based approach tends to conceive it as a population of people eligible to use (or at risk of using) the clinical or educational service. The planners assess population needs beyond those of the individuals who appear for illness or injury treatment, or beyond the people who turn out for educational events. Such groups of individuals may provide numerators against the denominator of the population.

This initial focus on the denominator or population at risk is the critical distinction made implicitly in the emergence of health maintenance organizations (HMOs) in the 1970s and later community-oriented primary care (COPC)[56] and managed care in the United States[57] and population health elsewhere. It is also the distinction made implicitly in the 1974 Canadian Lalonde report,[58] in the 1979 *Healthy People: The Surgeon General's Report on Health Promotion and Disease Prevention,*[59] and in the succession of countries adopting a planning-by-objectives approach to health promotion and disease prevention (United Kingdom, the Netherlands, Australia, and New Zealand).[60] Most of these countries built on the Lalonde report and after 1979 on the U.S. report and the World Health Organization's Primary Health Care and Health for All initiatives.[61] Efforts to prevent disease or injury and to promote health become more compelling when an organization assumes responsibility for the population's health needs, regardless of the prevailing medical care resources.

In the second phase of the population-based planning cycle (see Figure 1-3), one assesses the causes of the health needs. Such **assessments** typically reveal a set of causes common to several of the leading causes of death, disability, illness, and injury. Most countries and communities understandably make these common **risk factors**—for example, alcohol, tobacco, poor nutrition, and physical inactivity—their priorities for the focus of limited health promotion and disease prevention resources. In 1986, the First International Conference on Health Promotion produced the Ottawa Charter,[62] which helped reorient policy, programs, and practices away from these **proximal risk** factors. The shift that followed was to the more distal risk factors in time, space, or scope, which we shall call **risk conditions**. These also influence health, either through the risk factors or by operating directly on human biology over time, but they are less likely than risk factors to be under the control of the individuals at risk.

The risk factors and risk conditions, together with factors predisposing, enabling, and reinforcing them, are referred to collectively as the **determinants of health**. These include adequate housing; secure income; healthful and safe community and work environments; enforcement of policies and regulations controlling the manufacture, marketing, labeling, and sale of potentially harmful products; and the use of these products (such as alcohol and tobacco) where they can harm others.

In assessing the causes of health needs, one may need to take measures in such populations as patients of clinical services, students in a school, employees in a workplace, or people in a community. Measurement typically involves data collection from records or from observations or **surveys**, data reduction, and statistical analyses of the data. Following these steps, one first constructs profiles or descriptions of the risk factors and risk conditions in the population. These statistical distributions are then examined in relation to the factors predisposing, enabling, or reinforcing the development or incidence of the most important risk factors or risk conditions in the population.

The third phase of the population-based planning approach calls for the strategic application of data and knowledge about the causes identified in the second phase. These considerations lead to strategies or programs designed to influence change in the factors predisposing, enabling, or reinforcing the causes and thereby improve health outcomes. This and the second phase are usually the main subjects of textbooks and articles on program planning and implementation.[63]

The fourth phase in Figure 1-3 is the evaluation of the program or procedures implemented to meet the population needs. This phase leads logically in the long run to a reassessment of the needs of the population (Phase 1). It can also lead to the reassessment of assumptions or hypotheses in Phase 2 or of the program itself toward improving its construction or delivery. This, then, is the cycle of planning and evaluation that will be described in this book.

THE TYPES OF BEHAVIOR ADDRESSED BY HEALTH PROMOTION

One stereotype of **health promotion** views lean and ruddy people alone, grimly adhering to a regimen of **health-directed behavior** to reduce their risks of premature death, disease, and even aging. Such goal-oriented, risk-factor–reducing activity remains important for that minority of individuals, and health education can point to its development in recent years with pride. Health-directed or goal-oriented activity, however, is but a piece of the more pervasive and problematic web of **health-related behavior** of individuals, as well as whole families, groups, communities, and organizations. This more pervasive behavior has to do with patterns and **conditions of living**—housing, eating, playing, working, loafing—most of which lie outside the realm of the health sector and are not consciously health directed.

FROM HEALTH EDUCATION TO HEALTH PROMOTION

For a time, many defined **health education** as planned learning experiences to facilitate *voluntary* change in behavior, thereby limiting its scope to developing or bringing about change in consciously health-directed behavior.[64] Health education could be shown to work most directly, effectively, and humanely when people were clearly oriented to solve a discrete and immediate problem of importance to them. Patient education and self-care education (where people are motivated to cure or control a disease) offered the best evidence for health education practice, partly because they could be evaluated in highly controlled clinical trials, but mostly because people were predisposed, enabled, and reinforced to pursue purposeful actions. Immunization programs (where people wish to avoid a potential threat) and screening programs (where people seek a specific diagnosis or reassurance) also had relatively well established track records. Smoking-cessation programs (where people want to quit), family planning programs (where people want to prevent or delay a pregnancy), and other highly targeted programs were advanced by the idea of voluntary change.

CONTROVERSY CONCERNING THE GOALS AND METHODS OF HEALTH PROMOTION

In 1979, the *Surgeon General's Report on Health Promotion and Disease Prevention*[65] challenged the U.S. public and professional health community to examine more critically routine, usually unpremeditated, health-related behaviors. It also urged greater attention to community conditions of living. Together, these accounted for over 50% of the causes of premature death. The policies influencing such behavior and living conditions could be seen as prime opportunities for intervention. Among health-related behaviors, the most critical were substance misuse and addiction (including tobacco and alcohol), poor diet, sedentary work and leisure, and stress-related conditions (including suicide, violence, and reckless behavior). These behavioral and **lifestyle** risk factors accounted for 40–70% of all premature deaths, a third of all cases of acute disability, and two thirds of all cases of chronic disability. Already considered important in relation to teenage pregnancy and sexually transmitted diseases, sexual behavior took on much greater significance as a cause of death with the emergence of the HIV/AIDS epidemic.

The complexity and value-laden character of these proposed targets of health promotion policies were signaled by the language of the critiques and debates that greeted the Surgeon General's report. The controversy hinged on phrases like "individual versus social responsibility for health,"[66] "facilitating individual behavior change" versus "broader, institutional and social change approaches to health promotion,"[67] "behavioral" versus "ecological strategies,"[68] "healthy people" versus "healthy cities and healthy policies,"[69] and "blaming the victim" versus blaming "the manufacturers of illness."[70] From within the school health-education camp came expressions of concern that the emphasis on behavior was abandoning an educational perspective.[71]

The federal office that issued the Surgeon General's report published in the same year a quasi-official definition of health promotion as "any combination of health education and related organizational, political and economic interventions designed to facilitate behavioral and environmental changes conducive to health."[72] This did not silence the critics who continued to worry in subsequent years that conservative political leaders and policies would use a narrower concept of individual responsibility for health promotion to justify cuts in basic health services and government programs.

At the heart of the health promotion debates and in some of the contentious phrases and ideologies, one can find both positive and pejorative uses of the word *lifestyle*. As a target for health promotion policy and programs, *lifestyle* refers for some to the consciously chosen, personal behavior of individuals as it may relate to health. Others see the word as a composite expression of the social and cultural circumstances that condition and constrain behavior, in addition to the personal decisions the individual might make in choosing one behavior over another.[73] Both uses of the term acknowledge that lifestyle is a more enduring (some would say habitual) *pattern* of behavior or **socialization** than connoted by the terms **behavior** and **action**.

The **habituation** of behavior or prevention of "relapse" and "recidivism" became an increasingly important dimension of health as the chronic and degenerative diseases displaced acute, communicable diseases in the list of the leading causes of morbidity and mortality. Once, as we have seen, people had looked to magic bullets. A single act such as getting an immunization could provide a lifetime of protection against an infectious disease. After the Surgeon General's report, a lifetime of simple, seemingly harmless acts such as eating high-fat foods, smoking a few cigarettes each day, going to work in heavy traffic without seat belts, and driving home after a few drinks accounted for most of society's disease, injury, disability, and premature death. The focus of health education programs has needed to shift from predisposing factors—knowledge, beliefs, attitudes, and perception—to enabling and reinforcing factors.

Health education had demonstrated its success in the public health campaigns of the 1960s to change single, health-directed acts such as obtaining immunizations. It had demonstrated in the 1970s its ability to change medical care behavior through patient education and self-care initiatives. But many of the policy makers and public health officials of the 1970s were not confident that health education could bring about changes in the new public health targets—the more complex, lifetime habits and social circumstances associated with the term *lifestyle*.[74] With such elusive targets as socially imbedded lifestyles, public health education could significantly improve population health only if it joined other sectors and brought multiple social forces to bear on the problem. Some of these new forces, such as economic and regulatory measures to control tobacco, would go beyond the ethical definition, and most policy makers' understanding, of health education.

In the early 1980s, questions arose also about the effective reach of mass health education and the consequent issues of equity and social justice.[75] As James Mason, then the Director of the Centers for Disease Control, said:

Until now, most of the behavior changes we have promoted have involved the better-educated, upper-, and middle-class segments of our society. If health promotion is a good thing, it should be good for the whole society, not just that portion which is favorably predisposed. Unless we are able to reach all segments of the population, we will never meet the goals we have set for a national consciousness for wellness in America.[76]

Health education was drawn into the fray with the opportunity to provide leadership for an expanded public health policy of lifestyle priorities and objectives under the mantle of health promotion.[77] The quasi-official definition of health promotion from the U.S. federal government sought to position health education centrally in the new federal policies and programs. Here is a refined and simplified version of that definition, offered for the purposes of this book: *Health promotion is the combination of educational and environmental supports for actions and conditions of living conducive to health.* The actions or behavior in question may be those of individuals, groups, or communities; of policy makers, employers, teachers, or others whose actions control or influence the determinants of health. The purpose of health promotion is to enable people to gain greater control over the determinants of their own health.[78] When the determinants are ones over which he or she can exert personal control, this control ideally resides with the individual. But with some aspects of complex lifestyle issues, especially those that affect the health of others such as drunk driving, the control that people exercise must be through community decisions and actions.[79]

COMMUNITY AS THE CENTER OF GRAVITY FOR HEALTH PROMOTION

If the first *Surgeon General's Report on Health Promotion and Disease Prevention* seemed to put too much responsibility on the individual, some of the wishful thinking of some health promotion advocates has expected too much of national policy and centralized planning.[80] If the victim blaming implicit in policies that focused on individual behavior was unfair, the system blaming implicit in some of the more sweeping social-reform proposals offered as alternatives was unproductive. A unified middle ground must be found if health promotion is to be viable policy.[81] The value-laden, culturally and ethnically defined nature of many of the lifestyle issues such as diet make them impossible to dictate uniformly from a distant central government, especially in pluralistic, democratic societies.[82] The private nature of many of these practices, such as sexual and sedentary behavior, makes them inaccessible to effective surveillance and regulation. The constitutional and civil rights of citizens protect most individual behaviors, including bearing arms in the United States, sexual practices among consenting adults, advertising unhealthful products, or even producing pornography. Governments such as those of Australia, Canada, and the United States limit the powers of central government in favor of state or provincial rights to police power in matters of health. Most of these powers are ceded to local governments.[83]

Central governments retain their legitimate exercise of public health leadership by

- Establishing health policies and objectives
- Distributing and **allocating** resources according to national priorities and concerns with equity among regions or population groups
- Providing technical assistance
- Maintaining uniform data systems that allow for the monitoring of national progress and comparison among regions

One way some governments have coordinated these national roles has been to reach consensus on a set of health goals and targets, then gear their data systems to help track progress on achievement of the goals and allocate resources according to progress and gaps. For instance, once national policy settled on goals and objectives for health promotion in countries such as Australia, Finland, the Netherlands, Sweden, and the United States, the necessity of adapting those policies to the state or provincial and community levels became inescapable.[84] States in turn have found themselves unable to finance some of the programs previously financed by federal or national governments. They also have sought to decentralize their authority and allocation of resources to regional and local levels.

In the final analysis, the most appropriate center of gravity for health promotion is the community.[85] State and national governments can formulate policies, provide leadership, allocate funding, and generate data for health promotion. At the other extreme, individuals can govern their own behavior and control the determinants of their own health, up to a point, and should be allowed to do so. But the decisions on priorities and strategies for *social* change affecting the more complicated lifestyle issues can best be made collectively as close to the homes and workplaces of those affected as possible. This principle assures the greatest relevance and appropriateness of the programs to the people affected, and it offers the best opportunity for people to be actively engaged in the planning process themselves. This is more than a philosophical principle. Evidence from decades of research and experience on the value of participation in learning and behavior indicates that people will be more committed to initiating and upholding those changes they helped design or adapt to their own purposes and circumstances.[86]

The principle of participation, however, can be carried to excess. Specifically, many local agencies and professionals must demonstrate the commitment of multiple local organizations and agencies to support each program before they can qualify for state or national funding. The requirement for committed local **coalitions** has much to recommend it for the sake of **leveraging** outside funding and ensuring local coordination and minimal duplication. The requirement, however, must be tempered by a recognition of the limitations and complexities of community coalitions, especially as instruments of implementation.[87]

Community may be the town or county in sparsely populated areas; the school, work site, or neighborhood in more populous metropolitan areas. It is, ideally, a level of collective decision making appropriate to the urgency and magnitude of the problem, the cost and technical complexity of the solutions required, the culture and traditions of shared decision making, and the sensitivity and consequences of the actions required of people after the decision is made.

SHARING RESPONSIBILITY AMONG THOSE WITH INFLUENCE ON HEALTH

The evolution of health policy and programs for health education and health promotion, described earlier in this chapter, acts like a pendulum.[88] It swings from one era, with heavy reliance on centralized government and institutions for environmental and policy change, to the next era, with heavy reliance on individuals and families or local government to change behavior, and back. Ideological attempts to throw the responsibility more exclusively to one side or the other have met with a seemingly inexorable cycle of political swings. The reality of program planning and execution is that both sides must be engaged.[89]

The chapters that follow propose methods for health promotion planning that seek an optimum mix of responsibility. These methods require that individuals, families, professionals, private and government organizations, and local and national agencies must determine case by case how to divide and share the responsibility for each health problem or objective. For each, participants must determine its urgency, causes, variability, and distribution, as well as the degree to which individuals want and can exercise control over the determinants of the health problem or goal. Those directly affected should have a voice in negotiating this division of responsibility. Providing opportunities for that voice to be heard applies the principle of participation so central to learning theory and effective community organization.[90] It also assures a link to the philosophical and ethical underpinning of the professional commitment to supporting voluntary change where possible.

The World Health Organization (WHO) and UNICEF global initiatives reflected in the primary health care approach and the Ottawa Charter make the emerging concepts of health promotion relevant also to the developing nations. The case-by-case assessment of needs and tailoring of **strategies** to local circumstances apply particularly to the culturally distinct populations of developing countries. Finding the right balance between personal and societal responsibility and providing for the active participation of individuals and communities, of public and private sectors, in the assessment of needs and the division of responsibility all apply as much to the developing countries as to the so-called developed ones.[91] Both also require some **coercive strategies.**

Health promotion has apparently shifted the locus of initiative for health, and control over its determinants, from medical institutions and professionals to individuals, families, schools, and work sites. But it has done so in a context of growing community, social, and technological support for shared responsibility for health. Work-site health promotion has expanded rapidly, with notable provisions for institutional supports for employee participation.[92] Schools increasingly emphasize social and organizational factors in programs for the modification or development of diet and prevention of substance abuse.[93] In most communities, new emphasis is being placed on concerns with the environment and with housing and other conditions of living that shape the lifestyles, health, and quality of life of the community. All of this calls for more collaboration among sectors, organizations, and individuals.

THE LIFESTYLE CONSTRUCT

One ecological break from earlier emphases on health behavior has been the increased use of the term *lifestyle*. Health-related behavior is seen increasingly not as isolated acts under the autonomous control of the individual, but rather as socially conditioned, culturally imbedded, economically constrained patterns of living.

The lifestyle construct has its roots in anthropology, sociology, and clinical psychology, where it describes *patterns* of behavior that endure and are based in some combination of cultural heritage, social relationships, geographic and socioeconomic circumstances, and personality.[94] Initially, the behavioral pattern described in the lifestyle construct was assumed to be made up of a full range of daily routines within a social fabric of family, friends, and school- and workmates. Each behavior within the pattern was assumed to have some connection and possibly dependent relationship with each other behavior in the lifestyle.[95] In later usage by medical sociologists and psychologists,[96] there was a search for subsets of behaviors highly correlated to health protection, health promotion, and use of health services.[97]

These features made the lifestyle construct appropriate and useful for some analyses of health-related behavior, especially those that might have a synergistic or multiplier effect on each other in producing poor health outcomes, such as smoking coupled with consumption of high-fat foods, or drinking while driving combined with driving without seat belts. Unfortunately, such analyses have produced rather modest correlations among the presumably related behaviors. This leaves some doubt about the utility of the lifestyle construct in describing or explaining consistent patterns of interrelated health behavior in populations.[98]

The meaning of the term *lifestyle* has been further eroded by its widespread misuse in describing single acts, temporary practices, and behavior of any kind related to health. These and other criticisms of using the term in health promotion[99] should alert the student or practitioner to be cautious in its application and interpretation. In this book, *lifestyle* will be used only to describe a complex of related practices and behavioral patterns in a person or group, maintained with some consistency over time. It includes conscious health-directed behavior as well as unconscious health-related behavior and practices pursued for nonhealth purposes but with health consequences or risks.

This somewhat holistic view of lifestyle as a health-related construct justifies a more holistic approach to promoting health in communities and individuals. For example, a recognition that each behavior related to health is also related to other facets of a lifestyle should make program planners and professionals more aware of the need to include in the planning process the thoughts and perspectives of those whose behavior might be expected to change. Methods to do this are proposed in the next chapter. It also argues for a comprehensive approach to health promotion, with a combination of educational and organizational, economic, or other environmental supports rather than only persuasive appeals for change in each specific behavior. When a health-related behavior is seen as embedded in a complex web of lifestyle, changing that behavior will necessarily require attention to the social norms, the cultural values, and the economic and environmental circumstances surrounding and supporting that lifestyle.[100]

Considering the complexity of lifestyle, it will be prudent to stay with the terms *behavior, actions,* and *practices* to describe the intermediate targets of health education and health promotion. This helps one avoid the traps of arrogance and pretentiousness that accompany practical but simplistic strategies to change a lifestyle. Only the most ambitious, long-term, complex health promotion programs can be expected to affect lifestyle significantly,[101] and such programs are impractical for everyday health promotion planning.[102] At the same time, this does not diminish the importance of local health education and health promotion programs, which make a vital contribution to social and lifestyle change. In this book, helping just one person gain control over a single determinant of his or her health qualifies as health promotion.

While striving to be practical and down to earth, this book will not shrink from the larger tasks of social change and policy advocacy that each health professional should seek to support. As health professionals encourage citizens to participate and become empowered advocates for the health of their communities, so too should the health professional be a part of social and policy change. But these changes require the cooperative and sustained effort of many professionals, sectors, and public constituencies. Each individual who is helped to gain control over the determinants of health in his or her own life is one more voice added to the constituencies advocating social change. This cumulative effect is clearly illustrated by the development of social demand for clean air, which led to local ordinances for smoke-free environments. Each person who successfully adapts his or her own behavior becomes a source of help, inspiration, or influence for others to make similar changes. This process has been described as the **normative effect** of behavior change and health promotion in groups and communities.[103]

THE EDUCATIONAL APPROACH TO HEALTH PROMOTION

Our definition of health promotion reserves a place—as indicated by the subtitle of this book—for educational and ecological approaches. In this section, we say a bit more about the educational approach. In the next, we examine the ecological.

The commitment to an educational approach to health promotion is part practical necessity, part political expediency, and part philosophical commitment to provide for informed consent and voluntary change *before* attempting to change social structures and ecologies.

When Ilona Kickbusch was the director of the Division of Health Promotion, Education, and Communication of the World Health Organization, she gave the following reasons why health promotion emerged out of health education:

> First: health educators became more aware of the need for positive approaches in health education—enhancing health and creating health potential rather than focusing on disease prevention. Second: it became self evident that health education could only develop its full potential if it was supported by structural measures (legal, environmental, regulatory, etc.).[104]

As Milio said earlier, the task for health promotion beyond health education was how to make healthier choices the easier choices.[105] That policy, organizational, economic, regulatory, and other environmental interventions are necessary to accomplish the original intent of health education does not justify abandoning health education as the primary modality for democratic social and behavioral change.[106] Health education provides the consciousness-raising, concern-arousing, action-stimulating impetus for public involvement and commitment to social reform essential to its success in a democracy. Without health education, health promotion would be a manipulative social engineering enterprise. Health education of the public keeps the social change component of health promotion accountable to the public it serves. Without the policy supports for social change, on the other hand, health education is often powerless to help people reach their health goals even with successful individual efforts.

In short, health education aims primarily at the voluntary actions people can take on their own part, individually or collectively, for their own health or the health of others and the common good of the community. Health promotion encompasses health education, as defined in this book, and is aimed at the complementary social and political actions that will facilitate the necessary organizational, economic, and other environmental supports for the conversion of individual actions into health enhancements and quality-of-life gains.

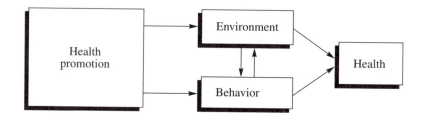

FIGURE 1-4

The essential relationships in an educational and ecological approach to health promotion consist of these few, which we shall explore in later chapters.

THE ECOLOGICAL APPROACH[107]

The interaction of behavior and **environment** in the middle of Figure 1-4 isolates the essence of the ecological approach to health promotion. The reciprocal, virtually inseparable, relationship of behavior and its environment is what makes the combination of educational and ecological approaches a defining feature of health promotion.

PRECEDENTS FOR ECOLOGICAL APPROACHES

One can find several streams of thought and action from which ecological perspectives have influenced health promotion. Before that, they influenced public health education, and public health before that. These disciplines converged with various social and behavioral sciences and other professional perspectives to form the ecological and behavioral foundations of health promotion.

Public Health. The ecological perspective has been central to public health concepts and methods from their earliest formulations and applications.[108] It was influenced by the 19th century development of biological, especially Darwinian, concepts of the "web of life" and the role of the environment and adaptation in the survival of species. Public health first sought to ensure the survival of human species by controlling the physical environment. John Snow's removal in 1854 of London's Broad Street pump handle to prevent people from using cholera-contaminated water is heralded as the first classic epidemiological study. By mapping the sources of drinking water of those who died of cholera, Snow identified the environmental source of the illness 30 years before Koch isolated the cholera organism. The host-agent-environment triad was central to the development of epidemiology, but this ecological analysis informed an effective public health intervention even before the discovery of the agent.

Epidemiology. Epidemiology remained almost exclusively preoccupied with the physical, chemical, and biological environments until the 1960s. Its host-agent-environment triad kept it tied to human ecology, but its avoidance of social science theory made it a diffident partner of social ecology. The refocusing of epidemiology on chronic diseases in the 1960s added a growing concern with behavioral determinants of health, accelerated in the 1980s with the advent of HIV and AIDS as the newest epidemic. The behavioral emphasis resulted in a narrowing of the focus and the methodologies of epidemiology. This has led to a growing clamour in other sectors of public health, especially public health education, to widen the focus to include social, economic, organizational, and political environments as determinants of health and points of intervention.[109]

Sociology. In 1921, Park and Burgess introduced the term *human ecology* in an attempt to apply the basic theoretical scheme of plant and animal ecology to the study of human communities.[110] The subdiscipline of demography had arisen earlier, when Malthus and others in the 19th century attempted to interpret population growth and movement in relation to environmental capacity to support the survival of populations. Borrowing a mathematical model of population growth and distribution from demography, rural sociology examined the patterns of social forces that could account for the diffusion and adoption of new farm practices and other innovations in agricultural communities or geographic areas. These ecological concepts of diffusion and adoption of innovations influenced the breadth of early thinking about mass health-education campaigns,[111] and later family planning[112] and chronic disease control in public health.[113] Medical sociology also applied ecological and diffusion frameworks in its examination of the social and cultural contexts in which health conditions and health behavior developed and distributed in populations.[114]

Psychology. Because of its interest in individual differences in behavior, psychology had an ecological awakening,[115] even in its most behaviorist areas of specialization, including behavior modification and analysis.[116] Psychology's focus on micro-ecologies offers as much to health promotion within settings (such as clinical settings, workplaces, and schools) as the public health and sociological analyses of wider-ranging environments (macro-ecology) offer community, state or provincial, and national health promotion planning and policy. Further, the subdisciplines of social, community, and environmental psychology have emerged to encompass ecological perspectives on individual behavior. They have influenced health education since World War II in the formulation of theories about how the mass media influence behavior through social networks.[117] They also have influenced health education's use of group dynamics in resolving social conflict and bringing social forces into play in the decision-making process.[118] These applications spilled over into early public health applications of community organization, community development, and planned change.[119]

Education. Learning theory has always given prominence to the interaction of learner and environment.[120] This has been elaborated in latter-day Social Learning Theory (more recently called Social Cognitive Theory) and its core concept of reciprocal determinism between person and environment.[121] Education formalized theories in which the role of the environment and its interdependency with the person were paramount considerations in the development of educational policies and programs.[122] These concepts extended into the development of the subspecialty of school health education and the broader field of school health, which encompassed health curriculum, school environment, school lunch programs, and school health services, among other elements in an ecological approach to the health of schoolchildren.[123] These ideas persist in the modern practice of school health promotion, in which ecological notions of school-community coordination[124] and multilevel interventions with students, faculty, school environment, school policy, and school districts have been studied.[125]

Other Disciplines and Professional Contributions. Human and medical geography have lent particular emphasis on place to the study of health and health behavior. This has blended with health promotion concepts of setting-specificity in the planning of interventions for schools, workplaces, neighborhoods, and clinical settings. Within the broader field of community health promotion, geography has provided critical analyses of the relation of environment and health.[126] Geography has teamed with social work and other professions in the development and critique of indicators of healthy communities.[127]

THE CENTRAL LESSONS OF ECOLOGY FOR HEALTH PROMOTION

Ecological approaches in health promotion view health as a product of the interdependence of the individual and *subsystems* of the ecosystem (such as family, community, culture, and physical and social environment).[128] To promote health, this ecosystem must offer economic and social conditions conducive to health and healthful lifestyles. These environments must also provide information and life skills so individuals can make decisions to engage in behavior that maintains their health. Finally, healthful options among goods and services offered must be available.[129] In the ecological model of health promotion, all these aspects are envisioned as determinants of health. They also provide essential support in helping individuals modify their behaviors and reduce their exposure to risk factors.[130]

Ecological perspectives have insinuated themselves into the consciousness of most health practitioners working outside the clinical setting because it is what distinguishes their work most from the one-to-one patient or client relationships of the more numerous clinical health professionals. Community health and public health textbooks make ecology one of the four or five scientific foundations on which they build the community or population approach to health analysis and planning.[131] Besides the descriptive aspects of ecology, what do the lessons of ecology have to say to health promotion practitioners?

Unanticipated Effects. Ecology cautions social reformers and practitioners in the applied sciences against tampering with change in smaller systems without considering and anticipating, before the intervention, their second- and third-order consequences, "not merely to rue them afterward."[132] The unintended consequences on smaller systems may be even greater from larger systems when policy makers fail to consider cultural, geographic, and demographic variations within their scope of influence with technological and legislative changes. This has clearly also been the admonition and the contribution of cultural anthropology and applied anthropology to the field of public health.[133]

Reciprocal Determinism. The ecological or transactional view of behavior holds that the organism's functioning is mediated by behavior-environment interaction. This has two implications for behavioral and social change:

1. Environment largely controls or sets limits on the behavior that occurs in it.
2. Changing environmental variables results in the modification of behavior.

These two points lead to the recognition that health promotion can achieve its best results by exercising whatever control or influence it can over the environment. But the reciprocal side of this equation also holds that the behavior of individuals, groups, and organizations also influences their environments. This leads to the credo of health promotion that seeks to "empower" people by giving them control over the determinants of their health, whether these are behavioral or environmental. By taking greater control themselves, rather than depending on health professionals to exercise the control for them, they should be in a better position to adjust their behavior to changing environmental conditions, or to adjust their environments to changing behavioral conditions.

Environmental Specificity. The same person will behave differently when observed in different environments.[134] This principal has led to a recognition in health promotion that environment modifies or conditions the more direct attempts to predispose, enable, and reinforce individual and collective behavior through persuasive or informative communications, training, rewards, or incentives. Its implication for health promotion planning and evaluation is that there is nothing *inherently* superior or inferior in any health promotion method or strategy. A method's **effectiveness** always depends on its appropriate fit with the people, the health issue at stake, and the environment in which it is to be applied. This gives further credence to the local or community focus of health promotion as its center of gravity, because it can be more adaptable and sensitive to particular traditions, cultural variations, and circumstances when planned at a community rather than a state, provincial, or national level.

Multilevel and Multisectoral Intervention. Because of its emphasis on the complex interdependencies of the elements making up an ecological web, an ecological approach would seem to demand interventions directed at several levels within an organizational structure or system and at multiple sectors (such as health, education, welfare, commerce, and transportation) of a social system. This is where most descriptions of ecological approaches take us and where most of them leave us. The specificity with which ecological guidelines can identify the particular levels and sectors in need of attention is inherently limited by the infinite variety of interactions that might apply in each idiosyncratic organization, community, or other social system. Following the first principle, "Do no harm," and falling back on the prior lesson of environmental specificity, one might best in some instances restrict one's interventions to selected levels and sectors of a complex system. At most, one should intervene where one can with certainty match interventions with need appropriately and where one can be accountable for side effects. The first calls for an assessment such as that offered by the Precede-Proceed model. The second requires restraint and a touch of humility.

LIMITATIONS OF THE ECOLOGICAL VIEW FOR HEALTH PROMOTION

Much as it forces a broader perspective on planning and practice that might otherwise drift into a **reductionist**, person-centered, or victim-blaming orientation, ecological thinking has its own traps and pitfalls. Because of their complexity, ecological approaches have not been worked out in great detail. Slobodkin complains that ecology is an intractable science, immature and not very helpful.[135] Others have reproached ecologists for not producing simple testable hypotheses. But the usual conclusion of such debates is that the scientific method requires the simplification of ecosystems, making artificial what is inherently complex. Health promotion is drawn to ecology because it enlarges the spotlight from a sharper focus on behavior to include the environment. But we are forced to retreat to behavior at some level. "We will have to learn that we don't manage ecosystems, we manage our interaction with them."[136] Ecological approaches in health promotion cannot have been as thoroughly evaluated as clinical interventions, because the units of analysis lend themselves neither to random assignment to experimental and control groups nor to manipulation as independent variables, given the interdependence of persons and environments. Here follow some particular limitations that ecological approaches will face in health promotion in the near future.

Complexity Breeds Despair. If the ecological credo that everything influences everything else is carried to its logical extreme, the average health practitioner has good reason to do nothing, because the potential influence of or consequences on other parts of an ecological system lie beyond comprehension, much less control. Some specific forms of this despair include the following questions:

1. *How much is enough?* When trying to set the parameters around any given program, health planners, administrators, or practitioners must ask if they are doing enough to make a difference, but they will always be subject to the criticism that they have not gone deeply enough to the root of the problem. For example, even after public health workers had disavowed more strictly educational approaches to alcohol control, Pittman challenged the field, stating,

    Environmental factors that impact alcohol problems are broader than such questions as alcohol availability, advertising, and the alcohol beverage industry's marketing practices. . . . It is much easier to mandate warning labels . . . or propose further restrictions on alcohol advertising or alcohol availability than to address and enact legislation to reduce social inequality, racism, discrimination, and inadequate health care in the United States.[137]

2. *Is everything that takes an educational approach, or attempts to help individuals, to be regarded as trivial and misguided?* Those health practitioners and teachers whose jobs are organized around helping or educating people in clinical, school, or workplace settings are made to feel by some of the academic and politically correct rhetoric that their efforts are a waste of time and, worse, part of the problem. The most vituperative epitaphs for such work are "victim blaming" and "Band-Aid" treatment of the symptoms rather than the cause.

The Level of Analysis in an Ecosystem Hierarchy Is Observer-Dependent. Neither a reductionist (small number, highly controllable), nor a holistic (large number, statistically described) approach suffices to study or describe an ecosystem, because neither captures the system-subsystem relationships. One must examine both the system as a whole and the component subsystems. The frustration and inevitable criticism comes when one must acknowledge that the ecosystem within which one was examining subsystems is itself a subsystem of a larger ecosystem. The observer must decide what to include and what to omit from the analysis—that is, what slice of the hierarchy of subsystems to take for analysis.[138] This necessarily subjective decision will be invariably too narrow or too broad for the tastes (or values) of some other observers. Combine this problem with the dynamic rather than static nature of ecosystems, making the chosen slice a time-dependent set of observations, and one is left unavoidably with a case study of limited generalizability.

Planners wondering which slice of complex systems to analyze and target for intervention can do well by choosing those close enough to reach the people whose needs are to be served. Further, planners should reach as far as they can beyond that to assure support for the more immediate environmental changes needed, but not so far that the unknown needs of others might be affected adversely. Again, some restraint and humility might be blended with the courage it took to undertake an ecological approach in the first place.

THE NOTION OF POSITIVE HEALTH

Another element in the current use of the term *health promotion* is that health is more than the absence of disease or disability. Some restrict their use of health promotion to refer *only* to the positive end of the illness-**wellness** continuum.[139] Nevertheless, the reduction of behavioral risk factors in individuals can be a legitimate and important task for health promotion. Recognition of this need provides considerable impetus to policy support for health promotion. In the short run, at least, reduction of health risks can be expected to accomplish greater reductions in morbidity than can a focus on health enhancement in those without significant behavioral risk factors. This becomes especially clear when one considers that the people most likely to respond to the appeal of wellness opportunities are more affluent, educated, and at lower risk of imminent disease, injury, or death. Though health is more than risk reduction, the people whose health is at greatest risk might warrant first priority in the allocation of resources.

The hope for **health enhancement** and "high-level wellness" captures the imagination of many. Most people who have responded personally to health promotion are interested in these kinds of promises—improved **quality of life,** efficient functioning, the capacity to perform at more productive and satisfying levels, and the opportunity to live out the life span with vigor and stamina. Such potential benefits also appeal to the other sectors whose support is needed for health promotion. Employers will sponsor work-site health promotion programs and facilities if they are assured of improved worker morale and productivity. School administrators will support a school-based program if they are convinced it will help children stay awake and alert in school, perform better on standardized tests, and generally achieve better educational outcomes. In each case, the proponent of health promotion is seeking practical, situation-specific results other than the traditionally defined health outcomes. There are, then, three options:

- Adopt a broader definition of health than conventional measures dictate.
- Abandon these other sectors as arenas in which health promotion can usefully operate.

- Retain the traditional definitions of health and the proposed definition of health promotion while explicitly identifying some of the other outcomes and potential benefits of health promotion.[140]

This third approach is depicted in Figure 1-5.

COMBINING EDUCATIONAL AND ECOLOGICAL APPROACHES

Health education is any combination of learning experiences designed to facilitate voluntary actions conducive to health. *Combination* emphasizes the importance of matching the multiple determinants of behavior with multiple learning experiences or educational interventions. *Designed* distinguishes health education from incidental learning experiences as a systematically planned activity. *Facilitate* means predispose, enable, and reinforce. *Voluntary* means without coercion and with the full understanding and acceptance of the purposes of the action. *Action* means behavioral steps taken by an individual, group, or community to achieve an intended health effect or to build their *capacity* for health.

Health promotion was defined in the earlier paragraphs of this chapter as the combination of educational and ecological supports for actions and conditions of living conducive to health. *Combination* again refers to the necessity of matching the multiple determinants of health with multiple interventions or sources of support. *Educational* refers to health education as defined in the foregoing paragraph. *Ecological* refers to the social, political, economic, organizational, policy, regulatory, and other environmental circumstances interacting with behavior in affecting health. *Ecology* is defined in the *Dictionary of Epidemiology* as "the study of relationships among living organisms and their environment."[141] The more restrictive terms, *human ecology* and *social ecology* apply here. They refer less to the physical environment than to the dynamic social forces operating on the situation and the population. In planning health promotion, physical environmental factors usually need to be considered, but one can distinguish health promotion from the other two major components of public health by leaving the engineering of the physical environment to health protection and the management of the medical environment to preventive health services.

Living conditions permit our definition of health promotion to range beyond the strictly behavioral into the more complex web of culture, norms, and socioeconomic environment associated with the broader historical meaning of *lifestyle* and *determinants of health.* Though the least well-defined or researched aspects of health promotion, these are the ones on which much has been written. Much of the writing about these dimensions of health promotion tends to be either descriptive, as in correlational studies of the relationship of poverty and health, or exhortatory, as in polemical critiques of health promotion policies attributed to a victim-blaming ideology. The two terms, *lifestyle* and *determinants of health,* are

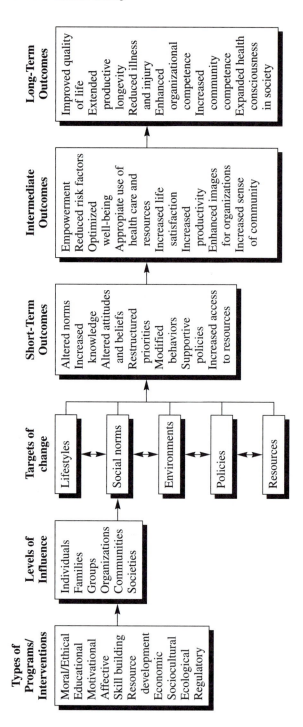

FIGURE 1-5

The approximate relationships among objects of interest to health and other sectors cooperating in health promotion are shown as causes and effects.

SOURCE: Reprinted by permission from *American Journal of Health Promotion* from "The Health Promotion Research Agenda Revisited," by L. W. Green, *American Journal of Health Promotion* Volume No. 6, pages 411–413. Copyright 1992 by *American Journal of Health Promotion*.

often contrasted with each other as if they were in a contest over which is more important to health. They are, in fact, inseparable and interdependent. Lifestyles are proximal determinants of health, while the other determinants considered important to health are usually more distal in time or space. They exert a distal influence because they produce the underlying predisposing, enabling, and reinforcing factors for lifestyle.

Educational approaches can attempt to influence the predisposing factors through direct communications, the enabling factors through training and organization, and the reinforcing factors through indirect communications in the social environment to create norms and values that support lifestyles conducive to health. Ecological approaches employ policy, organization, and regulation to influence the enabling and reinforcing factors for environmental and lifestyle changes supportive of health. Because behavior and environment have a fully reciprocal cause-effect relationship, what can be affected in one through either educational or ecological approaches will inevitably affect the other.

The Ottawa Charter's definition of health promotion as "enabling people to increase control over, and to improve, their health"[142] expresses the purpose and philosophy of health promotion. The definitions offered here emphasize the scope and methods as well as the purposes of health education and health promotion. They enable us to delineate which programs, activities, and methods may be characterized as educational or promotional. In practice, health education is usually embedded in health promotion or other programs (patient education in medical care programs, occupational health education in industrial safety and employee health promotion programs, school health education in school programs) rather than existing as autonomous activities.

The term *health promotion* itself emerged in U.S. health policy in its most recent incarnation as a last-minute substitute by Congress in 1975 for the term *health education.* As the legislative bills for a national health education act were readied to be referred to congressional committees, the term was replaced to avoid having the bills referred to the education committees. It was deemed likely that the bill would have died in the education committees of Congress for lack of interest in health within the education field.[143] The term *health promotion* did not receive a definition as it emerged in Public Law 94-317, The Health Information and Health Promotion Act. This act created the Office of Health Information and Health Promotion, which had no definition of health promotion until it fashioned an operational definition in 1979. This definition, much like the one from the Ottawa Charter, was expressly designed to seize the larger terrain of organizational and political interventions that enlightened health educators had always presumed were their responsibilities but that others usually assumed lay beyond the scope of health education.[144]

The most extensive exercise in delineating the elements of health education came with the Professional Role Delineation Project of the National Center for Health Education.[145] This project built on a foundation of previous work by national committees to specify the content and standards of professional training for health education specialists[146] and other health workers applying health education.[147]

The term *motivation,* as in *motivational programs,* has been used in fields such as family planning and social marketing to refer to the activities generally included in health education programs.[148] Motivational programs are often combined with "incentive schemes" designed to appeal to economic motives for changes such as consumption of products or services or family size limitation.[149] From a formal psychological standpoint, this usage is incorrect. Motivation is something that happens within a person, not something done *to* a person by others. It refers to the internal dynamics of behavior, not to the external stimuli. Thus, motivation programs are more correctly identified as programs based on the use of motive-arousing appeals. Strictly speaking, we can appeal to people's motives, but we cannot "motivate" them.

OF MEANS AND ENDS, CAUSES AND EFFECTS

If everyone were highly educated and held homogeneously common values about health-related matters, all that health promotion would require is late-breaking reports on the availability and appropriate uses of new health technologies and discoveries. For better or worse, the world is not like that. The voluntary nature of health education must confront the real world of self-destructive behavior, conflicting values, and actions by corporations and individuals that threaten the health of others. When the goals of a program matter enough to the community, some of the more coercive ecological features of health promotion, such as policies, organizational constraints, and regulatory restrictions on behavior, will be justified and acceptable. Drunk driving laws and laws that restrict smoking in public places, for example, have been deemed important enough in some societies to set very low limits on permissible blood alcohol levels in drivers and very restricted areas for smoking in restaurants or work sites. On the positive side of ecological approaches are incentives such as tax breaks for employers installing work-site health facilities for their employees, or prizes for people who stop smoking in quit-and-win contests.

The scope of health promotion is defined as much by its expected **health outcomes** as by its methods and forms. The changes in health-related behaviors and environments that can result from educational and ecological approaches to health promotion are numerous and varied. Some would seem trivial to people in another place or another time; some would seem draconian and even inhumane to people of another culture or era. Sir Godfrey Vickers once said, "The history of public health could be written as the successive redefinition of the unacceptable." Alternatively, one could write the history of health promotion as the successive and varied definition of what people want from health. The standards of acceptability for health and qualities of life vary across the age span, across communities, across eras, and within each of these.

The population control policies and programs of the People's Republic of China provide an example of ends justifying the means. Each married couple in China was offered the option of taking the "one-child pledge." They received extensive education through mass media, small groups, and counseling to develop their understanding of China's population problem, the country's economic and developmental goals as affected by population growth, and the advantages and disadvantages of small and large families. All of this is essentially educational. The government also offered bonuses and incentives to help offset the perceived disadvantages of having only one child and to reinforce the decision to do so. The couple could freely accept or reject the pledge. If they took it they received economic advantages, including special provisions for the firstborn child such as priority housing and preschool enrollment. If the couple subsequently had a second child, the bonuses were withdrawn. The economic aspect of this program is the promotional component that lies outside the scope of health education. The program had been judged a partial success in making progress toward the national goals of population control, improved maternal and child health, productivity, and, at least for urban couples, quality of life. It received little support in the West, where China's prerogatives to set its own social goals for development and quality of life were judged by Western values and where some sensibilities were inevitably offended by the means employed.[150] Where would you stand on the issues of means and ends in judging this program? Do the ends justify the means?

We can only judge the appropriateness of the ends—that is, the purpose of this policy—by applying our own values and societal norms. The values of most readers of this book arise from Western history and culture and the particular circumstances of Western countries. To apply them broadly is hazardous. The sole reliable criterion to use in judging a policy is the degree to which it meets the needs of the people it is supposed to serve. That criterion can be applied only if we know the needs of the people. Unless we ourselves are the focus of the policy, we are again limited in our ability to judge the people's needs, because the determination is made from our own perspective, filtered through our own perceptions. Our needs differ from the needs of the Chinese population, and need is relative to perceived or felt need. Felt need is a subjective reality. In short, we can only pass judgment on China's one-child policy if we know how the Chinese themselves feel about the population problem and the developmental problems created by population pressure.

So it is with any policy. Health professionals bring their own perception of the importance of health. They must consult with intended recipients of their programs and determine the recipients' perceptions of the needs, problems, and aspirations concerning quality of life. If they do not take this vital step, health policies remain sterile, technocratic solutions to problems that may not exist or that hold a low priority in the minds of the people. The danger is that such technocratic policies may waste resources on a "red herring" and so sabotage a real opportunity to address the people's true concerns. The Chinese family planning policy is an exotic example, easy to criticize on the basis of its means and ends. But the criticism of the means should be based on an understanding of the ends, and a criticism of the ends could appear sanctimonious coming from an outsider. Chapter 2 will introduce the concept of social assessment and suggest ways to ensure that the public's perception of its own problems, needs, or aspirations are taken into account as a first step in the planning process.

THE PRECEDE-PROCEED MODEL

The ideas of **intervention** and support are important for understanding the foregoing definitions of health education and health promotion. Organized health education activity or policies and regulations "intervene" in the process or flow of development and change. The purpose of intervention is to maintain, enhance, or interrupt a behavior pattern or condition of living that is linked to improved health or to increased risks for illness, injury, disability, or death (Figure 1-6). The behavior of interest is usually that of the people whose health is in question, either now or in the future. Equally important in the process of planning and developing the policies and programs are the behaviors of those who control resources or rewards, such as community leaders, parents, employers, peers, teachers, and health professionals.

Supports refer to the environmental conditions that health promotion seeks to leave in place following the intervention so that individuals, groups, or communities can continue to exercise their own control over the determinants of their health. New policies, regulatory provisions, and organizational arrangements represent environmental supports. Informed officials, committed legislators, concerned teachers, skilled parents, and understanding employers can all provide a supportive social environment, and each can be influenced by educational and political interventions. An increase in the proportion of the population who hold a favorable attitude toward the behavior that some individuals wish to adopt provides a supportive environment in the form of normative enabling and reinforcing supports. For example, mass media can be used to raise the level of public awareness of the need to reduce fat in the diet. This in turn can produce a consumer demand for low-fat products in the marketplace, which in turn can cause restaurants and grocers to place more healthful products on their menus and shelves. In the end, this can make the low-fat choice easier for those who wish to change their behavior.

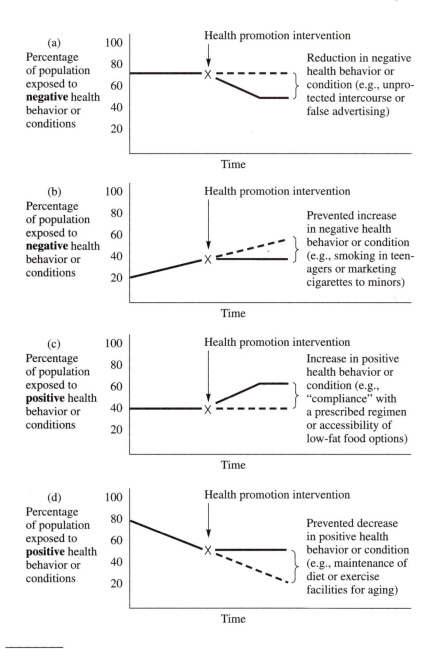

FIGURE 1-6

Examples in each chart illustrate how a type of health promotion intervention influences the prevalence or incidence of selected determinants of health.

Health promotion programs may operate at one of three stages of prevention: primary (hygiene and health enhancement), secondary (early detection), or tertiary (therapy to prevent sequelae or recurrence). In any of these, health promotion offers interventions intended to short-circuit illness or injury, increase health, and enhance quality of life through change or development of health-related behavior (control over the determinants of health) and conditions of living (see Figure 1-6). The Precede-Proceed model takes into account the multiple factors that determine health and quality of life. It helps the planner arrive at a highly focused subset of those factors as targets for intervention. PRECEDE also generates specific objectives and criteria for evaluation. Then PROCEED offers additional steps for developing policy and initiating the implementation and evaluation process (see Figure 1-7).

PRECEDE and PROCEED work in tandem, providing a continuous series of steps or phases in planning, implementation, and evaluation. The identification of priorities in one phase of PRECEDE leads to quantitative objectives that become goals and targets in the implementation phase of PROCEED. They then become the standards of acceptability or criteria of success in the evaluation phases of PROCEED. The progression within PRECEDE sets priorities in one phase that become the delimiting focus of assessment of causes at the next phase. Without this progressive narrowing of focus, the points in the causal chain where interventions would be designed would have so many predisposing, enabling, and reinforcing factors listed as targets that no program could afford to cover them all or to provide much population coverage on even half of them.

As you have seen, PRECEDE is an acronym for *p*redisposing, *r*einforcing, and *e*nabling *c*onstructs in *e*ducational/*e*cological *d*iagnosis and *e*valuation. *Diagnosis* is defined in *A Dictionary of Epidemiology* as

> The process of determining health status and the factors responsible for producing it; may be applied to an individual, family, group, or community. The term is applied both to the process of determination and to its findings.[151]

We used **diagnosis** in the original model[152] and in previous editions of this book to describe each stage of the Precede planning process (e.g., social diagnosis and epidemiological diagnosis). We have replaced this term with *assessment* in this edition, mainly in response to many users who feel uncomfortable with the term *diagnosis*. Though we still consider *diagnosis* to be an appropriate denotation for the processes described in each phase, its connotation tends to associate the model with clinical procedures. It also tends to imply that all the assessments must start with or find a problem. Positive approaches to health and assets-based approaches to community assessment call for at least part of the planning process to be concentrated on aspirations and strengths, not just on needs, weaknesses, deficits, problems, and barriers.

Recall that PROCEED stands for *p*olicy, *r*egulatory and *o*rganizational *c*onstructs in *e*ducational and *e*nvironmental *d*evelopment. PRECEDE and PRO-

PRECEDE

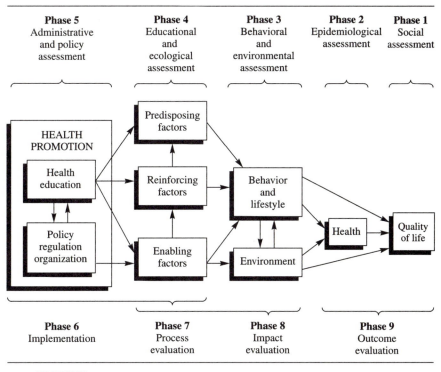

Phase 5	Phase 4	Phase 3	Phase 2	Phase 1
Administrative and policy assessment	Educational and ecological assessment	Behavioral and environmental assessment	Epidemiological assessment	Social assessment

Phase 6	Phase 7	Phase 8	Phase 9
Implementation	Process evaluation	Impact evaluation	Outcome evaluation

PROCEED

FIGURE 1-7

This generic representation of the PRECEDE-PROCEED model for health promotion planning and evaluation shows the main lines of causation from inputs to outcomes by the direction of the arrows, and it shows the order of analysis in planning and evaluation in the phases. This representation of the model does not show the feedback processes inherent in the theory underlying the model.

CEED work in tandem, providing a continuous series of steps or phases in planning, implementation, and evaluation. The identification of priorities and the setting of objectives in the Precede phases provide the objects and criteria for policy, implementation, and evaluation in the Proceed phases.

PRECEDE-PROCEED is not the only road to quality health promotion. Other models of health behavior, health education, health planning, and health promotion predate it, and many more have emerged since its first incarnation in 1974.[153] PRECEDE-PROCEED is, however, a theoretically "robust" model that addresses a major acknowledged need in health promotion and health education: comprehensive planning. This capability has increased with the more explicit representation of ecological aspects, which were implied in earlier versions. It is also robust in the sense that it applies to health promotion in a variety of situations.[154] It has served as a successful model in the planning of several rigorously evaluated, randomized clinical and field trials and has been formally tested in some of these.[155] Local health departments have used it as a guide to developing programs adopted by several state health departments.[156] It was widely distributed as a federal guide to the planning, review, and evaluation of maternal and child health projects.[157] It has been applied as an analytical tool for health education policy on a national and international scale.[158] Adaptations of it have been published and recommended by the National Committee for Injury Prevention and Control for planning and evaluating safety programs,[159] by the American Lung Association as a *Program Planning and Evaluation Guide for Lung Associations,*[160] and by the American Cancer Society and the National Cancer Institute as the framework for a school nutrition and cancer education curriculum.[161] It has served as an organizational framework for curriculum development or training in health education for nurses,[162] pharmacists,[163] allied health professionals,[164] physicians,[165] and interdisciplinary training for behavioral scientists and health educators.[166]

Other applications and validations of the model will be mentioned or illustrated in subsequent chapters. You can visit a web site (www.ihpr.ubc.ca) for a searchable bibliography of more than 750 published applications of the model. In an interactive software version of the model, available as a training package, we illustrate its application to planning a breast cancer detection program.[167] Various manuals and field guides for application of the model make it even more accessible to practitioners.[168]

The Proceed component of the model is of more recent vintage and has had less exposure and testing. It is essentially an elaboration and extension of the administrative assessment step of PRECEDE. In a later chapter, we shall explore the Proceed framework, which has emerged with increasing detail in work on health promotion planning,[169] policy,[170] evaluation,[171] and implementation.[172]

BEGINNING AT THE END

One of the motivations to create the first edition of this book came from the observation of two phenomena related to health education practice, both of which seem to apply to health promotion. First, many people responsible for planning health education programs had more or less predetermined what intervention strategy they were going to employ. Second, in some instances, there was no apparent reason for choosing either the health issue to be addressed or the target population to be reached. Usually, the practitioner seemed to select interventions

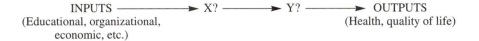

INPUTS —————————▶ X? —————————▶ Y? —————————▶ OUTPUTS
(Educational, organizational,   (Health, quality of life)
    economic, etc.)

FIGURE 1-8

A simplified schema of the causal chain expected to be set in motion by a health promotion program, where X and Y are some unknown combination of determinants of health that should be known before selecting the appropriate combination of program inputs.

based on which techniques he or she was most comfortable applying. Some were expert in mass media, some in community organization, and some in group work. Each tended to apply their preferred method even when it was not necessarily the most strategic or tactical choice.

That was then. Contemporary health education practice has far less of that kind of programming, primarily because demands for accountability require stronger justification for the expenditure of scarce resources. Health promotion today falls prey to this problem, however, because a much wider range of variously prepared professional, business, and commercial personnel find themselves planning programs in health promotion. The systematic and critical analysis of priorities and presumed cause-effect relationships will get the planner off on the right foot in health promotion today, as it has health educators in the past.

In Figure 1-8, *inputs* are interventions (processes) and *outputs* are the anticipated results of the interventions (changes in health or social conditions). Because of their activist orientation, health practitioners understandably tend to begin with inputs. Often, they take a quick glance at the general problem at hand and then immediately begin to design and implement the intervention, assuming that the outcome will occur automatically if they do what worked for them on their last assignment or what worked in some other place. The concept of "best practices" applies with greater reliability for medical and other clinical practices, because the human organism is relatively consistent in its biological functioning across the species. Human communities, organizations, and social behavior are far more variable, making "best practices" less certain of working in the ecological situation at hand.

The Precede framework directs initial attention to outcomes rather than inputs, forcing the planner to begin there. It encourages asking *why* before *how*. From the standpoint of planning, what at first seems to be the wrong end from which to start is in fact the right one. One begins with the desired final outcome and determines what causes it—that is, what must *precede* that outcome (X? or Y? in Figure 1-8). Stated another way, the determinants of health must be diagnosed before the intervention is designed; if they are not, the intervention will be based on guesswork and will run a greater risk of being misdirected and ineffective.

THE EIGHT PHASES OF PRECEDE AND PROCEED

Working through PRECEDE and PROCEED is like solving a mystery. One is led to think first inductively, then deductively; to start with the desired ends and work back to the original causes. Six basic phases comprise the procedure (see Figure 1-7). Evaluation of program impact and outcomes can extend it to seven or eight phases, depending on the evaluation requirements. As an overview, the phases are described in the following brief summary.

Phase 1: Social Assessment and Situational Analysis. Ideally, one begins with a consideration of quality of life by assessing some of the general hopes or problems of concern to the target population (patients, students, employees, residents, or consumers). This is best accomplished by involving the people in a self-study of their own needs and aspirations. The kinds of **social problems** a community experiences offer a practical and accurate barometer of its quality of life. Such problems can be ascertained by several methods, discussed in Chapter 2. Some of the indicators of these subjectively defined problems and priorities are listed in Figure 1-9 as social indicators.

Phase 2: Epidemiological Assessment. Phase 2 applies when the model is used by health professionals to plan a health program. A general community development program might apply this model to other problems or social goals identified in Phase 1, skipping Phase 2. The task of Phase 2 is to identify the specific health goals or problems that may contribute to the social goals or problems noted in Phase 1. Using available data, information generated by appropriate investigations and epidemiological and medical findings, the planner ranks the several health problems or needs. Based on methods outlined in Chapter 3, one selects the specific health problem most deserving of scarce resources. Examples of vital indicators or physiological measures of health factors and dimensions on which they might be measured are shown in Figure 1-9.

Many health professionals must develop a program assigned to them after someone else has concluded, with or without having employed Phases 1 and 2, that a particular health promotion intervention is needed. For example, a hospital administrator may order a smoking-cessation program, or a school principal may purchase an AIDS-oriented health education curriculum, but the developer initially has little idea if or how much the need and appropriateness for that particular intervention as been assessed. This may require starting the planning process at Phase 3 or even 4. When that situation prevails, practitioners need to determine what assumptions have been made in relation to the cause-effect linkages implied in the first two phases. This precautionary action ensures that the assumptions are valid, or at least explicit and understood. It familiarizes the practitioner with crucial information and the basis for the assumptions that have gone into the directive for a health promotion program.

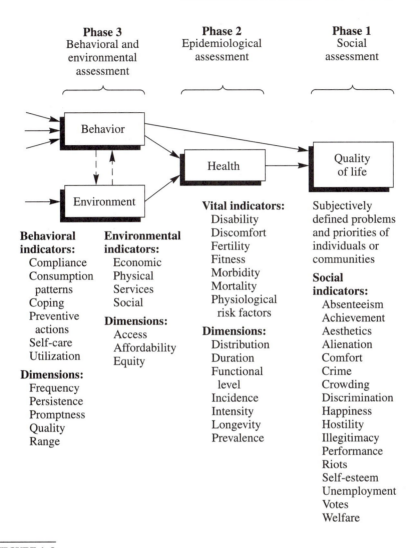

Phase 3
Behavioral and
environmental
assessment

Phase 2
Epidemiological
assessment

Phase 1
Social
assessment

Behavior

Health

Quality
of life

Environment

**Behavioral
indicators:**
Compliance
Consumption
  patterns
Coping
Preventive
  actions
Self-care
Utilization

Dimensions:
Frequency
Persistence
Promptness
Quality
Range

**Environmental
indicators:**
Economic
Physical
Services
Social

Dimensions:
Access
Affordability
Equity

Vital indicators:
Disability
Discomfort
Fertility
Fitness
Morbidity
Mortality
Physiological
  risk factors

Dimensions:
Distribution
Duration
Functional
  level
Incidence
Intensity
Longevity
Prevalence

Subjectively
defined problems
and priorities of
individuals or
communities

**Social
indicators:**
Absenteeism
Achievement
Aesthetics
Alienation
Comfort
Crime
Crowding
Discrimination
Happiness
Hostility
Illegitimacy
Performance
Riots
Self-esteem
Unemployment
Votes
Welfare

FIGURE 1-9

This more detailed representation of the output end of the model suggests relationships, indicators, and dimensions of factors that might be identified in Phases 1, 2, and 3 of the PRECEDE assessment process, or evaluated as outcomes in PROCEED Phases 8 and 9.

Phase 3: Behavioral and Environmental Assessment. Phase 3 consists of identifying the specific health-related behavioral and environmental factors that could be linked to the health problems chosen as most deserving of attention in Phase 2. If the model is applied to a problem other than health, skipping Phase 2, the outer arrows connecting lifestyle and environment to the quality-of-life box become the focus of this phase (see Figure 1-7). These are the risk factors or risk conditions the intervention will be tailored to affect. If the planners fail at this stage to become rigorous in identifying and ranking the lifestyle and environmental factors influencing the outcomes sought, the whole planning process will collapse under its own weight. The radiating cause-effect connections will proliferate beyond the capacity of most programs to encompass them. The process of setting priorities on the basis of causal importance, prevalence, and changeability is important at each phase, but most important in the early phases because of the potential for each factor selected in one phase to require dozens of causal factors to be considered in the next.

Environmental factors are those determinants outside the person that can be modified to support behavior, health, or quality of life. Being cognizant of such forces will enable planners to be more realistic about the limitations of programs consisting only of health education directed at the personal health behavior of the public. It also enables them to recognize that powerful social forces might be influenced when the principles of PROCEED are translated into organizational strategies applied by coalitions on the community, state, or national level. Even at the local level, health-related behaviors influenced by health education can include collective behavior directed at economic or environmental factors through voting or other social action.

Phase 4: Educational and Ecological Assessment. On the basis of cumulative research on health and social behavior, and on ecological relationships between environment and behavior, literally hundreds of factors could be identified that have the potential to influence a given health behavior. The Precede model groups them according to the educational and ecological approaches likely to be employed in a health promotion program to bring about behavioral and environmental change. The three broad groupings are predisposing factors, reinforcing factors, and enabling factors (Figure 1-10).

　　Predisposing factors include a person or population's knowledge, attitudes, beliefs, **values**, and perceptions that facilitate or hinder motivation for change. Predisposing factors could also include genetic predisposition and the early childhood experiences that created the attitudes, values, and perceptions in the first place. These are not included in Figure 1-10 because they are not typically the targets of health promotion programs, but early childhood nurturing truly should be part of a comprehensive policy of health promotion. For that purpose, we would place it in social factors under Phase 1 of the Precede model and direct all of the other arrows at childhood nurturing as a social goal that would produce health reciprocally in the long run.

　　Enabling factors are those skills, resources, or barriers that can help or hinder the desired behavioral changes as well as environmental changes. One can view them as vehicles or barriers, created mainly by societal forces or systems. Facilities and personal or community resources may be ample or inadequate, as might income or health insurance, and laws and statutes may be supportive or

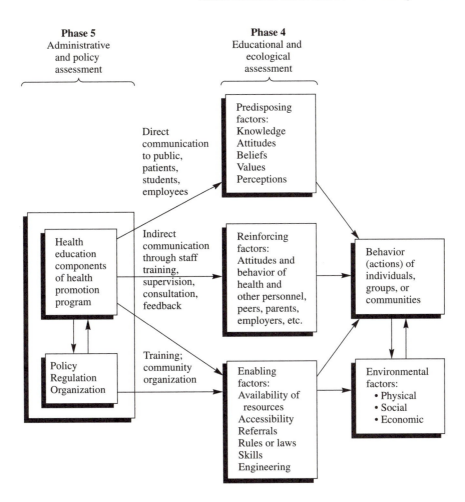

Phase 5
Administrative
and policy
assessment

Phase 4
Educational and
ecological
assessment

Direct
communication
to public,
patients,
students,
employees

Predisposing
factors:
Knowledge
Attitudes
Beliefs
Values
Perceptions

Health
education
components
of health
promotion
program

Indirect
communication
through staff
training,
supervision,
consultation,
feedback

Reinforcing
factors:
Attitudes and
behavior of
health and
other personnel,
peers, parents,
employers, etc.

Behavior
(actions) of
individuals,
groups, or
communities

Policy
Regulation
Organization

Training;
community
organization

Enabling
factors:
Availability of
   resources
Accessibility
Referrals
Rules or laws
Skills
Engineering

Environmental
factors:
• Physical
• Social
• Economic

FIGURE 1-10

Phases 4 and 5 of PRECEDE address the strategies and resources required to influence the predisposing, reinforcing, and enabling factors influencing or supporting behavioral and environmental changes.

restrictive. The skills required for a desired behavior to occur also qualify as enabling factors. These factors thus include all those that *make possible* a change in behavior or in the environment that people want.

Reinforcing factors—that is, the rewards received and the feedback the learner receives from others following adoption of a behavior—may encourage or discourage continuation of the behavior. Reinforcing behavior produces lifestyles (enduring patterns of behavior), which in turn influence the environment through political advocacy, consumer demand, or cumulative actions.

The fourth phase thus consists of sorting and categorizing the factors that seem to have direct impact on each behavioral and environmental target according to the three classes of determinants just cited. Study of the predisposing, enabling, and reinforcing factors automatically helps the planner decide exactly which of the factors making up the three classes deserve highest priority as the focus of intervention. The decision is based on their relative importance and any evidence that change in the factor is possible and cost-effective.

Phase 5: Administrative and Policy Assessment. Armed with the pertinent and systematically organized assessment information, the planner is ready for Phase 5, the assessment of organizational and administrative capabilities and resources for the development and implementation of a program. Limitations of resources, policies, abilities, and time are assessed through methods suggested in Chapter 6. Some of these limitations and constraints can be offset by cooperative arrangements with other local agencies or larger organizations at state, provincial, or national levels or through the development of coalitions and political alliances at the local level. All that remains then is to select a good combination of methods and strategies, to deploy an intervention staff, and to launch the community organizational process.

The planning and launching considerations specific to each of the major settings for health promotion—communities, work sites, schools, and health care settings—will be discussed and illustrated in Chapters 8 through 11, respectively.

Phases 6, 7, and 8: Implementation and Evaluation. Listing evaluation as the last phase is misleading, for evaluation is an integral and continuous process from the beginning through all phases of implementation. Although Chapter 7 presents a methodological discussion of the evaluation component of PROCEED, the criteria for evaluation fall naturally from the objectives defined in the corresponding steps in PRECEDE during the assessment process. These criteria are highlighted in Chapters 2–6. For example, the expositions of the social assessment in Chapter 2 and the epidemiological assessment in Chapter 3 emphasize the importance of stating program objectives clearly, so that the standards of acceptability are defined before, rather than after, the evaluation. Indeed, PRECEDE was first developed as an evaluation model,[173] evolving later into the planning framework presented in this book.

FIRM FOUNDATIONS IN MANY DISCIPLINES

The Precede-Proceed model for planning and evaluation is an outgrowth of the professional disciplines of epidemiology, health education, and health administration. These, in turn, lean heavily on cognate sciences including statistics, social and behavioral sciences, biomedical sciences, economics, and management sciences. The successful completion of Phases 1 and 2, and portions of Phase 3, depends heavily, therefore, on the use of epidemiological and social science methods and information. Working effectively through Phases 3 and 4 requires familiarity with social and behavioral theory and concepts. Handling the complex task of designing and implementing a health promotion program demands knowledge of political, educational, and administrative theory as well as experience. The Proceed phase calls for some understanding of political and administrative science and community organization in order to enter the advocacy and implementation process. It also calls for a knowledge of evaluation methods. In presenting this framework, we assume that you have had some basic exposure to these scientific foundations of health promotion.

Throughout the work with PRECEDE and PROCEED, we shall emphasize two fundamental propositions: (1) health and health risks have multiple determinants and (2) because health and health risks are determined by multiple causes, efforts to effect behavioral, environmental, and social change must be multidimensional or multisectoral. The multidimensional nature of health promotion requires the kind of professional preparation and collaboration that can integrate several scientific and professional disciplines. Not surprisingly, planners occasionally become discouraged and even disenchanted as they wade through and try to synthesize the literature of biomedical science, behavioral science, economics, social and political science, education, and administration. Involving others in a multidisciplinary effort is the best antidote to such disciplinary indigestion. The Precede model can give direction and focus to such attempts. The challenge is to pull together a variety of rapidly developing disciplines as a basis for understanding and in some way contributing to improvements in the quality of life. The ultimate interdisciplinarity, however, lies between the academic and professional disciplines and their counterparts in the community in the spirit of participatory research. It is this challenge that sustains commitment and hope for health education and health promotion.

EXERCISES

1. What trends have you noticed in recent years, in your community or among your friends, in health behavior, conditions of living, and health concerns? Can you find any objective data to support your observations? If not, how would you go about verifying your subjective view of these trends?
2. Identify at least three national or international health campaigns or programs spanning several years. How do you account for the public concern with these different health problems at different times? What were the major features of the health promotion component of these programs? Why have different

programs of problems at different times required different health promotion methods?

3. Identify and describe the demographic characteristics (geographic location, size, age and sex distribution, etc.) of a population (students, patients, workers, residents) whose quality of life you would like to improve. Follow the population you choose through most of the remaining exercises in this book. Look ahead at the upcoming exercises and make sure the population you choose is appropriate for the assessment and planning steps that will be required.

NOTES AND CITATIONS

1. Parts of this chapter were adapted from Green, 1997c, 1998, in press.

2. Terms introduced in boldface type are defined in the glossary.

3. Lalonde, M., 1974. See also Buck, 1986; Raeburn & Rootman, 1988.

4. Green, Richard, & Potvin, 1996; McLeroy, Bibeau, Steckler, & Glanz, 1988; Stokols, 1992.

5. R. M. Goodman, Steckler, Hoover, & Schwartz, 1993; Pearce, 1996.

6. For an early discussion of how this problem of the trade-offs among precision, control, and relevance affected evaluations of health education, Green, 1977. More recent examinations of this issue have emphasized the need for more extensive and systematic use of qualitative and participatory research methods in health promotion planning and evaluation: Green, George, et al., 1995; McGowan & Green, 1995; Wallerstein & Bernstein, 1996.

7. Gold, Green, & Kreuter, 1997 (Sudbury, MA: Jones & Bartlett, 1997); Green, Tan, Gold, & Kreuter, 1994; Schwab & Syme, 1997.

8. Green, 1994.

9. Schauffler, 1994. For an exception to this rule that might be developing, see Schauffler & Rodriquez, 1996.

10. U.S. Preventive Services Task Force, 1996.

11. Fortmann, et al., 1995; Krieger, 1994; Pearce, 1996; Susser, 1985; Terris, 1987.

12. Green, 1990.

13. Green & Frankish, 1996; Harvey, 1990; Wilshire, et al., 1997.

14. Berger, 1997; Chu & Simpson, 1994.

15. For an early account of the recognition of this creeping tendency in health planning, see H. L. Blum, 1981, 1983.

16. Hochbaum, 1956, 1959; Rosenstock, 1974.

17. Rosenstock, Derryberry, & Carriger, 1959.

18. Rosenstock, 1966. See also Harrison, Mullen, & Green, 1992; Janz & Becker, 1984.

19. We shall use lower-case letters in "Precede-Proceed" when it is followed by another word such as *model* or *framework*, sparing the use of all capital letters in the acronyms except when they stand alone to imply some combination of the theory, methods, procedures, model, concepts, steps, or other features of the model. The name PRECEDE was first attached to the model in the first edition of this book (1980), 6 years after its first publication.

20. Green, 1974. See also Green, Werlin, Schauffler, & Avery, 1977.

21. Andersen, 1968.

22. L. W. Green, Fisher, Amin, & Shafiullah, 1975; Green & Krotki, 1968.

23. Green, 1986f; Steuart, 1965.

24. Somers, 1976; Steckler & Dawson, 1978; Steckler, Dawson & Williams, 1981.

25. Moynihan, 1969.

26. Morone, 1990, p. 285.

27. *Report of the President's Committee on Health Education,* 1973.

28. Viseltear, 1976.

29. Mullen, Kukowski, & Mazelis, 1979; P. D. Mullen & Zapka, 1981, 1982.

30. For example, see De Friese, 1989.

31. Kronenfeld, 1986; Levin, 1982; Levin & Idler, 1983; Levin, Katz, & Holst, 1978.

32. L. W. Green, Werlin, Shauffler, & Avery, 1977; Schiller & Levin, 1983.

33. Bosin, 1992; Kreuter, 1993; Oxman, Thomson, Davis, & Haynes, 1995.

34. Devine & Cook, 1983; Green & Kansler, 1979; Posavac, 1980.

35. The research of the 1970s on "compliance" with prescribed medical regimens was assembled and reviewed in Haynes, Taylor, & Sackett, 1979; the patient education research organized by PRECEDE in Green & Kansler, 1979.

36. Green, 1978a; Vickery & Fries, 1981; Vickery, Kalmer, Lowry, et al., 1983.

37. Bibeau, Mullen, McLeroy, et al., 1988; Orleans & Shipley, 1982; Schwartz, 1978, 1987.

38. Green, Rimer, & Bertera, 1978.

39. Green, 1993; cost-benefit analysis also gave credence, Green, 1974.

40. Abelin, Brzezinski, & Corstairs, 1987; DeVries, Dijkstra, & Kok, 1992; DeVries & Kok, 1986.

41. Green, Mullen, & Stainbrook, 1986; Mullen, Green, & Persinger, 1985.

42. Kok, 1992; Kok, van den Borne, & Mullen, 1997.

43. Maiman, Green, Gibson, & Mackenzie, 1979; Mamon, Green, Gibson, Gurley, & Levine, 1987.

44. Gerstein & Green, 1994; Orlandi, 1986; Pentz & Trebow, 1991.

45. Hingson, et al., 1996. For "best practices," see B. G. Simons-Morton, Brink, Parcel, et al., 1989.

46. California Department of Health Services, 1995; University of Michigan, 1995.

47. E. B. Fisher, 1995; Green, 1997a; L. Hancock et al., 1997; Susser, 1995.

48. P. D. Mullen et al., 1995; Poland, Green, & Rootman, in press.

49. British Columbia Ministry of Health, 1994; Flynn et al., 1992, 1997.

50. Langille, Mann, & Gailiunus, 1997; Vincent, Clearie, & Schluchter, 1987.

51. Committee on Trauma Research, 1989; Klitzner, 1989.

52. Flay, 1986; Ramirez & McAlister, 1989; Winett, Altman, & King, 1990.

53. Chapman & Lupton, 1995; Ryan, 1991; Wallack, Dorfman, Jernigan, & Themba, 1993.

54. Flynn, 1995; Fortmann, et al., 1995; L. Richard, Potvin, Kishchuk, Prlic, & Green, 1996.

55. Gilbert & Sawyer, 1996; Kann, 1987; Lehrmann & Wolley, 1998.

56. Garr, 1989; F. Mullen, 1982; Nutting, 1987, 1990.

57. Schauffler & Rodriguez, 1993, 1996; cf. Terris, 1998.

58. Lalonde, 1974. Although the Canadian Minister of Health, Marc Lalonde, deserves the credit for putting health promotion on the policy map with his positioning of the **health field concept** in a major national policy document, it was his deputy, Hubert Laframboise, who developed the concept in a paper the previous year: Laframboise, 1973. An identical formulation of the determinants of health had been put forward in 1968, formally published in the same year as the Lalonde report, by Henrik Blum, 1968, 1974.

59. U.S. Department of Health, Education and Welfare, 1979.

60. Nutbeam & Harris, 1995; Ratner, Green, Frankish, Chomik, & Larsen, 1997.

61. Nutbeam & Wise, 1996; World Health Organization, 1979.

62. First International Conference on Health Promotion, 1986.

63. Gilmore & Campbell, 1996; Kok, 1992; Skinner & Kreuter, 1997.

64. We defined it this way in the first edition of this book. Green, Kreuter, Deeds, & Partridge, 1980.

65. U.S. Department of Health, Education and Welfare, 1979.

66. Allegrante, 1986; cf. Green, 1979a.

67. Minkler, 1989; cf. Frankish & Green, 1994; Green, 1986b. From the opposite end of the political spectrum came critiques of government overstepping its intrusion on individual behavior, e.g., M. H. Becker, 1986; cf. book review by Green 1992b.

68. Kickbusch,1989; McLeroy, Steckler, & Bibeau, 1988; cf. Green, Potvin, & Richard, 1996.

69. Duhl, 1986; T. Hancock, 1985; Milio 1983; cf. Wharf Higgins & Green, 1994.

70. Allegrante & Green, 1981; Green, 1994a; Holtzman, 1979; McKinlay, 1975.

71. Green, 1985a; Lohrmann & Fors, 1986; Williams, 1993.

72. Green, 1979b. See also Green, 1980a, p. 28: "Health promotion is a combination of health education and related organizational, political and economic programs designed to support changes in behavior and in the environment that will improve health." This was abandoned in the federal initiative, because its reference to environment encompassed **health protection,** which was designated a strategy separate from health promotion in the government's environmental initiatives such as sanitation, fluoridation, toxic agent control, and occupational safety.

73. *Health Promotion,* 1984; Kickbusch, 1986b; Nutbeam, 1985. WHO headquarters published the latest edition of Nutbeam's Glossary in 1998 with consultation from a wider geographic spectrum than the European Region: Nutbeam, 1998.

74. Green, 1978a, 1993; Green, Cargo, & Ottoson, 1994.

75. Kreuter, 1989; Wallerstein & Bernstein, 1988.

76. Mason, 1984.

77. Catford, 1983; Dwore & Kreuter, 1980; Freudenberg, 1978; Green, 1981, 1984c; Kreuter, 1984; Parlette, Glogow, & D'Onofrio, 1981; Steckler, Dawson, Goodman, & Epstein, 1987.

78. First International Conference on Health Promotion, 1986.

79. Gerstein & Green, 1993; Green & Ottoson, 1999; Green & Raeburn, 1988; Jenny, 1993; Mosher & Jernigan, 1989; Wallack, 1985.

80. Faden, 1987; L. E. Goodman & Goodman, 1986; Green 1986b; Green & Frankish, 1996.

81. Green, 1994b; McLeroy, Bibeau, Steckler, & Glanz, 1988; Minkler, 1989; Roberts, 1987.

82. Green & Frankish, 1996; Kreuter, 1984.

83. Green & Ottoson, 1999.

84. Eklundh & Pettersson, 1987; Evers, 1989; Green, 1991, 1995; Ingledew, 1989; Leppo & Melkas, 1988; McGinnis, 1982, 1990; Nutbeam & Wise, 1996.

85. Bracht, 1990; Green, 1990; Green & Raeburn, 1988; C. F. Nelson, Kreuter, Watkins, & Stoddard, 1987; R. D. Patton & Cissell, 1989; Wickizer, Wagner, & Perrin, 1998.

86. Freire, 1970; Green, 1982, 1986f; Minkler, 1980–1981; Minkler, Frantz, & Wechsler, 1982–1983; Steckler, Dawson, & Williams, 1981; Tonin, 1980; Zapka & Dorfman, 1982.

87. Altman, 1995; Altman et al., 1991; Fawcett et al, 1997; R. M. Goodman & Wandersman, 1994; Green & Ottoson, 1999; Kreuter & Lezin, 1998; McKinney, 1993; Plough & Olafson, 1994.

88. See the second edition of this book for more on this evolution: Green & Kreuter, 1991.

89. Frankish & Green, 1994; Green, 1978b, 1980c; 1986b; Roberts, 1987.

90. Green, 1986f; Green, George, et al., 1995; Minkler, 1997; Morgan & Horning, 1940.

91. Kickbusch, 1997b; Pollitt, 1994; World Health Assembly, 1985.

92. R. L. Bertera, 1990a; Fielding & Piserchia, 1989; National Resource Center on Worksite Health Promotion, 1992; *National Survey of Worksite Health Promotion Activities,* 1987.

93. R. Y. Cohen, Felix, & Brownell, 1989; Ellison et al., 1989; Flay, 1985; Gerstein & Green, 1993; Parcel, Simons-Morton, & Kolbe, 1988; B. G. Simons-Morton, Parcel, & O'Hara, 1988a.

94. Epstein, 1979; Mechanic, 1979.

95. Handel & Rainwater, 1964.

96. Mattarazzo, 1984.

97. Andersen, 1968; Green, 1970c; Langlie, 1977; A. F. Williams & Wechsler, 1972.

98. N. H. Gottlieb & Green, 1984; Kannas, 1982; Nutbeam, Aaro, & Wold, 1991.

99. Aaro, Laberg, & Wold, 1995; Coreil & Levin, 1985.

100. J. Allen & Allen, 1986; Krieger, 1994; Pearce, 1996.

101. P. Hawe, Noort, King, & Jordens, 1997; Kickbusch, 1997a.

102. Green, 1988e.

103. Dwore & Kreuter, 1980; London, 1982; Love, Davoli, & Thurman, 1996.

104. Kickbusch, 1986a.

105. Milio, 1983.

106. Green, 1978a, 1978b, 1979a, 1979b, 1979c, 1980b, 1980c; Morone, 1990.

107. Parts of this section are taken by permission of *American Journal of Health Promotion* from "Ecological Foundations of Health Promotion," by L. W. Green, L. Potvin and L. Richard, *American Journal of Health Promotion* Volume 10, pages 270–281. Copyright 1996 by *American Journal of Health Promotion.*

108. Green & Ottoson, 1999, chap. 2; E. S. Rogers, 1960; Rosen, 1958; Sydenstricker, 1933.

109. E. R. Brown & Margo, 1978; Freudenberg, 1978; Green, 1979b; Pearce, 1996; Schwab & Syme, 1997.

110. Park, Burgess, & McKenzie, 1925.

111. Griffiths & Knutson, 1960; M. A. C. Young, 1967.

112. Green, 1970a; E. M. Rogers, 1973.

113. Green, 1975; Green, Gottlieb, & Parcel, 1991.

114. Anderson, 1957.

115. Barker, 1965.

116. Baer, 1974.

117. Flay, 1987; Hovland, Janis, & Kelley, 1953; Worden et al., 1988.

118. Lewin, 1943; Nyswander, 1942.

119. Mico, 1982; Morgan & Horning, 1940; Steuart, 1965.

120. N. E. Miller, 1984.

121. Bandura, 1977b; N. M. Clark, 1987; Parcel & Baranowski, 1981.

122. Dewey, 1946.

123. Creswell, & Newman, 1997.

124. Kolbe, 1986.

125. Parcel, Simons-Morton, & Kolbe, 1988.

126. Poland, Green, & Rootman, in press.

127. Hayes & Willms, 1990.

128. Macdonald & Bunton, 1992; McLeroy, Bibeau, Steckler, & Glanz, 1988.

129. Thorogood, 1992.

130. Green & Raeburn, 1988; Minkler, 1989.

131. Green & Ottoson, 1999.

132. Eisenberg, 1972, p. 123. See also Foster, 1962; Paul, 1955.

133. Foster, 1962; Paul, 1955.

134. Sells, 1969.

135. Slobodkin, 1988.

136. Kay & Schneider, 1994, p. 39.

137. Pittman, 1993, p. 169.

138. A. W. King, 1993.

139. Jasnoski & Schwartz, 1985; Terris, 1975.

140. Green, A. L. Wilson, & Lovato, 1986.

141. Last, 1995, p. 52.

142. First International Conference on Health Promotion, 1986, p. i.

143. Viseltear, 1976.

144. Green, 1979b.

145. H. P. Cleary, 1995; Henderson, 1987; Henderson, Wolle, Cortese, & McIntosh, 1981; *National Conference for Institutions Preparing Health Educators,* 1981; *Preparation and Practice of Community, Patient and School Health Educators,* 1978.

146. Society for Public Health Education, 1977; World Health Organization, 1979b.

147. World Health Organization, 1979b.

148. Frederiksen, Solomon, & Brehony, 1984; Manoff, 1987.

149. Green, 1988d.

150. Ibid.

151. Last, 1995, p. 46.

152. Green, 1974.

153. For summaries of planning models in health promotion, see Bates & Winder, 1984; Breckon, 1982, 1997; Breckon, Harvey, & Lancaster, 1998; Dignan & Carr, 1992; Ewles & Simnett, 1985, chap. 6 and 7; Gilmore & Campbell, 1996, esp. pp. 12–18; Greenberg, 1987; Longe, 1985; Manoff, 1985; Marsick, 1987; Parkinson et al., 1982; Pollock, 1987; H. S. Ross & Mico, 1980; Simons-Morton, Greene & Gottlieb, 1995; Strehlow, 1983, chap. 6; Tones, 1979.

154. In the past, PRECEDE was called a framework. This was a caution against claiming too much for it as a model or a theory. A theory is "a set of interrelated constructs (variables), definitions, and propositions that presents a systematic view of phenomena by specifying relations among variables, with the purpose of explaining natural phenomena," from Kerlinger, 1979, p. 64. The primary purpose of PRECEDE was not to explain "natural phenomena" but to organize existing theories and constructs (variables) into a cohesive, comprehensive, and systematic view of relations among those variables important to the planning and evaluation of health education. Given the extensive application and validation of the framework in practice and in research during the 1970s and 1980s, we have felt confident in calling it a model for the past decade or more. Continuing research and application of the model in the 1990s has begun to take form as a theory of health promotion. For further discussion of models and theories see Glanz, Lewis, & Rimer, 1997; Green, 1986; Green & Lewis, 1986; Kar, 1986; Lorig & Laurin, 1985; P. D. Mullen, Hersey, & Iverson, 1987; Rothman & Tropman, 1987.

155. Some of the early trials that helped validate and shape the representation of the model in the first and second editions of the book were Cantor et al., 1985; Green, 1974; Green, Fisher, Amin, & Shafiullah, 1975; Green, Levine, Wolle, & Deeds, 1979; Green, Wang, & Ephross, 1974; Hatcher, Green, Levine, & Flagle, 1986; D. M. Levine et al., 1979; Maiman, Green, Gibson, & Mackenzie, 1979; Morisky et al., 1980, 1983, 1985; Morisky, Levine, Green, & Smith, 1982; Rimer, Keintz, & Fleisher, 1986; Sayegh & Green, 1976; Wang et al., 1979. Some of the more recent clinical trials and other tests and applications of the model will be cited or described in later chapters of this edition.

156. Brink, Simons-Morton, Parcel, & Tiernan, 1988; Gielen & Radius, 1984; Health Education Center, 1977; Newman, Martin, & Weppner, 1982; *PATCH,* 1985.

157. Green, Wang, et al., 1978.

158. Danforth & Swaboda, 1978; Green, 1986d; Green, R. W. Wilson, & Bauer, 1983.

159. National Committee for Injury Prevention and Control, 1989. For specific applications in injury prevention and control, see also Eriksen & Gielen, 1983; Sleet, 1987.

160. Green, 1987b.

161. Light & Contento, 1989. See also the broader ACS Plan for Youth Education: Corcoran & Portnoy, 1989.

162. Ackerman & Kalmer, 1977; Berland, Whyte, & Maxwell, 1995; Shine, Silva, & Weed, 1983.

163. Fedder & Beardsley, 1979.

164. B. I. Bennett, 1977; Simpson & Pruitt, 1989.

165. Green, 1984d, 1987a; Green, Eriksen, & Schor, 1988; R. S. Lawrence, 1988; D. M. Levine & Green, 1983, 1985; Mann, 1994; Oxman, Thompson, Davis, & Haynes, 1995; Wang et al., 1979.

166. Altman & Green, 1988; L. W. Fisher, Green, McCrae, & Cochran, 1976; D. M. Levine & Green, 1981.

167. Gold, Green, & Kreuter, 1997.

168. M. W. Kreuter, Lezin, Kreuter, & Green, 1998.

169. Green, 1980b, 1987b; Iverson & Green, 1981; Kolbe et al., 1981; Kreuter, 1984; Kreuter, Christenson, & DiVincenzo, 1982; *Strategies for Promoting Health in Special Populations,* 1987.

170. Green, 1979b, 1986d, 1988c.

171. R. Bertera & Green, 1979; Bibeau et al., 1988; Cantor et al., 1985; H. Cohen, Harris, & Green, 1979; Green, 1986a, 1986e; Green & Lewis, 1986; Green, George et al., 1995; Kreuter, 1985a; Kreuter, Christenson, & Davis, 1984; Kreuter, Christianson, Freston, & Nelson, 1981.

172. Cataldo et al., 1986; deLeeuw, 1989; Green, Simons-Morton, & Potvin, 1997; Kreuter, Christenson, & DiVincenzo, 1982; C. F. Nelson, Kreuter, & Watkins, 1986; Ottoson & Green, 1987; Powell, Christenson, & Kreuter, 1984.

173. Green, 1974.

Chapter 2

Social Assessment
and Participatory Planning

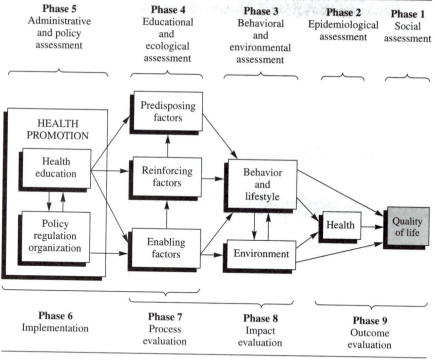

PRECEDE

| **Phase 5**
Administrative
and policy
assessment | **Phase 4**
Educational
and
ecological
assessment | **Phase 3**
Behavioral
and
environmental
assessment | **Phase 2**
Epidemiological
assessment | **Phase 1**
Social
assessment |

HEALTH PROMOTION

Health education

Policy regulation organization

Predisposing factors

Reinforcing factors

Enabling factors

Behavior and lifestyle

Environment

Health

Quality of life

| **Phase 6**
Implementation | **Phase 7**
Process
evaluation | **Phase 8**
Impact
evaluation | **Phase 9**
Outcome
evaluation |

PROCEED

This chapter begins with the rationale and assumptions that justify social assessment and participatory planning. It describes the reciprocal relationship between health and the **social indicators** that reflect quality of life and explains the importance of interpreting "health" as an instrumental rather than ultimate value. The chapter also describes tested methods and tools for conducting a social assessment and for promoting participation in planning.

SOCIAL ASSESSMENT AND PARTICIPATION: THE RATIONALE

Health promotion typically occurs in community or organizational settings that require policy decisions to support the programs.[1] The *ecological* perspective tells us that the factors influencing people's health status and their perceptions of what is important are shaped, modified, and maintained by the interaction of people with the community or organizational environments in which they live. The *educational* perspective tells us that people learn continuously from their environmental and social surroundings and can develop the knowledge and skills to modify them. Understanding the social context of communities and organizations from the perspective of those who live or earn their living there is both a pragmatic and moral imperative. First, it is pragmatic because the actions necessary to resolve contemporary health problems require joint participation from multiple community institutions and individuals. It is also pragmatic insofar as people living day-to-day with the issues to be addressed will have knowledge and insights that professionals might not have. Without some mutual understanding that the issue at hand is worthy of attention, joint participation is unlikely. Second, the imperative is moral, based on the principles of informed consent and respect. People should be informed and their views acknowledged, if not honored. It would be both undemocratic and disrespectful to deny them the opportunity to register their concerns on matters that effect their health and quality of life.

Social assessment is grounded in these two imperatives. **Social assessment** is the application, through broad participation, of multiple sources of information designed to expand the understanding of people regarding their own quality of life and aspirations for the common good.

HEALTH AND SOCIAL CONDITIONS: A RECIPROCAL RELATIONSHIP

Most diagrammatic representations of the Precede and Procede model present it as a linear, cause-and-effect process where *inputs* (health education, policy, regulation, and organization) cause certain changes that will eventually lead to *outcomes* (improved quality of life). Of course, some of these linkages, especially

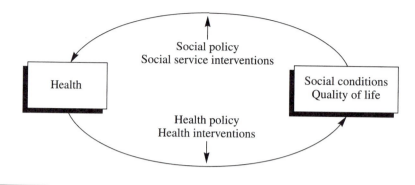

FIGURE 2-1

The relationships between health and social conditions are reciprocal.

the relationships between health and the social or personal quality of life, are not actually one-way streets. A more realistic view is suggested in Figure 2-1, representing the relationships between health problems and quality of life at the individual and community levels. The arrows indicate that health problems influence quality of life at the same time that quality of life affects health.

The top arrow implies that social conditions and quality of life can lead to health problems or the capacity and will to cope with health problems. Health workers can effectively address this aspect of the reciprocal relationship only in cooperation with social workers, recreation professionals, law enforcement, and those in other sectors who shape social policy and social service programs.

The bottom arrow indicates that social conditions and quality of life are themselves influenced by health problems or concerns amenable to modification by policies and interventions for health improvement or maintenance. PRECEDE-PROCEED emphasizes the aspect of the reciprocal exchange represented by the bottom arrow. The feedback loop from quality of life produced by health can make the job of the health professional easier. That is, people will appreciate and support health innovations and policies, even regulations, if they can see clearly how such efforts address their concerns and contribute to their quality of life.[2]

HEALTH: AN INSTRUMENTAL VALUE

The social assessment phase of the Precede-Proceed model is more than a step in a planning and evaluation framework—it is also a way of thinking. This becomes evident when we ask, "Among the many things in life we value, where does health fit?" Health is certainly a good thing. Music, art, work, and play are also good, as parenting or friendship, as well as eating. We value many good things in life, things that compete with each other for our investment of time, interest, and energy. In day-to-day affairs, it is probably rare for people to engage in a given "health-related behavior" primarily because they believe the behavior is going to make them live longer. More likely, actions we deem to be healthful[3] can be explained in terms of how those actions make us feel, function, or look. In some cultures, health behaviors are tied to religious and spiritual tenets. Generally, health seems to be cherished because it serves other ends. The 1986 Ottawa Charter for Health Promotion puts it this way: "Health is seen as a resource for every-day life, not the objective of living."[4] The sociologist Talcott Parsons defines health as "the ability to perform important social roles."[5] These functional views of health see it as a means to other ends and define health in terms of a person's ability to adapt to social and environmental circumstances.[6]

Planners who acknowledge that health is an instrumental value use that insight quite practically, whether at the population or the individual level. When seeking collaboration with nonhealth organizations, health promotion planners first identify the priority values of those organizations and then show how strategic health improvements can enhance those values. For example, corporate decision makers are more likely to support health promotion initiatives for their employees, or even their communities, if they can see how those initiatives relate to their corporate missions—that is, the extent to which they might affect such tangible things as work performance, absenteeism, or excessive medical claims.

Through the application of "tailored communications," computer technology has given health professionals the opportunity to apply our understanding of ultimate and instrumental values at the individual level while taking a population approach.[7] In tailored health communications, a computer generates specific, personalized messages based on an assessment of an individual's characteristics, including those things he or she values and enjoys.[8] For instance, suppose a large work site wants to implement a health promotion program, a part of which includes a tailored communication component designed to increase the level of physical activity across the entire workforce. Brief questionnaires are given to 450 employees. Communication messages are created for all possible combinations of responses to the various questions. The responses of one of those employees, a 32 year-old woman named Ellie Watson, reveals that she has a keen interest in classical music and a passion for gardening. Among the hundreds of messages designed for the subsequent communication back to the 450 employees, Watson will receive those framed within the context of her self-declared interests: listening to classical music while exercising, and earning physical activity points through gardening. In contrast to messages encouraging Watson to increase her level of physical activity because science says it will yield cardiovascular benefits over time, tailoring constitutes a planned effort to connect the *ultimate values* of music and gardening with the *instrumental value* of physical activity.

QUALITY OF LIFE: A MANIFESTATION OF ULTIMATE VALUES

When people undertake efforts to be productive and try to make their conditions of living safe and enjoyable, they are seeking to improve their quality of life. Like most concepts, *quality of life* is measurable to the extent that it can be operationally defined. We define it as *the perception of individuals or groups that their needs are being satisfied and that they are not being denied opportunities to pursue[9] happiness and fulfillment.*

ELICITING SUBJECTIVE ASSESSMENTS OF COMMUNITY QUALITY OF LIFE

Subjective assessments that elicit information from community members about their quality-of-life concerns provide the yeast for health promotion planning. Surveys, structured interviews, or focus groups are frequently used to gain insight on such concerns. The subjective assessment of quality of life offers a view of a particular situation through the eyes of the community residents themselves,[10] who share what matters to them and show where health lies in the context of their lives. Health promotion seeks to promote healthful conditions that improve quality of life as seen through the eyes of those whose lives are affected. Though health promotion might have instrumental value in reducing risks for morbidity and mortality, its ultimate value lies in its contribution to quality of life.

For example, when the Kaiser Family Foundation conducted a social reconnaissance with the state of Mississippi, prior to making health promotion grants in that state, structured interviews revealed that the main concerns of the population centered on quality of housing and economic development, which they related in part to the quality of schooling. These became central themes in the subsequent analysis of health problems and led to the coordination of planning with the housing and economic development sectors of the state government and with the school boards of local communities.[11]

CAN QUALITY OF LIFE BE MEASURED?

A variety of questionnaires or "tools" have been used to assess quality of life as it pertains to specific health outcomes,[12] physical therapy outcomes,[13] leisure activities,[14] mental health,[15] unemployment rates, and descriptions of such environmental features as housing density and air quality. Some quality-of-life scales are designed for individual assessment based on the assumption that quality of life can only be determined by each person's unique values and experiences. The Ferrans and Powers Quality of Life Index is such a scale. It measures four quality-of-life domains: health and functioning, psychological and spiritual, social and economic, and family, and has been effectively applied cross-culturally.[16] In 1992, Stewart and Ware reported on ten years of validation studies for the SF-36, a widely used instrument for assessing patients' views of well-being and ability to function.[17] In medical or nursing care, the counterpart of community social indicators or quality-of-life measures are health outcome measures other than biomedical. These may include ability to perform tasks of daily living, the tolerance for side-effects of medications, energy level, and other indicators of well-being associated with but not identical to the medical condition.[18]

A Caveat on Beginning. Emphasizing quality of life can give rise to unexpected problems. If health administrators have not been briefed on the rationale for focusing on the association between health and quality of life, some may resist allocating organizational support, because they believe that finite health resources will be spent on nonhealth objectives. Thus, effort should be made to make certain that agency directors and all health stakeholders understand that health promotion, more than health services and health protection, will depend on the cooperation of other sectors. Unless the health sector can buy into the broader social goals of primary concern to the community and the other sectors, one may find one's agency on the sidelines of the mainstream of community action and energy, isolated from community resources—unable to attract the interest of the community to the agency's mission, and unable to gain the cooperation of other nonhealth organizations.

A Caveat on Data. Some worry that efforts to make explicit and to generalize perceptions of quality of life will necessarily ignore the subtle differences in perceptions among individuals within a population. They rightfully contend that it is inappropriate to impose one person's perception of wellness and satisfaction on another whose values and priorities are different. Aggregating individual data and reporting averages can seem to suck out the soul of what is most precious in people's lives. Respect for the diversity inherent in communities justifies seeking greater insight about local values and interests through a social assessment phase of planning for health promotion. At the individual level, we have tools that enable us to identify individual interests and perceived quality of life. At the group or community level, we have access to numerous sources of information-gathering methods that allow people the opportunity to hear each other and increase the chances of identifying priorities that reflect the common concerns of all and the variability of concerns among individuals and groups. The social assessment phase of PRECEDE-PROCEED is designed to help planners (1) identify and interpret the social conditions and perceptions shared at the community or organizational level and (2) make the connection between those conditions/ perceptions and health promotion strategies.

THE PRINCIPLE AND PROCESS OF PARTICIPATION

An effective social assessment applies the principle of participation to ensure the active involvement of the people intended to benefit from a proposed program. The importance of this principle, echoed for decades in various applied behavioral sciences, has been confirmed in community experience in three fields: technical assistance, including public health (health education), family planning, and agricultural extension;[19] community and rural economic development from around the world, especially India;[20] and the concern with community involvement through *concientación*,[21] a process largely of Latin-American origin in the 1960s and early 1970s. Figure 2-2 presents a rationale for participation based on the differing perspectives professionals and laypeople have concerning health.[22] Professionals tend to have a sharper focus on the objective indicators of health, whereas laypeople tend to have a more diffuse perception of health, with greater emphasis on subjective indicators such as social, emotional, and metaphysical or spiritual dimensions of health.

FORMS OF PARTICIPATION

The extreme forms of participation are contrasted in Freire's discussion of two theoretical approaches to community change. He characterizes the first as "cultural invasion," the second as "cultural synthesis." In cultural invasion, the actors draw the thematic content of their action from their own values and ideology; their starting point is their own world, from which they enter the world they invade. In cultural synthesis, the actors who come from "another world" do not come as invaders. They come not to teach or transmit or give anything, but rather to learn about this new world along with the people in it.[23]

He contends that those who are "invaded," irrespective of their level in society, rarely go beyond or expand on the models given them, implying that there is no internalizing, no growth, and seldom much adoption and incorporation into their social fabric. In the synthesis approach, there are no imposed priorities: Leaders and people collaborate in the development of priorities and guidelines for action.

According to Freire, resolution of the inevitable contradictions between the views of leaders or outsiders and the views of the local people is only possible

The lenses of health professionals and laypeople

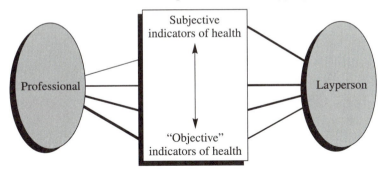

FIGURE 2-2

The public views health through a different set of lenses than do professionals and scientists. The public lens has greater acuity at the subjective end of the spectrum, while professionals have greater acuity at the objectively measured end.

SOURCE: Adapted from an unpublished manuscript by the Yukon Bureau of Statistics, Whitehorse, and the Institute of Health Promotion Research, University of British Columbia, Vancouver, 1995.

where the spirit of cultural synthesis predominates. "Cultural synthesis does not deny differences between the two views; indeed it is based on these differences. It does deny invasion of one by the other, but affirms the undeniable support each gives to the other."[24]

PARTICIPATION IN SETTING PRIORITIES

Given the reality that resources for health promotion and disease prevention are limited, one must prioritize to avoid the debilitating bind of trying to do too much with too little. The need to engender community participation and the need to set program priorities constitute mutually reinforcing reasons for putting the social assessment at the beginning of the Precede-Proceed process. As you will discover in Chapter 3, the careful analysis of statistical information on mortality and morbidity plays a critically important part in determining how resources will be allocated for health improvement efforts at the national, regional, provincial, state, or local level. Political experience demonstrates, however, that priorities will not be determined solely on the basis of the statistical analysis of data indicating the pervasiveness of the problems, or even on their human and economic costs. If planners set priorities based on objective health data without involving the community in the process, the priorities, judged to be "lower" based on statistical criteria, will come back to haunt them on the grounds that the public's perceptions

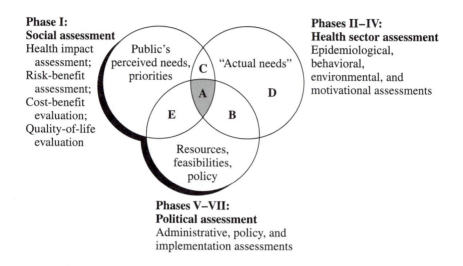

Phase I:
Social assessment
Health impact
    assessment;
Risk-benefit
    assessment;
Cost-benefit
    evaluation;
Quality-of-life
    evaluation

Public's
perceived needs,
priorities

"Actual needs"

C

A

D

E   B

Phases II–IV:
Health sector assessment
Epidemiological,
behavioral,
environmental, and
motivational assessments

Resources,
feasibilities,
policy

Phases V–VII:
Political assessment
Administrative, policy, and
implementation assessments

FIGURE 2-3

Finding the common ground among the public's perception of needs, the health sector's assessments, and political assessments. The potential for action is greatest where public, professional-scientific, and policy perspectives match (A).

of what constitutes a priority was ignored. The community will ask not "Why are you doing A?" but "Why aren't you doing C?" We are not calling for the abrogation of scientific evidence and professional judgement in favor of incorrect public understanding. Nor are we advocating political decisions by public polls. We *are* advocating a sincere synthesis and search for common understanding.[25]

PUBLIC PERCEPTION AND PROFESSIONAL ASSESSMENT: COMMON GROUND

Figure 2-3 illustrates the need to discover "common ground" (area A) by bringing together the three key factors that influence planning: the public's perceived needs, "actual" needs as indicated by scientific data, and resources, feasibilities, and policy. Usually, the public perceives its needs in ways that only partially accord with what epidemiologists and other health professionals might view as "actual needs" (area C). Yet, the view through the lay lenses often carries more weight with policy makers (elected legislators, appointed officials) than do the scientific data brought to the table by health professionals, except in public health crises. Priorities expressed by the public will influence the extent to which resources (the lower circle) are brought to bear on issues of common concern.

Formal planning at national and state levels is generally broader in scope than planning at the local level and tends to rely heavily on quantitative, epidemiological health information.[26] One might therefore assume that the principle of participation, so critical at the local level, is of lesser or even no importance at these more central levels. Not so. When policies and priorities set at one level depend on persons or institutions at another, planners must make every effort to solicit active participation, input, and even endorsement, from that second level. Without such collaboration, the support and cooperation needed from the second level will be unlikely to appear.

Failure to attend to this simple principle, even at the highest levels, is at once a foolish and serious oversight. It is foolish because participation requires mostly simple acts of courtesy and respect, along with the time needed to foster dialogue and, ultimately, trust. The oversight is serious because it often produces a threat to the proposed program. Continued failure to consult and reconcile differences fosters mistrust and undermines collaboration. This sentiment of mistrust explains much of the tension frequently observed between agencies at the national and state or state and local levels.[27] It is also what marks a weakened democracy, as Rose describes:

> Political decisions are for the politicians. Their agenda is complex and mostly hidden from public scrutiny. This is unfortunate, because often the public would give higher priority to health than those who formulate health policies. Anything which stimulates more public information and debate on health issues is good, not just because it may lead to healthier choices by individuals but also because it earns a higher place for health issues on the political agenda. In the long run, this is probably the most important achievement of health education . . . [that] in a democracy the ultimate responsibility for decisions on health policy should lie with the public.[28]

A VISION TO CONSIDER

Figure 2-4 presents an admittedly ideal characterization of health promotion planning. Although ideal, it is meant to provide a graphic vision of what health promotion planners are trying to achieve through participatory planning. The steps fall into two broad categories of actions separated by the vertical divider: community functions and official agency functions. In this instance, we view *community functions* as those closest to where the people whose needs are in question live or work. This could be a work team in a factory, a department or a floor of workers in an office building, an industrial plant, a classroom, a school, a neighborhood, a town, a county, or a district. *Official agency functions* refer to those taken by organizations operating under the auspices of government policies or public mandates at either the local, state or provincial, or national levels. Most often, this will be an official health agency or department, but it may also include a foundation or the headquarters of a private or voluntary health organization. Ideally, the entire sequence would be triggered by the needs and interests expressed at the local level.

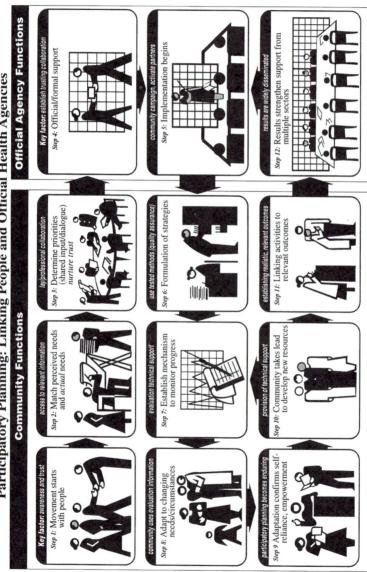

FIGURE 2-4

The ideal sequence of steps in a systematic process of community social assessment, leading to official agency or centralized support, intersectoral cooperation, and ultimately self-reliance.

SOURCE: Adapted from *Health Promotion Planning: An Educational and Environmental Approach*, by L. W. Green and M. W. Kreuter, 1991, Mountain View, CA: Mayfield.

EXAMINING THE STEPS OF ASSESSMENT

Two Functional Levels. The steps to the left under community functions are those initiated, implemented, and controlled by local people. These community functions are placed side by side with official agencies rather than at the bottom of a vertical structure to challenge the perception of hierarchical relationships characteristic of bureaucracies. The relationship between the communities and official agencies, regardless of their "level," should not be viewed or approached as bureaucratic, with implicit top-down command and bottom-up reporting. In planning for health promotion, the ideal is for the initiative and the control to be vested at the most local level and for official agencies or legislatures to seek common elements of local needs and priorities that would benefit from policy, regulatory, organizational, financial, or technical support.

Technical Support. All this talk about local initiative, autonomy, participation, and empowerment would seem to imply that the necessary skills and technical knowledge to carry out a systematic social assessment and planning process are extant in the local group or community. Clearly, communities do indeed possess many of the skills and resources (although often untapped) needed to plan and implement an effective community-based health promotion program. At the same time, however, gaps exist, sometimes quite substantial, in local capacities and skills.[29] With sufficient searching and encouragement, one can find indigenous skills and resources in the community, but they will remain dormant without concerted efforts to identify and bring those resources into play. When health promotion planners nurture community participation, they test their command of the predisposing, enabling, and reinforcing functions of the Precede-Proceed model: (1) *to arouse indigenous community awareness, concern, and initiative,* (2) *to provide technical assistance to those who wish to take initiative,* and (3) *to connect them with the sources of moral and tangible support needed from other levels of organization.* These are implicit in all of the "community functions" depicted in Figure 2-4.

Tasks Common Across Precede Phases. In Figure 2-4, the community functions are expressed in 12 steps. Cutting across all 12 are three essential elements that are applied, with some variation, in the first four phases of PRECEDE—the social assessment, the epidemiological assessment, the behavioral and environmental assessment, and the educational and ecological assessment. Those three steps are

1. Self-study by the community (with or without technical assistance) of its needs, aspirations, and resources or assets
2. Documentation of the presumed causes of the needs, or determinants of the desired goals

3. Decision on the priorities to be assigned among the problems, needs, or goals, based on perceived importance and presumed changeability, and formulation of quantified goals and objectives

These three tasks become more technical as the planning proceeds through the epidemiological, the behavioral and environmental, and educational assessments. For example, the work a professional staff must do in reviewing the scientific literature to document the causes or determinants of health, behavioral, and environmental problems increases in the phases after social assessment; this is because the answers lie more in scientific fact than in values and local insight, which predominate at the level of social and quality-of-life assessment. Failure to engage the community actively in these three steps in the social assessment phase, however, can be most costly in the long-term effectiveness and viability of the health promotion program.

Step 3 in Figure 2-4 will reveal a good deal about the level of collaboration and sensitivity between professionals and lay participants. Hawe astutely calls our attention to the reality that planners can take two routes to change.[30] They can either base a proposed change in the needs of the community or consumer, or they can focus primarily on the needs of the managers or organization(s) they serve. In the former, community members or consumers must play a critical role, but not in the latter. This distinction made, Hawe warns those engaged in community-based planning of the political temptation to seek community "endorsement" to support the planner's agenda: "They should recognize the danger in sublimating community interests in an orchestrated process of consensus building and priority setting, which has a high risk of having its deliberations ignored."[31]

Armed with factual data on a community's problems and trends, professionals will come face-to-face with the felt needs of community members and their natural desire to acknowledge the strengths of their community—often the felt needs either won't show up or will rank low on routine data charts.

Official Functions. In Step 4, an official health organization formalizes the plans or proposals received from one or more local community groups and generates a strategic plan for allocating its resources. Official agency resources include funding, material support, and technical assistance. Step 5 suggests the need for centralized agencies to coordinate their assistance to communities so that a harmonized flow of resources reaches the community. Too often, the state and national organizations seeking to carry out their separate missions at the local level compete unwittingly for the time and effort of precious talent and energy in needy communities. Intersectoral and interagency coordination at the central levels helps reduce the confusing and often redundant signals communities receive.

Implementation and Evaluation. Steps 6 through 8 require central agencies to return selected implementation and evaluation functions to the community. Information and technical assistance number among the supports communities need to be able to carry out these functions, as in some of the earlier assessment and planning functions. We are getting ahead of the social assessment phase here, but it should serve you at this stage to have a picture of how the whole process of community organization and development for health promotion might play out.

The Self-Reliance Cycle. Steps 7 through 10 engage the community in a progressively greater degree of responsibility for managing and evaluating their own progress. By Step 10, the "competent community"[32] will have unearthed or developed its own indigenous resources to maintain the program[33] or to move on to solve other problems on its priority list.[34] Rather than turning back to central agencies for more support at that point (Step 10), the community is "empowered" and returns to Step 7, continuing the self-reliance cycle outlined in Figure 2-4.

Demonstration and Diffusion. Often, the payoff of central support to local community projects, from the point of view of the official or central agencies, is not solving a local problem, but rather demonstrating the problem-solving process by a typical community. The hope of most grant-making organizations is that their grants will inspire other communities or groups to emulate the example demonstrated by the grantees. To maximize this potential, evaluation of project impact and outcomes (Step 11) becomes a central priority. Evaluation results can inspire other communities. They can also help the funding organizations by providing documented examples of how they can improve their coordination with other central organizations (Step 12) and their technical assistance and support to other communities.

KEEPING PERSPECTIVE ON PARTICIPATION AND PARTNERSHIP

Total community participation in developing good polices or plans should be neither expected nor targeted. As George Bernard Shaw put it:

> Every citizen cannot be a ruler any more than every boy can be an engine driver or a pirate king. . . . If you doubt this—If you ask me "Why should not the people make their own laws?" I need only ask you "Why should not the people write their own plays?" They cannot. It is much easier to write a good play than to make a good law. And there are not a hundred men in the world who can write a good play enough to stand the daily wear and tear as long as a law must.[35]

Nevertheless, broad participation through a representation process should be sought in the assessment of needs, because some of the people least "skilled" at planning or "making laws" will bring other valuable assets to the planning table.

Globally, the terms *community, participation, empowerment,* and *collaboration* have become virtual shorthand for health promotion. Although professional health practitioners can take great pride in working in a "people oriented health promotion,"[36] they should not lose sight of the technical insights and scientific data and skill they can share with communities. Counsel offered in the 1983 WHO Expert Committee Report remains valid in the new millennium.

> While health care workers should not compel communities to accept the health technologies they propose, they should also not allow themselves to be forced into a situation where they have to abdicate their views on technical matters. The common ground between the two groups should serve as a basis for fruitful dialogue, which may lead to change, provided health workers keep in mind that sociocultural factors and beliefs are not necessarily for development.[37]

This point deserves careful attention: Professionals should take care not to abdicate their responsibilities while engaging the community in dialogue. In working hard to avoid being manipulative, one can go too far and be so fearful of falling into the trap of Freire's "cultural invasion," of imposing one's own agenda, that one cannot offer constructive assistance. As a planner, you can do two things to avoid this situation. First, keep in mind the fact that you, the lay community, and your collaborators in other agencies and sectors are *partners*. Each can contribute technical or cultural experience and capacities to the task of making a difference. Secondly, make every effort to ensure that all the partners understand what you do and whom you represent. People are more willing to collaborate with you when they know what agency or group you represent and what its mission or agenda is. They need to understand what you can and cannot do—the technical capacities you have to offer as well as the limitations placed on you by your agency or employer. An understanding of these issues, which at first glance may seem irrelevant, helps all parties clarify boundaries and roles and set realistic expectations.

Partnership implies complementarity of roles and contributions. Each partner can magnify the contribution of others and through the partnership can leverage his or her own capabilities and resources. In the end, the partnership should evolve into "delegated power," relinquished by the outside helping agencies, and eventually into full control by the community and its own professional and lay leadership. This will not happen easily if the partnership starts out with a "senior partner" from the outside, with the community in the role of "junior partner."

In summary, social assessment should begin with more than token participation from the community, and it should lead toward full citizen control of the process with helping agencies providing information and technical assistance as requested by the community.

STRATEGIES FOR SOCIAL ASSESSMENT

In seeking ideas, methods, and strategies for planning, implementing, and evaluating health promotion programs, one should look to the literature of public health, social and behavioral sciences, community development, and health education as a first and continuing resource. By carefully examining the findings and methods of others, one gains insights and sharpens one's thinking on social assessment.[38] The literature illustrates the ways diverse methods of data collection have been used in social assessments, including key informant interviews, community forums, focus groups, nominal group process, and surveys. Because time and resources are precious, it is wise to retrieve existing information whenever possible; sources of routinely collected data exist and most of these are in the public domain and easily accessible. A thorough social assessment, however, will always require at least some new and tailored information, or it will tend to reinforce the status quo.[39] We offer the following descriptions of procedures and methods as options for obtaining such information.

ASSESSING ASSETS: COMMUNITY RESOURCES

Communities differ on virtually any demographic parameter one can think of: population size, ethnicity, culture, history, industry, employment, geography, and so on. However, just as they differ demographically, communities vary in terms of their resources and capacities, including past experience with implementing community-based health promotion programs.

The North Karelia Cardiovascular Disease Prevention Project is one of the most successful and well documented of such programs. Analysis of 20 years' data and experience revealed that the combination of their multiple intervention strategies achieved a 50% decline in cardiovascular mortality among Finnish men.[40] In a publication describing their methods and strategies, the investigators offered this advice: "To the greatest extent possible, the community analysis ('community assessment') should provide a comprehensive understanding of the situation at the start of the program."[41] Adhering to the principles of social assessment, they systematically obtained data to understand better the people's perceptions about the problems and how they felt about the possibility of solving those problems, but they did not stop there.

> Because the program would depend upon the cooperation of local decision-makers and health personnel, these groups were surveyed at the outset. *The community resources and service structure were also considered before deciding on the actual forms of program implementation.*[42] [Italics ours]

The last sentence highlights the commonsense notion that before taking action, one should determine what resources critical to the planning process one has at hand. Travel anywhere in the world and you will see this simple truth played out in architecture—wooden structures predominate in forested regions, rock structures prevail near quarries, and igloos dot the arctic. In a computerized application of the Precede-Proceed model called *EMPOWER*,[43] we refer to this general process as a "situation analysis." The results of such an analysis gives planners useful information about the resources (human and economic) and

---
TABLE 2-1

Situation analysis: some key questions to be addressed before planning

Stakeholders
(all those who have an investment in the health of the community organization)
    1 Who are they?
    2 Are they aware of the program?
    3 Are they supportive or apprehensive?

Potential Organizational Collaborators and Key Informants
    1 Who are they?
    2 Have they been invited to participate?
    3 Are they supportive or apprehensive?

Staff/Technical Resources
    1 Are experienced personnel available for this planning?
    2 Will the staff require special training for planning?
    3 What existing data and systems resources are available to plan a program or strategy?

Budget
    1 Have planning costs been estimated?
    2 Are the facilities and space necessary to conduct the program available?
    3 Are there opportunities to apply for funds to meet staff, equipment, and space needs?
    4 What is the time line for the planning process before the program must begin?

---

conditions currently in place. Part of the situational analysis follows from pursuing answers to routine questions like those presented in Table 2-1.

ASSESSING CAPACITY: COMMUNITY COMPETENCE/READINESS

In their critical examination of the multiple determinants of health, Evans, Barer, and Marmor ask the provocative question: "Why are some people healthy and others not?"[44] Changing the focus from individuals to communities, we pose a similar question: "Why are some communities healthier than others?" Studies testing the effectiveness of community-based public health programs reveal that even with the application of sound theory, tested methods that are adequately supported, and rigorous evaluation, some programs may fall short of their expected goals. We believe that at least some portion of so-called program failures is likely to be attributable to preexisting social factors that mediate the planning and execution of those programs. One such factor may be a given community's past experience and capacity—its *social capital*.[45] We define **social capital** as the processes and conditions among people and organizations that lead to accomplishing a goal of mutual social benefit. Those processes and conditions are manifested by four interrelated constructs: trust, cooperation, civic engagement, and reciprocity.

Studies of the Effects of Social Relationships on Human Health. Discussions about social support are often framed in terms of three factors, first described by House:[46] characteristics of individuals, properties of the relationships among individuals, and community contexts. In the area of "community contexts," the idea of social support becomes critical. The practical implications for determining a community's level of social capital are quite significant for the development of social support. Given a sound plan and the resources to implement it, communities with high levels of social capital would be well positioned to move forward. Those with lower levels of social capital would likely require a focused, preimplementation effort to strengthen their existing collaborative capacities.

The "constructs" or components of social capital (trust, civic participation, social engagement, and reciprocity) have been independently measured.[47] Although not rigorously tested, the *Civic Index*[48] offers a practical approach that is likely to give planners a sense of the level of a community's capacity for undertaking a community-based health promotion program. Devised by the National Civic League and applied in numerous settings,[49] the Civic Index addresses ten categories, each of which has just a few questions or probes designed to elicit information about the community's strengths and weakness for that domain (see Table 2-2).

ASSET MAPPING

Some have correctly observed that a good deal of social and health policy seems to be driven by a focus on health "problems," with outsiders and professionals calling attention to "deficiencies." This problem-oriented approach is inherently negative,

---

TABLE 2-2

The ten categories of the Civic Index are measured by the National Civic League

Citizen participation	Civic education
Community information sharing	Capacity for cooperation and consensus building
Community leadership	Community vision and pride
Government performance	Intercommunity cooperation
Volunteerism and philanthropy	Intergroup relations

especially for low-income populations. To balance this perspective, McKnight and Kretzmann[50] advocate a strategy called *asset mapping,* which is an assessment of the capacities and skills of individuals and the existing assets in a neighborhood or community. The process of asset mapping is divided into three tiers called primary building blocks, secondary building blocks, and potential building blocks. The most accessible, primary building blocks can be discovered by assessing individual capacities and those assets *controlled within the neighborhood or community.* Secondary building blocks refer to those assets located in the neighborhood or community but *controlled by those outside that area* (see Table 2-3).

Potential building blocks, which are the least accessible, refer to potential assets *located and controlled outside of the community.* Examples include state and federal grant programs, corporate capital investments, and public information campaigns. The lists of specific assets in a community can be visually reflected using the metaphor of a map, an architectural metaphor as suggested by the notion of "building blocks," or as a balance scale showing assets on one side and needs and problems on the other.

Given the diversity of communities and cultures, experienced health promotion planners may be inclined to devise their own simple surveys to identify community assets and individual abilities within the areas they serve. Before doing that, however, we urge them to review existing survey instruments such as the Civic Index, mentioned earlier, or the Community Capacity Inventory checklist, developed by Kretzmann and McKnight for identifying community assets.[51]

THE SOCIAL RECONNAISSANCE METHOD
FOR COMMUNITY SOCIAL ASSESSMENT

Social reconnaissance is a method for determining relevant aspects of the social structure, processes, and needs of a community using leaders (general, local, and specialized) as informants or interviewees.[52] Developed by Sanders,[53] and elaborated on by Nix,[54] social reconnaissance was adapted and applied by the Henry J. Kaiser Family Foundation from 1988 to 1991 for use in engaging state government and voluntary agencies in the southern region of the United States in a process of assessing community health promotion needs and priorities.[55] The Kaiser staff recognized that in the poorest communities of the South, technical and financial assistance would inevitably have to come from outside the communities, thereby risking Friere's "cultural invasion." To engage the state-level bureaucrats and agency workers in more of a "cultural synthesis" and to give greater play to the assets of communities with limited economic means, foundation officials insisted on a partnership in which they would offer funds in support of collaboration between state and local agencies if the state officials would participate in a social reconnaissance process.

TABLE 2-3

The primary and secondary "building blocks" of a community represent assets that can facilitate planning and should be acknowledged in the planning process to balance the negative connotation associated with assessing needs or problems

Primary Building Blocks	
Individual Assets	Organizational Assets
Skills, talents, and experiences of residents	Associations of businesses
Individual businesses	Citizens associations
Home-based enterprises	Cultural organizations
Personal income	Communications organizations
Gifts of labeled people	Religious organizations
Secondary Building Blocks	
Individual Assets	Organizational Assets
Private and nonprofit organizations	Public institutions and services
Institutions of higher education	Public schools
Hospitals	Police
Social services agencies	Libraries
	Fire departments
	Parks
Physical Resources	
Vacant land, commercial and industrial structures, housing	
Energy and waste resources	

SOURCE: "Mapping Community Capacity," by J. L. McKnight and J. P. Kretzmann, 1997, in M. Minkler (Ed.), *Community Organizing and Community Building for Health,* New Brunswick, NJ: Rutgers University Press, pp. 163, 165.

Kaiser Foundation staff recognized that changes in the determinants of health must be preceded by changes in the "social structure . . . the prevailing attitudes, values, aspirations, beliefs, behavior, and relationships in the community."[56] The community in this case was the larger state community in which relationships between state- and local-level organizations had to be rebuilt to replace a legacy of suspicion and grievances. The host community was assisted in the social reconnaissance process, through its own agencies and organizations, to

1. Identify the felt needs or problems of the community (and other elements of social structure)

2. Rank in priority the needs and problem areas to be dealt with
3. Organize or mobilize the community to deal with chosen needs or problems
4. Study the identified needs or problems to determine specific goals or recommendations
5. Develop a plan of action to accomplish locally determined goals
6. Find the resources needed to accomplish goals
7. Act or stimulate action to accomplish goals
8. Evaluate accomplishments

Application at the State Level. In this chapter, we shall focus on the first four of these objectives of social reconnaissance. The Kaiser Family Foundation's application of the reconnaissance method in the South engaged the governor's office, the state health department, other state-level social service agencies, state legislators, local or regional foundations, the United Way, the Chamber of Commerce, and other organizations in working through the first four functions. The foundation then provided a planning grant to a selected state agency or coalition to complete the process down to the community level, where projects would be developed (Step 5) and funded by grants from the foundation, other cooperating national and state organizations, and sometimes federal agencies (Steps 6–8). The process was designed to assure greater support for the community projects from state-level organizations than would have materialized if Kaiser had funded community health promotion projects directly without state involvement or simply had made the grants to the states with the expectation that they would in turn distribute funds to localities.

Application at the Community Level. The same process and advantages apply at the community level and even within large organizations such as schools, work sites, or hospitals where health promotion planning calls for broad participation. The steps in applying the method can be delineated as follows:

Step 1: *Identify an entry point.* Choosing the point of entry to a host community can be crucial, affecting all subsequent information and relationships. The official health agency is the logical starting point, but in some communities that agency may be part of the community's greatest concern and perhaps a cause of some of the problems. The preferred entry point, where possible, is the chief executive official of the community: the governor, the mayor, the chair of the town council, the county board of supervisors. Usually, the chief policy maker is an elected official. Though an appointed official, the city manager tends to have the public's confidence. Entry at this level helps open doors at all levels and in all sectors. By making their first task to understand the structure and concerns of their community, planners can avoid a premature focus on health problems.

Step 2: *Identify local cosponsors.* An existing organization or an ad hoc group needs to support the study in one or more of the following ways, which various authors drawing on decades of experience in community development and participatory research have identified:

1. Provide the opportunity for a representative group of local residents to participate in an initial session to explore common concerns and possibilities for collaboration and sharing of expertise and resources to study the issues.

2. Organize representative sponsoring organizations, or a community steering committee or "coalition" made up of representatives from different organizations and groups.[57]

3. Support the participatory research group as they carry out the study. This support should include
   a. Assisting in the legitimization process
   b. Designing the instruments and sampling procedure for data collection
   c. Providing news releases that share the proposed study's purpose, sponsors, and schedule
   d. Contacting each person to be interviewed
   e. In some cases, schedule the interviews in a central place

4. Pay for or share the cost of publication of the study

5. Facilitate the public release of the findings through various media such as newspapers, public meetings, and publication

6. Assure the use of the findings to stimulate study groups, program planning, policy decisions, and other community developmental efforts[58]

Step 3: *Development of research and briefing materials.* Background data usually need to be compiled from discursive sources in the community—its leaders, demography, and current affairs (based on content analysis of newspaper stories). Such a compilation of data provides an archival account of the community's structure, assets, and trends. A summary of these analyses in a briefing book to be shared with participants puts everyone on an equal footing in regard to factual data. Ideally, this briefing book is produced by the host community group. With this archival analysis, one can formulate questions to be asked of community leaders and bring them for discussion and pretesting before the sponsoring group. These questions may form the basis of an interview schedule for private meetings with community leaders or an agenda for public meetings with community groups.

Step 4: *Identification of leaders and representatives.* Planners need to select interviewees who can speak either for the community's power structure or for the population at large and segments of the population, especially underrepresented segments. The **positional** approach to identifying leaders selects those who hold key positions in government, political, business, and voluntary organizations. The **reputational** approach tends to identify the more socially active among this same group of influential leaders; it also picks up "activists" and "opinion leaders" who do not hold official positions. A combination of these two is recommended, with a careful eye to ensuring the inclusion of minority and women's organizations and reputational polling among underrepresented groups.[59]

Step 5: *Field interviews.* An intensive period of actual interviews and meetings with influentials, specialized leaders, subcommunity leaders, and leaders of underrepresented categories comes next. Planners should avoid spreading this phase out over too many weeks, because local events could intervene to invalidate any comparisons between those interviewed early and those late. The number of individuals that should be included in the sample of leaders ranges from 50 to 125, depending on the size and diversity of the community. External helping agencies must restrain themselves from turning an assessment of needs and assets into an academic research project that the community may view as a burden on their time and resources as well as something that might delay the action they desire.[60]

Step 6: *Analysis, reporting and follow-up.* Ideally, the local sponsoring group would carry out this step, with technical assistance as needed from the helping agency. The report should by made public through open meetings, the news media, and broad distribution of the written report. Community organizations or groups are encouraged to select their own priorities among the broader community priorities defined; this leads to task groups that pursue specific issues of organizing a coalition or task force to pursue the interest to them and mobilize resources in relation to those issues. Criteria and procedures for setting priorities among multiple needs (identified through the community self-studies) have been suggested in the health promotion literature; these criteria, and variations thereof, will be applied in each of the next three chapters.[61]

OTHER ASSESSMENT METHODS

Nominal Group Process. The **nominal group process** is a method for assessing community perceptions of problems in a way that overcomes many of the difficulties arising from the usual unequal representation of opinions. The method consists of a series of small-group procedures designed to compensate for the dynamics of social power that emerge in most planning meetings. Those who use the method should keep in mind that its central purpose is to identify and rank problems, not to solve them. This process, described as it applies to public health by Van de Ven and Delbecq,[62] should be the method of choice when the task at hand is generating ideas, getting equal participation from group members having unequal power or expertise, and ranking the perceived importance of ideas or problems. Delbecq[63] has summarized the method for human services in general. More recently, Gilmore and Campbell have provided a detailed accounting of the steps in applying the method specifically for health promotion needs assessment.[64]

The Delphi Method. The **Delphi Method** is also useful at the social assessment phase, especially if face-to-face meetings are impractical. Linstone and Turoff developed the method most fully,[65] and Leo has recently applied it in an assessment of stress in the workplace.[66] In this method, one mails a series of questionnaires to a small number of experts, opinion leaders, or informants. The Delphi Method offers several advantages. First, differences of opinion among various key people can be resolved by the planner without forcing confrontation. Second, the method enables planners to work from a distance with a variety of target-group representatives who are informed about the issue of concern. Third, large numbers can be managed at a relatively low cost, although having more than 30 respondents may not enhance results. Finally, throughout the process, participants remain anonymous, thus protecting the generated ideas from the influences of group conformity, prestige, power, and politics. Gilmore and his colleagues have provided a detailed description of the steps required to apply the Delphi Method in social assessments in health education and health promotion.[67]

Focus Groups. Marketing groups have used **focus groups** as a means of obtaining target-group perceptions and testing marketing ideas and products. In recent years, focus groups have become the most popular qualitative interview strategy used in the application of social and behavioral sciences to practical enterprises. Focus groups last for one to one and a half hours. They are usually small in number (8 to 12 persons per group), with particular emphasis placed on recruiting people who represent the community or target group of interest. In a comfortable, informal session, a trained moderator asks representatives of a target population to discuss their thoughts on a specific issue or product. In the health promotion planning process, focus groups are typically used to help planners zero in on what should be the content, delivery, and appeal of the message of a given program. Nevertheless, the flexibility of the method enables planners to employ it as a means to assess social concerns and consequences.[68] Recent published applications of focus-group methods applied this way include work with African-American women,[69] an assessment of the social consequences of tuberculosis,[70] mothers in the Women, Infants and Children (WIC) Program,[71] and perceptions of physical activity and rest among African-American workers.[72] Krueger offers a practical step-by-step guide to conducting focus groups.[73]

Central Location Intercept Interviews. **Central location intercept** interviews, or intercept interviews for short, offer the advantage of obtaining information from large numbers of people in a short time. Such interviews are typically conducted where there are high levels of pedestrian traffic, such as at shopping malls, churches, and special community events. This method also provides a low-cost opportunity to obtain the opinions and interests of so-called hard-to-reach target populations.

A manual of methods for improving health communications describes intercept interviews as follows:

> A typical central location interview begins with the intercept. Potential respondents are stopped and asked whether they are willing to participate. Specific screening questions are then asked to see whether they fit the criteria of the target audience for the pretest. If so, they are taken to the interviewing station—a quiet spot at a shopping mall or other site—and are shown the pretest materials. Respondents are then asked a series of questions to assess recall, comprehension, and reaction to the items.[74]

Although the respondents intercepted through central location interviews may not statistically represent the entire target population, the sample is larger than that used in focus groups or individual in-depth interviews. Program planners often use the central location technique at the message development stage, when assessments of comprehension, attention, believability, and other reactions are essential. Unlike focus groups or in-depth interviews, this method uses a highly structured questionnaire that contains primarily closed-ended questions. Open-ended questioning, which allows for free-flowing answers, should be kept to a minimum, because it takes too long for the interviewer to record responses. As in any type of research, the questionnaire should be tested before it is used in the field. An example of the combined use of data generated from mall intercept interviews and focus groups is found in the National Cancer Institute's use of the Precede-Proceed model to develop a national nutrition program.[75]

Surveys. Surveys are perhaps the principal means used by health workers or any other group whose work depends on a better understanding of the **beliefs**, perceptions, knowledge, and attitudes of the people they serve. The quality of a survey is determined by several factors, including the validity and reliability of the instrument (Does it consistently measure what it is supposed to?), how representative the sample is (Can you generalize your results to the entire community or group?), and how the survey is administered (Are the questions asked and coded in the same way for all the subjects interviewed?). Schultz and her colleagues offer a thorough and practical description of the steps and methods used to develop and implement a participatory community-based survey. Especially relevant are their insights on creating collaborative roles for community members, representatives of community-based organizations, service providers, and researchers.[76]

Some notable examples of using survey methods for social assessments specifically within the context of applying the Precede-Proceed model, include

- Work in El Paso, Texas, on the perception of quality of life for those with bowel dysfunction among Hispanic and non-Hispanic whites[77]
- A work-site survey of employees to assess their preferences for self-help or group approaches to smoking cessation[78]
- An award-winning project in Houston, Texas, that used surveys and focus groups with adolescent patients and their parents concerning their lives with cystic fibrosis[79]
- A survey of staff nurses in eight British Columbia hospitals concerning their perceptions of health promotion in their professional role and of the assets, resources, and needs of hospitals to support nurses in this role[80]
- The development of the Du Pont employee health promotion program, one of the largest work-site employee health promotion programs in the world, which started with social and economic assessment through surveys of managers to understand their expectations of benefits to the company and of some 1,200 employees, spouses, and pensioners[81]
- A combined use of focus groups and surveys with adolescents in Manaus, on the Amazon in Brazil, to assess social and economic aspects of their nutrition[82]
- Canada's first health promotion survey, which applied the Precede-Proceed model in expanding the range of variables included in a national health survey beyond the usual health status and health risk factors[83]

Public Service Data. Data on perceived needs and problems are more readily available than one might realize. For example, a rich source of this kind of data, and one that is often overlooked, is broadcast media. The Federal Communication Commission requires television and radio broadcasters to ascertain community needs and concerns regularly and to offer public service programming to address such problems. In some communities, members of the print media along with radio and television broadcasters have formed coalitions with universities and foundations to conduct public opinion surveys periodically to identify the needs and problems of the population in their service area.[84] When asked to do so, most organizations will share their data unless they have proprietary value.

ANALYZING INFORMATION FROM A SOCIAL ASSESSMENT

Throughout this chapter, we have referred to the importance of obtaining multiple sources of information to help develop an understanding of people's perceptions of their own needs. Regardless of how sophisticated, valid, or plentiful, information matters only to the extent that one uses it. To maximize the probability that data gathered will indeed be used, we offer the following practical guidelines.

1. *Stay focused on the purpose.* Anyone with responsibility for collecting data, regardless of the subject area, should repeatedly ask and answer two simple questions: Why do we need this information? How will we use it? In the social assessment phase of the Precede-Proceed model, we seek to improve our insight into the following: (1) the ultimate values and perceived needs of a specific population; (2) existing human and resource assets, within a population, that would support a health promotion program or strategy; and (3) program, organizational, or policy barriers that might inhibit program planning or implementation. When health promotion planners gather only those data they need and can use, analysis becomes more efficient and less burdensome.

2. *Look for connections.* Social scientists use a method of analysis called *data source triangulation,* analogous to navigation and surveying. For one trying to locate one's position on a map, a single landmark can only provide the information that one is situated somewhere along a line in a particular direction from that landmark. With two landmarks, however, one can pinpoint one's position by taking bearings on both.[85]

If health promotion planners make judgments on a single piece of information, they run the risk that their source of information, and consequently their analysis, could be incorrect. Data source triangulation is possible when planners use different methods or reach different target groups to assess a common issue.

3. *Identify themes.* Once gathered, both objective data and information about perceived needs should be studied to identify the factors that constitute the most formidable barriers to a desired quality of life. Some objective indicators can be calculated, such as frequency counts, incidence rates, utilization rates, and frequency distributions. These *quantitative data* can be compared with previous measures of the same indicators to ascertain trends or changes. Information about personal opinions and interests based on open-ended interviews or focus groups are examples of *qualitative data.* Although some qualitative data can be characterized by measurement on a variety of categorical scales, the strength of such data lies in the descriptive richness, depth, and insight they provide. Qualitative data collected from open-ended questions are most often analyzed by seeking out categories of responses or recurrent themes. For example, Boston and her colleagues used interviews, participant observation, and field notes as the primary sources of data in a study to understand how Canadian aboriginals (the James Bay Cree) perceived the problem of noninsulin diabetes within the context of their cultural beliefs about health. Their data were "organized electronically and analyzed according to emerging themes and categories relevant to the aims of the study."[86] One of the major categories, "Health and Illness Beliefs," included the Cree's association between "going into the bush" and feelings of rejuvenation and energy. The following excerpt from one interview exemplifies how qualitative data reflects a theme or a category: "If you're here at that time of the year,

the town just empties out and the people have this urgency to get ready and go [in the bush]. Everybody's talking about it. It's just a feeling of rejuvenation. One of the best times of the year, really."[87]

4. *Promote trust.* "Taking the temperature and pulse" of the community is a consciousness-raising activity not only for the planner, but also for others in his or her organization involved in the overall health promotion program, as well as for the patients, students, workers, and residents. For this reason, results of an analysis of information from the social assessment process should be translated and shared with the community. Through the sharing of such information, one strengthens the community's trust in one's endeavors to promote health.[88]

During this important first step in assessment, the main resource for health planners involves critical observation and good professional judgment. The final determination of quality-of-life concerns must be made by careful consideration of the available evidence, including the sentiments of community members—and especially those patients, students, workers, or residents who will participate in the health promotion program.

A SOCIAL ASSESSMENT "AFTER THE FACT"

In many instances, those responsible for implementing health education and health promotion activities will receive that task after a social assessment, or something like it, has already been done by someone else (if only in the minds of an administrator or decision-making board). In fact, an epidemiological assessment, or at least some general aspects thereof, may also have been completed (see Chapter 3). In some instances, educational programs are instituted to address a need that has caused sufficient concern. For example, in schools, "units" or classes on alcohol and drugs or HIV/AIDS are driven by the public's judgment about the dangerous effects of these problems on society. National and international population and family-planning education programs receive money because funders expect them to help reduce the social maladies that often accompany overpopulation and problem pregnancies. Self-care health education efforts are currently offered in the hope that program outcomes will include not only better health but also decreased medical costs, less sick leave from work, and increased self-esteem and personal control.[89] Indeed, most health education programs with any significant support from the general public are likely addressing health problems already identified as potentially detrimental to quality of life.

Those practitioners who find themselves in this situation should, if at all feasible, make it a priority to recapture and become familiar with the information used by others in the assessment process. Such a review provides the crucial information and orientation needed to keep perspective on the ultimate goal of the program. In addition, it may also reveal gaps that are not too late to fill, such as failure to engage the participation of the target population and/or key organizational partners.

SUMMARY

The identification and analysis of the social or economic problems and aspirations of a population is a valuable, if not essential, first step in thorough health promotion planning. Health is not an ultimate value in itself except as it relates to social benefits, quality of life, or an organization's "bottom line." Health takes on greater importance—both to those who must support the program and those expected to participate in it—when they can see clearly the connection between the health objective and some broader or more compelling social objective. This chapter has described a series of steps and a variety of strategies and techniques the planner can use to gather and analyze information about social problems and perceived quality of life, as well as to seek out maximum feasible participation.

One can summarize the objectives of social assessment (Phase 1 of health promotion planning) as follows:

1. To *engage* the community as active partners in the social diagnostic process
2. To *identify* ultimate values and subjective concerns with quality of life or conditions of living in the target population
3. To *verify* and clarify these subjective concerns either through existing data sources or new data from surveys or interviews
4. To *demonstrate* how social concerns and ultimate values can serve to heighten awareness of and motivation to act on health problems
5. To *assess* the capacities and assets of a community
6. To *make explicit* the rationale for the selection of priority problems
7. To use the documentation and rationale from social assessment as one of the variables on which to *evaluate* the program

EXERCISES

1. List three ways you could (or did)[90] involve the members of the population you selected in Exercise 3 of Chapter 1 in identifying their quality-of-life concerns. Justify your methods in terms of their feasibility and appropriateness for the population you are helping.
2. How did (or would) you verify the subjective data gathered in Exercise 1 with objective data on social problems or quality-of-life concerns?
3. Display and discuss your real or hypothetical data as a quality-of-life assessment, justifying your selection of social, economic, and health problems to become the highest priority for a program.

NOTES AND CITATIONS

1. Our use of the term *community* henceforth will refer to the larger geographically defined community (neighborhood, town, city, county, district, or occasionally, a whole state, region, or country), or to the organizationally defined community (school, work site, industry, church, hospital, or nursing home) through which communication and decisions flow. (See the glossary.) *Community,* however, appears in some writings as a reference to a group of people who share a common interest. This use may apply in patient education, self-help groups, and health promotion for dispersed groups. Electronic bulletin boards and satellite television open new possibilities for the interactive engagement of dispersed populations in health promotion planning to address their common concerns. Such electronic meetings have been held, for example, to involve chief executive officers of major companies in discussions of the potential for work-site health promotion programs in their industries.

2. Buck, 1986; Dane, Sleet, Lam, & Roppel, 1987; Sanders-Phillips, 1991, 1996.

3. We avoid the misnomer "healthy" in describing actions, policies, or programs conducive to health (e.g., "healthy behavior" or "healthy public policy") because these objects of the adjectives are means, not ends; they are not living organisms that can be healthy. At best they can enhance health.

4. First International Conference on Health Promotion, 1986, p. iii.

5. Parsons, 1964, p. 433.

6. Green & Ottoson, 1999.

7. For reviews of the methods and research on the use of tailored communications, see M. K. Campbell et al., 1994; Kreuter, Lezin, Kreuter, & Green, 1998; chap. 6; Kreuter, Vehige, & McGuire, 1996; Mann, 1989; Rimer, Orleans, Fleisher, et al., 1994.

8. Assessing "things people value and enjoy" can be determined by using the following tools. For the Valued Life Activities (VLA) index, see Jette, 1993. For the STARLITE scale see Wilshire et al., 1997.

9. Recalling the phrase in the U.S. Constitution, "life, liberty, and the pursuit of happiness," we acknowledge here that happiness and fulfillment are elusive concepts. The wisdom of most philosophical systems suggests that we can help people find the freedom and capacity to pursue those elusive states, but we cannot expect to achieve them for others. Furthermore, happiness and fulfillment are *states* of being, not permanent *traits*. As states, they are variable and, therefore, can serve as positive and appropriate goals for promotion. The Canadian variation on the theme of "life, liberty, and the pursuit of happiness" is "peace, harmony, and good government." This phrase reflects a cultural difference in ultimate values that conditions how the people of neighboring countries might judge their quality of life.

10. Green, George, et al., 1995; Schultz, et al., 1998; Wallerstein & Bernstein, 1994.

11. Butler et al., 1996; Governor of Mississippi, 1989. Cf. Eng & Parker, 1994.

12. Carr, Thompson, & Kirwan, 1996; Fryback, Lawrence, Martin, Klein, & Klein, 1997.

13. Jette, 1993.

14. Hu, 1990; McGuire, O'Leary, Alexander, Dottavio, 1987; Plante & Schwartz, 1990.

15. Berwick et al., 1991; Pahkala, Kivela, & Laippala, 1991; Plante & Schwartz, 1990.

16. The Ferrans and Powers Quality of Life Index is a 68-item instrument designed to measure satisfaction with and importance of health juxtaposed to psychological, spiritual, and family-life factors. See Ferrans, 1996.

17. Stewart & Ware, 1992.

18. Bergner, 1985; J. W. Bush, 1984; Kaplan, 1988; Lohr et al., 1985.

19. Bivens, 1979; G. P. Cernada, 1982; Green, 1986f; Macrina & O'Rourke, 1986–1987; Minkler, 1997; Morgan & Horning, 1940; Nyswander, 1942; Steuart, 1965.

20. Arnstein, 1969; Dore & Mars, 1981; Eng, 1993; Green, George, et al., 1995; Soen, 1981.

21. *Concientación* is a Spanish word that refers to consciousness raising for a process whereby persons with limited means become conscious of the political realities and root causes of their situation and take collective action to address them. Shor & Freire, 1987.

22. The importance of taking these perceptions into account through participation in planning is developed formally as a theory of participation in Green, 1986f.

23. Freire, 1970, p. 181.

24. Ibid., p. 183. See also Wallerstein & Sanchez-Merki, 1994.

25. We would have to temper this sentiment in the areas of health protection such as water and food safety, as well as preventive health services such as immunizations, where whole populations may be at more extreme risk if the values and misunderstandings of a small but vocal group were to override scientific evidence.

26. Bosin, 1992; Green, 1978a, 1979b; Green & Frankish, 1994.

27. Ottoson & Green, 1987.

28. Rose, 1992, pp. 123–124.

29. R. M. Goodman, Spears, McLeroy, et al., 1998; Kreuter & Lezin, 1998.

30. Hawe, 1996.

31. Ibid., p. 477.

32. Cottrell, 1976; Eng, Hatch, & Callan, 1985; Eng & Parker, 1994; Goeppinger & Baglioni, 1985.

33. R. M. Goodman & Steckler, 1987–1988; Shediac-Rizkallah & Bone, 1998; Steckler & Goodman, 1989a, 1989b; Steckler, Orville, Eng, & Dawson, 1989.

34. Green, 1989.

35. Shaw, 1930, pp. xiv–xv.

36. Raeburn & Rootman, 1997; Rimer, 1997; Runyon, et al., 1998.

37. World Health Organization, 1983, p. 17.

38. Gilmore, Campbell, 1996; Tillgren, Hoglund, & Romelsjo, 1996.

39. Hawe, 1996; Papenfus & Bryan, 1998.

40. E. Vartiainen et al., 1994.

41. P. Puska et al., 1985, p. 164.

42. Ibid., p. 165. See also Grunbaum, Gingiss, & Parcel, 1995.

43. *EMPOWER (Enabling Methods of Planning and Organizing Within Everyone's Reach)* is a software application of the Precede-Proceed model to develop programs for the early detection of breast cancer. It contains an interactive segment entitled "Situation Analysis," in which prompts help the user identify existing resources and conditions likely to be relevant to planning an effective breast cancer early detection program. See Gold, Green, & Kreuter, 1997.

44. R. G. Evans, Barer & Marmor, 1994.

45. For reviews of the theory of social capital, see Coleman, 1978, p. 119; E. Cox, 1995; Putnam, 1995; Tarrow, 1996.

46. House, 1981. See also Israel, 1985; Minkler, Frantz, & Wechsler, 1982–83.

47. For ideas and references for measuring social capital and/or constructs related to social capital, see Eng & Parker, 1994; Kawachi, Kennedy, Lochner, & Prothro-Stith, 1997; Louis Harris & Associates, 1996; Runyan et al., 1998; Sampson, Raudenbush, & Earls, 1997.

48. A copy of the *Civic Index* can be obtained from the National Civic League, 1445 Market Street, Suite 300, Denver, CO 80202.

49. Gates, 1991; W. J. McCoy, 1991.

50. McKnight & Kretzmann, 1997. For a review see R. M. Goodman, Speers, et al., 1998.

51. The complete survey can be found in Kretzmann & McKnight, 1993, pp. 19–25.

52. Nix, 1977, p. 140

53. Sanders, 1950.

54. Nix & Seerly, 1971.

55. The Kaiser Foundation's experience in the southern states was documented in many unpublished reports, but the only published accounts so far are in the annual reports of the Foundation (1989, 1990), in the second edition of this book (1991), and in an article in the Council on Foundations magazine: R. M. Williams, 1990. See also Butler et al., 1996.

56. Nix, 1977, p. 141.

57. Bibeau, Howell, Rife, & Taylor, 1996; Kreuter & Lezin, 1998.

58. Nix, 1997, pp. 143–144.

59. Gold, Green, & Kreuter, 1997; Michielutte & Beal, 1990; Mico, 1965; Nix, 1969, 1970; Nix & Seerly, 1973; Shoemaker & Nix, 1972.

60. R. M. Goodman, Steckler, Hoover, & Schwartz, 1993; Wickizer, Wagner, & Perrin, 1998.

61. W. J. Brown & Redman, 1995; Conway, Hu, & Harrington, 1997; Milewa, 1997.

62. Van de Ven & Delbecq, 1972.

63. Delbecq, 1983.

64. Gilmore & Campbell, 1996. See also Sarvela & McDermott, 1993, p. 146.

65. Linstone & Turoff, 1975.

66. Leo, 1996.

67. Gilmore & Campbell, 1996. Hunnicutt, Perry-Hunnicutt, Newman, Davis, & Crawford, 1993, provide a Precede-Proceed model application of the Delphi Method in planning a campus alcohol abuse prevention program. See also Sarvela & McDermott, 1993, pp. 147, 197.

68. G. A. Williams, Abbott, & Taylor, 1997.

69. Ibid; Danigelis, et al., 1995; Dignan, Michielutte, Shap, et al., 1990.

70. Liefooghr, Michiels, & De Muynck, 1995.

71. Shefer, Mezoff, & Herrick, 1998. See also a PRECEDE-PROCEED application of focus groups in this population by Reed, 1996; and in Brazil by Doyle & Feldman, 1997.

72. Airhihenbuwa, Kamanyika, & Lowe, 1995.

73. Krueger, 1988. See also Basch, 1987; Gilmore & Campbell, 1996, pp. 73–78.

74. Arkin, 1989, p. 40.

75. Lefebvre et al., 1995.

76. Schultz et al., 1998.

77. Zuckerman, Guerra, Drossman, Foland, & Gregory, 1996.

78. Bertera, Oehl, & Telepchak, 1990.

79. L. K. Bartholomew, Seilheimer, Parcel, Spinelli, & Pumariega, 1988. See also Bartholomew, Czyzewski, & Seilheimer, 1997; Bartholomew et al., 1991.

80. Berland, Whyte, & Maxwell, 1995.

81. Bertera, 1990b, 1993.

82. Doyle & Feldman, 1997.

83. Rootman, 1988.

84. Washington Post/Kaiser Family Foundation/Harvard University Survey Project, 1996.

85. Hammersley & Atkinson, 1995. See Keintz, Rimer, Fleisher, Fox, & Engstron, 1988 for a PRECEDE example.

86. P. Boston et al., 1997, p. 6.

87. Ibid., p. 10.

88. Laraque, Barlow, Durkin, & Heagarty, 1995. The most effective means of sharing data is to engage the community actively in the collection, analysis, and interpretation of data through participatory research. See Green, George, et al., 1995; McGowan & Green, 1995.

89. Green, Werlin, Shauffler, & Avery, 1977 [this contains a description of the first study testing an early version of the Precede model]; Squyres, 1985; Vickery et al., 1983.

90. We suggest that these exercises be carried out on a real population accessible to the student or practitioner, but if this is impracticable, the exercises can be applied to a well-described hypothetical population using actual census data and vital statistics from similar populations.

Chapter 3

Epidemiological Assessment

PRECEDE

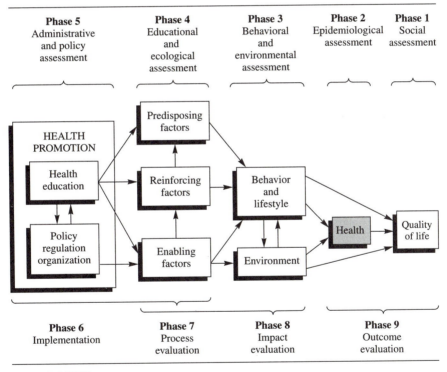

Phase 5
Administrative
and policy
assessment

Phase 4
Educational
and
ecological
assessment

Phase 3
Behavioral
and
environmental
assessment

Phase 2
Epidemiological
assessment

Phase 1
Social
assessment

HEALTH
PROMOTION

Health
education

Policy
regulation
organization

Predisposing
factors

Reinforcing
factors

Enabling
factors

Behavior
and
lifestyle

Environment

Health

Quality
of life

Phase 6
Implementation

Phase 7
Process
evaluation

Phase 8
Impact
evaluation

Phase 9
Outcome
evaluation

PROCEED

The Precede-Proceed model is grounded in the assumption that effective health promotion planning starts by carefully examining two, equally important, types of information:

- The social, health, and quality-of-life concerns as perceived by the population
- The specific health problems, measured objectively, that pose the greatest threat to the health and quality of life of the population.

Chapter 2 described various approaches to gathering the former. This chapter turns now to the latter, the second phase of the Precede-Proceed framework: **epidemiological assessment.** The primary task in this phase is to determine for a given target population which health problems, measured objectively, pose the greatest threat to health and quality of life. We begin by reaffirming the importance of connecting and reconciling social and epidemiological information in the planning process. We then describe two methods of logic that planners can apply in making that connection. These will apply equally in working out the linkages, at each later phase of planning, between causes and effects, means and ends. The remainder of this chapter reviews the key elements of epidemiology that are particularly relevant to this phase of the model.[1] We examine how epidemiological analyses help in determining which health problems deserve the highest priorities in a health promotion program. Finally, we review the process of establishing measurable health objectives.

THE RELATIONSHIP BETWEEN SOCIAL PROBLEMS AND HEALTH

Cost-benefit, social impact, and environmental impact assessments have led health planners and policy makers to use data on a community's perceived quality of life and social goals or problems as a formal basis for deciding which health problems deserve attention. Reciprocally, planners in other sectors have been led by health impact assessments to consider how the policies of their sectors influence health. As highlighted in Chapter 2, quality-of-life information often comes from surveys, polls, or interviews that have been routinely conducted by various public, private, and voluntary agencies with mandates other than health. By linking their priorities more systematically with the community's quality of life or social concerns, official agencies elicit greater public support for programs and initiatives.

In studying the Global Burden of Disease (GBD), Murray and Lopez[2] provide an example of how planners can weave social concerns into the process of identifying and setting health priorities. With input from over 100 international collaborators, these researchers developed a measure reflecting the impact of premature death *and* disability, regardless of the cause: Disability Adjusted Life Years or (DALYs). Specifically, this calculation expresses both the years of life lost to premature death and the years lived with a disability of a specified severity and duration. One DALY equals a year of healthy life lost. The new measure is especially relevant to the issue of connecting social concerns with health status, because one cannot calculate DALYs without addressing social values. Consider the following questions:

1. How long should people live? To estimate years of life lost at any given age, we have to know the number of years for which a person at that age should be expected to survive under ideal conditions for that population. Not only do life expectancy rates differ among countries (e.g., Japan and Somalia), they also differ within countries (e.g., Utah and Nevada, neighboring states with vastly different death rates) and among more localized regions, counties, or prefectures. For that reason, the determination of ideal life expectancy cannot be made by mathematics alone; it must involve value choices and social input.
2. Are years of healthy life worth more in young adulthood than in childhood or middle age?
3. Is a year of healthy life now worth more to society than a year of healthy life in 30 years' time?
4. Are all people equal? For example, should one socioeconomic group's year of healthy life count more than another's? Is a housekeeper's year worth more or less than her or his working spouse's?
5. How do you compare years of life lost to premature death and years of life lived with disabilities of differing severities?

In the GBD project, answers to these questions were sought, country by country, through discussions using a method akin to the nominal group process described in Chapter 2. The authors' search for ways to incorporate human perceptions and preferences in determining health priorities is poignantly reflected by this observation:

> Health researchers developing a measure of disease burden must recognize their responsibility to reflect societies' preferred answers to these five questions, but also to guard against and "filter out" unjustifiable preferences such as racism, sexism, or economic discrimination that may be institutionalized in certain societies. It is unlikely that any measure can reflect a perfect vision of the ideal society; but its choices should be acceptable to as many people of as many different cultures as possible.[3]

STARTING IN THE MIDDLE

Chapter 2 argued that the ideal place to begin planning is with a social assessment, working back from people's perceptions of their needs to health and other causes of the social or quality-of-life concerns of a population. Ideal, maybe, but practical? Often, planners find themselves invited to develop programs after the first steps have been taken or the ultimate outcomes already decided. Sometimes, they are given a health problem to solve or a health outcome to achieve without much, if any, thinking having gone into the social or quality-of-life issues to which it might relate. We recognize that, for some practitioners and some organizations, the health issue is the *starting point,* not a second phase of planning as the Precede-Proceed model portrays it. The Cancer Society is committed to work on cancer; its staff, volunteers, and contributors have joined in its efforts on that assumption. They have done their own prior calculations as to the importance of this disease to them, their families, or their communities. In short, they are prepared to start their planning in the middle of the model rather than at the end.

Another way to view this typical circumstance is to acknowledge that for some people or agencies, the health issue *is* the end, not a means to some other end. Even then, however, it may be useful for them to cast an eye back over their shoulders to understand why this health problem or issue matters—to look for reasons beyond just the numbers of people who experience the health problem or want the selected health improvement. As soon as they ask, for example, what benefits might accrue to the population, they are addressing broader social concerns and issues. It is perfectly appropriate, then, to start in the middle of PRECEDE and work in both directions.

Some health problems, for example, come with birth. They have immediate social and economic consequences for the newborn and for the family. Genetic and congenital anomalies produce birth defects with health conditions that must be addressed as lives are physically, mentally, socially, and economically compromised. Injuries resulting in spinal cord damage or other trauma may leave people physically or mentally damaged with social and quality-of-life consequences. The International Classification of Impairments, Disabilities, and Handicaps (ICIDH), developed by the World Health Organization,[4] offers a framework that acknowledges the *nonfatal consequences* of disease or injury as they might affect quality of life or social condition. The ICIDH divides the consequences of disease or injury into three categories:

- *Impairment* (any loss or abnormality of structure or function)
- *Disability* (any restriction or lack of ability to perform an activity in a manner or range considered normal)
- *Handicap* (a disadvantage for a given individual resulting from an impairment or disability that prohibits that individual from fulfilling a role deemed normal)

The World Health Organization has translated the ICIDH into 14 languages. The ICIDH has served as an organizational framework for assessment of a wide range of social and environmental issues or consequences related to health status.[5]

Figure 3-1 displays the sequence of the three categories as they are connected to the disease or disorder (health problem) and to social and quality-of-life out-

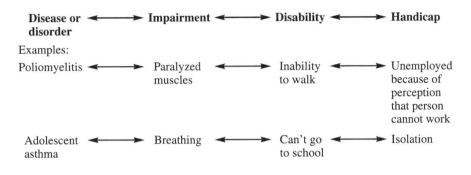

FIGURE 3-1

The ICIDH schema for assessment of nonfatal consequences of disease and injury defines the terms *impairment, disability,* and *handicap* as degrees of health, social, and quality-of-life outcomes, shown here with examples for poliomyelitis and adolescent asthma.

SOURCE: Figure adapted from "Non-Fatal Health Outcomes: Concepts, Instruments and Indicators," by A. Goerdt, J. P. Koplan, J. M. Robine, M. C. Thuriaux, and J. K. van Ginneken, 1996, in J. L. Murray and A. D. Lopez (Eds.), *The Global Burden of Disease,* Cambridge, MA: Harvard University, p. 101.

comes. Although depicted in a linear progression, the relationships among the three dimensions are much more complex and interdependent, just as the association between health and social problems in the Precede-Proceed model is reciprocal, as characterized in the previous chapter.

A review of the scientific and professional literature helps the health professional assess the relationships between health and social problems in both directions of causation. For example, the relationships between health problems and the social problem of poverty are analyzed in a variety of works.[6] Figure 3-2 suggests how poverty, health, lifestyle, and environmental factors can be viewed in an ecological perspective of reciprocal relationships. Such a categorization of factors can help one plan health promotion programs directed at health-related factors but designed within a broader ecological context.

Health factors include fertility rates, as well as morbidity and mortality rates. Those that contribute to a social problem will also vary depending on the makeup of the target population and its location. For example, migrant workers and their families might suffer from poor access to organized social support systems such as education and welfare. Poor roads or geographic isolation might contribute to poverty, as might lack of jobs. In addition, social biases regarding racial or ethnic minority status frequently contribute to social and health problems. Adolescent pregnancy is more common in rural than in urban areas, and it plays a major role in holding some urban and rural families in an intergenerational cycle of poverty.[7]

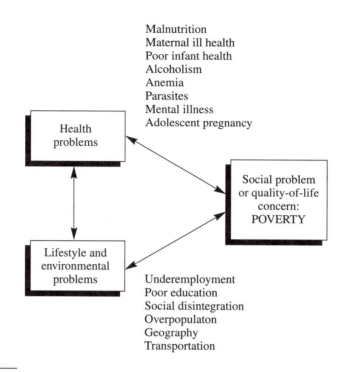

Malnutrition
Maternal ill health
Poor infant health
Alcoholism
Anemia
Parasites
Mental illness
Adolescent pregnancy

Health problems

Social problem
or quality-of-life
concern:
POVERTY

Lifestyle and
environmental
problems

Underemployment
Poor education
Social disintegration
Overpopulaton
Geography
Transportation

FIGURE 3-2

The examples here of health, lifestyle, and environmental factors interacting with poverty
in reciprocal relationships support an ecological approach to assessment that cannot be
rigidly linear or unidirectional in addressing causes and effects.

Figure 3-3 shows declining rates for all the major racial and ethnic groups in the
United States, but vast differences still exist among the groups. While the teenage
birth rates declined, the percentage of births to teenagers who were unmarried
increased in the United States from less than 20% in 1950 to more than 75% in
1996.[8]

Unfortunately, health professionals seldom have a specific mandate to
address such social-environmental factors that affect quality of life; in some
instances, they may not be allowed to devote agency resources to do so. Nonetheless, it helps to be aware of the potential effect of the physical environment and of
socioeconomic factors on potential solutions to a reciprocal poverty-health problem. Recent interest in population health determinants and in recasting health
objectives in relation to the broad social determinants of health has brought these
relationships into greater focus for the health sector.[9]

Connecting an already selected health problem back to its social impact
is particularly useful when one is assigned an oversimplified problem. Suppose

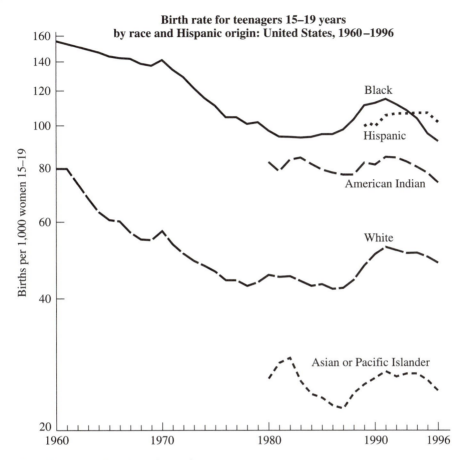

**Birth rate for teenagers 15–19 years
by race and Hispanic origin: United States, 1960–1996**

Note: Rates are plotted on a log scale.

FIGURE 3-3

Birth rates for teenagers age 15–19 declined for all major racial and ethnic groups in the United States between 1960 and 1996, but the differences among groups remain proportionately the same.

SOURCE: "Teenage Births in the United States. National and State Trends, 1990–96," by S. J. Ventura, S. C. Curtin, and T. J. Mathews, 1998, in *National Vital Statistics System,* Hyattsville, MD: National Center for Health Statistics.

a newspaper article announces an alarming comparison between the local infant mortality rate and the statewide rate. A statement on the newspaper's editorial page denounces the quality of infant care in local hospitals, and the city council calls for a corrective program directed at neonatal care in the community hospital. Faced with this situation, a health professional might analyze the following information:

- The two-county rural area within which the community lies is populated mainly by a low-income minority agricultural group with a high rate of teenage pregnancy.
- The infant mortality rate in this community has remained at 24.9/1000 live births while there has been an overall decline in the state rate to 14.6/1000.
- The identified pregnancy outcome problems include premature birth, low birth weight, respiratory distress at delivery, and failure to thrive. The visiting nurse service also reports a high prevalence of maternal anemia and a high incidence of gastrointestinal infection and respiratory diseases in infants.
- Many mothers are at risk because of age (a disproportionate number between age fourteen and seventeen), poor nutrition, lack of medical care, multiple pregnancies, and preeclampsia during pregnancy.
- Childhood health is poor: Injuries are common; children look malnourished and report for school with handicapping conditions and no immunizations.

This information challenges the validity of the assumption that the relatively high infant mortality rate in the area is due chiefly to deficiencies in the quality of neonatal care in community hospitals. Rather, the data strongly suggest that the cause may lie in poor prenatal care, poor maternal and infant nutrition, and lack of infant immunizations. Therefore, a decision to buy new, improved hospital equipment to care for neonates may actually be a more costly and less effective solution to the problem than would be a program of community outreach for prenatal health care, nutritional support, and childhood immunizations. By expanding his or her understanding of the problem and seeing the statistics in the broader context of relationships between health and social problems, the health professional can help the community address the problem more comprehensively and productively through prevention and health promotion rather than through high-technology medical care, or in addition to medical care improvements.

This example illustrates two additional points. First, the relationship of health problems to quality of life can be readily discerned. High rates of adolescent pregnancy lead to high rates of school absenteeism and dropouts as well as of single-parent homes, often in lower income brackets and in need of proportionately greater social services.

Second, the example suggests the vital importance of developing data for significant subgroups. In this population, these are the low-income, minority, rural, teenage girls and their infants. In other populations, data might reveal a high prevalence of hypertension among African-American men or of lung cancer among middle-aged European-American men. Without such data, the health professional with a preassigned target problem could not possibly know which sub-

populations should receive special attention and which health problems deserve higher priority than the assigned one.

EPIDEMIOLOGY

A thoughtful analysis of the information generated from social and epidemiological assessments enables health promotion planners to understand how their work to mitigate specific health problems is connected to desired social benefits. As implied by its title, the epidemiological assessment phase relies heavily on the principles and practice of epidemiology.

Epidemiology[10] is the study of the distribution and determinants of health-related conditions or events in defined populations and the application of this study to control health problems. A closer examination of the components of this definition reveals its relevance for all phases of the health promotion planning process.

First, the word *study* implies a planned examination of health problems through a combination of methods: (1) observation and surveillance and (2) interpretive analysis. *Distribution* is an important concept because health problems are not distributed equally within or across populations. Not everyone is at the same risk of having a given health problem. *Determinants* are all the physical, biological, social, environmental, cultural, and behavioral factors that influence health; the complexity implied by the multiplicity of these determinants justifies the need for careful analysis and planning. For example, planners in Community X gain valuable practical insight from knowing that alcohol-related auto crashes among teens tend to occur Friday through Sunday, between 10:00 P.M. and 2 A.M., and that the events tend to occur most often in two locations.

Health-related conditions refers to specific, measurable events such as diseases, causes of death, behavior such as use of tobacco, reactions to preventive regimens, and provision and use of health services. *Specified populations* refers to those who either have, or are at risk for having, one or more health-related conditions. Finally, the phrase *application to control* refers to the ultimate aim of epidemiology—to promote, protect, and restore health.

Epidemiologists work to discover this kind of information by seeking the answers to three unambiguous questions:

1. What is the problem?
2. Who has the problem?
3. Why do those with the problem have it?

We shall address the first two questions in this chapter, and the third in Chapter 4, where we show how one can use epidemiological methods to assess the behavioral and environmental determinants of selected health problems. In epidemiological assessment, one has a three-fold task. First, one must *gain access* to existing epidemiologic data (for answers to the three previous questions).

Second, one *combines those data* with information documenting the social concerns and needs of that population. Finally, one *uses both sources of information* as the basis for discussion and negotiation for establishing program priorities and, eventually, program strategies.

ASSESSING THE IMPORTANCE OF HEALTH PROBLEMS

By showing the magnitude and distribution of health problems in the population, descriptive epidemiological data suggest the relative importance of the health problems as measured and compared in terms of vital statistics such as fertility, morbidity, disability, or mortality. Such data also suggest how the importance of health problems varies among subgroups of the population. To determine which health problems should receive priority, one has to describe and quantify health problems in sufficient detail. Going through this process serves three principal functions:

- To establish the relative importance of various health problems in the target population as a whole and in population subgroups
- To provide a basis for setting program priorities among the various health problems and subgroups
- To help allocate responsibilities among collaborating professionals, agencies, or departments

It has long been the tradition of the health professional to interpret local data in the light of medical and epidemiological knowledge about cause-and-effect relationships and the natural history and distribution of the health problems in the wider population. Numerous documents describe in detail the nature, scope, and burden of health problems at the national level: See, for example, *Canada's Health Promotion Survey* and the *Canadian Health and Disability Survey;*[11] see also the U.S. Department of Health and Human Services' annual publication, *Health, United States;*[12] its monthly *Vital and Health Statistics;* and its weekly *Morbidity and Mortality Weekly Reports* series. These and similar series in Canada, Australia, and other countries provide national, regional, and state or provincial incidence, prevalence, mortality, and fertility data for the major health events by age, gender, race or ethnic group, and location.[13] Some also provide long-term care, hospital, and ambulatory care statistics. The World Health Organization publishes an annual report that summarizes comparable statistics compiled by each country.

ONLINE DATA AND ITS USES

Until recently, the main barrier to retrieving data from these various documents has been logistics—having the time to track down the source through libraries or by contacting the source agency directly. With the advent of information retrieval through the Internet, virtually all of the information just referred to, as well as a rapidly growing amount of local area health data, is now readily available.

For instance, to illustrate how existing epidemiological data can provide important clues in determining health priorities, we went directly to the web site for the Missouri State Department of Health[14] and downloaded the most recent mortality data for Boone County, Missouri. Table 3-1 presents a portion of the mortality data for all residents of this county. The H or L designation in the "significantly different" column indicates whether a rate for a given cause of death is significantly higher or lower than the state rate. The column headed "ranking quintile" reveals the ranking, among Missouri's 115 counties, for a given cause of death. If the ranking quintile is "1" then it means it is in the highest 20% with 23 other counties. If it is "2" it is in the second-highest 20%, and so on, with "5" indicating that the rate for a given cause of death is in the lowest 20% of all counties. Suppose a coalition of planners in Boone County has been asked to submit a list of health priorities for use in the development of their 5-year county health plan. As a part of their charge, they are told that priorities should be tied to key social problems, one of which is that some minorities feel their problems are not given serious attention. What insights can the planning team gain from the data in Table 3-1?

Here is an example. Note that while the age-adjusted rate for Diabetes Mellitus for all residents in Boone County is 12.4 (not significantly different from the state rate of 10.8), the ranking quintile is "1." On the computer screen, we could then select hypertext designated "African American," which enabled us to retrieve the same selected mortality data for African Americans in Boone County (Table 3-2). These data reveal that for these African Americans, the age-adjusted rate for diabetes mellitus is 43.7, twice as high as the state rate for African Americans and more than three times greater than the overall rate for Boone County—this constitutes a problem that deserves priority attention. The ability to retrieve data electronically, at virtually no cost, has significant implications for participatory planning. In Chapter 12, we shall provide more details on the role of technology in health promotion planning.

INDICATORS OF HEALTH STATUS IN POPULATIONS

The classic indicators of health problems are **mortality** (death), **morbidity** (disease or injury), and **disability** (dysfunction). Sometimes, discomfort and dissatisfaction are added, making a list of "five D's" extending into quality-of-life measures. In addition, there are positive indicators of health status, such as life expectancy and fitness.[15] Mortality has been expressed increasingly in recent years as *years of potential life lost* (YPLL) to give greater weight to deaths at younger ages. This measure is more sensitive to the preventable mortality in

TABLE 3-1

This tabulation of leading causes of death for all residents of Boone County, Missouri (1985–1995), was downloaded directly from a web site of the Missouri State Health Department

Indicator	Number of Events	Age-Adjusted Rate	Significantly Different (H, L)	Ranking Quintile	State Rate
All causes	7,425	470.6	L	5	535.1
Heart disease	2,161	126.7	L	5	161.5
Cancer (malignant neoplasms)	1,689	129.6	L	3	137.7
Lung cancer	478	40.2		3	43.6
Breast cancer (female)	151	22.4		2	22.3
Stroke (cerebrovascular disease)	488	23.4	L	5	29.0
Chronic pulmonary obstructive disease (COPD)	309	20.8		4	21.9
Accidental deaths	340	23.6	L	5	35.0
Motor vehicle	179	13.1	L	5	20.6
Work-related injury	15	2.1		4	2.5
Pneumonia and influenza	230	10.0	L	5	13.8
Diabetes mellitus	193	12.4		1	10.8
Suicide	143	11.8		4	12.8
Kidney disease (nephritis and nephrosis)	99	5.0		3	4.7
Homicide and legal intervention	49	3.9	L	3	10.5
Liver disease and cirrhosis	58	5.0		2	6.1
AIDS	48	4.0	L	1	5.5
Septicemia	86	4.9			4.0
Alzheimer's disease	90	3.7	H		2.1
Smoking-related deaths	1,055	74.7	L	4	86.7
Alcohol and substance abuse	91	8.2			8.2
All injuries and poisonings	559	41.4	L	5	59.9
Firearm-related deaths	115	9.1	L		16.7

NOTE: Causes of death at the left margin are listed in order from most to least prevalent statewide, excepting smoking-related deaths, alcohol and substance abuse, all injuries and poisonings, and firearm-related deaths. These causes include deaths from other causes; e.g., some deaths due to heart disease and cancer are included in the count for smoking-related deaths. All rates are per 100,000 population and are adjusted for age using the U.S. 1940 population as the standard.

Rates based on fewer than 20 deaths are unstable; comparisons based on them should be made with extreme caution.

SOURCE: Center for Health Information Management and Epidemiology, Missouri Department of Health.

TABLE 3-2

Leading causes of death for African-American residents of Boone County, Missouri (1985–1995), from the same web site show the excessively high age-adjusted diabetes death rates for this population

Indicator	Number of Events	Age-Adjusted Rate	Significantly Different (H, L)	Ranking Quintile	State Rate
All causes	599	723.1	L		814.3
Heart disease	167	193.5	L		222.4
Cancer (malignant neoplasms)	115	173.7			196.2
Lung cancer	32	51.7			58.2
Breast cancer (female)	9	21.6			27.9
Stroke (cerebrovascular disease)	23	25.6	L		46.5
Chronic pulmonary obstructive disease (COPD)	14	18.0			18.7
Accidental deaths	27	27.6			37.9
Motor vehicle	11	12.9			14.0
Work-related injury	1	3.0			2.0
Pneumonia and influenza	12	12.6			17.3
Diabetes mellitus	31	43.7	H		24.3
Suicide	3	2.6	L		7.9
Kidney disease (nephritis and nephrosis)	13	12.3			10.5
Homicide and legal intervention	18	17.3	L		56.0
Liver disease and cirrhosis	4	7.1			10.8
AIDS	10	11.4			13.6
Septicemia					
Alzheimer's disease					
Smoking-related deaths	65	91.1			102.4
Alcohol and substance abuse					
All injuries and poisonings	57	59.4	L		104.5
Firearm-related deaths					

NOTE: Causes of death at the left margin are listed in order from most to least prevalent statewide, excepting smoking-related deaths, alcohol and substance abuse, all injuries and poisonings, and firearm-related deaths. These causes include deaths from other causes; e.g., some deaths due to heart disease and cancer are included in the count for smoking-related deaths. All rates are per 100,000 population and are adjusted for age using the U.S. 1940 population as the standard.

Rates based on fewer than 20 deaths are unstable; comparisons based on them should be made with extreme caution.

SOURCE: Center for Health Information Management and Epidemiology, Missouri Department of Health.

children, youth, and the adult "productive" years.[16] Fertility measures among the vital statistics collected in virtually every jurisdiction in the world provide another measure used in health planning. Indirect measures of health, including environmental, behavioral, and social indicators, also serve in lieu of direct measures. These are becoming increasingly important as public health and medical care confront prevention issues related to chronic diseases for which direct measures may not show up for many years after the onset of the condition.

Comparative data on these indicators are available from a variety of sources, all of which have online web sites. These include the National Center for Health Statistics, Centers for Disease Control and Prevention, and other agencies of the Department of Health and Human Services (or the ministries of health in other countries). Local and state or provincial health departments and ministries, the Bureau of the Census (see the annual *Statistical Abstract of the United States*) and Statistics Canada, professional journals and associations, voluntary health associations, and the World Health Organization all have web sites. One can easily search these for statistical information on specific diseases, injuries, vital statistics, and survey data. Some of these include charts and graphs one can download to use in local planning meetings, bringing the data to life for community groups.

MAKING COMPARISONS

To determine the relative importance of health problems, one makes comparisons. One can compare the data of interest to Community X with those of other communities, the state, or the nation; one can compare data for different health problems within the same community; and one can compare data for various subgroups of the community, based on age, race, or gender. Such comparisons allow identification of health problems that are greater in this community than in other places, are most important within the community, and characterize specific subgroups.

RATES

One can make data comparisons only between like data—apples with apples, oranges with oranges. For example, expressing rates of death and disease uniformly as "number per thousand population per year" allows direct comparisons between populations of different sizes over different periods. It does not mean much to say, "In 1999, County Z had 48 fatal injuries, and its state had 1,712." Because the state is much bigger than the county and the size of neither is given, one cannot compare the numbers. One must first turn them into rates. A *rate* is the number of events (in this case, fatal injuries) per 1,000 or 100,000 population.

To generate rates in our example, one could do the following:

- First, divide the number of deaths in the county by the population of the county
- Then, divide the number of deaths in the state by the population of the state
- Finally, multiply the results by a multiple of ten to obtain a value between 1 and 100

This calculation enables one to compare data with common properties: The injury death rate in County Z within the United States is 55.8 deaths per 100,000, and that of the state is 36.4 deaths per 100,000. Because the county has a higher rate of fatal injuries than does the state as a whole, further examination is warranted to determine what factors might explain the differences. For example, knowing that fatal injuries are more common among younger age groups, planners might want to see if the age distribution of the county might explain a portion of the difference observed. Summary descriptions of the epidemiological rates commonly used to support planning are presented in Table 3-3.

As another example, see Figure 3-4 to compare firearm injury death rates among men 15–24 years of age in selected countries. Note that the firearm death rate in the United States was 54 per 100,000, about five times that in Norway, Israel, and Canada, and 60 times that in England and Wales.

Offering an example from a smaller population, Table 3-4 provides an in-depth view of death rates due to firearm-related injuries among white and African American men and women age 15–24.[17] These data provide a compelling justification for actions to discover the root causes underlying the disproportionate mortality rates among young African-American men.

INCIDENCE AND PREVALENCE

Two rates deserve particular discussion: incidence and prevalence. Though both measure morbidity (disease or injury) in the population, they have important differences. **Incidence** measures *new* cases of the disease within a certain period, whereas **prevalence** measures the total number of continuing or surviving cases or people with the disease at a particular *point* in time.

Incidence. Although incidence rates for population groups are hard to find, especially for chronic diseases, they can reveal important insights for planners. For example, Figure 3-5 shows the incidence of cervical cancer among Canadian women, by age group for the years 1969–1993. Figure 3-6 shows cervical cancer mortality among Canadian women by age group for the years 1950–1995.

Collectively, these data show that the steady decline in the incidence and mortality was similar for all age groups, but greatest in the 50–64 group. Note that in both cases, the decline reached a plateau around 1985, with only modest declines evident thereafter. These patterns might be explained by a plateau in cervical cancer screening activity or perhaps a change in the prevalence of risk

TABLE 3-3

Common epidemiological measures for comparison purposes; their numerators, denominators, and multipliers for standardized expression of number at risk

Natality Measure	Numerator	Denominator	Expressed per Number at Risk
Crude birth rate	# live births reported during a given time interval	estimated total population at midinterval	1,000
Crude fertility rate	# live births reported during a given time interval	estimated number of women age 15–44 years at midinterval	1,000

Morbidity Measure	Numerator	Denominator	Expressed per Number at Risk
Incidence rate	# new cases of a specified disease reported during a given time interval	average or midpoint population during time interval	variable: $10x$ where $x = 2, 3, 4, 5, 6$
Attack rate	# new cases of a specified disease reported during an epidemic period of time	population at start of the epidemic period	variable: $10x$ where $x = 2, 3, 4, 5, 6$
Point prevalence	# current cases, new and old, of a specified disease at a given point in time	estimated population at the same point in time	variable: $10x$ where $x = 2, 3, 4, 5, 6$
Period prevalence	# current cases, new and old, of a specified disease identified over a given time interval	estimated population at midinterval	variable: $10x$ where $x = 2, 3, 4, 5, 6$

Morbidity Measure	Numerator	Denominator	Expressed per Number at Risk
Crude death rate	total number of deaths reported during a given time interval	estimated midinterval population	1,000 or 100,000
Cause-specific death rate	# deaths assigned to a specific cause during a given time interval	estimated midinterval population	100,000
Neonatal mortality rate	# deaths under 28 days of age during a given time interval	# live births during the same time interval	1,000
Infant mortality rate	# deaths under one year of age during a given time interval	# live births reported during the same time interval	1,000

SOURCE: Adapted from *Self-Study Course 3030-G: Principles of Epidemiology,* 1992, 2nd ed., Atlanta, GA: Centers for Disease Control and Prevention.

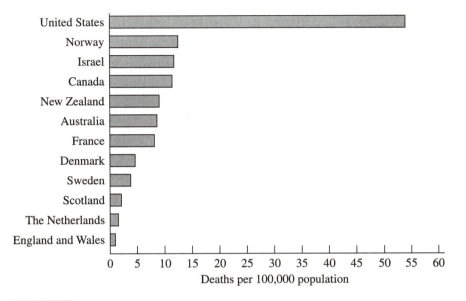

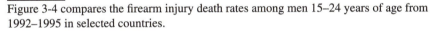

FIGURE 3-4

Figure 3-4 compares the firearm injury death rates among men 15–24 years of age from 1992–1995 in selected countries.

factors (age of first intercourse, number of sex partners, infection with human papilloma virus, smoking, and low socioeconomic status). Clearly, such information will be crucial to Canadian health officials and community planners as they frame their cervical cancer prevention and control strategies.[18]

Prevalence. Prevalence rates and incidence rates give health planners complementary, but different, information. Prevalence reflects both the incidence and the duration of disease. Suppose diseases A and B have equal incidence rates, but disease A is mild and unlikely to be life threatening, while B is severe and causes early death. Disease A will have a higher prevalence in the population, because those who died from Disease B are no longer around to be counted when the prevalence survey is done! Just looking at the prevalence rates could mislead you in determining which disease affects a population most.

This is illustrated by comparing common allergies with AIDS. Because of both a higher incidence and a much milder disease course, allergies have a much higher prevalence than does AIDS. It would certainly be incorrect to deduce from the higher prevalence that allergies are more important, because here the one with the low prevalence causes death. In another example, the prevalence of Type 1 (insulin dependent, juvenile onset) diabetes is much higher today than it was early in this century, because improved treatment now allows those diabetics to live

TABLE 3-4

Death rates due to firearm-related injuries within the U.S. have varied widely among European- and African-Americans age 15–24 for the years between 1970 and 1995

15–24 Year Age Group	1970	1980	1985	1990	1993–95
White Males	16.9	28.4	24.1	31.4	32.9
Black Males	97.3	77.9	138.0	140.2	162.8
White Females	3.4	5.1	4.4	4.6	4.9
Black Females	12.2	12.3	8.3	13.3	15.8

SOURCE: *Health United States 1996–97 and Injury Chartbook,* by National Center for Health Statistics, 1998, Washington, DC: Public Health Service.

longer (and thus be counted). These examples illustrate that when one compares prevalence rates, one needs additional information about severity and duration to determine which diseases matter most. Although prevalence rates combine information about incidence and duration, and so must be interpreted with care, they are important for planning health resources and programs.

Prevalence: A Caveat. From a health promotion perspective, the prevalence rates of chronic diseases can be misleading when one is setting priorities for the future. They may identify the people whose behavior and living conditions 20 years ago caused the disease from which they died the previous year, when the disease-specific rate was calculated. We can say that "smoking is the number-one preventable cause of deaths" because we are reaping the lung cancers, lung diseases, and heart attacks of people who started smoking as many as 20 years ago. Considering the dramatic declines in smoking in the past two decades, we might be more accurate in saying that "smoking that began 10 to 20 years ago is the number-one cause of deaths today." Today's true main cause of deaths, the one that will cause the most deaths in the future, is the proper criterion for setting a mortality-based priority in health promotion. This might still be tobacco, or it might be alcohol, or most likely it will be a combination of dietary fat and physical inactivity. In Chapter 4, we take up these and other issues concerning the etiology and determinants of disease, death, injury, and health.

Sensitivity and Specificity. Sensitivity analysis in epidemiological assessments pertains to the use of mass screening results as the basis for generating estimates of prevalence of a disease or condition in a population. If the test can detect virtually every case without fail, it is said to have high **sensitivity.** To take two extreme examples, death reporting by death certificates has high sensitivity, whereas physician reporting of communicable diseases has low sensitivity because it

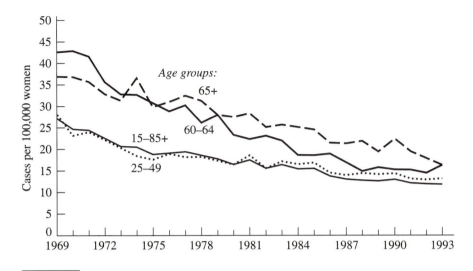

FIGURE 3-5

Incidence of cervical cancer among Canadian women, by age group for the years 1969–1993, shows an apparently steady decline in the number of new cases over the three decades, especially in older women.

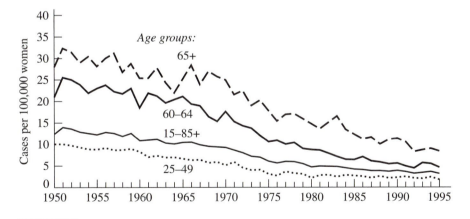

FIGURE 3-6

Cervical cancer mortality among Canadian women, by age group for the years 1969–1993, shows an even greater decrease than in Figure 3-5, apparently attributable to some combination of primary prevention (see Figure 3-5, accounting for most of the decrease here), screening for early detection and treatment, and more effective treatment.

misses many of the cases of some diseases. Sensitivity applies mostly to laboratory and clinical tests such as mammograms and pap smears for cancer, blood tests for serum cholesterol and sexually transmitted diseases, or blood pressure measures for hypertension. Some of these tests may yield normal readings when in fact the person tested has the condition. To that degree they lack sensitivity.

The related concept, **specificity,** rules out the degree to which a screening test yields results that may be wrong in the other direction—positive when the case is negative. The false positive case (detected in a test lacking specificity) might be better off than the false negative case (from a test lacking sensitivity), insofar as he or she has not been missed when a treatable disease is present. Yet, health officials tend to eschew tests with low specificity because of the high cost in following up on large numbers of false positives and because of the fear and shame aroused in those who have been told their test was positive. The latter has been referred to as the "labeling" problem of mass screening. It applies to both false and true positives in that these people often overreact to being labeled as having a condition that they consider dangerous or shameful.

Issues of sensitivity and specificity surround the use of mass screening to determine population prevalence rates and to detect cases early enough to be most effectively treated. Cost-benefit considerations also enter the debate on mass screening when the cost of the tests run high relative to the yield in number of treatable cases. These debates reach a crescendo when the disease in question is one that has social stigma and possible hiring, firing, or promotion consequences. HIV testing and drug testing in the workplace, as well as the possibility of genetic testing, have come to this juncture. Issues of sensitivity, specificity, cost-benefit, and labeling all pertain to the work-site debate on these as well as blood pressure screening and even fitness testing. Confidentiality of test results and assurances that they will not be used in personnel decisions help overcome some resistance but lack credibility in some corporate settings.

Surveillance. Most of the public health data systems that monitor health trends over time were designed many years ago for **surveillance** of communicable disease outbreaks. A large portion of such surveillance is based on information provided by physicians when they complete forms required when they encounter a patient with a "reportable" disease.[19] The word *surveillance* is derived from French term *surveiller,* which means "to watch over."[20] Last[21] defines *surveillance* as the "continuous analysis, interpretation, and feedback of systematically collected data." In the United States, many states require physicians to report some specific noncommunicable diseases such as occupational lung diseases or lead toxicity so that health officials can intervene on environmental health threats.

The emergence of survey tools and systems to identify and "watch over" the prevalence of risk factors (behavioral, environmental) known to influence chronic disease morbidity and mortality has added an important dimension to health promotion planning. We shall deal with these more in the next chapter, but because some behavioral risk factors, such as drug abuse, can also be defined as health problems, they add to the surveillance of disease. Two systems addressing such problems are prominently used in the United States. The Behavioral Risk Factor Surveillance System (BRFSS) is a national, population-based telephone survey, managed and conducted by individual states to assess the prevalence of health-related behavioral risk factors associated with leading causes of premature death and disability. For the most part, BRFSS data concern the state level, and most communities do not have good surveillance systems in place to monitor the risk factors on a continuous or periodic basis.[22] However, the Youth Risk Behavior Surveillance System (YRBSS) monitors health risk behaviors among high-school youth. Because information for this system is collected at the school level, YRBSS can provide comparable national, state, and local data.

SPECIFIC RATES

Rates may need other kinds of adjustment to make them equivalent for comparison. For example, data from different years or locations may need to be **age-adjusted** to account for different age distributions in the populations. Figure 3-7 shows the age-adjusted death rates for the United States from 1950 through 1995. Because the rates are age-adjusted, the trends for decreasing death rates must be ascribed to some factor or factors other than the changing age structure of the nation. The differences between the races and sexes can also be ascribed to factors other than the different age structures between them.

To compare rates among various subgroups or for different diseases, a **specific rate** is used. This rate is calculated for a specified population subgroup based on age, race, or sex. For example, a rate for 55–60 year olds is an **age-specific rate.** If the rate is further broken down by race, it becomes an age-race–specific rate, such as a rate for African-American 18–24 year olds. Going a step further, we can break the rate down by sex to obtain an age-race-sex–specific rate: African-American 55–60-year-old men. Rates can also be calculated for particular causes of death: the rate of cancer deaths and the rate of lung cancer deaths are examples of cause-specific rates.

Comparing the rates of different groups can provide a clearer picture of the relative importance of health problems among those groups. If we examine the differences in cause-specific death rates among socioeconomic groups, we can identify causes of death that are more important for the poor or for the affluent. Comparison of rates within a group also can be instructive.

At this point, you may ask if all this attention to data is truly applicable in the real world of the practitioner. An affirmative response to this question can be seen in Table 3-5, prepared by staff of the North Carolina Department of Health in 1986. These data on mortality rates and their social costs were assembled to support legislation that would establish a permanent, state-funded health promotion and disease prevention program. The report was prepared and presented to the North Carolina General Assembly to inform them of important, preventable

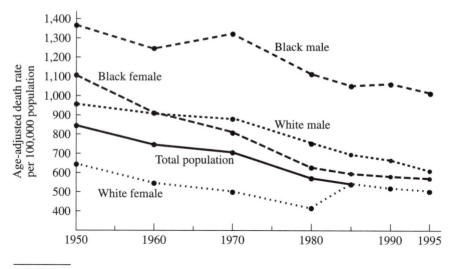

FIGURE 3-7

Age-adjusted death rates for all causes by sex and race, 1950 to 1995, United States, show trends typical of most countries, except that the gradients by socioeconomic and ethnic factors are greater for the U.S. than for most other Western countries.

problems. In July 1987, the assembly passed the legislation and provided a program budget.

SETTING PRIORITIES FOR HEALTH PROGRAMS

Setting sound program priorities for health promotion depends on objectively constructed descriptions of prevailing health problems and how they manifest in the target population. To select one problem from several, one should answer the following questions:

1. Which problem has the greatest impact in terms of death, disease, days lost from work, rehabilitation costs, disability (temporary and permanent), family disorganization, and cost to communities and agencies for damage repair or loss and cost recovery?
2. Are certain subpopulations, such as children, mothers, ethnic minorities, refugees, indigenous populations, at special risk?
3. Which problems are most susceptible to intervention?
4. Which problem is not being addressed by other agencies in the community?

TABLE 3-5

Mortality and social cost data assembled by North Carolina public health staff to make a case to the state legislature for permanent funding of health promotion

Cause of Death	1985 Total Number of Deaths (Ages 18–64)	1985 Years of Life Lost (Below Age 65)	Lifetime Lost Wages, $[a]	Lifetime Lost State Income Tax, $[b]	Lifetime Lost General Sales Tax, $[c]
Cardiovascular disease	5,436	52,941	725,291,700	36,254,585	9,317,616
Cancer	4,475	47,353	648,736,100	32,436,805	8,334,128
All accidents	2,013	58,943	807,519,100	40,375,955	10,373,968
Subtotal	11,924	159,237	2,181,546,900	109,077,345	28,025,712
All other causes[d]	4,679	79,351	1,087,138,700	54,355,435	13,965,776
Total	16,603	238,588	3,268,685,600	163,432,780	41,991,488

NOTE: Total population in North Carolina age 18–64 is 3,928,097 based on extrapolation from 1970–1980 census data, N.C. Office of State Budget Management.

[a] Based on 1982 average yearly income of $13,700. *Statistical Abstract for State Government, 1984.* Figures in this column represent what could have been contributed if these persons had lived to age 65.

[b] 5% derived from net income tax paid, 1982. Ibid. Figures in this column represent what could have been contributed if these persons had lived until age 65.

[c] For a family of three (average in N.C., 1980), $176 is the estimated sales tax paid, 1982 (Federal Income Tax Form). Figures in this column represent what could have been contributed if these persons had lived until age 65.

[d] Includes diabetes mellitus, pneumonia/influenza, chronic obstructive pulmonary disease, chronic liver disease/cirrhosis, nephritis/nephrosis, suicide, homicide, all other causes.

SOURCE: Adapted from North Carolina Department of Health, unpublished data.

5. Which problem, when appropriately addressed, has the greatest potential for an attractive yield—in improved health status, economic savings, or other benefits?
6. Are any of the health problems highly ranked as a regional or national priority? (State health agencies develop priorities among health problems, often based on local epidemiological data.)

Elaborating on the scope and impact of the health problems helps the planner focus clearly on the problems of the target population and its subgroups. With sufficiently detailed information, the process can also help one select the strategies to be used and decide whether a program is to be preventive, curative, rehabilitative, or some combination thereof.

Consider the complex problem of motor vehicle injuries. Prevention efforts might consist of trying to reduce drunk driving, increasing the use of seat belts in combination with consistent enforcement of a legislated speed limit, or employing strategies to improve road markings and conditions in areas where crashes are most common. A curative program would emphasize immediate emergency medical services (including the transportation of injury victims to the appropriate facility). A rehabilitative effort would deal with disabilities resulting from injuries, increasing the number of victims who regain productive lives and the speed with which they do so. Epidemiological information will provide insights on which facets of the problem will or will not yield to intervention and on which focus—preventive, curative, or rehabilitative—should predominate.

DEVELOPING HEALTH OBJECTIVES

When the health problem has been specifically defined and the risk factors identified, the next step is to develop the program objectives. This vital phase in program planning is often treated quite superficially, with unfortunate consequences for program implementation and evaluation.

Objectives are crucial. They form a fulcrum for converting diagnostic data into program direction. Objectives should be cast in the language of epidemiological or medical outcomes and should answer these questions:

- *Who* will receive the program? (On whose health does it focus?)
- *What* health benefit should they receive?
- *How much* of that benefit should be achieved?
- *By when* should it be achieved, or *how long* should the program run?

Consider the hypothetical maternal and child health data presented earlier in this chapter. The following program objective could be developed, based on those diagnostic data, and consonant with the mission or resources of the given agency:

> The infant mortality rate in Counties A and B will be reduced by 10 percent within the first two years and an additional 51 percent over the next three years, continuing to decline until the state average is reached.

The target population *(who)* is demographically implied (pregnant women) and geographically explicit (within counties A and B). *What* is reduced maternal mortality. *How much* benefit is to be achieved by when is stated in stages: a 10-percent reduction in two years, a 25% reduction over five years, to continue until the state average rate is achieved. (Note that the average rate for the state will probably go down concurrently, so the program has tackled a moving target.)

In developing program objectives, the planner should strive to set up the plan so that (1) progress in meeting objectives can be measured; (2) individual objec-

tives are based on relevant, reasonably accurate data; and (3) objectives are in harmony across topics as well as across levels.

The third of these conditions implies *consistency*. It means that objectives dealing with various aspects of a health problem (for example, the objectives of a maternity program to improve nutrition, prenatal appointment compliance, weight and blood pressure control, and percentage of hospital deliveries) should be consistent with each other. *Healthy Communities 2000: Model Standards*[23] was developed to provide both exemplary standards and a practical process for establishing objectives for community health programs consistent with the disease prevention and health promotion objectives for the year 2000 and beyond.

Objectives should also be *coherent* across levels, with objectives becoming successively more refined and more explicit, level by level. In the usual language of health planners, goals are considered to be more general than are objectives. For example, the maternal and child health program objective just presented is in reality part of a three-tier hierarchy of concordant objectives consisting of an overall program goal, a set of more specific program objectives, and several even more specific objectives stated in behavioral terms. Health objectives arise from epidemiological assessment; **behavioral objectives** are developed in the next phase of PRECEDE, the behavioral and environmental assessment:

1. *Program Goal:* The survival rate of mothers, infants, and children will be raised through the optimal growth and development of children.
2. *Health Objectives:*
   a. The maternal mortality rate within Counties A and B will be reduced by 10 percent within the first two years and an additional 51% the next three years, with reductions continuing until the state average rate is reached.
   b. The infant mortality rate will be reduced to the state average within ten years. Perinatal mortality rate will be reduced by 94%. Fetal death will be reduced from x to y percent in the same period.

Note that the objectives in this example, ranging from the broadest statement of program mission to the most immediate and precise target, are coherent. Achievement of each of the more specific and more immediate objectives will contribute causally to the achievement of the more general and the more distant objectives and goals.[24]

ENSURING COOPERATION

Detailing the health problem helps harmonize the activities of the various individuals and groups involved in the program. Health education is usually part of a larger endeavor, engaging a variety of disciplines and perhaps several units within an agency. Hospital-based health programs, for example, might function in both inpatient and outpatient units and involve social service and nutrition departments. Programs based in a health department will often deploy staff from various personal health service units as well as from environmental protection and other sections.

The more heterogeneity among participants (and, therefore, perspectives), the greater the utility of sharply delineated statements of the problem. All participants in the activity need to share a full understanding of it. Understanding is further facilitated when program goals and subobjectives are thoroughly spelled out. A coalition of disparate agencies will stick through difficult negotiations and disagreements on methods if they can be reminded of a common goal that all agree is worth the effort. We address this important issue in more detail in Chapters 6 and 8.

SUMMARY

This chapter highlights (1) the relationship between health problems and social problems, (2) methods by which health problems are quantified and prioritized, and (3) assessment of determinants of health.

Though health professionals usually do not address social problems directly, it is instructive to analyze the relationship between quality of life and each health problem addressed by a program. One should describe health problems in detail, using data from local, regional, state, and national sources interpreted against a background of current epidemiological knowledge as reflected in the literature. Health promotion planners will gain critical insight by analyzing existing data on who is most affected (age, sex, race, residence), the ways they are affected (mortality, disability, signs, symptoms). This information will lead to the identification of most likely routes to improvement (impact of immunizations, treatment regimens, environmental alterations, behavioral changes). The program's health priorities are expressed as objectives by specifying *who will benefit how much of what outcome by when*. A thorough epidemiological assessment is basic to the next phase of the Precede framework: identifying the behavioral and environmental components of the health problem.

EXERCISES

1. List the health problems related to the quality-of-life concerns identified in your population in Exercise 3, Chapter 2.

2. Rate (low, medium, high) each health problem in the inventory according to
   (a) its relative importance in affecting the quality-of-life concerns and
   (b) its potential for change.
3. Discuss the reasons for your giving high-priority ratings to health problems in Exercise 2a in terms of their prevalence, incidence, cost, virulence, severity, or other relevant dimensions. Extrapolate from national, state, or regional data when local data are not available.
4. Cite the evidence supporting your ratings of health problems in Exercise 2b. Refer to the success of other programs and/or to the availability of medical or other technology to control or reduce the high-priority health problems you have selected.
5. Cite two uses for data generated by epidemiological assessments other than for program planning, and give an example of each.
6. Write a program objective for the highest-priority health problem, indicating who will show how much of what improvement by when.

NOTES AND CITATIONS

1. We are indebted to Denise Simons-Morton, M.D., M.P.H., Ph.D., for her special contributions to this chapter in the previous edition, some of which were carried over to this edition.
2. Murray & Lopez, 1996.
3. Ibid., p. 8. See also Kaplan & Lynch, 1997, Winkleby, Kraemer, & Varady, 1998.
4. World Health Organization, 1980. See also *Statistics Canada,* 1995.
5. Bezzaoucha & Dekkar, 1990; Gomez-Rodriguez, 1989; Minaire, 1992.
6. Blane, 1995; Krieger et al., 1993; National Center for Health Statistics, 1996a; Pollitt, 1994.
7. Abma, Chandra, Mosher, Peterson, & Piccinino, 1997; Edet, 1991; Schorr, 1988.
8. Ventura, Curtin, & Mathews, 1998. See also Chung & Elias, 1996.
9. Federal, Provincial and Territorial Advisory Committee on Population Health, 1996; Frank, 1995.
10. Last, 1995, p. 55. The definition and explanation of epidemiology has been paraphrased from pp. 55–56. For variations on this definition, see Green & Ottoson, 1999, p. 70; Timmerick, 1998, pp. 2–3. See also Krieger, 1994; Pearce, 1996.
11. Health and Welfare Canada, 1993; Statistics Canada and Department of the Secretary of State of Canada, 1995.
12. National Center for Health Statistics, 1998. This annual publication, in addition to its detailed tables comparing health status and health behavior statistics among regions, states, and demographic groups, contains a detailed description of the sources and limitations of vital and health data systems of the federal government and various other national organizations, as well as a glossary of social and demographic terms used in health statistics. The text and tables of all *Vital and Health Statistics* reports can be viewed and downloaded from www.cdc.gov/nchswww/ on the world wide web. For sources particularly relevant to health promotion, see also Green & Lewis, 1986, pp. 128–45.
13. Australian Bureau of Statistics, 1987; Better Health Commission, 1986.
14. The data used in this example are the actual data for Boone County, Missouri, for the years given and were downloaded directly from the Missouri Health Department website:

http://www.health.state.mo.us/cgi-bin/uncgi/ShowProfile?CountyName=Boone&Profile=Cause-OfDeath. Throughout the world, public and private health organizations have web sites that make data like these openly accessible.

15. Abelin, Brzezinski, & Carstairs, 1987; Andresen, Rothenberg, & McDermott, 1998; Bergner & Rothman, 1987; Carr, Thompson & Kirwan, 1996; Fries, Green, & Levine, 1989; Green, 1985b; Pate, 1983; World Health Organization Quality of Life Group, 1996.

16. In use since 1982, years of potential life lost (YPLL) measure the impact of diseases and injuries that kill people before the customary age of retirement. It is computed as the sum of products over all age groups up to age 65, sometimes 75, each product being the annual number of deaths in an age group multiplied by the average number of years remaining before the age of 65 for that age group. See Centers for Disease Control, 1986; McDonnell & Vossberg, 1998.

17. National Center for Health Statistics, 1998, pp. 161–163.

18. The information and tables illustrating how incidence data can be applied were taken from "Cervical Cancer in Canada," *Cancer Updates,* March 1998, published by the Cancer Bureau, Laboratory Centre for Disease Control, Health Protection Branch, Health Canada. Web site: http://www.hc-sc.gc.ca/hpb/lcdc/bc

19. Green, R. W. Wilson, & Bauer, 1983.

20. N. J. Thomson, 1900, p. 15.

21. Last, 1995, p. 163.

22. Arday, Tomar, & Mowry, 1997; Green, R. W. Wilson, & Bauer, 1983; Mergenhagen, 1997.

23. *Healthy Communities 2000,* 1991.

24. Some applications of PRECEDE illustrating epidemiological assessments and setting of health objectives include Antoniades & Lubker, 1997; Gielen, 1992; Green, Mullen, & Friedman, 1991; Green, Wilson, & Bauer, 1983; Livingston, 1985; Simons-Morton, Parcel, Brink, Harvey, & Tiernan, 1991; Stevenson, Jones, Cross, Howatt, & Hall, 1996; Timmerick, 1998, pp. 338–340; Walter, Hoffman, Connelly, et al., 1985.

Chapter 4

Behavioral and Environmental Assessment

PRECEDE

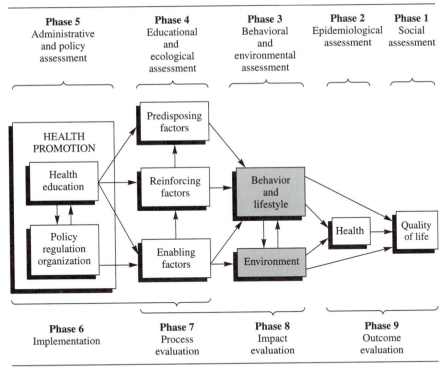

Phase 5
Administrative
and policy
assessment

Phase 4
Educational
and
ecological
assessment

Phase 3
Behavioral
and
environmental
assessment

Phase 2
Epidemiological
assessment

Phase 1
Social
assessment

HEALTH
PROMOTION

Health
education

Policy
regulation
organization

Predisposing
factors

Reinforcing
factors

Enabling
factors

Behavior
and
lifestyle

Environment

Health

Quality
of life

Phase 6
Implementation

Phase 7
Process
evaluation

Phase 8
Impact
evaluation

Phase 9
Outcome
evaluation

PROCEED

"When I use a word it means just what I choose it to mean—neither more nor less."
—Humpty Dumpty to Alice, courtesy Lewis Carroll

DEFINITIONS

The Ottawa Charter's definition of *health promotion* as "enabling people to increase control over, and to improve, their health"[1] implies that people can at least partially control some of the determinants of their health. The First International Conference on Health Promotion, from which this definition emerged, addressed a wide range of behavioral and environmental determinants of health, including economic and social determinants. Subsequent international conferences have given further attention to environmental,[2] policy,[3] and participatory determinants.[4] This has widened the lens of health promotion from a focus on the behavioral determinants that educational approaches had become increasingly effective at changing, but mostly in selected segments of the populations of most countries. We have defined the strategy of health promotion for this book as any combination of educational and ecological supports for actions and conditions of living conducive to health. These actions may be the personal health behavior and lifestyle adaptations of individuals and families, the advocacy of organizational or public policies to assure healthful living conditions, or direct intervention by individuals or groups to improve environmental living conditions. This range of possibilities for behavioral and environmental changes encompasses the determinants addressed in recent efforts to integrate health promotion and population health concepts.[5]

Phase 3 of the Precede planning process calls for an analysis of those personal and collective actions most pertinent to controlling the determinants of health or quality-of-life issues selected in the preceding phases. It also calls for an analysis of the immediate environmental circumstances that may be constraining or conditioning behavior or that may be directly influencing the selected health and quality-of-life issues from the previous phase. This chapter will review the major determinants in the **etiology** of the leading causes of death and disease. These comprise the most likely behavioral and environmental targets for health promotion. The chapter will then outline the steps to conduct a behavioral assessment and those to conduct an environmental assessment. Finally, we shall discuss how to set priorities among the assessment data to determine a program's objectives for change.

Behavioral assessment is a systematic analysis of the behavioral links to the goals or problems identified in the epidemiological and social assessments. The **environmental assessment** is a parallel analysis of factors in the immediate social and physical environment, other than specific actions, that could be causally linked to the behavior identified in the behavioral assessment or directly to the outcomes of interest (health or quality of life).

In these definitions, we depart from the distinction made by some between health promotion and health protection. On the surface of U.S. federal health policy documents, health promotion appears to address only the lifestyle and behavioral determinants of health (for both individuals and communities), whereas health protection is directed at the physical environment to control potential threats to health and safety, especially through engineering and regulation. Because health promotion components exist in health protection, and vice versa, we shall abandon this rigid distinction, choosing instead the World Health Organization's use of the term *health promotion* as encompassing both the behavioral and environmental determinants of health. The feature that distinguishes it from other medical care, disease prevention, and public health strategies is its emphasis on enabling people to exercise control over health determinants.[6]

ETIOLOGY: ASSESSING THE DETERMINANTS OF HEALTH

Once one has identified the most important health problems (Phase 2), one can try to identify the factors that contributed to them. The widely used term, **determinants of health**, is something of a misnomer insofar as most of the evidence linking so-called determinants with health outcomes is mostly correlational or relative risk data. In most branches of science, such estimates do not achieve the status of "determinants." We use the term broadly to refer to the forces predisposing, enabling, and reinforcing lifestyles, or shaping environmental conditions of living, in ways that affect the health of populations. This broad use treats them as a group of factors with aggregate effects that one could count as deterministic, even though each of them individually could at best account for a small proportion of the variance in health outcomes. Determinants of health, then, will include all the factors to be considered in this chapter and the next.

As you saw in Chapter 1, *risk factor* is the more formal and precise term for a factor that increases the probability of developing a disease or health problem. Some population health circles object to this term because risk factors are measured at the individual level and tend to focus the planner's attention on interventions directed at individual behavior rather than ecological conditions. In contrast to such factors, recall the class of factors called *risk conditions*. These are the determinants of health that are more distal in time, place, or scope from the control of individuals than are the more proximal and malleable risk factors such as current behavior. By this definition, epidemiologists would see risk conditions as a subclass of risk factors. The International Epidemiological Association's *Dictionary of Epidemiology* defines *risk factor* as "an aspect of personal behavior or life-style, an environmental exposure, or an inborn or inherited characteristic, which on the basis of epidemiologic evidence is known to be associated with health-related condition(s) considered important to prevent."[7]

The following descriptions reflect the main differences we shall maintain among these classes of factors:

- *Risk factors* are characteristics of individuals; even if they refer to environmental conditions, when measured as a risk factor they refer to the exposure of the individual to that environmental condition.
- *Risk conditions* are characteristics of the environment that may contribute to health problems, disease, or injury.
- *Determinants of health* refer to broad classes of more distal factors considered powerful in their cumulative and aggregate effects on the health of populations, primarily because they shape behavioral and environmental risk factors.

Most health problems have some combination of behavioral, environmental, and genetic or biological causes (risk factors). Table 4-1 shows the associations of the most commonly targeted behavioral and environmental risk factors with the leading causes of death. Although the behavioral and environmental assessment for health promotion is directed toward changeable factors, one must also consider unchangeable factors such as genetic predisposition, age, gender, race, ethnicity, existing disease, physical or mental impairment, and climate. These factors do not lend themselves to intervention, but one must take them into account to keep a perspective on the multiple determinants of the health problem being addressed and to identify high-risk population groups.[8]

Through educational and ecological approaches, health promotion programs attempt to modify the behavioral, biological, social, and environmental risk factors over which people can exert control by individual or collective action. Examples on the behavioral side include smoking cessation, "heart healthy" eating, seat belt use, and exercise. On the environmental side, they include living conditions such as housing, transportation, food policies, and social norms or regulations. Such causes can be influenced by the behavior of health professionals, of the public, of employers and teachers, or of individuals at risk. Communities, neighborhoods, or special-interest groups can organize, vote, boycott, lobby, or otherwise support or prevent certain environmental and technological changes.

These paths to health improvement, then, can include *direct* behavioral influence on health through change in personal behavioral risk factors or actions building fitness and host resistance, as suggested by Arrow 2 in Figure 4-1. Behavior also can *indirectly* affect health by influencing environmental factors. People can exercise some control in exposing themselves to environmental risks (such as solar radiation), and in using health services (Arrow 3), and they can work through community channels to change some of the environmental risk factors, including the health care environment.

TABLE 4-1

The most common priorities for health promotion programs are the 12 leading "causes of death" and the changeable risk factors and conditions associated with them

Risk Factors and Conditions	Leading Causes of Death										
	Heart Disease	Cancers	Stroke	Injuries (nonvehicular)	Influenza, Pneumonia	Injuries (vehicular)	Diabetes	Cirrhosis	Suicide	Homicides	AIDS
Behavioral risk factors											
Smoking	•	•		•	•						
High blood pressure	•		•								
High cholesterol	•										
Diet	•	•					•				
Obesity	•	•					•				
Lack of exercise	•	•	•				•				
Stress	•		•	•		•					
Alcohol abuse		•		•		•		•	•	•	
Drug misuse	•		•	•		•			•	•	•
Seat-belt nonuse						•					
Handgun possession				•					•	•	
Sexual practices											•
Biological factors	•	•	•				•	•			
Environmental risk											
Radiation exposure		•									
Workplace hazards		•		•		•					
Environmental contaminants		•									
Infectious agents		•			•						
Home hazards				•							
Auto/road design						•					
Speed limits						•					
Medical care access	•	•	•			•	•	•	•	•	
Product design				•							
Social factors[a]	•		•	•			•	•		•	•

[a]This residual category of risk factors includes a variety of less well defined lifestyle factors and conditions of living related to social relationships, social support, social pressures, and socioeconomic status.[9]

SOURCE: Adapted from unpublished material, Centers for Disease Control, U.S. Department of Health and Human Services.

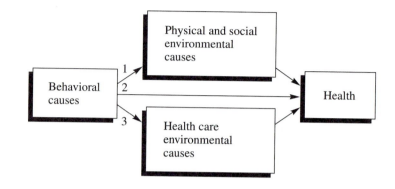

FIGURE 4-1

Behavior can influence health along one direct pathway (Arrow 2), representing actions that change behavioral risk factors such as smoking, and two indirect pathways (Arrows 1 and 3) by which actions are directed at or through environmental and health care influences on health.

ASSESSING THE CAUSAL IMPORTANCE OF RISK FACTORS

One of the purposes of epidemiology is to discover and calibrate the strength of risk factors for health problems. After much research, a consensus often develops about the strength of the association between given risk factors and a specific health problem. Although epidemiological methods are used in these analyses, we place these steps in the flow of the Precede phases within the behavioral and environmental assessment. Besides assessing which risk factors are causally important, this phase determines which of those risk factors are present, and at what level, in the target population or community.

Planners can identify the known risk factors for the health problems prioritized in the epidemiological assessment. They can find relevant epidemiological literature on the relative importance of specific risk factors (see Table 4-1) summarized in consensus documents published by leading health science journals or in government publications. Planners can search for key data about most of the health problems likely to turn up as priorities.[10]

Overall, the risk factors that will appear most frequently in behavioral and environmental assessments are those accounting for the greatest burdens of death and disease. For deaths, these will tend to be the ones associated with the leading "causes of death" which means the causes as written on death certificates. The real causes of these causes, the behavioral and environmental risk factors, have been estimated to account for total deaths in the United States as follows:[11]

Risk Factors	Percentage of Total Deaths
Tobacco	19
Diet/activity patterns	14
Alcohol	5
Microbial agents	4
Toxic agents	3
Firearms	2
Sexual behavior	1
Motor vehicles	1
Illicit use of drugs	<1
Total for this set of risk factors	50

These estimates for total proportions of all deaths are drawn from studies using different methods, including actual counts in the case of microbial agents and firearms, and population-attributable risks calculations in the case of tobacco, diet, and alcohol. These calculations have no specific use in the behavioral and environmental assessments for any given health problem except to anticipate which risk factors will most likely arise in relation to the leading causes of death. The same factors tend to account for the diseases that precede deaths.

For specific conditions such as cardiovascular disease, the planner begins by consulting consensus documents or reviews to produce a list of risk factors such as those shown in Table 4-2. This table presents the known risk factors for cardiovascular disease, categorized as behavioral or not. Some are easy to classify this way, some more difficult. Smoking, heavy alcohol consumption, high-fat diet, and sedentary lifestyle are clearly behavioral, whereas gender, age, and family history of heart attacks are clearly nonbehavioral. Although not strictly behavioral, other factors—high serum cholesterol, obesity, high blood pressure, and

TABLE 4-2
Risk factors for cardiovascular disease

Nonbehavioral	Behavioral	Related to Behavior
Gender	Smoking	High blood pressure
Age	High-fat diet	Elevated serum cholesterol
Family history of disease	Heavy alcohol consumption Sedentary	Stress Obesity
Diabetes		

stress—are associated with behavior. High blood pressure, serum cholesterol level, and obesity are all linked to eating habits; stress is associated with behaviors like overworking, not taking time to relax, and inactivity.

Such lists of known risk factors help the planner determine which risk factors might be appropriate targets of change for a health promotion program. In the behavioral and environmental assessment, the planner assesses the prevalence and causal importance of these potential targets so he or she can set priorities among them for intervention.[12]

ASSESSING STRENGTH OF ASSOCIATION
BETWEEN RISK FACTORS AND HEALTH

After identifying risk factors or conditions, the behavioral and environmental assessment weighs their relative strength in relation to the health problem. Epidemiological studies employ measures of disease association to assess risk factors. There are two types of such measures: (1) ecological correlations between environmental factors and the health status of whole populations and (2) individual risk-factor data associated with individual symptoms or indicators of health status. Your familiarity with these measures will enable you to understand epidemiological findings on the relative importance of the risk factors and conditions.

Ecological Correlations. Ecological studies can measure the relative strength of association between risk conditions in environments and rates of disease, injury, or death in populations without having data on individual risk factors. Ecological correlations require large numbers of census tracts, schools, or other local data units from which to draw aggregate data for comparison. They have the advantage of being relatively available through census and other routinely collected community-level descriptors of neighborhoods, political districts, census tracts, blocks, postal code zones, school districts, and so forth.

One can produce ecological correlations by correlating aggregate statistics for a large number of population units with data on health status measures for the same group of units. An ecological correlation tells us the characteristics of the social or physical environment or aggregate behavioral norms of a place that are associated with the health measures of the same place. The ecological analysis connects these environmental conditions with population health outcomes so that it can suggest public health interventions on the social or physical environment.

The disadvantage of the ecological correlation is that it does not say whether individuals affected by a given feature of the place where they live are the same people who have the health problem associated with the feature. For example, the "fallacy of the ecological correlation" could lead us to conclude from such aggregate data that the people who died from lung cancer in one group of counties with high rates of beer consumption got their cancer because of their beer consumption. The correlation would tell us correctly that people drink much beer in areas where the disease rates are high, and this might be useful data for planning population-based programs. The correlation does not say, however, that those who died from lung cancer drank beer, nor that those who abstained from beer drinking did not develop lung cancer. Beer drinking might merely have been associated with the large numbers of blue-collar workers, who also had higher smoking rates and higher rates of exposures to carcinogens at their workplaces in neighboring counties. In short, ecological correlations can be useful and efficient ways of drawing attention to social and environmental conditions associated with health conditions, but they should be interpreted cautiously to avoid spurious correlational interpretations at the level of individual characteristics.

Relative Risk Measures. Measures of risk-factor association relate individuals' exposure to a factor (a possible risk factor) to the development of the health problem of interest (e.g., disease or death) in the same people. The most commonly used measure is **relative risk**, which compares the risk of developing the health problem for people exposed to a factor and for people not exposed. This is done by dividing the incidence of the health problem in the exposed population by that in the nonexposed:

$$\text{Relative risk} = \frac{\text{Incidence of the problem in those exposed to the risk factor}}{\text{Incidence of the problem in those not exposed to the risk factor}}$$

When the incidence of the disease is greater in the exposed group, the relative risk will be greater than one. A relative risk tells you how many *times* greater the risk is in persons exposed to the risk factor. For example, the relative risk of developing coronary heart disease (CHD) in smokers compared with nonsmokers is about 2. This means that smokers have twice the nonsmokers' risk of CHD. Stated another way, they are 100% more likely to develop the disease than are nonsmokers.

The size of the relative risk indicates the comparative importance of the factor to the development of disease. If factor A has a relative risk of 10 for a particular disease and factor B has a relative of risk of 2, then you conclude that factor A is the stronger risk factor. Table 4-3 shows the relative risks of developing CHD for several risk factors. Evidence that the risk factors have about the same impact on disease occurrence, and that the presence of more than one risk factor in the same people further increases the risk of disease, provides a rationale for interventions addressing multiple risk factors.

Relative risk also indicates the importance of a factor in different population groups. For example, as seen in Table 4-4, the relative risk of CHD death due to cigarette smoking for people who smoke 1–2 packs per day depends on the age of the smoker: the older the smoker, the less the relative risk. Understanding this principle provides a rationale for allocating resources or directing program focus to younger age groups.

Stronger epidemiological evidence that a factor increases risk is provided when there is a **dose-response relationship.** Such a relationship is shown in

TABLE 4-3

Relative risk for each of the major risk factors for coronary heart disease in middle-aged men are compiled from various sources

Risk Factor	Relative Risk
Smoking[a]	2.0
Hypertension	2.4
Elevated serum cholesterol	2–3 (depending on level of elevation)
Diabetes	2.5
Obesity	2.1
Physical inactivity[b]	1.9

[a]See ref. 13 in References and Notes at the end of this chapter.
[b]See ref. 14 in References and Notes at the end of this chapter.
SOURCE: Compiled by Denise Simons-Morton, M.D. Smoking and physical inactivity relative risk estimates are from the references cited. The other relative risk estimates are from "Report of the Inter-Society Commission for Heart Disease Resources," by W. B. Kannel, et al., 1984, *Circulation,* 70(1), 155A–205A.

Table 4-5 for smoking and CHD death: the higher the number of cigarettes smoked per day, the higher the relative risk.

You may see other terms in the epidemiological literature. **Risk ratio,** *odds ratio* (OR), and *standardized mortality* or *morbidity ratios* (SMRs) are other terms used to refer to relative risk. These estimates of the relative risk are also used as measures of association, and they can be interpreted in the same way. They offer a major advantage over other measures of association, such as correlation coefficients, used extensively in the social sciences: Epidiological relative risk measures can be translated directly to a meaningful statement about how much more risk is incurred in a population (or by a leap of inference, for an individual) with increased exposure to the risk factor. A relative risk or odds ratio of 1.2, for example, is a 20% increase in risk.

PREVALENCE OF RISK FACTORS IN THE POPULATION

After causal importance, the second indicator of the relative importance of risks is a measure of prevalence. In addition to the relative risk, which measures strength of the causal importance for exposed individuals, the prevalence of a risk factor in a population indicates the impact the factor has on a population.

As noted in the previous chapter, the prevalence rates of chronic diseases themselves or of deaths can be misleading in relation to setting health promotion priorities for the future. They may identify the people whose behavior and living

TABLE 4-4

Relative risks for coronary heart disease death vary systematically by age, shown here for men and women, 40–79 years old

Age Group (years)	Relative Risk	
	Men	Women
40–49	3.76	3.62
50–59	2.40	2.68
60–69	1.91	2.08
70–79	1.49	1.27

SOURCES: Adapted from "Cardiovascular and Risk Factor Evaluation of Healthy American Adults," by S. M. Grundy et al., 1987, *Circulation, 97,* 1340A–1362A. Data are from "Coronary Heart Disease, Stroke, and Aortic Aneurysms," by E. C. Hammond and L. Garfinkel, 1969, *Archives of Environmental Health, 19,* 167–182.

TABLE 4-5

Relative risks for coronary heart disease death vary systematically by number of cigarettes smoked per day, shown here for men and women, 40–79 years old

Number of Cigarettes Smoked Daily	Relative Risk	
	Men	Women
Nonsmoker	1.00	1.00
1–9	1.45	1.07
10–19	1.99	1.81
20–39	2.39	2.41
40+	2.89	3.02

SOURCES: Adapted from "Cardiovascular and Risk Factor Evaluation of Healthy American Adults," by S. M. Grundy et al., 1987, *Circulation, 97,* 1340A–1362A. Data are from "Coronary Heart Disease, Stroke, and Aortic Aneurysms," by E. C. Hammond and L. Garfinkel, 1969, *Archives of Environmental Health, 19,* 167–182.

conditions 20 years ago caused the disease from which they died last year when the disease-specific prevalence rate or relative risk ratio was calculated. The data become available much too late to plan for primary prevention and often too late for secondary prevention for such people. Prevalence data on chronic disease or even deaths this year are of limited utility for targeting health promotion priorities to prevent the future diseases and deaths that will be associated with today's lifestyles and conditions of living. Relative risks can tell us which risk factors among today's population might account for future deaths; however, viewing the prevalence of today's risk factors together with relative risk ratios allows one to make more reliable indicators of chronic disease prevention priorities. As we saw in Chapter 3, most communities unfortunately do not have good surveillance systems in place to monitor the risk factors effectively.

POPULATION ATTRIBUTABLE RISK

A partial solution to the mortality-based and relative-risk priority-setting problem just described is provided by the prevalence of those risk factors in the particular population for which one is planning a health promotion program. Where the prevalence of risk factors is known or can be estimated, the projected number of deaths in the population can be estimated. Conversely, the number of deaths in each mortality category can be used to work back to an estimate of the number of those deaths attributable to each of the major risk factors. Table 4-6 illustrates a set of such calculations by the Michigan Department of Public Health's Center for Health Promotion. Take, for example, the smoking example in the first row of the table. A statewide survey showed that 32.4% of Michigan adults were smokers. As shown in Table 4-5, smokers have a 10 times greater risk of getting lung cancer, and a relative risk of 2 of cardiovascular death, compared with nonsmokers. By combining the prevalence rate for smoking with the mortality from cancer, heart disease, lung diseases, stroke, and fires, each multiplied by a relative risk statistic, one generates a product known as Population Attributable Risk (PAR). This represents the mortality attributable to smoking. One can express this as the total number of deaths, the number of deaths before age 65 (responding to those policy makers who say, "Ya gotta go sometime"), or total years lost before age 65 (for those policy makers who worry most about "productive" years lost).

COST-BENEFIT ANALYSIS FROM PAR

Once the mortality data have been interpreted in relation to risk factors of known prevalence, the population attributable risk data can be related back to the social diagnosis in a form that has additional meaning to policy makers—namely, cost-benefit analysis. The health department, for example, knows the cost of starting and maintaining a smoking-cessation program. The cost-per-person-enrolled is easily calculated from the experience of the agency in maintaining such programs. On the benefit side, the medical costs associated with all diseases linked to a risk factor (e.g., smoking) and the lost income due to premature death before age 65 can be added up for a dollar estimate of the losses associated with each risk factor. These losses can be interpreted as the potential benefit of controlling the risk factor in question.

TABLE 4-6

Population Attributable Risk (PAR) estimates[a] for six risk factors in the State of Michigan

Risk Factor	Michigan Adult Prevalence, %	PAR Deaths Before Age 65	PAR Life Years Lost Before 65
Smoking	32.4	3,444	38,106
Drinking	7.5 (heavy) 20.5 (moderate)	1,751	51,493
Seat belts[b]	86.5+ (use less than always)	546	17,736
Hypertension	20.6 (uncontrolled)	1,422	15,549
Exercise	65.1 (no regular exercise)	1,024	10,647
Nutrition/weight	17.7 (120% of ideal) 15.0 (111–119% of ideal)	4,088	45,485
Total		12,275	179,016

[a]These estimates show a wider range of ratings on relative importance of the risk factors than do the risk ratios in previous tables. This is because the risk ratios are multiplied by the prevalence of the risk factors. For prediction of future rates of death or disease, they also can be adjusted for trends in risk factors and for the latency period between the onset of risk factors and the onset of disease.

[b]Before seat-belt law took effect

SOURCE: *Health Promotion Can Produce Economic Savings,* by Michigan Department of Health, 1987, Lansing: Center for Health Promotion, Michigan Department of Health, p. 7; used with permission of the publisher.

To obtain a cost-benefit ratio, the potential benefits in dollars can be divided by the costs of interventions needed to achieve those benefits. As in Table 4-7, the ratio is expressed as the return on each dollar invested in the risk-factor intervention.

The bottom line on smoking, then, appears to be that smoking is important not just because of high current death rates for past smokers, as shown by the relative risk estimates from exposures in the past. PAR tells us also that with recent smoking prevalence and related death rates projected into the future, smoking could cause thousands of needless deaths and illnesses in the 21st century.[15] Cost-benefit analyses also tell us that because of all the attendant costs following from smoking, the preventable deaths and illnesses would cost 10 to 21 times more than the cost of interventions to prevent them. (We shall refer back to Table 4-6 when we get to Chapter 6, on policy assessment.)

Using the data in the previous tables as reference points, and adding some new knowledge of trends in the prevalence of risk factors, consider how the relative importance ratings might change if we restrict the planner's health objective to reduce cardiovascular disease (CVD) mortality. We know that all of the behavioral

TABLE 4-7

Return on dollar invested in health risk-factor interventions over working lifetime (age 20–64) of those at risk, State of Michigan

Risk-Factor Intervention	$ Discount at 0%	$ Discount at 4%	$ Discount at 8%
Smoking	21.01	15.26	10.88
Hypertension	0.99	0.92	0.84
Nutrition/weight			
Moderate	0.34	0.26	0.18
Severe	0.62	0.48	0.36
Drinking			
Drinking/driving	1.40	1.30	1.19
Heavy drinking	3.17	2.68	2.24
Binge drinking	1.41	1.30	1.19
Sedentary (exercise)	0.42	0.35	0.27
Seat belt	105.07	105.07	105.07
Combined (nutrition/hypertension/exercise)	2.74	2.07	1.50

SOURCE: *Health Promotion Can Produce Economic Savings,* by Michigan Department of Health, 1987, Lansing: Center for Health Promotion, Michigan Department of Health, p. 9; used with permission of the publisher.

risk factors presented have relative risk values of about 2. But smoking rates have declined dramatically in some places (to less than 16 percent in California, for example). Sedentary living has not changed significantly for the population at large, and has increased for children, so that it is now the most prevalent risk factor. Suppose a report on the health risk factors for residents age 18 years and older revealed the following estimates of prevalence: smoking 22%, diabetes 4%, uncontrolled hypertension 12%, and physical inactivity 55%. How might this added information influence priority risk-factor targets to be featured in a CVD prevention campaign? By using PAR, we can take the prevalence of the risk factor in the population into account along with relative risk for those exposed to the risk factor.

AN EXAMPLE: COAL MINERS IN APPALACHIA

The following is an example of the use of health status indicators and measures of association in a project in which the behavioral and environmental assessment procedures of PRECEDE were applied systematically.[16] The Mineworkers Union wanted to sponsor a health promotion program for a population of coal miners in two northern Appalachian counties of West Virginia. Population data clearly suggested that the incidence of lung disease in coal miners in this area was greater than in other areas of the state, a situation they wanted to change. An important risk factor for lung disease in this area was, not surprisingly, frequent exposure to coal mining.

The behavioral, environmental, and biological determinants of the health problem were studied. Certain epidemiological questions were pursued: Do all miners get lung disease? Who does and does not get lung disease? Are all mineworkers male? Do those who get lung disease have a family history of the disease? Answers to questions about these nonbehavioral factors (age, gender, and family history) identified the high-risk groups.

In general, once one has identified the high-risk groups, one asks questions about behavioral and environmental factors: Is there a higher incidence of disease in workers exposed to different levels of coal dust because of working, for example, in different mine locations? Do some mines have better air circulation, associated with lower rates of lung disease? Is there a higher incidence of disease in smokers than in nonsmokers? These types of questions helped project leaders select the behavioral and the environmental factors warranting further attention.[17]

PROTECTIVE FACTORS FOR POSITIVE HEALTH

The relationships between risk factors and disease illustrated thus far (e.g., smoking causes lung and heart diseases) can be construed as negative, driven by a preoccupation with disease. This raises the concern of some who believe that too much attention to epidemiological aspects results in a disease or health-problem approach (negative) rather than a health and wellness (positive) approach. We wonder how valid or productive this concern really is.

Attention to and a working knowledge of the complex factors that compromise our health and quality of life do not dictate that the subsequent effort to resolve the problem has to be accompanied by a negative tone. The epidemiological data that pinpoint the causes of a health problem, or the points of intervention to achieve a health goal, need not form part of the message to the public about their role in improving their health.

Data drive policy, and policy generates resources. The use of "negative" information (AIDS is a disease caused mainly by unprotected sex and sharing of needles; smoking causes lung cancer and heart disease), has been instrumental in helping pry loose resources needed for comprehensive school, community, and work-site programs. The availability of these resources has enabled wonderfully talented teachers, nurses, physicians, physical educators, and others to develop upbeat wellness programs in schools, communities, and work sites.

Most epidemiological data derive from someone focusing on a problem. On the positive side, epidemiological risk-factor studies like the classic research of Belloc and Breslow can be turned around to emphasize the factors that can *improve* health. Analyzing data from large-scale surveys of adults in Alameda County, California, they found at least seven personal health practices that were highly correlated with physical health and cumulative in their effect. These included sleeping seven to eight hours daily, eating breakfast most days, rarely or never eating between meals, being at or near the recommended height-adjusted weight, being a nonsmoker, using alcohol moderately or not at all, and participating in regular physical activity.[18]

These findings lent support to the lifestyle construct discussed in Chapter 1, showing that a combination of factors, rather than any one behavior alone, was associated with good health. The study also showed a correlation between positive health practices and physical health, rather than the usual relationship between negative risk behavior and mortality and disease. Further analyses also showed that social support and association memberships accounted for a large part of the lifestyle and positive health variations.[19]

The California investigators followed up the people originally interviewed in 1965, examining mortality records 5.5 and 9.5 years later. They found, for both men and women in all age groups, that those who had practiced more of the health behaviors were less likely to have died than were those who practiced fewer of them. Indeed, at 9.5 years, men who were engaging in all seven practices in 1965 had experienced 72% lower mortality than those who practiced zero to three of the behaviors; for women, the figure was 57%. Most of these relationships held when adjusted for 1965 income level and health status.[20]

These data on positive health practices or lifestyle lend credibility to estimates that at least 50% of all mortality is attributable to health behavior. They also lend scientific justification to an emphasis on lifestyle determinants of health, especially if lifestyle is interpreted to encompass conditions of living. For those whose mission is not primarily mortality control and for those who seek a more comprehensive or holistic approach to health, the evidence of improved physical health status associated with combined health actions and social relationships provides a rationale for the emphasis on behavior and lifestyle.

Health workers of all disciplines and professional roles share the long-term goal of improving the health and quality of life of the people they serve. To succeed, these workers must have the active and effective participation of such people. Behavior is a pivotal variable in the relationship between professional or program interventions on the one hand and health or quality-of-life outcomes on the other. Virtually all members of a target population, other than terminally comatose patients, can play an active role in improving their health. Even bedridden postsurgical patients can make a major difference in postoperative recovery outcomes—for example, by following specific instructions for breathing, coughing, and moving while in bed.[21] At the other end of this continuum, some people participate in or donate to political action to bring about legislation for environmental reforms or enforcement of laws regulating tobacco advertising. Human behavior inescapably influences most of medicine and all of health promotion.

The extent of behavioral influence on years of potential life lost can only be inferred from the association of behavior with the leading causes of death (Table 4-1). Distinct from environmental, genetic or biological, and technological (medical) influences, it has been roughly estimated at 50 percent or more.[22] At least half of the mortality in the United States and Canada, by this estimate, is attributable to behavioral or lifestyle causes. This estimate is derived by working backwards from the distribution of annual deaths in a population to the risk factors associated with each of those causes, a process parallel to PRECEDE. What this estimate does not address are the causes of behavior and the interaction of behavior and environment in their influence on health.

The data presented in Chapter 3 support the estimate that at least 50% of premature mortality is attributable to health behavior. Although some question the precision of this estimate, they cannot escape the dominant count of behavioral risk factors associated with the twelve leading causes of death, summarized here in Table 4-8. Most of the risk factors shown for these twelve causes of death, which account for the vast majority of all deaths and medical care costs in Western countries, are directly controllable through the behaviors of individuals,

TABLE 4-8

Prominent controllable risk factors for leading causes of death in North America, Europe, and Australia

Cause of Death	Risk Factors
Heart disease and stroke	Smoking, high blood pressure, elevated serum cholesterol, diabetes, obesity, lack of exercise
Cancer	Smoking, alcohol misuse, diet, solar radiation, ionizing radiation, pollution
Unintentional injuries	Alcohol misuse, smoking (fires), product design, home hazards, handgun availability
Motor vehicle injuries	Alcohol misuse, lack of safety restraints, excessive speed, automobile design, roadway design
Pneumonia and influenza	Smoking, infectious agents
Diabetes mellitus	Obesity (for adult-onset diabetes)
Cirrhosis of the liver	Alcohol ingestion
Suicide	Handgun availability, alcohol or drug misuse, stress
Homicide	Handgun availability, alcohol or drug misuse, stress
AIDS	Sexual practices, drug misuse, exposure to blood products

NOTE: The causes of death listed above account for the vast majority of all mortality and morbidity in the more developed societies.

families, organizations, and communities, as well as through social policies and environments supporting such behaviors.

MEASUREMENT OF BEHAVIORS IN POPULATIONS

Recognition of the role of behavior in determining health has inevitably produced a rapid growth of survey activity to assess the distribution patterns of health behavior in populations. For example, to provide a means of monitoring progress on the U.S. Objectives for the Nation, the National Center for Health Statistics initiated a major health promotion supplement to the National Health Interview Survey in 1979. Periodic national surveys together with other data sources now enable planners to construct detailed trend analyses on key health-related practices of the U.S. public and many of its high-risk subpopulations. Among other things, the surveys assess all the principal behavioral risk factors associated with the leading causes of death, disease, and disability in the United States.[23] A similar survey was developed by the Canadian Health and Welfare Department, using PRECEDE as part of the conceptual framework.[24] Comparisons of the U.S. and Canadian adult populations were made possible by the standardization of some risk factor definitions and measures between the two countries.[25] These data, together with periodic follow-up surveys, now provide a series of baselines and norms for comparison of community survey results. Most communities, however, cannot afford to administer the full questionnaire. They can, nevertheless, use the national and regional data as a source of estimates of population differences and trends when they plan local health promotion programs.

Shorter or more specialized behavioral surveys are conducted at state, provincial, and local levels.[26] The U.S. Centers for Disease Control has developed a national data collection system designed to enable states to assess health risk behaviors and selected nonbehavioral factors (e.g., health conditions, medical/dental insurance coverage) known to contribute to or increase the risk of chronic disease, acute illness, injury, disability, and premature death. Although the Behavioral Risk Factor Survey System (BRFSS) was originally created to gather state-level data, many states now stratify their sampling to estimate prevalence for regions within their respective states.[27] School-based surveys to obtain similar data on children and youth have been conducted nationally in Canada and the U.S.[28]

NONBEHAVIORAL CAUSES OF HEALTH PROBLEMS

Behavioral assessment is directed toward specific modifiable behaviors, but health problems have nonbehavioral causes that must also receive careful consideration. These include the personal factors that are least controllable by individual or collective action but that do contribute to health problems. Among the least modifiable or controllable personal factors are genetic predisposition, age, gender, congenital disease, physical and mental impairment, and places of work and residence that encompass various social and environmental factors beyond the control of the individual.

Some nonbehavioral risk factors lend themselves to community intervention and, to a lesser degree, individual action to avoid or limit exposure to environmental risks such as solar radiation, lead-based paint, and ambient smoke. Some can be addressed in the long term through systematic reproductive health and early childhood development programs to prevent the problems from developing over time. We shall discuss some of these later in this chapter and in the next chapter, where we examine the causes of behavioral and environmental determinants of health. Their significance here is that they contribute to the goals and problems of health and quality of life.

The health practitioner who takes into account the contribution of nonbehavioral factors to health problems will be better able to

- Maintain perspective on the multiple determinants of the health problem or goal
- Isolate and rank behavioral and environmental determinants to become the targets of the program
- Identify factors for which strategies other than health education (e.g., political or regulatory interventions directed at social or physical environment) may be developed and concurrently used as part of the total health promotion strategy

Ignoring the influence of nonbehavioral factors, placing all the responsibility for health protection on the individuals whose health is threatened, produces programs or policies vulnerable to the charge of "blaming the victim." Recognizing the nonbehavioral causes of health problems acknowledges other threats to health besides the behavior of the victim. It may also encourage a long-range view of population health promotion insofar as it directs attention now to the needs for intervention on the very young to avoid repeating the damage already done to the older individuals in the population.

Of the modifiable, nonbehavioral, direct causes of health problems, most are either environmental (air, water, food, roads, fluoridation) or technological (adequacy of medical care, health facilities). These factors can be influenced by the behavior of the public or the victim but especially by collective action. Communities, neighborhoods, or special-interest (e.g., self-help) groups can organize, vote, boycott, lobby, or otherwise support or prevent certain environmental and technological changes. In short, behavior can influence health in the three ways shown in Figure 4-1, where one is direct and two are indirect.

FIVE STEPS IN BEHAVIORAL ASSESSMENT

Here is an illustration of the steps in behavioral assessment. A local health department has just completed a quality-of-life and an epidemiological assessment. On the basis of the findings, the director wants to allocate some of her resources to fight cardiovascular disease. She gives a planning team, which includes community representatives, the task of developing a demonstration project that will reduce the incidence of cardiovascular disease in the community. Epidemiological diagnosis has suggested that the intervention should include a component aimed at asymptomatic youth and young adults. The behavioral assessment now begins.

STEP 1: DELINEATING THE BEHAVIORAL AND NONBEHAVIORAL CAUSES OF THE HEALTH PROBLEM

At some level of ecological theory, separating the behavioral and nonbehavioral causes is admittedly an artificial dichotomy. Because behavior is so intertwined with biological, genetic, and environmental causes, the partitioning of behavior for planning purposes is partly an exercise in considering the degree to which important actions and circumstances affecting the health problem or need can be influenced or controlled by people. One can begin this exercise by reviewing the known risk factors for the disease in question, as described in Tables 4-1 and 4-2. Smoking, heavy alcohol consumption, and a high-fat diet and sedentary lifestyle are clearly behavioral, whereas gender, age, and family history of heart attacks are more clearly (at least from now into the future) nonbehavioral. High serum cholesterol, obesity, high blood pressure, and stress are physiological, not strictly behavioral factors, yet they are obviously closely tied to behaviors. High blood pressure, serum cholesterol, and obesity are linked to eating habits; stress is associated with behaviors like working in a chaotic environment, having interpersonal conflicts, and not getting enough physical activity.

STEP 2: DEVELOPING A CLASSIFICATION OF BEHAVIORS

The second step in behavioral assessment is to divide the list of behavioral factors into (1) preventive behaviors (primary, secondary, and tertiary) and (2) treatment procedures:

   a. Identify the behaviors associated with promoting health, preventing the health problem, or maintaining self-care and controlling the sequelae of the health problem. A useful typology is presented in Table 4-9, which

TABLE 4-9

This typology of health-related behaviors is classified according to how the social and behavioral sciences have constructed theory and research in relation to health behavior and lifestyles associated with health

Behaviors	Definitions
Wellness behavior	Activity undertaken by an individual, who believes himself to be healthy, for the purpose of attaining an even greater level of health.
Preventive health behavior	Activity undertaken by an individual, who believes herself to be healthy, for the purpose of preventing illness or detecting it in an asymptomatic state.
At-risk behavior	Activity undertaken by an individual, who believes himself to be healthy but at greater risk of developing a specific health condition, for the purpose of preventing that condition or detecting it in an asymptomatic state.
Illness behavior	Activity undertaken by an individual, who perceives herself to be ill, to define the state of her health and discover a suitable remedy.
Self-care behavior	Activity undertaken by an individual, who considers himself to be ill, for the purpose of getting well. It includes minimal reliance on appropriate therapists, involves few dependent behaviors, and leads to little neglect of one's usual duties.
Mutual-aid behavior	Activity in which people support each other in relation to their common health problems or aspirations.
Sick-role behavior	Activity undertaken by an individual, who considers himself to be ill, for the purpose of getting well. It includes receiving treatment from appropriate therapists, generally involves a whole range of dependent behaviors, and leads to some degree of neglect of one's usual duties.
Family-planning behavior	Activity undertaken by an individual or couple to influence the occurrence or normal continuation of pregnancy.
Parenting health behavior	Wellness, prevention, at-risk, illness, self-care, or sick-role actions performed by an individual for the purposes of ensuring, maintaining, or improving the health of a conceptus or child for whom the individual has responsibility.
Health-related social action	Activity undertaken by an individual singularly or in concert with others (i.e., collectively) through organizational, legal, or economic means, to influence the provision of medical services, the effects of the environment, the effects of various products, or the effects of social regulations that influence the health of populations.

SOURCE: Adapted from L. J. Kolbe, in *Health Education and Youth: A Review of Research and Development,* in G. Campbell, ed. (Philadelphia: Falmer Press, 1984), as printed with permission in L. W. Green, *Annual Review of Public Health* 5 (1984): 215–36.

shows a broad classification of various types of health behaviors.[29] Each type of behavior associated with the health problem, need, or goal would then need to be analyzed further by specifying the particular actions undertaken for its accomplishment.

b. Identify and list sequentially the actions or treatment procedures for the health goal or problem. What are the steps that people have to go through to reach their goal or to "comply" with the recommended method of prevention or treatment? Each step in a procedure can be identified as a particular action or behavior.

The major aim of Step 2b is to generate an inventory of highly specific actions that can be used as the basis for specifying the behavioral objectives of the program. Table 4-10 shows such a list. Notice that many actions appear as both preventive and treatment behaviors. This is not at all unusual, and the information is valuable. If a single behavioral problem, such as smoking, appears in both parts of the inventory, a change in the behavior (stopping smoking) increases the probability of health improvement through both primary and secondary pre-

---

TABLE 4-10

This example of an inventory of behaviors lists specific actions associated with reduction of mortality from cardiovascular disease

Preventive behaviors
1. Maintain or attain desirable weight.
2. Stop smoking (or don't start).
3. Stop heavy drinking (or don't start).
4. Continue or begin regular exercise.
5. Reduce consumption of foods high in saturated fats.
6. Avoid excessive, constant stress and/or do relaxation exercises.
7. Participate in high-blood-pressure and cholesterol-screening programs.

Treatment behaviors
1. Make informed decisions regarding medication and surgery.
2. Keep scheduled appointments with health care providers.
3. Take medications as prescribed.
4. Maintain or reduce weight as prescribed.
5. Stop smoking.
6. Cut down alcohol consumption as prescribed.
7. Continue or begin regular exercise as prescribed.
8. Reduce consumption of foods high in saturated fat or sodium, as prescribed.

vention. Primary prevention consists of actions taken in the absence of signs or symptoms; secondary prevention is directed toward early detection and treatment.

Though Table 4-10 consists of several distinct behaviors, it is still crude and relatively nonspecific with respect to the actual steps one would have to take for each. Some of the behaviors comprise several specific behaviors and so can themselves be further broken down into lists of behaviors. For example, "achieving or maintaining desirable weight" results from such behaviors as buying low-calorie foods, cooking with less fat, serving smaller portions, eating fewer portions, and minimizing sugary desserts.

For Steps 2b, 3, and 4, the list in Table 4-10 is specific enough, but to translate the behaviors into behavioral objectives, one usually needs to break them down into the actual steps or stages that people will go through to achieve each behavioral goal. One approach to analyzing behavior in more specific terms is to develop a systems analysis flowchart of causation or transition from the beginning to the end of a behavioral process or event. For example, taking a prescribed medication (see Table 4-10) is preceded by other discrete behaviors such as seeking medical care, obtaining a prescription, and seeing that the medication is modified as necessary, as in the control of high blood pressure. This behavioral cycle could be sabotaged at many points along the way, for example, if the patient fails to keep an appointment at which prescriptions might be renewed or changed (see Chapter 11). The "broken appointment cycle" itself can be analyzed into a series of causes and effects (Figure 4-2). This level of specificity makes it possible to isolate concrete behavioral events from nonbehavioral factors so that educational and administrative interventions can be highly targeted. Training of staff, adjustment of appointment schedules, and child-care or transportation provisions all could become relevant interventions identified by the behavioral assessment reflected in the broken-appointment cycle.

This cycle illustrates a causal and sequential chain of behavior. The broken appointment means the patient will miss the medical assessment and advice needed to stay on a preventive or therapeutic course. The planner must ask, "Why are appointments made but not kept?" The motivation was there, but the behavior was somehow thwarted. At this phase of PRECEDE, rather than leaping to the motivational question we shall focus on the behavior of other actors, including physicians, receptionists, and clinic administrators. The environmental circumstances surrounding the broken-appointment problem will also be assessed.

Chapter 11 presents a related example (Figure 11-2). The flowchart there shows several paths the individual can follow from recognition of symptoms to seeking medical diagnosis to obtaining a prescription to using, misusing, or not using the prescribed treatment. Each step involves one or more specific behaviors for which behavioral objectives and interventions can be designed, some for the public at large, some for patients, and some for the drug manufacturers, physicians, nurses, pharmacists, and other professionals and sectors relating to the issue.

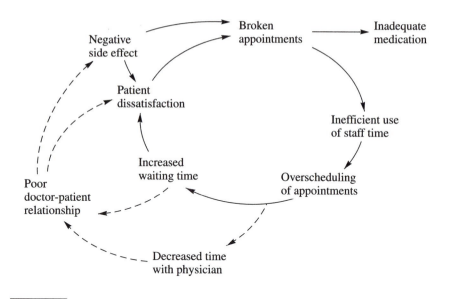

FIGURE 4-2

A systems view of the behavior of keeping appointments can be delineated as a broken-appointment cycle with a sequence of actions and reactions, decisions and choices, branching toward or away from further broken appointments.

STEP 3: RATING BEHAVIORS IN TERMS OF IMPORTANCE

On the understanding that no program has sufficient resources to do everything that might be done, the extensive list of behaviors identified in Step 2 now needs to be reduced to a manageable length. This is done first by establishing which behaviors are the most important and eliminating (or at least deferring) the least important. The following broad criteria provide guidelines for this task. The importance of a behavior is indicated when data are available showing that (1) it occurs frequently and (2) it is clearly and potently linked to the health problem. One can consider a behavior important if a strong theoretical case can be made for its being causally related to a health problem. In the absence of firsthand data, the strength of such a relationship may be inferred from a review of the literature. Based on these tests, a rationale is developed for selecting the behavior as a target of intervention.[30]

Using data such as the relative risk ratios in Table 4-3 and prevalence data from surveys, one can estimate the relative importance and prevalence of each behavior. In Table 4-11, eight key behaviors are ranked in terms of their importance as behavioral targets for a primary prevention program to reduce the inci-

TABLE 4-11

Rating the relative importance of behaviors associated with cardiovascular disease prevention can be based on prevalence (number of people affected) and on strength of association with the health outcome

Important	Basis for rating behavior
Smoking	Very strong risk ratio, medium prevalence
Eating high-fat foods	Strong risk ratio, very high prevalence
Sedentary living	Low risk ratio, very high prevalence
High stress	
Less important	All unrelated to the desired outcome: primary prevention
Not monitoring blood pressure	
Not adhering to medical prescription	
Not keeping medical appointments	
Making uninformed decisions about treatment	

dence of cardiovascular disease. The basis for these ratings is information on their incidence in the target population and the strength of their association with the disease.

STEP 4: RATING BEHAVIORS' CHANGEABILITY

The fourth step in a behavioral assessment is rating behaviors' relative changeability. How susceptible to change are the behaviors that have been selected? Even if a behavior is extremely important to a health problem, it will not be a suitable target unless developers can reasonably expect it to change through health promotion. For example, many claim that excessive stress is associated with cardiovascular disease. A health promotion program directed at stress reduction would need to alter the major sources of stress, including the home and the workplace. How feasible is that for a health promotion program? The answer to such questions about environmental changes needed to support behavioral risk-factor changes will be deferred until the environmental assessment later in this chapter.

Resource Considerations. Judgments about changeability must also include careful consideration of the time factor—in how much time must the program show change? Deeply rooted and widespread behaviors are likely to take a while to change, making the time factor quite important. Like other resource questions, how much time is needed can be answered more definitively at a later stage (see Chapter 6). At this stage, the judgments on changeability can be based primarily on evidence that the behavior has responded to interventions in previous studies and programs. Here, the professional and scientific literature is the best guide. The most recent critical or quantitative review of previous research can be found in journals such as *Health Education and Behavior, American Journal of Public Health, Canadian Journal of Public Health, American Journal of Preventive Medicine, Annual Review of Public Health, American Journal of Health Promotion, Health Education Research, International Quarterly of Community Health Education, Journal of School Health, Family and Community Health, Health Promotion International, Patient Education and Counselling, Journal of Community Health, Nursing Research,* and others cited in the bibliography of this book.[31]

Rules of Thumb. A few rules of thumb can help one determine the potential for behavioral change. High changeability is probable when behaviors

- Are still in the developmental stages
- Have only recently been established
- Are not deeply rooted in cultural patterns or lifestyles
- Have been found to change in previous attempts

Most resistant to change, or subject to the highest relapse rates, are those behaviors that have an addictive component (tobacco, alcohol, drug misuse), those with deep-seated compulsive elements (compulsive eating, compulsive work), and those with strong family patterns or routines surrounding them (eating patterns, work and leisure).

Attribute Method. Behaviors not ruled out by applying the simple criteria in the previous paragraph can be further analyzed for changeability using another approach. The *attribute method* examines the characteristics of the behavior that make it more or less easy to adopt, using criteria from the literature on the adoption of innovations.[32] The method is illustrated for the behaviors associated with cardiovascular disease in Table 4-12. Note that a total changeability score can be obtained by adding horizontally across the columns, scoring +1 for a plus sign and −1 for a minus sign. A more refined score can be obtained if the relative importance of the criteria can be estimated, allowing weighting factors to be applied. This procedure recognizes that not all criteria are equally important in determining the changeability of a behavior.[33]

By testing behaviors for changeability, we come a step closer to an informal decision on which behaviors we should slate or recommend for intervention. Table 4-13 illustrates changeability ratings for cardiovascular disease, based on data in the foregoing tables. The table implies that reducing high-fat food intake and smoking prevention will reduce cardiovascular disease more than will eating

TABLE 4-12

Relative changeability based on perceived attributes of selected preventive health behaviors, as illustrated here for heart-health behaviors

Health Behavior	Relevance	Social Approval	Advantages	Complexity	Compatibility with Values, Experiences, and Needs	Divisibility or Trialability	Observability
1. Quitting smoking	+	+	+	−	−	+	+
2. Controlling weight	+	+	+	−	+	+	+
3. Controlling blood pressure	+	+	−	−	−	+	−
Taking medication	+	+	−	−	−	+	−
Maintaining low-sodium diet	+	+	−	−	−	+	−
4. Maintaining low-cholesterol diet	+	+	+	−	+	+	+
5. Exercising	+	+	+	−	+	+	+
6. Having preventive medical examinations	+	+	+	−	+	−	+

+ = positive, − = negative. Changes since the first edition in 1980 reflect changes in social norms and technologies. The only change in a negative direction has been in the complexity dimension of having preventive medical examinations. This is a manifestation of decreased support for indigent care and inaccessibility of health services to the rural and disadvantaged segments of the population in the United States.

SOURCE: Adapted from L. W. Green, "Diffusion and Adoption of Innovations Related to Cardiovascular Risk Behavior in the Public," by L. W. Green, 1975, in A. Enelow and J. B. Henderson (Eds.), *Applying Behavioral Sciences to Cardiovascular Risk,* New York: American Heart Association.

and exercising the right amount. Although one can argue against such a conclusion, findings in the literature on primary prevention of cardiovascular disease are, in fact, insufficiently consistent to place the latter behaviors in the high changeability category with complete confidence.

STEP 5: CHOOSING BEHAVIORAL TARGETS

With the behaviors ranked on importance and changeability, the planner is ready to select the focus of the program or interventions. To facilitate this selection, we

TABLE 4-13

Rating the changeability of behaviors associated with cardiovascular disease follows from consideration of research and evaluation literature and past experience

Changeability	Basis for Rating Behavior
More changeable	Recent trends and new research
Smoking	
Eating foods with high fatty-acid content	
Less changeable	These practices are deeply rooted in culture, social relationships, and lifestyle. Previous attempts to change them have had limited success for populations.
Overeating	
Exercise	

recommend that the ratings for importance and changeability be arranged in a simple fourfold table, as shown in Figure 4-3.

Depending on the program objectives, the behavioral objectives will most likely originate in Quadrants 1 and 2. Evaluation is crucial when one is uncertain about whether change will occur. Behaviors in Quadrant 3 will be unlikely candidates. Two exceptions to this might arise. One involves a political need to address a lower priority behavior. For instance, a community group might insist on their

	More important	**Less important**
More changeable	High priority for program focus (Quadrant 1)	Low priority except to demonstrate change for political purposes (Quadrant 3)
Less changeable	Priority for innovative program; evaluation crucial (Quadrant 2)	No program (Quadrant 4)

FIGURE 4-3

The rankings of behaviors on the two dimensions of importance and changeability leads to at least four categories of possible action.

preference for a behavior that scientific review has deemed less important. The other exception might arise when an administrator or steering committee needs to see "evidence" of some change before investing in more costly behavioral interventions. When such a need exists, the behaviors should be given priority on a temporary basis only, and only if the planner can proceed with assurance that no harm will be done. If no behaviors appear in Quadrant 1, but the health problem is urgent, then extensive educational and behavioral research and experimental program evaluation are justified. These procedures merely make explicit and systematic what most good practitioners and planners, agencies and foundations, do intuitively and implicitly in determining their own research or program priorities.

Figure 4-4 shows how the behaviors generated in the sample problem would be placed in the matrix. Only smoking and high-fat foods appear in Quadrant 1. Quadrant 2 shows two behaviors important in preventing cardiovascular disease; however, neither has produced consistent, conclusive evidence of significant, lasting change in response to large-scale program interventions. Imagine the following likely scenario for the planning meeting to select behaviors as the focus of the program:

- A team member cautions against spreading limited resources too thinly by choosing several behaviors.
- The coalition agrees that *one* behavior must be chosen.
- During the discussion that follows, smoking, fat consumption, and physical activity surface as possible targets.

	More important	Less important
More changeable	Smoking Eating foods with high fatty-acid content	Medical treatment, related behaviors
Less changeable	Overeating Lack of exercise	Not relaxing

FIGURE 4-4

This final matrix of health behaviors in the sample problem, cardiovascular disease prevention, suggests program priorities for smoking and high-fat intake, as well as evaluation priorities on innovative approaches to reducing overeating and increasing physical activity.

- Members cite research evidence indicating that lack of physical activity, smoking, and high cholesterol are equally important as cardiovascular risks.
- Someone points out that, in the general population, twice as many people are physically inactive as smoke or have high cholesterol, and that cholesterol consumption is continuing to decline in the general population.
- The group discusses the notorious difficulty of inducing sedentary adults to undertake appropriate physical activity.
- An informed and reasoned discussion of the available evidence ensues. The group debates the relative merits of investing in program efforts in relation to each behavior. Then, one of the community representatives on the panel asks, "What about the community residents themselves? What do they see as the most important or interesting behavior?"
- This leads to a discussion of the feasibility of a community survey to determine the actual prevalence of the key behaviors and their perceived importance to the community.

CAVEATS

Here, we need to offer some caveats. Surveys can be expensive in money and time. Putting off action to raise funds for, and to plan, execute, analyze, and interpret a survey, may only delay other effective work. Besides the delayed action, the cost of the survey will have taken resources that might otherwise have gone to program activity. Another caution is that surveys will not yield definitive answers in a matter of scientific choice in program priorities for the whole population; rather, they will yield different priorities for different subpopulations according to interests and readiness. If a marketing type of survey is to be used in setting priorities, decisions should be made in advance as to how the data will be used and as to the limits on departing from the scientific analysis of importance and changeability. We have argued for extensive use of public perceptions and subjective data in the social assessment and quality-of-life considerations in Phase 1 of the Precede model. As one progresses through subsequent phases of planning, however, more technical, scientific, professional, and resource-based considerations must come into play in deciding on actions.

EVALUATION CONSIDERATIONS

Beginning with the placement of some priority on social and health outcomes in the previous phases, and on behavioral outcomes in this phase, the planning of **evaluation** has begun. By setting objectives on the highest-priority social and health objectives in previous phases and on behavioral outcomes in the next, planners can establish criteria of success for the eventual program evaluation. The placement of some priority on those behavioral outcomes that are deemed important but less changeable puts more weight on the need for systematic evaluation of new program ideas in those areas. The consideration of a population survey at this point also raises possibilities for making the most of such a survey for evaluation purposes. A diagnostic-baseline survey can serve both the diagnostic purposes of program planning and the baseline purposes of evaluation. A survey conducted at any stage of the planning process should be designed with evaluation in mind. It probably should not be conducted if its only purpose is political justification of decisions that could be made much less expensively and more expeditiously with existing data. If action has been delayed for the sake of a survey, evaluation will be all the more important.

STATING BEHAVIORAL OBJECTIVES

Once one has identified a target health behavior, one can take the final step in this stage of planning: stating behavioral objectives. In this, specificity is vital. The efficiency and effectiveness of health promotion efforts are jeopardized when behavioral objectives are too vague or generic. Given the scarcity of health promotion resources, vagueness is a luxury one cannot afford. Instances of "intangible" and unmeasurable target behaviors generally reflect inadequacy in how the behavioral components of the health problem have been delineated. Phrases such as "improve health habits" and "increase the use of health services" cannot stand as useful behavioral objectives. Program efforts aimed at such diffuse targets will likely be scattered, with too little effort directed at any one behavior to make a difference for the individuals reached and with too few individuals reached to make a difference on the population level.

For this reason, when behavioral change is possible and appropriate, one must take the utmost care in stating the objectives with specificity. Each behavioral objective should answer the following questions:

- *Who?* The people expected to change
- *What?* The action or change in behavior or health practice to be achieved
- *How much?* The extent of the condition to be achieved
- *When?* The time in which the change is expected to occur

In our sample problem of cardiovascular disease, what might be the behavioral objectives? Recall the target behavior of smoking. In addition, suppose the planning team has determined that the program should be implemented initially in District A because it demographically represents the state or province and resembles several other districts. The "who" (for at least this pilot program) will consist of all residents age 20–35 in District A. The "what" will be a reduction in the prevalence of cigarette smoking. "How much" will be established as 20%.[34] "When" is defined as the proposed time of follow-up evaluation, such as two years for the pilot program discussed here. Concisely stated, then, the behavioral objective will read, "District residents age 20–35 will show a 20% reduction in the prevalence of cigarette smoking within two years of program implementation."

WHY EMPHASIZE ENVIRONMENT?

Besides behavioral and biological factors that determine health, a complex array of environmental influences must also be assessed with procedures similar to those for behavioral assessment. The manageability of environmental assessment depends on having a good epidemiological diagnosis from Phase 2 of PRECEDE. One can identify and manage a finite number of important environmental risk factors for a given health problem, but if the question is "What environmental influences on health exist?" then the analysis becomes at least a lifetime undertaking.

If the scope of environmental determinants on health becomes so encompassing and complex as to be impractical for health promotion planning, we recommend concentrating attention on those aspects of the environment that are

1. More social than physical (e.g., organizational and economic)
2. Interactive with behavior in their impact on health
3. Changeable by social action and health policy

Such environmental determinants deserve first consideration in health promotion planning. The more strictly physical environmental factors can be addressed more directly through engineering and ergonomic solutions. Those that interact with behavior, especially the social environmental factors, are ones over which people might exert individual or collective control, which is a defining goal of health promotion.

Figure 4-5 shows three levels at which the environment interacts with or influences other determinants of health and disease or injury. It also identifies some primary determinants within the social environment, including social network (formal and informal memberships and ties, social support, social norms), culture, and family history. The physical environment makes its greatest impact on living conditions and directly on some risk factors for disease brought about by exposures through air, water, soil, housing, transportation vehicles and barriers, climate, noise, and radiation. The health care environment could be classified as part of the social environment, but it is separate in Figure 4-5 to show its specific points of potential contribution to the causal chain of determinants of health.[35]

The relation of the social environment to health has emerged as an important area for research and a priority for health promotion. The World Health Organization has proposed two important objectives: (1) to try to control not only phys-

Determinants of health and disease

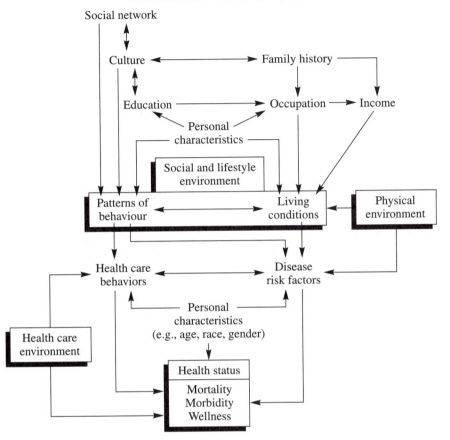

FIGURE 4-5

The interactions of lifestyle and environment are shown here with environmental influences made up of three components: social environment, physical environment, and health care environment.

SOURCE: Adapted from "Educational and Life-Style Determinants of Health and Disease," by L. W. Green, D. G. Simons-Morton, and L. Potvin, 1997, in R. Detels, W. W. Holland, J. McEwen, and G. S. Omenn (Eds.), *Oxford Textbook of Public Health* (3rd ed.), New York: Oxford University Press, p. 134; used with permission of the publisher and authors.

ical and environmental risks but also risks arising from the social environment and (2) to encourage and support those factors in the environment that "cushion" individuals and help them cope with the social structure.[36]

One other distinction will help narrow the health promotion focus of this book. Much of health promotion, unlike health education, concerns the passage of laws and organizational changes to regulate or constrain behavior that threatens the health of others. We consider the initial stimulation of public interest and support for such legislation or regulation to be a function of health education, especially through media advocacy and community organization. The political and organizational efforts to gain passage of such legislation falls to aspects of health promotion that lie beyond health education. The enforcement of such laws may be considered the role of health *protection*. In short, the promotion of health policy is health promotion (including health education); the enforcement of those health policies that require the restraint of individual behavior is health protection.

In general, the priority of most health education professionals is to plan a solid health education program for a classroom or a group of students, workers, residents, or patients within a supportive institutional or community context. For them, the environmental diagnosis is an additional burden on PRECEDE that may be the straw that breaks the planner's back. We recommend detailed consideration of this assessment phase, therefore, only for those who carry the responsibility for implementing, organizing, and evaluating broad-scale population health promotion programs. This puts the environmental assessment more squarely into the framework of PROCEED. If the environmental assessment is to be used later, it must precede the development and implementation of policy, regulation, and organization; therefore, we keep it in PRECEDE as an optional step, recommended for those with broad health promotion responsibilities.

FIVE STEPS IN ENVIRONMENTAL ASSESSMENT

STEP 1: IDENTIFYING WHICH ENVIRONMENTAL CAUSES OF THE HEALTH PROBLEM ARE CHANGEABLE

This first step follows Step 1 in behavioral assessment, in which nonbehavioral factors were identified but set aside for behavioral factors. We now revisit that list to sort out the genetic and historical factors in which little if any change can be expected, even with sweeping policy reforms. The list is now narrowed to a subset of organizational, economic, and environmental factors known to contribute to the health or quality-of-life problem or goal either indirectly (through behavior) or directly.

STEP 2: RATING ENVIRONMENTAL FACTORS ON RELATIVE IMPORTANCE

As with the behavioral assessment, the inventory of environmental factors influencing the health goal or problem will likely be too long to be manageable within the scope of a health promotion program or policy change. Some of the factors will matter more than others because of one or both of the following criteria: (1) strength of the relationship of the environmental factor to the health or quality-of-life goal or problem; (2) incidence, prevalence, or number of people affected by the environmental factor.

STEP 3: RATING ENVIRONMENTAL FACTORS ON CHANGEABILITY

This differs from Step 1 only in narrowing the list down still more, based on relative changeability. In the first step, one eliminates those nonbehavioral factors that are not subject to change at all because they do not fall in the environmental category. Now you narrow the list further by eliminating those environmental factors that have the least chance of yielding to intervention through policy, regulation, or organizational change. One can make this step more efficient by applying it only to those environmental factors that survived the importance rating in Step 2. There is little to be gained from a critical analysis of the changeability of an environmental factor that has been deemed relatively unimportant in its causal link to the health or quality-of-life goal or problem.

Alternatively, the changeability criterion could be applied first and time saved on Step 2 by applying it only to those environmental factors that survive Step 3. This would amount to a more technocratic approach insofar as importance has taken into consideration the subjective importance the population attaches to the environmental factors. Figure 4-6 suggests that consultation by "risk assessors" (you, the planner) with "risk managers" (practitioners, policy makers, and others responsible for the environmental or ecological risks) and with "stakeholders" (the community) should occur at two points in the planning process. At the early point of formulating the problem or issue (upper left in Figure 4-6) and at the point of analyzing the results (lower center), discussion should assess views of changeability as a matter of assessing political will and costs associated with change. Views of importance as a matter of subjective quality-of-life concerns and lifestyle priorities can be factored into these discussions, but most of the analysis of importance is part of the technical ecological risk assessment itself (the center of Figure 4-6).

Assessing political will to make changes is essential to changeability analysis, because environmental factors, like lifestyle factors, will often prove to be important to the community for purposes other than health. For example, a common dilemma is the occupational hazard that can only be eliminated at the risk of losing the industry that supplies jobs for the community. Recall the West Virginia mining example discussed earlier in this chapter. The lung disease might be largely attributable to the mining work, and so there might be no way to eliminate that hazard without eliminating the jobs. When the hazard cannot be eliminated, we usually resort to behavioral solutions, such as wearing protective equipment, stopping one's smoking, and going for periodic screening.

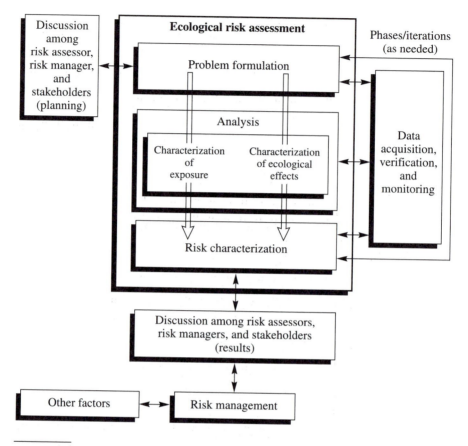

FIGURE 4-6

The Environmental Protection Agency's framework for ecological risk assessment was adapted by the Commission on Risk Assessment and Risk Management for the U.S. Congress to include the particular points at which public consultation or community "stakeholders" would be most important.

STEP 4: CHOOSING THE ENVIRONMENTAL TARGETS

The analytic method used in selecting behavioral targets can be applied here. See Figure 4-3. The same four quadrants in the two-by-two table would yield a distribution of environmental factors that would be more or less important and more or less changeable. The policy implication for action on factors in each quadrant would pertain equally to the environmental factors.

The only exception might be the greater weight one could give to Quadrant 3, where the environmental factor is apparently changeable but relatively low in objective importance. As Slovic and others have pointed out in their research on risk perception, the subjective importance of an environmental factor for the community is often greater than the objective evidence for its relationship or causal link to the health goal or ecological problem.[37] This might call for some priority for working with the community (the **stakeholders** identified in Figure 4-6) to discuss the formulation of the problem and the results of the risk assessment and eventually to help bring about change in that environmental factor. These steps will ensure their greater acceptance of the results of the assessment (which necessarily will involve technical procedures for data acquisition, verification, and monitoring). It will also help build their confidence and experience in making policy and organizational, economic, or environmental change.[38]

STATING ENVIRONMENTAL OBJECTIVES

With the priorities established among environmental factors to be changed, the final step in this phase of the assessment-planning process is to state the objectives for environmental change in quantitative terms. The main departure from the formula for behavioral objectives here is that the "who" in the behavioral objective would be eliminated for most environmental objectives. For example, the coalition of agencies working to reduce air pollution might set as its environmental objective, "The amount of carbon monoxide released into the atmosphere in our community will be reduced by 20% by the year 2010."

If the environmental or social change objective requires for its accomplishment the action of specific groups of people, behavioral objectives might be set for their actions as well. This relationship between environmental and behavioral objectives is reflected in the vertical arrows in the diagrams of the Precede-Proceed model (see Chapter 1) and by the ecological acknowledgement of the overlapping spheres of lifestyle, environment, health, and quality of life in Figure 4-7. This latter representation of the model also suggests the complex that comprises these interacting spheres could be viewed as an ecosystem. Within it, the combination of lifestyle and environmental risks found to be associated with the health and quality-of-life "vision" or goals could be referred to as risk characterization (Figure 4-6) or risk management products (Figure 4-7) when they are specified as behavioral and environmental objectives.

SUMMARY

By working through the first phases of the Precede model (Chapters 2 and 3), we laid three foundations of program planning:

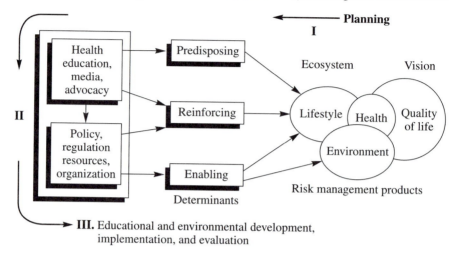

Proceed: policy, regulating or resourcing, and organizing for. . .

Precede: predisposing, reinforcing, and enabling constructs in ecosystem diagnosis and evaluation

FIGURE 4-7

This representation of the Precede-Proceed model acknowledges the overlapppng spheres of behavioral, environmental, and health components, which together make up quality of life.

1. The first step in health promotion planning should be an assessment of the quality of life or social goals and needs of the target population or client system, together with a situational analysis of the capacity of the community for participation in planning.
2. Epidemiological assessment based on the quality-of-life or social assessment can identify specific health problems and risk factors that impede or compromise quality of life.
3. Program objectives should be based on findings of the behavioral and environmental assessments and an extension of the quality-of-life and epidemiological assessments. The integration of these produce an ecological vision for the program.

This chapter took you through the third phase of the Precede planning framework, showing you how to identify the most fruitful behavioral and environmental targets for intervention. Since each chosen behavior generates an educational assessment and each environmental factor generates an ecological assessment, the planner must be parsimonious in selecting problems. Concentrating on only the most fruitful areas curbs the multiplication of subsequent planning steps and their associated costs. This is facilitated by the use of rigorous criteria and the application of critical judgment in the epidemiological assessment. Strict and realistic examination of the importance and changeability of each potential target behavior and environmental condition will cut down on the need for subsequent diagnostic efforts. Finally, the concise statement of objectives will lead to greater specificity in program development and will simplify the evaluation process.

EXERCISES

1. For the highest priority health problem identified in your program objective (Exercise 6, Chapter 3), list the specific behaviors that might be causally related to achieving that objective in your population or client system.
2. Rate each behavior in your inventory as low, medium, or high according to (a) prevalence (using population data where possible), (b) epidemiological or causal importance (using relative risk ratios where possible), and (c) changeability (using evidence from previous research where possible).
3. Write a behavioral objective for your population *(who)*, indicating to what extent *(how much)* they will exhibit the behavior *(what)* at a given point in time *(when)*. Note that you can state *what proportion* of the population will exhibit the behavior as a measure of *how much.*
4. Repeat Exercises 1–3 for the environmental assessment (substituting *environmental* for *behavioral*).

NOTES AND CITATIONS

1. *Health Promotion,* 1998.
2. *Supportive Environments for Health,* 1998. See also *Conference Proceedings,* 1998; St. Leger, 1997.
3. *Conference proceedings,* 1995; *Healthy Public Policy,* 1988; *The Jakarta declaration on leading health promotion into the 21st century,* 1997. To view some of the international declarations from the Ottawa, Adelaide, Sundsvall, and Jakarta conferences, visit http://www.who.ch/hep
4. Windsor et al., 1988.
5. Dean & Hancock, 1992; Green, 1994; Hamilton & Bhatti, 1996; Minkler, 1994.
6. U.S. Department of Health and Human Services, 1990, and the 1990 objectives that proceeded from *Healthy People* (U.S. Department of Health, Education, and Welfare, 1979). The separate category for health protection, which contained the environmental-regulatory objectives, gave the impression that health promotion was concerned only with behavior, not with the environment. The health promotion objectives themselves provide ample evidence to the contrary. They included numerous "service and protection" objectives under health promotion that addressed policy, regulatory, and organizational interventions required to reduce smoking, alcohol and drug misuse, and violent behavior; improve diet; increase exercise and fitness; and improve the vitality and independence of older people. For more on the evolution and debates about definition of health promotion terms, see Modeste, 1996; Nutbeam, 1998.

7. Last, 1995, p. 148.

8. For discussions and applications of the determinants of health and the health field concept in health promotion, see Green & Ottoson, 1999, chap. 2; Raeburn & Rootman, 1988.

9. For examples of these social factors as risk factors for disease and premature death, see Butler et al., 1996; N. H. Gottlieb & Green, 1984, 1987; Keil, 1984; Polissar, Sim, & Francis, 1981.

10. Examples of consensus documents include Canadian Task Force on the Periodic Health Examination, 1996; Castro, Valdiserri, & Curran, 1992; Committee on Trauma Research, 1989; Food and Nutrition Board, National Research Council, 1989; Gerstein & Green, 1993; Institute of Medicine, 1997; U.S. Preventive Services Task Force, 1996.

11. McGinnis & Foege, 1993, p. 2208.

12. For examples of the application of PRECEDE in behavioral risk factor assessment in cardiovascular disease, see Arbeit et al., 1992; P. H. Bailey, Rukholm, Vanderlee, & Hyland, 1994; Downey, Butcher, et al., 1987; Green, Lewis, & Levine, 1980; Mantell, DiVittis, & Auerbach, 1997, pp. 199–203; Morisky et al., 1981; Morrison, 1996; Nguyen, Grignon, Tremblay, & Delisle, 1995; Nguyen et al., 1995; O'Loughlin et al., 1995; Paradis et al., 1995.

13. Office on Smoking and Health, 1987.

14. Powell et al., 1987.

15. L. F. Ellison, Mao, & Gibbons, 1995.

16. Terry et al., 1981; Wang et al., 1979.

17. For more detail and results on similar epidemiological and behavioral assessments applying PRECEDE to chronic obstructive lung disease, see Windsor, Green, & Roseman, 1980.

18. Belloc, 1973; Belloc & Breslow, 1972.

19. Berkman, 1986; Berkman & Breslow, 1983. For more on the social support factor, see Cwikel, Dielman, Kirscht, & Israel, 1988; Dean, 1992; Minkler, 1986; Power et al., 1997; Runyan et al., 1998.

20. Breslow & Egstrom, 1980.

21. Devine & Cook, 1983.

22. Centers for Disease Control, 1978, 1986; Lalonde, 1974; McGinnis & Foege, 1993.

23. A. Friede et al., 1994; R. W. Wilson & Elinson, 1981. For a copy of the survey questionnaire, adapted for local use, see Green & Lewis, 1986, Appendix A; *Toward a Healthy Community,* 1980.

24. Rootman, 1988.

25. Stephens & Schoenborn, 1988.

26. Chen & Bill, 1983; Green, R. W. Wilson, & Bauer, 1983; Steckler, Goodman, & Alciati, 1997.

27. For a detailed description of the BRFSS and accounts of its published applications going back to the early 1980s, go online at the web site for the National Centers for Disease Control at http://www.cdc.gov; once you are into the CDC home page, select "Data and Statistics"; once there, click on "Surveillance" and you will discover many options for exploring BRFSS further. Also, if you wish to go directly to the individual state applications and reports specifically related to the BRFSS, the most convenient approach is to go to the web site for the Association of State and Territorial Health Officers (ASTHO): http://www.astho.org; once there, click on "State and Territorial Health Agencies on the Web." This will produce a map of the United States and Territories. By clicking on the state or territory of interest, you will immediate access that state's web site for public health. BRFSS data are accessible in most of those sites.

28. Kann et al., 1995; A. J. C. King & Coles, 1986, 1992.

29. Kolbe, 1997.

30. An example of a form for making such ratings, applied to injury control, can be found in Kreuter, Lezin, Kreuter, & Green, 1998; a more detailed example of the scientific rationale for ratings of importance in a community diabetes program can be seen in Daniel & Green, 1995.

31. Recent books that compile, review, and integrate the best of these bodies of research and theory for behavioral and environmental assessment in health promotion include Airhihenbuwa, 1995; Cramer & Spilker, 1991; Glanz, Lewis, & Rimer, 1997; Gochman, 1997; Leviton, Needleman, & Shapiro, 1997; Poland, Green, & Rootman, 1998; Tones & Tilford, 1994.

32. Basch, Eveland, & Portnoy, 1986, esp. p. 18; Green & Johnson, 1996; E. M. Rogers, 1995, esp. pp. 15–16 for definition of the characteristics of innovations.

33. Green, 1975.

34. The "how much" could also be set in terms of number of cigarettes consumed, on an individual basis (reducing each smoker's consumption by 20%) or on a population basis (reducing the average or overall smoking consumption by 20%). In addition, such quantitative aspects of program goals should be adjusted for secular trends, such as the steady national decline in smoking prevalence of about 1% per year. For a comprehensive analysis of related trends, see National Center for Health Statistics, 1996b, and for Canada, the population health surveys following Health and Welfare Canada, 1993. For related considerations in setting behavioral and environmental objectives, see Caulkins & Reuter, 1997; Reuter & Caulkins, 1995.

35. Green, Simons-Morton, & Potvin, 1997.

36. Health Education Unit, Regional Office of Education, WHO Regional Office for Europe, 1986.

37. Commission on Risk Assessment and Risk Management, 1996; Covello, von Winterfeldt, & Slovic, 1986; Slovic, 1986.

38. A commitment to change environmental factors is a commitment to engage the political forces in the community or target area. The issues in taking on that responsibility as a health professional are discussed in Chapters 6 and 8. The issues tend to be most explosive in matters of environmental control. See, for example, Freudenberg, 1984b.

Chapter 5

Educational and Ecological Assessment of Factors Affecting Health-Related Behavior and Environments

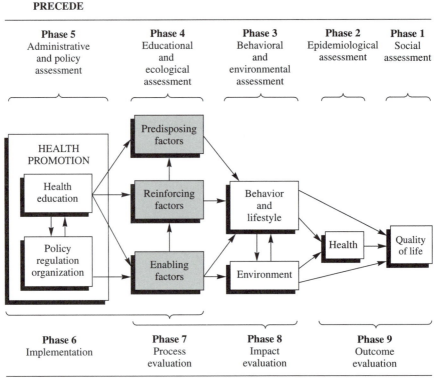

A n orderly sequence of social, epidemiological, behavioral, and environmental assessments produces a clear understanding of the actions and conditions of living affecting a population's aspiration, problem, or need. The next phase of the Precede model—the educational and ecological assessment—examines those behavioral and environmental conditions linked to health status or quality-of-life concerns to determine what causes them. The educational and ecological assessment identifies factors that require change to initiate and sustain the process of behavioral and environmental change. The determinants of health and social conditions identified in this phase will become the immediate targets or objectives of a program. Planners may see them as the processes of change that must be activated or set in motion if the necessary behavioral and environmental changes are to occur.

The educational and ecological assessment in health promotion is concerned with factors influencing the health-related behavior and conditions of living identified in Chapter 4. It also begins a process of behavioral assessment on those people who can influence environmental conditions. This assessment phase of PRECEDE helps planners untangle the complex forces shaping health-related behavior and environmental conditions.

FACTORS INFLUENCING BEHAVIOR

We begin by identifying three general categories of factors affecting individual or collective behavior: predisposing, enabling, and reinforcing factors. Each exerts a different type of influence on behavior.

Predisposing factors are antecedents to behavior that provide the rationale or *motivation* for the behavior.

Enabling factors are antecedents to behavior that allow a motivation to be realized.

Reinforcing factors are factors following a behavior that provide the continuing *reward* or incentive for the persistence or repetition of the behavior.

THE THEORY UNDERLYING THIS PART OF THE MODEL

One can explain any given behavior as a function of the collective influence of these three types of factors. The notions of *collective causation* and *contributing causes* represent behavior as a multifaceted, multidetermined, probabilistic phenomenon. Any one behavior, or action, is not caused by just one factor. "'Tis a tangled web we weave" of causal factors, each increasing or decreasing the probability the action will be performed and each potentially affecting the influence of other factors. Even so, there are exceptions. For example, a highly motivated behavior can sometimes overcome some deficit of resources and rewards. A highly rewarded behavior might occur in the absence of personal beliefs about its value or correctness. For the average person, however, the three conditions—predisposing, enabling, and reinforcing—must be aligned for the behavior to occur and persist. Any plan to influence behavior must consider not just one, but all three sets of causal factors. For example, a program disseminating health information to increase awareness, interest, and knowledge, without recognizing the influence of enabling and reinforcing factors, will most likely fail to influence behavior except in that segment of the population that has resources and rewards readily at hand—usually, the affluent.

Of the hundreds of theories that attempt to explain human behavior, each explains a useful portion of reality for different purposes. No single theoretical model has been universally accepted as sufficient to encompass the range of human experience in all circumstances. Models undergo modification in response to new situations. The classification of predisposing, enabling, and reinforcing determinants of behavior offers a broad framework within which one can organize more specific theories and research. The rationale of this framework is based on several common theoretical themes that have proven especially applicable and appropriate to health promotion.[1] PRECEDE merely organizes the multitude of precursors into three categories. Within these three categories, the various concepts and models can be used in planning the details (e.g., messages, incentives, policies) of a particular component of a health promotion program.

Figure 5-1 shows in more detail some relationships among the three types of factors and how these factors can effect behavior through various pathways. For example, an adolescent may have a negative attitude toward smoking and believe that smoking is harmful (predisposing factors), which causes her not to smoke (the behavior); her nonsmoking may then be rewarded by her parents (reinforcing factors). Strong enforcement of local ordinances prohibiting the sale of cigarettes to minors may lead to unavailability of cigarettes in her immediate environment (an enabling factor). On the other hand, an adolescent may perceive peer pressure to smoke (a reinforcing factor) and notice the availability of cigarettes in vending machines (an enabling factor), both of which can result in a positive attitude toward smoking (a predisposing factor), which then causes her to smoke (the behavior), which is then reinforced by her peers (a reinforcing factor).

Figure 5-1 illustrates how the three types of factors interact with the environment to affect behavior through various pathways. The interdependence of these factors and the circumstances and conditions of living defines behavioral assessment as an ecological process.

Normally, we would expect the sequence to be as follows: (1) A person has an initial reason, impulse, or motivation (predisposing factor) to pursue a given course of action. This first factor (Arrow 1 in Figure 5-1) in the causal chain may suffice to start the behavior, but it will not complete it unless the person has the resources and skills needed to carry out the behavior. The motivation, then, is followed by (2) the deployment or use of resources to enable the action (enabling

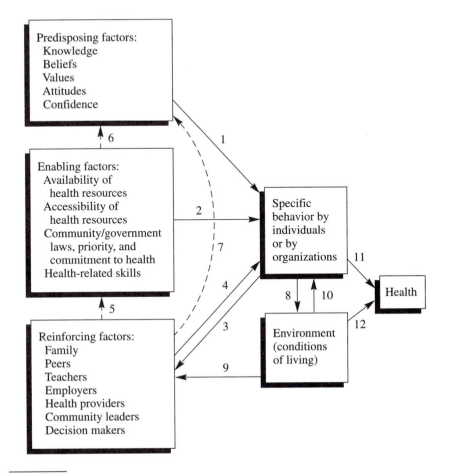

FIGURE 5-1

This portion of the Precede-Proceed model includes additional lines and arrows to outline a theory of causal relationships and order of causation for the three sets of factors influencing behavior.

factor). This usually results in at least a tentative enactment of the behavior, followed by (3) a reaction to the behavior that is emotional, physical, or social (reinforcing factor). Reinforcement strengthens (4) behavior, (5) the search for, mobilization, or commitment of future resources, and (6) motivation. The ready availability of enabling factors provides cues and heightens awareness and other factors predisposing the behavior. An exercycle in your home will more likely prompt you to use it than will one at the YMCA. (7) Similarly, rewards and satisfactions from behavior make that behavior more attractive on the next occasion; today's reinforcing factor becomes tomorrow's predisposing factor. Finally, perhaps most relevant to the social ecological perspective of health promotion, building up social reinforcement for a behavior can lead to the enabling of behavior in the form of social support and assistance (Arrow 5). This sequence of developmental steps and presumed cause-effect relationships in behavior change and maintenance uses language and concepts related to, but distinct from, those of the Transtheoretical Model,[2] the Health Belief Model (see later in this chapter), and other similar models and theories.

In seeking to uncover the factors that influence behavior (smoking in the recent example), planners must take into account the circumstances and conditions of the population of interest (adolescents). Fisher and his colleagues used the Precede-Proceed model as the organizing structure for a community-based pediatric asthma-control program in a low-income African-American neighborhood in St. Louis. Key to their approach was the clear delineation of parental behaviors associated with selected preventive actions, the early detection of a potential asthma attack, and prompt seeking of appropriate care as needed. In selecting the predisposing, reinforcing, and enabling factors influencing the behaviors of interest, Fisher and his colleagues were guided in part by existing data from the literature on surveys of parents of children with asthma. More importantly, they had data that enabled them to compare survey findings on adult patients from a clinic that served their neighborhood population with data on patients from a predominantly middle-class, suburban practice. They found that patients in their target population

> rated asthma as less of a concern and indicated that they were less careful to take their asthma medications, more satisfied with over-the-counter medications for asthma, and more likely to try to fight asthma attacks on their own without medical help. . . . These observations have led us to identify several key curricular concepts for the NAC education activities: (i) take asthma seriously, (ii) take asthma medications for asthma symptoms, (iii) when symptoms persist or worsen, follow an asthma action plan developed with your doctor, (iv) when symptoms continue or worsen, get help.[3]

THE UTILITY OF THIS COMPONENT OF THE MODEL

Besides its theoretical value in explaining and predicting behavior, the classification of factors that affect behavior into predisposing, reinforcing, and enabling categories makes it possible to group the specific features of the situation according to the types of interventions available in health education and health promotion. *Direct communications* to the target population strengthen the predisposing factors. *Indirect communications* through parents, teachers, clergy, community leaders, employers, peers, and others strengthen the reinforcing factors. *Community organization,* political interventions, and training strengthen the enabling factors.

Educational and ecological assessment identifies the prevalence or intensity of specific factors of each type while keeping in mind that there may be complex interactions among the factors. These interactions need not be delineated in precise

detail or for each person in a target population: The average or prevailing configuration of factors will suffice to plan an effective health promotion program for any relatively homogeneous group such as residents, students, patients, or employees. In recognizing that personal factors differ among individuals, that each average has a range and a distribution of values within a population, and that these variations have their covariations or interactions with other factors, one can maintain a statistical or probabilistic perspective rather than a simple deterministic one.

One other caveat before plunging more deeply into individual factors: for practical, program planning purposes, the exact placement of a factor believed to be important need not become a matter of paralyzing debate or indecision. As shown in the next section, some types of knowledge and skills may serve both predisposing and enabling functions in supporting different types of behavior. Further, as stated earlier, today's reinforcement becomes tomorrow's predisposition. The decision to place a factor in one category or another is less important than ranking the factor as an influence or determinant of behavior worthy of attention and finding a way to address it in the program. It is preferable also to think of the predisposing, enabling, and reinforcing factors as capacities to be strengthened, rather than deficits or problems to be overcome.

PREDISPOSING FACTORS

The predisposing factors of immediate concern—including knowledge, attitudes, beliefs, values, and perceived needs and abilities—relate to the motivation of an individual or group to act. Falling mostly in the psychological domain, they include the cognitive and affective dimensions of knowing, feeling, believing, valuing, and having self-confidence or a sense of efficacy. Personality factors could also predispose a given health-related behavior, but we set these into a special subcategory of predisposing factors that do not lend themselves readily to educational or other health promotion interventions besides psychotherapy. Predisposing personality factors and deep-seated values may not yield to change within the context of a health promotion program, but marketing companies use them in "psychographic" profiles to pitch or "spin" the advertisement of products and services.[4] These less changeable factors may serve health promotion similarly as planning indicators in the short run, but they might also indicate the need for early childhood interventions and broad cultural change in the long run.

Sociodemographic factors—such as socioeconomic status, age, gender, ethnic group, and family size or history—predispose health-related behavior through a variety of mechanisms.[5] Social status (based on income, education, occupation, area of residence, and other census data), age, and gender all can be used to segment a target population or individuals for planning purposes.[6] In planning short-term programs, though, we set these aside from the predisposing factors that will become targets for change, because these cannot be readily and directly influenced by most health promotion programs. The identification of socioeconomic and demographic factors can help the planner determine whether different interventions should be planned for different groups. For example, predisposing factors for smoking cessation in women include attitudes and concerns about weight control, whereas those concerns are not so important in men.[7] Without attempting to change these perceptions or the values underlying them, a health promotion program can take them into account when planning different smoking-cessation messages and supportive services for women and men. In the long term, again, or at broad national or policy levels, these can and sometimes should be the targets of health promotion programs.

CAPACITY-BUILDING CYCLE OF PREDISPOSING AND ENABLING FACTORS

Besides enabling behavior, existing skills and resources can predispose people to take action. This loop (shown in Figure 5-1 as Arrow 6) operates through the self-efficacy factor, which we shall examine later in this chapter.[8] The extent to which people, organizations, or communities possess certain skills or capacities may predispose them to take certain actions, but for most purposes, we classify skills as enabling factors. Similarly, some types of knowledge could be seen as enabling, rather than predisposing, insofar as knowledge serves the individual or group less as a stimulus to than a facilitator of action. Knowing where to go for a desired service, for example, enables one to obtain it. Generally, we can think of predisposing factors as the motivation, desires, or preferences that an individual or group brings to a behavioral or environmental choice or to an educational, political, or organizational experience. These preferences may pull the person or group either toward or away from specific actions.

One can view these capacity-building processes as operating through a natural history of health (Figure 5-2), whereby people adapt to their inherited environmental, biological, and health circumstances. Their successful adaptation results in learning through a process of reinforcement. The learned behavior is reinforced, which means it repeats itself in response to further challenges or opportunities presented by the environment and biological aging process. This is the simple cycle of health and health behavior that might apply to most species and might have prevailed in prehistoric human species before social organization.

AWARENESS AND KNOWLEDGE

Cognitive learning results from awareness and produces knowledge. An increase in knowledge alone does not always cause behavioral or organizational change, but positive associations among changes in these variables have been found in countless studies over decades of educational research before and since health

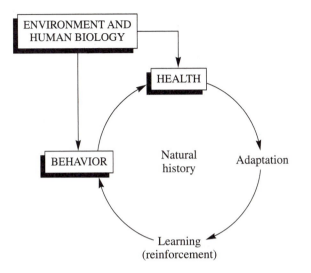

FIGURE 5-2

This simple cycle representing the natural history of health places the learning process, however unconscious, as a response to successful adaptation to inherited environmental and biological circumstances as they affect health.

SOURCE: Adapted from *Community and Population Health,* by L. W. Green and J. M. Ottoson, 1999, New York: WCB/McGraw-Hill; used with permission of the publisher.

education emerged as a discipline or profession.[9] Health knowledge of some kind, at least at the level of some awareness of a need and an action that can be taken to meet that need, is probably necessary before a conscious personal health action will occur—necessary, but not sufficient. The desired health action will probably not occur unless a person receives a cue strong enough to trigger the motivation to act on that knowledge. A threshold of knowledge may need to be met for some actions to occur, such as recognizing a symptom as abnormal before one will go for a medical check, but after that amount of knowledge is attained, additional information will not necessarily promote additional behavioral change.[10]

Cognitive learning also accumulates as experience, which produces beliefs, which combine over time to produce values, which in turn produce attitudes. Figure 5-3 shows these processes of shaping personal experience and behavior through the predisposing factors; we shall unfold this process more fully in the sections that follow. First, we shall discuss more on the foundation that knowledge provides.

Specific knowledge requirements for the person or population to carry out an intended behavior can often be identified through simple logic. Before people will act, they need to know *why* they should act, *what* actions are needed, *when* or

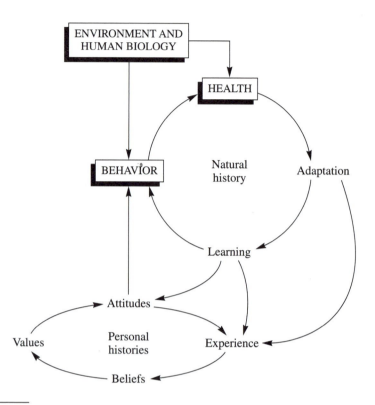

FIGURE 5-3

The development of predisposing factors shows the interaction of experience with learning in natural human history and with beliefs, values, attitudes, and behavior in personal histories.

SOURCE: Adapted from *Community and Population Health*, by L. W. Green and J. M. Ottoson, 1999, New York: WCB/McGraw-Hill; used with permission of the publisher.

under what circumstances, *how* to do it, and *where*. For example, some essential informational components of asthma education include

- How to recognize asthma symptoms and their severity
- When to administer medications (recognize symptoms, know how to measure airflow)
- What avoidance strategies to employ and what minimum of medication to use
- Where to avoid allergens or triggers of asthma attacks
- How to maintain self-management and control through normal daily activities[11]

The same considerations influencing health behavior in people whose health is at risk also influence the behavior of health professionals and even organizations. Knowledge influences decisions by those in charge, but other strategic and political considerations must come into play in the implementation of those decisions. The applications of PRECEDE-PROCEED to professional and policy decisions and to regulatory and organizational behavior will be addressed in Chapter 6. That chapter also will address how to use the results of the foregoing stages of the planning process to produce the final plan for implementation.

Motivation usually comes from sources other than, or in addition to, factual knowledge. School health curricula, for example, are frequently justified by reference to the simple, commonsense notion that knowledge is the best road to good health. Opponents argue that goals of knowledge are too "soft" and intangible to be used as criteria for program effectiveness in school health curricula. They also view students as bored by facts. A more accurate assessment might be that students are turned off not by facts, but by moralization, superficial coverage of subject matter, scare tactics, and tedious methods of presentation. Some health teachers may be abandoning information and facts in favor of armchair moralization about how one should behave to be healthy. We believe that both colorfully presented facts and sensitivity to values, such as those reflected in the social and quality-of-life assessment, are essential to predisposing behavioral change.

To say knowledge makes no difference is as ludicrous as to say it makes all the difference. The appropriate, balanced perspective is that knowledge is a necessary but usually not a sufficient factor in changing individual or collective behavior.[12] The same could be said for every other factor in the predisposing category. To recapitulate: a *combination* of factors defines motivation, and combinations of interventions define health promotion.

Like any other change in the complex system of predisposing factors, a change in awareness or knowledge will affect other areas because of the human drive for consistency.[13] Behavior may not change immediately in response to new awareness or knowledge, but the cumulative effects of heightened awareness, increased understanding, and greater command (recognition and recall) of facts will seep into the system of beliefs, values, attitudes, intentions, self-efficacy, and eventually behavior.

BELIEFS, VALUES, AND ATTITUDES

Beliefs, values, and attitudes are independent **constructs,** yet the differences between them are often fine and complex. As this book is directed primarily to practice rather than research, we shall forgo technicalities and examine these factors in a practical way, trusting that those interested in more detailed analysis will look further in the theoretical research literature.[14]

Beliefs. A *belief* is a conviction that a phenomenon or object is true or real. *Faith, trust,* and *truth* are words used to express or imply belief. Health-oriented belief statements include such statements as "I don't believe that medication can work"; "Exercise won't make any difference"; "When your time is up, your time is up, and there's nothing you can do about it." If beliefs such as these are strongly held, to what extent will they interfere with good health? Can they be changed? Will changes facilitate health-promoting behavior?

The **Health Belief Model,** developed and widely employed over the past half century,[15] attempts to explain and predict health-related behavior from certain belief patterns.[16] The model is based on the following assumptions about behavior change:

1. The person must believe that his or her health is in jeopardy. For an asymptomatic disease such as hypertension or early cancer, the person must believe that he or she can have it and not feel symptoms. This constellation of beliefs is referred to generally as *belief in susceptibility.*
2. The person must perceive the *potential* seriousness of the condition in terms of pain or discomfort, time lost from work, economic difficulties, and so forth.
3. On assessing the circumstances, the person must believe that benefits stemming from the recommended behavior outweigh the costs and inconvenience and are indeed possible and within his or her grasp. Note that this set of beliefs is not equivalent to actual rewards and barriers, which fall under enabling and reinforcing factors in the PRECEDE model. In the Health Belief Model, these are *perceived* benefits and costs.
4. There must be a "cue to action" or a precipitating force that makes the person feel the need to take action.

Specific applications and experimental tests of the Health Belief Model for **educational assessment** and evaluation can be found in studies of the following health actions or health problems,[17] with citations to the most recent publications found in each category:

- HIV/AIDS and sexually transmitted diseases[18]
- Contraceptive practices and sex education[19]
- Diabetes[20]
- Alcohol, driving, and injury control[21]
- Child care and child health behavior[22]
- Participation in screening programs[23]
- Use of clinical health services[24]
- Dietary behavior[25]
- Asthma[26]
- Genetic counseling and screening[27]
- Breast self-examination[28]
- Immunization[29]

- Skin cancer and sun protection behavior[30]
- Patient adherence to medical regimens[31]
- Smoking[32]
- Hypertension[33]
- Physician behavior in patient education and health promotion[34]
- Cardiac rehabilitation[35]
- Tuberculosis[36]
- Dental health behavior[37]
- Occupational therapy[38]
- Toxic shock syndrome[39]
- Exercise and physical activity[40]
- Correlated preventive health practices[41]
- General guidelines for development of measurement instruments[42]
- Other predisposing factors correlated with beliefs[43]

The Health Belief Model relates largely to the predisposing factors in the Precede-Proceed Model and serves as a useful tool to carry out that part of the educational assessment in PRECEDE.[44] Several authors have suggested ways of integrating this and other specific cognitive and affective models with PRECEDE-PROCEED.[45] Others have related beliefs to other factors in the Precede model without using the Health Belief Model.[46]

Fear. Two of the dimensions of the Health Belief Model—belief in susceptibility and belief in severity of consequences—could be interpreted as fear of the disease, condition, or behavior. **Fear** is a powerful motivator, and it contains the additional dimension of anxiety beyond the belief. The source of such anxiety is the belief in susceptibility and severity *in combination with* a sense of hopelessness or powerlessness to do anything about a vague or diffuse threat. This combination produces a flight response that often manifests as denial or rationalization of the threat as unreal. Thus, arousal of fear in health education messages can backfire, unless the fear-arousing message is accompanied by an immediate course of action the person can take to alleviate the fear.[47]

Values. The cultural, intergenerational perspectives on matters of consequence reflect the values people hold. Values tend to cluster within ethnic groups and across generations of people who share a common history and geography. They come down ultimately to the basis for justifying one's actions in moral or ethical terms. Values underpin the right and wrong, the good and bad dimensions of people's outlook on specific behaviors. Consider this brief exchange between two people:

He: Did I hear you say that you are going to try skydiving?
She: Absolutely not!
He: Why not?

She: Because I value my life, that's why not!

He: Then why do you smoke cigarettes?

She: Because I enjoy smoking and it helps me relax.

He: If that's the case, can you honestly say that you really value your life?

She: Sure I can. It's not that I don't value my life and health but that I value other things too, among them the pleasure of smoking. What's wrong with that?

Obviously, personal values are inseparably linked to choices of behavior. In the scenario just presented, the person who values life and health—and cigarettes, too—reveals a conflict of values. Values often conflict with each other, as the former Minister of Health for Canada has reported: "Most Canadians by far prefer good health to illness, and a long life to a short one but, while individuals are prepared to sacrifice a certain amount of immediate pleasure in order to stay healthy, they are not prepared to forgo all self-indulgence nor to tolerate all inconvenience in the interest of preventing illness."[48]

We do not set out in short-term health education or health promotion programs to *change* values. We seek instead to help people recognize inconsistencies between their values (usually pro-health) and their behavior or environment (often anti-health). Recognizing deeply held values within ethnic groups, age groups, and other demographically defined subpopulations provides an immediate and efficient indicator of starting points for the analysis of predisposing factors in segments of the population.[49]

Attitudes. After *motivation,* one of the vaguest yet most frequently used and misused words in the behavioral sciences lexicon is **attitude.** To keep matters short and simple, we offer two definitions that, in combination, cover the principal elements of attitude. Mucchielli describes attitude as "a tendency of mind or of relatively constant feeling toward a certain category of objects, persons, or situations."[50] Kirscht viewed *attitudes* as a collection of beliefs that always includes an evaluative aspect.[51] Attitudes can always be assessed as positive or negative. They differ from values in being attached to specific objects, persons, or situations and being based on one or more values. In the hierarchy posited by Rokeach, values are more deeply seated and therefore less changeable than are attitudes and beliefs.[52]

Keep in mind the two key concepts: (1) Attitude is a rather *constant* feeling that is *directed toward an object* (be it a person, an action, a situation, or an idea). (2) Inherent in the structure of an attitude is *evaluation,* a good-bad dimension. We gain further understanding of the structure of an attitude by examining one technique frequently used to measure attitudes: the semantic differential.[53] In this technique, one responds to concepts by making a mark on a continuum between antonyms. Suppose we want to measure the attitudes toward skydiving and cigarette smoking expressed by the woman in the dialogue. Having heard her conversation with the man, we already have an idea about what her attitudes are, but let's measure them just the same.

Concept: Skydiving

good   : __ : __ : __ : __ : X : __ : bad

pretty   : __ : __ : __ : __ : X : __ : ugly

happy   : __ : __ : __ : X : __ : __ : sad

Concept: Cigarette smoking

good   : __ : X : __ : __ : __ : __ : bad

pretty   : __ : __ : X : __ : __ : __ : ugly

happy   : X : __ : __ : __ : __ : __ : sad

From the conversation and from what we can see now in her response, her attitudes toward skydiving and smoking are consistently in opposite directions. Insofar as they are constant, they are probably also strong. We can also see the woman's evaluation of the concepts (in terms of good and bad). The woman avoided neutral responses on the continuum.

Though not completely understood, the relationships between behavior and constructs such as attitudes, beliefs, and values exist, given the ample evidence of their association. Analysis will show, for example, that attitudes are to some degree the determinants, components, and consequences of beliefs, values, and behavior. This alone gives sufficient reason to be concerned with attitudes, beliefs, and values as interrelated predisposing factors. Let us now see how these personal psychological characteristics relate to behavior and to the more basic learning process suggested by the natural history of health in Figure 5-2.

SELF-EFFICACY AND COGNITIVE LEARNING THEORY

When first introduced, the concept of self-efficacy as a determinant of behavior found immediate acceptance in health education and health promotion because of its emphasis on learning and on the empowerment of people to have a sense of control over their health. This concept from social learning theory, later called *cognitive learning theory,* has held a special fascination for health educators[54] and others in health promotion[55] and in patient education.[56] The concept of self-efficacy is attractive probably because it expresses so succinctly the dominant purpose ascribed to health promotion. As declared by the Ottawa Charter, health promotion is "the process of enabling people to increase control over, and to improve, their health."[57] Self-efficacy implies a mental or cognitive state of taking control.[58]

"Inherent in the social learning conception is the idea that people self-regulate their environments and actions. Although people are acted upon by their environments, they also help create their surroundings."[59] This concept of reciprocal determinism is social learning theory's major departure from *operant conditioning theory,* which tends to view all behavior as a one-way product of the environment. Reciprocal determinism, with its associated concepts of self-management and self-control, make social learning theory ideally suited to the integration of the Precede and Proceed frameworks and the development of an educational approach to health promotion.

Learning takes place through three processes: (1) direct experience, (2) indirect or vicarious experience from observing others (modeling), and (3) the storing and processing of complex information in cognitive operations that allow one to anticipate the consequences of actions, represent goals in thought, and weigh evidence from various sources to assess one's own capabilities. Out of this last process comes a situation-specific self-appraisal that makes the individual more or less confident in taking on new behavior in situations that may contain novel, unpredictable, or stressful circumstances. Self-efficacy, then, is a perception of one's own capacity for success in organizing and implementing a pattern of behavior that is new, a capacity based largely on experience with similar actions or circumstances encountered or observed in the past.

In addition to its influence on behavior, self-efficacy also affects thought patterns and emotional reactions that may alleviate anxiety and enhance coping ability. These interactions make self-efficacy particularly useful in studies of smoking[60] and other addictive and compulsive behavioral patterns where high rates of relapse are experienced,[61] including weight loss.[62]

The self-efficacy variable has proved particularly useful in planning health promotion programs using mass media with role models for the vicarious learning and modeling process and for instruction in self-control.[63]

Measurement instruments to assess self-efficacy have been developing gradually in recent years. Self-efficacy scales have been validated, for example, for health-related diet and exercise behaviors[64] and for weight loss.[65] A review of the literature to identify the latest measurement advances is always advisable before one embarks on a survey to assess any of the predisposing factors.

BEHAVIORAL INTENTION

Central to the theory of reasoned action[66] is the concept of behavioral intention. The theory of *reasoned action* holds that the final step in the predisposing process, before actual action takes place, is the formulation of a **behavioral intention.** This step is influenced by attitudes toward the behavior and by perception of social norms favorable to the behavior. These attitudes, in turn, are influenced both by beliefs concerning the efficacy of action in achieving the expected outcomes and by attitude toward those outcomes. Perception of social norms is influenced by beliefs about the strength of others' opinions about the behavior and the person's own motivation to comply with them.

Applications of the theory of reasoned action in health behavior studies can be found in the literature on dental health,[67] tobacco control,[68] recycling behavior,[69] alcohol,[70] drug abuse and HIV prevention,[71] seat-belt and helmet use,[72] and contraceptive practices.[73] A school-based smoking prevention project in the Netherlands specifically integrated the theory of reasoned action with PRECEDE to design interventions that proved effective in reducing the uptake of smoking.[74] Longitudinal data from two cities in which surveys were conducted before and after the national HealthStyle campaign provided for a comparative analysis of the predictive power of several models, including the theory of reasoned action.[75]

EXISTING SKILLS

A person may come to an educational situation already possessing the skills to take certain actions. Such skills may predispose the person to act in a particular way. For example, an experienced mother may already possess the skills for breast-feeding. When she gives birth to another child, those skills may predispose her to breast-feed that child. The mother has a high self-efficacy about breast-feeding because she has successfully breast-fed in the past; she has formulated a behavioral intention to breast-feed because of her prior acquisition of skills. Thus, existing skills are closely tied to self-efficacy and behavioral intention.

Self-confidence and self-efficacy can be linked to skills that are already present for a specific health-behavior situation and thus do not need to be learned. For example, the ability to resist peer pressure is associated with nonsmoking in adolescents.[76] If a person does not possess the skills for a certain action, then the acquisition of those skills becomes an enabling factor for performing the action. Several smoking-prevention programs have included skills training in resisting peer pressures to smoke, in order to aid those students who do not already have those skills.[77]

ENABLING FACTORS

Often conditions of the environment, enabling factors *facilitate* the performance of an action by individuals or organizations. These conditions include the availability, accessibility, and affordability of health care and community resources. They also include conditions of living that act as barriers to action, such as availability of transportation or child care to release a mother from that responsibility long enough to participate in a health program. Enabling factors also include *new* skills that a person, organization, or community needs to carry out a behavioral or environmental change.

Enabling factors become the immediate targets of community organization or organizational development and training interventions in one's program. They consist of the resources and new skills necessary to perform a health action and of the organizational actions required to modify the environment. Resources include the organization and accessibility of health care facilities, personnel, schools, outreach clinics, or any similar resource. Personal health skills, such as those discussed in the literature on self-care and school health education, can enable specific health actions.[78] Skills in influencing the community, such as those used to promote social action and organizational change, can enable actions directed toward influencing the physical or health care environment.[79]

In a position paper on enabling factors, Milio contended that the health behaviors of a population may be limited by the degree to which health resources are made available and accessible: "Organizational behavior . . . sets the range of options available to individuals for their personal choice-making."[80] To plan interventions directed at changing enabling factors, the health promotion planner assesses the presence or absence of enabling factors in the community of interest. This calls for an organizational assessment of resources and an educational assessment of required skills.

THE HEALTH CARE ENVIRONMENT

Enabling factors for health care or medical care behaviors include health care resources such as outreach clinics, hospitals, emergency treatment rooms, health care providers, classes in self-care, and other facilities, programs, or personnel. Cost, distance, available transportation, hours open, and so forth are enabling factors that affect the availability and accessibility of the health care services.

Suppose a well-intended educational effort were successful in appealing to the motivation of members of a target group to make greater use of medical services in their area, but the health care providers in the area were not consulted. If they had been, they would have warned that existing facilities were overcrowded and that providers were overworked and unwilling to take on more work without an expansion of facilities and additional personnel.

What will the outcome likely be? Deprived of services they need and were promised, participants in the program may become discouraged and feel they have been "let down." Because they were not considered and were made to look bad for not delivering promised services, health care providers may become angry and alienated from health education efforts. A broken-appointment cycle like that shown in Figure 4-2 would likely develop.

As emphasized throughout this book, a health behavior has many causes, so unidimensional efforts to affect behavior rarely produce the desired results. In this example, health education for better utilization of medical services would fail to achieve its desired outcome because it paid no attention to the enabling factors for that utilization.

OTHER ENVIRONMENTAL CONDITIONS
THAT AFFECT HEALTH-RELATED BEHAVIOR

Many environmental conditions adversely influence health-related behavior. For example, the availability, accessibility, and low cost of unhealthful consumer products adversely affect health behavior in the United States today. Examples include cigarette machines, which enable smoking by adolescents even where laws prohibit sale to minors; laborsaving devices, which foster sedentary lifestyles; "fast food," which is convenient but often high in salt and fat; and alcoholic beverages sold at sports events, which puts intoxicated fans in the driver's seat on the road home. Examples of environmental enabling factors that can counteract such influences include the availability and low cost of smoking-cessation programs, exercise facilities, and healthful food, as well as the enforcement of laws prohibiting alcohol sales to minors or during the second half of a sporting event.

For each priority behavioral risk factor or capacity identified in the behavioral assessment, one can identify environmental enabling factors. For example, many such factors have been found to affect smoking: cost of cigarettes, accessibility of cigarettes, smoking restrictions and bans, availability of smoking cessation and smoking prevention programs, and smoking cessation aids such as nicotine gum.[81]

In a second example, the following enabling factors can discourage alcohol misuse among youth: leisure-time alternatives such as sports and recreation programs, after-school activities, and alcohol-free social events; adult supervision; and regulation of alcohol sales through retail outlets.[82] Project Graduation demonstrated that chemical-free graduation celebrations can reduce the number of fatalities, alcohol or drug-related injuries, and arrests for driving under the influence of alcohol.[83] Figure 5-4 shows the dramatic decline in teenage highway deaths associated with alcohol following the initiation of Project Graduation in one state.

For physical activity in adults, the following environmental enabling factors pertain: programs that emphasize moderate exercise and increases in daily physical activity; accessibility of an exercise facility; low cost; and environmental opportunities for physical activity.[84]

NEW SKILLS

The term *skills* here refers to a person's ability to perform the tasks that constitute a health-related behavior. Skills for health promotion include abilities to control personal risk factors for disease, skills in appropriate use of medical care, and

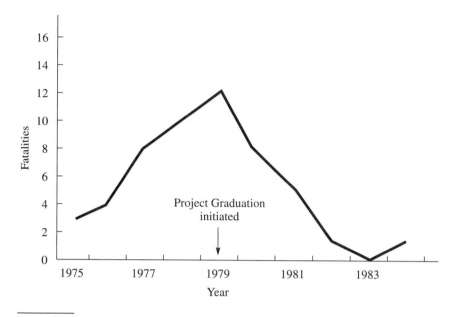

FIGURE 5-4

Motor vehicle–related fatalities among 15–19-year-old residents involving teenagers driving under influence of alcohol during graduation period, May 15–June 15, 1975–1984, in the State of Maine.

SOURCE: "Project Graduation: Maine," by C. Mowatt, J. Isaly, and M. Thayer, 1985, *Morbidity and Mortality Weekly Report, 34,* 233–235.

skills in changing the environment. Examples include knowing how to use relaxation techniques, to exercise properly, to use the variety of medical instruments and diagnostic procedures frequently required in self-care programs, and to tap one's voting power and potential for coalition-building and community organizing to bring about change in one's neighborhood or community.

For each specific behavioral priority identified in the behavioral assessment, one should identify needed skills. For smoking prevention, such skills include resisting peer pressures to smoke; for smoking cessation, skills in coping and relaxation.[85] For physical activity, skills in flexible goal-setting can increase adherence to an exercise program.[86]

Health promotion programs working to increase the ability of the people to change their environment need to know whether the people possess skills for influencing organizations or their community. Such skills might include community organizing, coalition building, fund-raising, negotiating, working with the media, writing, and speaking.[87]

Assessing the extent to which members of the target population possess enabling skills can give the planner valuable insight into possible program components. Failure to consider the impact of enabling factors on the achievement of behavioral goals can lead to serious problems that threaten program success.

REINFORCING FACTORS

Reinforcing factors are those consequences of action that determine whether the actor receives positive (or negative) feedback and is supported socially afterward. Reinforcing factors thus include social support, peer influences, and advice and feedback by health care providers. Reinforcing factors also include the physical consequences of behavior, which may be separate from the social context. Examples include the alleviation of respiratory symptoms following the correct use of asthma medication and feelings of wellbeing or pain caused by physical exercise.

Social benefits—such as recognition; physical benefits such as convenience, comfort, relief of discomfort, or pain; tangible rewards such as economic benefits or avoidance of cost; and imagined or vicarious rewards such as improved appearance, self-respect, or association with an admired person who demonstrates the behavior—all reinforce behavior. Reinforcing factors also include adverse consequences of behavior, or "punishments," that can lead to the extinction of a positive behavior. Rewards also can reinforce behavior that is not conducive to health. For individuals, these might include the "high" that rewards the drug abuser, the relief of tension that rewards the smoker, or the masking of emotions that accompany compulsive eating. For organizations, these might include the profits that accrue from promoting a harmful product or the savings that accrue from using a pollutant in the manufacturing process. Tax incentives that support nonpolluting products and penalties or fines that discourage polluting ones can positively and negatively reinforce changes in organizational behavior, respectively.

For each of the priority behaviors from the behavioral diagnosis, important reinforcing factors can be determined. For example, for smoking cessation, one may seek support from peers and spouse or advice from health care providers.[88] Cigarette and alcohol advertising provides vicarious reinforcement for continuing to smoke or drink.[89] Family support and recommendations from health care providers reinforce adherence to physical activity programs.[90]

Social reinforcements, as well as social images created by the mass media, set up norms of behavior transmitted from one generation to another as *culture*. Culture shapes our institutions, which in turn organize themselves to meet our cultural expectations. By organizing resources institutionally, we can as communities and

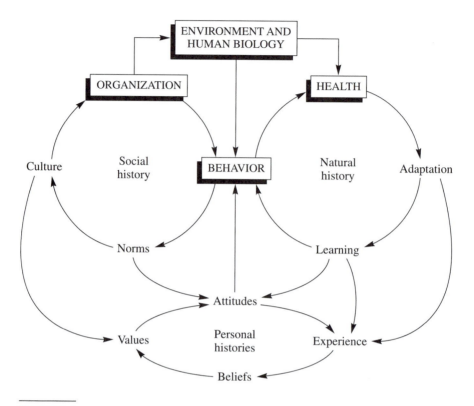

FIGURE 5-5

The social history of health includes the dimensions of social norms, culture, and organization because these influence behavior directly and indirectly through values, attitudes, and the environment.

SOURCE: Adapted from *Community and Population Health,* by L. W. Green and J. M. Ottoson, 1999, New York: WCB/McGraw-Hill; used with permission of the publisher.

societies exert much more extensive and effective control over the environment. The cycle is thus closed with the third cycle, shown in Figure 5-5, the social history of health, as related to natural history and personal histories. Culture influences personal values; norms influence personal attitudes. Organizations directly affect behavior through the enabling and reinforcing factors discussed in the preceding paragraphs.

One can anticipate reinforcement—negative or positive—prior to a behavior. Such *anticipated* reinforcement will influence the subsequent performance of the behavior. Social acceptance or disapproval thus can be reinforcing factors. Some such factors that provide social reinforcement can become enabling ones if they generate ongoing social support, such as financial assistance or transportation, or even friendly advice. Reinforcement can also be *vicarious* in the form of modeling a behavior after a television personality or after an attractive person in an advertisement who seems to be enjoying the behavior.

In developing a health promotion program, the source of reinforcement will, of course, vary depending on the objectives and type of program, as well as the setting. In occupational health promotion programs, for example, co-workers, supervisors, union leaders, and family members may provide reinforcement. In patient education settings, reinforcement may come from nurses, physicians, fellow patients, and, again, family members.

Whether the reinforcement is positive or negative will depend on the attitudes and behavior of significant people, some of whom will more greatly affect behavior than will others. For example, in a high-school health education program, where reinforcement may come from peers, teachers, school administrators, and parents, which group will likely have the most influence? Research in adolescent behavior indicates that adolescent smoking, drinking, and drug-taking behavior is most influenced by approval from friends, especially a best friend.[91] Parental attitudes, beliefs, and practices, especially those of the mother, hold second place among social influences affecting the health status of adolescents.[92]

Which people are significant may vary not only according to the setting but also by growth and development stages. For smoking, younger adolescents (grades 6, 7, and 8) appear to be influenced more by parents. That of older adolescents (grades 9–11) is influenced more by peers and siblings.[93]

Incremental and easily reversible changes in behavior are more likely to be reinforced by success than are drastic changes. For example, to decrease salt consumption, people tolerate small steps of a low-salt diet more easily, and these are more apt to be reinforced through their successful implementation than are large steps toward the goal. Consider, for example, the steps one can use for low-salt diets. The following could be added one at a time after success in the previous steps: salting only after tasting, cutting salt in cooking, eliminating table salt, buying low-salt food products, and, finally, eliminating cooking salt.

Behaviors that influence environmental or health care conditions also respond to reinforcing factors. Community or social support can reinforce actions to influence these changes. Such support can be provided by community residents, health-care providers, and health education or health promotion practitioners. The community change agent who does not have such support becomes discouraged, experiences "burnout," and consequently abandons his or her efforts.

Program planners must carefully assess reinforcing factors to make sure that program participants have maximum opportunities for supportive feedback for new behaviors. Without such feedback, programs have a reduced chance of sustained momentum and eventual success.

SELECTING DETERMINANTS
OF BEHAVIOR AND ENVIRONMENTAL CHANGE

The core of PRECEDE's educational and ecological assessment phase is selecting those predisposing, reinforcing, and enabling factors that, if modified, will
help bring about the targeted health-related behavior and environmental change.
The three basic steps in this process are (1) identifying and sorting factors into
the three categories, (2) setting priorities among the categories, and (3) establishing priorities within the categories. Specific factors selected by this process form
the basis for both educational and community organization objectives, which
then lead to the selection of materials and methods for program implementation.
If the program is well designed and carefully implemented, the probability is
high that objectives will be met and target behaviors and environments modified.

STEP 1: IDENTIFYING AND SORTING

The list of causal factors initially identified for each behavior and environmental
target should be as comprehensive as possible to help the planner avoid overlook-
ing crucial determinants. Both informal and formal methods can be used to
develop the list.

Informal Methods. The team assigned the responsibility for designing the intervention plan usually have educated guesses and hypotheses about the reasons why
people behave in the desired manner. At this point, it can be helpful to involve
members of the group at risk (the consumers or target population) in the planning
again. Their information and insight on their own behavior, attitudes, beliefs, values, and barriers to reaching the stated objectives are quite relevant. Intensive
interviews, informal group discussions, nominal groups, focus groups, panels,
and questionnaires can provide useful data.[94]

The same methods of eliciting information can be used with staff who will be
involved in the delivery of the intervention and with people in agencies providing
related services. They might suggest potential causes of behavior based on
insights from personal experience or unrecognized effects of agency or community resources, services, and operations. Systematic recording of the data will
make this information useful and retrievable.

Brainstorming and nominal group process are useful techniques for generating data on barriers to behavioral change.[95] A vital step in this phase of PRE-
CEDE is sorting factors according to whether they have negative or positive
effects. The negative effects must be overcome, and the positive effects can be
built on and strengthened.

Planners must be critical in accepting health care providers' assumptions
about the predisposing factors of patients or clients. Some providers may judge

behavior that differs from expectations as lazy, apathetic, or ignorant. Generalizations of this sort do not help explain the behavior at issue but merely describe it. "Blaming the victim" may arise out of misunderstanding, poor communication, "burnout," or rationalization: The system may be at fault, rather than the population or patient.[96] On the other hand, "system blaming" may arise out of frustration with the organizations and management of services, and this can be just as unproductive as putting all the responsibility for change on individuals.[97] The purpose of the assessment at this stage is not to fix blame or responsibility, but rather to take inventory of all the potential targets of change that might improve the situation.

Formal Methods. A search through relevant literature can yield information on cultural and social attitudes and descriptions of studies defining the impact of specific factors on health-related behavior.[98] For example, a market segment analysis to examine those beliefs and perceptions of adults that may influence their exercise behavior found that (1) people are generally misinformed about the frequency, intensity, and duration of activity needed to obtain a cardiovascular benefit; (2) one's doctor is the most important referent regarding exercise; and (3) subjects did not think health benefits of exercise were as critical as the intrinsic, psychological, or emotional benefits.[99] Such a search may also yield items that can be used in surveys or being a record-keeping system that will eventually become the basis for evaluation of the program.

Checklists and questionnaires are structured ways of collecting and organizing information from important individuals and groups. These can be used to measure knowledge, attitudes, and beliefs as well as perceptions of services. Zapka and Mamon conducted a formal study of the predisposing, enabling, and reinforcing factors associated with breast self-examination among college women on a university campus. Their analysis illustrates the formal application of survey methods to the sorting process.[100] Other formal surveys applying the Precede model have been published and can therefore be used in future assessments as a source of developed survey instruments and comparative data.[101]

Planning agencies often compile directories of available community resources. These directories are particularly helpful when enabling factors are being examined. Utilization data from health care organizations and attendance records from agencies may also be available.[102] Surveys of community organizations can also be conducted, as recommended and detailed in a series of CDC community intervention handbooks.[103]

If planners have trouble deciding whether a factor is predisposing, enabling, or reinforcing, they should list it in whichever categories might apply. As you have seen, the three categories are not mutually exclusive; a factor can appropriately be placed in more than one. A family may be predisposed to dieting, for example, and reinforce (negatively or positively) that behavior once it has been undertaken. We do not wish to define the categories so rigidly that PRECEDE becomes an academic debating point. The categories are meant to sort the causal factors into three classes of targets for subsequent intervention according to the three broad classes of intervention strategy: (1) direct communication to change the predisposing factors, (2) indirect communication (through family, peers, teachers, employers, health care providers) to change the reinforcing factors, and (3) organizational or training strategies to change the enabling factors.

Later in the planning process, the specific educational and organizational activities and messages for each factor will be devised based on judgment of their importance as determinants of the desired outcomes. Then, the category in which the factor falls *will* make a difference. For example, the design of messages, learning opportunities, and organizational strategies directed at families will differ according to whether a family seems most important in creating rewards to *reinforce* the behavior or in providing financial support to *enable* the behavior.

A list at this point might look something like the one in Table 5-1, which shows both positive and negative factors related to reducing the sequelae of streptococcal throat infections in a preschool population. At the end of this chapter, you will convert some of these factors into learning and resource objectives, which are statements of the immediate goals of a health promotion program. One must achieve such objectives in order to obtain behavioral and environmental changes, which are the intermediate goals of the program. In turn, one must meet the behavioral and environmental objectives if one hopes to achieve health improvements or improvements in quality of life—the ultimate goals of the program.

STEP 2: SETTING PRIORITIES AMONG CATEGORIES

All the causes in a complete inventory for several behaviors cannot be tackled simultaneously. One therefore needs to decide which factors are to be the objects of intervention first and in what order.

One possible basis for establishing priorities among the three kinds of factors is development. For example, an HIV screening service must have its facility in operation and services available before it creates a demand for the services. The organizational enabling factors that provide the services and make them accessible will have to precede the educational efforts to predispose people to use them. People will not adopt a set of behaviors to reduce a health risk if they are not aware that there *is* a risk. Belief in the immediacy of the risk and its implications will have to be developed for the enabling resources to be utilized. Finally, reinforcing factors cannot come into play until behaviors have taken place. Thus, for a community program, enabling, then predisposing, then reinforcing factors would be translated into interventions in that order. Different situations may require a different order of development, depending upon the factors that already exist.

Some enabling factors may have to be developed over a long period by means of community organization efforts, legislative pressure, and reallocation of resources. If so, the concerns of the basic target group may have to be postponed for months. In such cases, the population so predisposed might be mobilized to support legislation or organizational development.

TABLE 5-1

An example of classifying the determinants of behavioral and environmental factors in relation to parents' actions on sore throat symptoms in young children

Behavioral objectives

Within three days of the initial manifestation of sore throat, 80% of the children in Hobbit's Preschool Program will have a throat culture done based on a swab taken by a parent.

The target group for the learning objectives will be the parents of the preschoolers, the parents' employers, relatives, and physicians, and the preschool personnel.

Predisposing factors

Positive	Negative
Attitudes, beliefs, and values: Mothers value child's health; mothers have been willing to use health services regularly. Knowledge: Mothers can read thermometers and determine temperatures; children are old enough to report sore throats.	Attitudes, beliefs, and values: Sore throats are not important; mothers feel that sore throats are temporary; mothers feel that sore throats do not have serious consequences and that there is no relationship between strep throat and sequelae.

Reinforcing factors

Positive	Negative
Teachers relate well to parents; physician has set up positive interaction with group; teachers and medical personnel encourage and support parents in taking throat swabs.	Mother's employers are not generous about time off for child's illness; grandmothers (or baby sitters) consider sore throats inconsequential and temporary.

Enabling factors

Positive	Negative
Mothers have thermometers in homes; clinic is close by; insurance reduces cost of follow-up visit. Throat swab kit for home use is available; clinic provides culture and analysis in three days; skill in swabbing is easily learned.	Cost of prescription penicillin regimen; teachers cannot take child to doctor; parent has to stay home with child or arrange for sitter because there is no preschool isolation room.

Some factors may be difficult to work with because of agency policies or mandates. An agency may be restricted to activities related to one set of factors. A hospital may not have the personnel to contact families at home and may have to depend on another agency to undertake the task. A school system may have to follow a board of education ruling that AIDS information can be taught only within classes on marriage and the family and that discussion and provision of contraception is not a school responsibility.

Work on several factors can and should proceed simultaneously, however. Cooperation with the appropriate agency to establish a rehabilitation service for alcoholics, for example, can coincide with the mounting of a general information campaign on the costs of alcoholism and the efficacy of treatment. By the time the service is operational, the climate is set for specific information about the type and availability of services.

STEP 3: ESTABLISHING PRIORITIES WITHIN CATEGORIES

Within the three categories of behavioral causes, factors can be selected for intervention. One uses the same criteria as those used for selecting high-priority behaviors: importance and changeability.

Importance. Importance can be estimated by judging *prevalence, immediacy,* and *necessity* according to logic, experience, data, and theory. **Prevalence** asks, "How widespread or frequent is the factor?" If the factor identified is very widespread or occurs often, it should qualify for priority consideration. For example, if 80% of the students in a school system believe smoking is glamorous, then addressing that belief in an antismoking campaign should have much higher priority than if only 10% of students hold that belief.

Immediacy asks, How compelling or urgent is the factor? Knowing the symptoms of a heart attack and what is needed to save a victim's life is one example of knowledge that has immediate consequences for people at high risk of heart attacks. Another type of immediacy has to do with how close the connection is between the factor and the group at risk. If a certain group of adults believes no connection exists between strep throat and rheumatic heart disease, changing that belief is a high priority if the adults are the parents of young children, who are at high risk. It is not a high priority if the adults are the parents of graduating seniors.

Necessity is based on the consideration of factors that have a low prevalence but still must be present for the change in behavior or environment to occur. If an outcome cannot be achieved without a certain factor, that factor deserves priority. Knowledge is often necessary though insufficient to bring about an action. It is difficult to envision an intravenous drug user giving up drugs to avoid AIDS without understanding how dirty needles can transmit HIV. Or a person committing himself or herself to a patient role, for example, without at least a minimal awareness of the illness. Knowledge of the unavoidable need for exercise is necessary for a person to join an aerobics program in response to a physician's referral. Certain beliefs can also be considered necessary. People who are supposed to present themselves for medical services must have some belief (however faint) that the health professional can help alleviate the problem. A person who is attempting to stop smoking must believe smoking is harmful, at least to his or her social relationships if not to health.

Changeability. One can gather evidence of the changeability of a factor by looking at the results of previous programs. Assessments of changeability can also be made using techniques set forth in the literature. Rokeach, for example, posits a hierarchy in which beliefs are easier to change than are attitudes, and attitudes are easier to change than are values.[104] One also can analyze changeability and the priority of factors according to a theory on stages in adoption and diffusion of innovations. This theory is based on work in communications and extensive experience in agriculture, education, family planning, and public health.[105]

Behavior change is analyzed over time, and the stages by which one adopts behavior are observed at the individual and societal levels. Individuals pass through stages labeled awareness, interest, persuasion, decision, and adoption. When these stages are charted in a population or social system, they follow a pattern of prevalence or cumulative diffusion that looks like a series of increasingly flattened S-shaped curves.

In Figure 5-6, the five stages of adoption and the four groups of adopters identify points in time when different communication methods and channels are more or less effective. Identification of the stages allows the health promotion planner to match the most appropriate intervention strategy with the stage of the program recipients. For example, mass media are most efficient with **innovators** and **early adopters,** but outreach methods such as home visits are necessary with

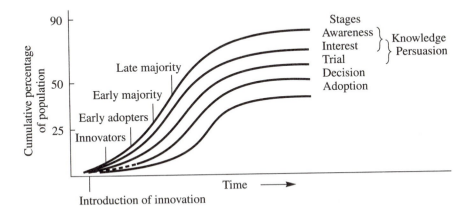

FIGURE 5-6

Five stages of adoption for four groups of adopters show increasing time lags among awareness, interest, trial, decision, and adoption stages as time passes from introduction of the innovation.

late adopters. Depending on the percentage of the population who have already adopted the health behavior at a given point in time, the relative changeability of the behavior in the remaining population is defined by this theory of diffusion.

Observability also influences changeability. If one can demonstrate the factor, one can set a climate for others and reinforce their efforts. As an example, consider the growing emphasis on nonsmoking in public meetings. Mass communications often can be utilized to promote reinforcing messages that support certain behaviors. The function of media, in such instances, is not to motivate but to reinforce.

LEARNING AND RESOURCE OBJECTIVES

Writing learning and resource objectives is similar to writing behavioral objectives, as presented in Chapter 4. Learning objectives define the targeted predisposing factors and skills in the targets of intervention at the end of a program. Resource objectives define the environmental enabling factors that should be in place at the end of a program.

Examples of learning objectives are shown in Table 5-2. The predisposing and enabling factors analyzed in Table 5-1 have been restated in terms of learning objectives for parents. Note the variations in the "how much" in these examples. One can usually create a high level of knowledge. Often, over 90% of a given population can be made aware of a given fact. A smaller percentage of those who are aware will believe the fact is relevant, important, or useful. Not all of these will develop the requisite skill to carry out recommended actions. Hence, if 60% of the population is expected to adopt a behavior, it is necessary to develop skills in 70%, establish health beliefs in 80%, and to create knowledge of the problem or recommendation in 90% or more.

Learning objectives may be developed not only for the target population but also for those people who will reinforce the target population. For the example of throat cultures in preschool children, the preschool personnel might also be targets of intervention to teach them how to reinforce the parents. In addition, information about environmental enabling factors provides the basis for developing resource objectives.

Examples of learning objectives for reinforcement and of resource objectives for environmental enabling factors are shown in Table 5-3. Note that the objectives address the reinforcing and environmental enabling factors that were defined in Table 5-1. Learning objectives for reinforcers and resource objectives are important components of a health promotion program that addresses all three categories of determining factors. Achievement of ongoing reinforcement and environmental resources can create a situation where the effect of the health promotion program can continue even after the program ends.

Diffusion theory also provides a framework for assessing reinforcing and enabling factors. For example, the presence of "No Smoking" sections in restau-

TABLE 5-2

These examples of learning and resource objectives are based on reinforcing and enabling factors analyzed in Table 5-1

Problem	Teaching parents to swab sore throats and submit swabs for throat cultures

Target Group: Parents

Knowledge	By the end of the program, 90% of the parents will be able to
	(a) Identify sore throat and fever as potential strep throat
	(b) Identify throat swabs as necessary to determine whether strep accompanies sore throat
	(c) State the cure for strep throat
	(d) State that prescriptions are available at the clinic
Beliefs	By the end of the program, 80% of parents will believe
	(a) The consequences of strep throat can be serious
	(b) A cure is available
	(c) They can take action leading to identification and treatment of strep throat
	(d) This series of steps will reduce the potential for further illness
Skills	By the end of the program, 70% of the parents will be able to
	(a) Swab the child's throat
	(b) Return the swab to the clinic laboratory

rants—an enabling factor for nonsmoking—has undoubtedly followed a diffusion curve. Analyses of smoking support the view that "nonsmokers' rights" are an extremely important influence on current trends of decreasing smoking in the population. Reactions to smokers by nonsmokers—fueled by the nonsmokers' rights movement—can be considered reinforcing factors for nonsmoking. Attitudes and behaviors that support nonsmokers' rights have probably also followed a diffusion curve.

SUMMARY

This chapter examines the factors affecting behavior and the environment as these relate to health. We call this phase of PRECEDE the educational and ecological assessment because we identify those factors on which health education and community organization can have a direct and immediate influence and thereby an indirect influence on behavior or environment. Three sets of factors are identified—predisposing, reinforcing, and enabling. Each plays an important role in health-related behavior and organization. After identifying the factors, we suggest

TABLE 5-3

These examples of learning and resource objectives are based on reinforcing and enabling factors analyzed in Table 5-1

Problem	Teaching preschool personnel to reinforce and enable parents to swab sore throats of children

Target Group: Preschool Personnel

Learning objectives for reinforcement	By the end of the program period, 90% of the preschool personnel will (a) Verbally reinforce mothers for swabbing their children's throats within 3 days of the initial manifestation of sore throat (b) Verbally reinforce mothers for returning swabs to the clinic laboratory (c) Inquire of parents about the results of throat swabs (d) Inform parents that prescriptions are available at the clinic (e) Administer prescribed medication according to parents' and physicians' instructions (f) Inform other parents when a positive throat culture occurs in a preschool child
Resource objectives for environmental enabling factors	By the end of the program period, 100% of the time the following will be made available by preschool personnel for parents' use: (a) Throat swab kits (b) Thermometers (c) Laboratory slips for throat cultures

how to assess their relative importance and changeability. Use of these two criteria allows one to prioritize the various causes of health behavior. Then, related learning and organizational objectives can be stated so that health promotion programs can focus where they will do the most good in facilitating development of or changes in behavior and environment.

Formulation of learning objectives follows from the identification of predisposing factors and skills; development of organizational and resource objectives follows from the identification of reinforcing and enabling factors.

EXERCISES

1. For one of the high-priority behaviors you selected in the previous chapter, make an inventory of all the predisposing, enabling, and reinforcing factors you can identify. For a priority environmental condition, list the enabling factors.

2. Rate each factor believed to cause the health behavior or environmental condition according to its importance and changeability. Give each factor a rating of low, medium, or high on each criterion.
3. Write learning or resource objectives for the highest-priority predisposing factor, enabling factor, and reinforcing factor.

NOTES AND CITATIONS

1. Andersen, 1968; Green, 1974, 1984a, 1984b; Green, Rimer & Elwood, 1981. See the first and second edition of this book for other historical and theoretical roots of the Precede model. For a searchable bibliography of more than 750 published applications of this framework, visit http://www.ihpr.ubc.ca/preapps.html.

2. Prochaska, 1994; Prochaska, DiClemente, & Norcross, 1992; Prochaska, Norcross, & DiClemente, 1994; For an application of the Stages of Change in conjunction with the Precede-Proceed model, see Grueninger, 1995; Grueninger, Duffy, & Goldstein, 1995. For critiques of the theory and its application, see Bandura, 1997; Lechner, Brug, & Mudde, 1998.

3. E. B. Fisher et al., 1996, p. 371. For other Precede analyses of educational and ecological determinants of behavior and environments influencing asthma, see W. C. Bailey et al., 1987; Boulet, Belanger, & Lajoie, 1996; Boulet, Chapman, Green, & FitzGerald, 1994; H. Cohen, Harris, & Green, 1979; Fireman, Friday, Gira, Vierthaler, & Michaels, 1981; Green, 1974; Green & Frankish, 1994; Hindi-Alexander & Cropp, 1981; Maiman, Green, Gibson, & Mackenzie, 1979; Mesters, Meertens, Crebolder, & Parcel, 1993; Taggart et al., 1991.

4. Heath, 1996.

5. N. H. Gottlieb & Green, 1987; Green, Simons-Morton, & Potvin, 1997; G. A. Kaplan & Lynch, 1997; Tillgren, Haglund, & Romelsjo, 1996.

6. Pasick, 1997.

7. French & Jeffery, 1995; Gritz, Nielsen, & Brooks, 1996.

8. Bandura, 1982; Baranowski, Perry, & Parcel, 1997, esp. p. 164; Parcel et al., 1995; Sallis et al., 1988; Strecher, DeVellis, Becker, & Rosenstock, 1986; Thomas, Cahill, & Santilli, 1997.

9. For a discussion of the converging research and philosophical perspectives on the ways knowledge and knowing relate to health promotion, see Weare, 1992.

10. M. H. Becker & Joseph, 1988; Wang, Ephross, & Green, 1975.

11. Boulet, Chapman, Green, & FitzGerald, 1994.

12. Awareness or new knowledge sometimes appear to be the only thing required to get a change in behavior in those situations where the other predisposing, enabling, and reinforcing factors are already in place. A case study of the Ford Motor Company's medical screening and surveillance program notes, "Although there is little evidence that information alone achieves behavior change . . . considerable evidence exists to indicate that, in some kinds of situations, information is all that is needed to provide behavior change. . . . This was such a case." Quotation from Ware, 1985, p. 321.

13. Abelson et al., 1968.

14. For reviews of the various theories of intrapersonal or psychological dynamics in health education and health promotion, see P. Bennett & Hodgson, 1992; Rimer, 1997; B. G. Simons-Morton, Greene, & Gottlieb, 1995; K. Tones & Tilford, 1994, esp. pp. 87–103.

15. The classic study that put this model on the health education map was reported in Hochbaum, 1956, 1959. The model soon changed shape when applied to another set of problems concerning immunization, substituting belief in susceptibility for belief that one could have a disease and

not know it, which had been featured as the most important belief accounting for seeking screening examinations. See Rosenstock, 1974; Rosenstock, Derryberry, & Carriger, 1959.

16. Becker, 1974; Janz & Becker, 1984; Maiman et al., 1977. For a review and critique of studies testing the Health Belief Model, see J. A. Harrison, Mullen, & Green, 1992. For a validation of its predictive power in relation to other models, including PRECEDE, which encompasses the Health Belief Model, see P. D. Mullen, Hersey, & Iverson, 1987.

17. Most recent examples are cited here. For more extensive and earlier bibliographic references on applications and tests of the Health Belief Model in each of these areas, see the previous edition of this book or Harrison, Mullen, & Green, 1992; Strecher & Rosenstock, 1997.

18. Bakker, Buunk, & van Den Eijnden, 1997; Basen-Enquist, 1992; Lollis, Johnson, & Antoni, 1997; Lux & Petosa, 1994; Rosenstock, Strecher, & Becker, 1994.

19. Brock & Beazley, 1995.

20. Daniel & Green, 1995.

21. Webb, Sanson-Fisher, & Bowman, 1988; T. Y. Wong & Seet, 1998.

22. Deeds & Gunatilake, 1989.

23. Haber, 1994; Padilla & Bulcavage, 1991.

24. Mirotznik, Ginzler, & Baptiste, 1998; Ureda, 1993.

25. Neumark-Sztainer & Story, 1996.

26. W. C. Bailey et al., 1987; Green & Frankish, 1994.

27. Black, 1980.

28. Calnan & Moss, 1984.

29. Rundall & Wheeler, 1979b.

30. Marlenga, 1995.

31. Richardson, Simons-Morton, & Annegers, 1993.

32. Ellickson & Bell, 1990b.

33. Salazar, 1985; See also Haynes, Taylor, & Sackett, 1979; Table 5 (pp. 458–459) and pp. 103–109 for a summary of the early studies supporting and those not supporting relationships between the Health Belief Model and various compliance outcomes.

34. Green, Eriksen, & Schor, 1988. See also Chapter 11 for related applications of the Health Belief Model.

35. Tirrell & Hart, 1980.

36. Wurtele, Roberts, & Leeper, 1982.

37. Rayant & Sheiham, 1980.

38. Kielhofner & Nelson, 1983.

39. Riggs & Noland, 1983.

40. Mullen, Hersey, & Iverson, 1987; Sommers, Andres, & Price, 1995.

41. Langlie, 1977.

42. Green & Lewis, 1986.

43. King, 1984.

44. Lux & Petosa, 1994.

45. Airhihenbuwa, 1995; Neumark-Sztainer & Story, 1996; Skinner & Kreuter, 1997, esp. pp. 56–59.

46. H. Becker, Hendrickson, & Shaver, 1998; Risker & Christopher, 1995; Szykman, Bloom, & Levy, 1997.

47. Berman & Wandersman, 1990; Botvin, Schinke, & Orlandi, 1995; Keesling & Friedman, 1995; Rosen & Schulkin, 1988; Rowe, 1988; van der Pligt, 1998; Witte, 1994.

48. Lalonde, 1974, p. 8.

49. This approach to audience segmentation and analysis is central to the marketing and social marketing fields. For examples of this application within the Precede model, see Bonaguro & Miaoulis, 1983; De Pietro, 1987; esp. pp. 105–107; Glanz & Rimer, 1995; Kotler & Roberto, 1989, pp. 282–294; Lefebvre et al., 1995; Miaoulis & Bonaguro, 1980–1981; J. A. Smith & Scammon, 1987.

50. Mucchielli, 1970, p. 30.

51. Kirscht, 1974.

52. Rokeach, 1970.

53. Osgood, Cuci, & Tannenbaum, 1961.

54. Baranowski, Perry, & Parcel, 1997; Bowler & Morisky, 1983; N. M. Clark, 1987; Green, Levine, & Deeds, 1975; Parcel & Baranowski, 1981; Strecher, DeVillis, Becker, & Rosenstock, 1986.

55. Clarke, Patrick, & Durham, 1995; Maibach & Murphy, 1995; McAuley, Mihalko, & Bane, 1997; Peterson & Stunkard, 1989; K. W. Smith, McGraw, & McKinlay, 1996.

56. Barlow, Williams, & Wright, 1996; Burglehaus, Smith, Sheps, & Green, 1997; J. A. Johnson, 1996; Lev & Owen, 1996; F. M. Lewis, 1987; Lorig, 1996; Lorig & Laurin, 1985; Parle, Maguire, & Heaven, 1997; Schwarzer & Scroder, 1997; Taal, Rasker, & Wiegman, 1996.

57. First International Conference on Health Promotion, 1986.

58. Bandura, 1982.

59. Schunk & Carbonari, 1984, p. 230.

60. Condiotte & Lichtenstein, 1981; Glasgow, Schafer, & O'Neill, 1981.

61. Marlatt & Gordon, 1985; Strecher, DeVillis, Becker, & Rosenstock, 1986.

62. Kingsley & Shapiro, 1977; Love, Davoli, & Thurman, 1996; Parcel, Green, Bettes, 1989.

63. Buller et al., 1989; Chung & Elias, 1996; De Vries, Dijkstra, & Kuhlman, 1988; R. I. Evans et al., 1981; Jaffe, 1997. However, more skeptical conclusions about this application have been drawn from critical reviews of the literature and his own effectiveness study in southern California by Flay, 1987, esp. pp. 159–161.

64. Brug, Glanz, & Kok, 1997; DuCharme & Brawley, 1995; Love, Davoli, & Thurman, 1996; Sallis et al., 1988; Shannon, Kirkley, Ammerman, & Simpson, 1997.

65. Bernier & Avard, 1986; S. M. Glynn & Ruderman, 1986.

66. Ajzen & Fishbein, 1980; Ajzen & Madden, 1986.

67. Sogaard, 1988.

68. Bauman & Chenoweth, 1984; Chassin, Presson, et al., 1984; DeVries, Dijkstra, & Kuhlman, 1988; Flynn, Goldstein, & Dana, 1998; A. O. Goldstein, Cohen, & Munger, 1997; Jaccard, 1975; Newman & Martin, 1982; Page & Gold, 1983; Secker-Walker, Flynn, & Solomon, 1996.

69. Kok & Siero, 1985.

70. Rise & Wilhelmsen, 1998; London, 1982; McCarty, Morrison, & Mills, 1983.

71. Budd, Bleiner, & Spencer, 1983; Buunk, Bakker, & Yzer, 1998; Godin, Lambert, & Locker, 1997; Lacy, 1981.

72. Budd, North, & Spencer, 1984; Farlay, Haddad, & Brown, 1996.

73. Jaccard, 1975, p. 158.

74. DeVries & Kok, 1986.

75. P. D. Mullen, Hersey, & Iverson, 1987. Other applications of the behavioral intention concept within PRECEDE include Liburd & Bowie, 1989; Ostwald & Rothenberger, 1985; Padilla & Bulcavage, 1991; Salazar, 1985; J. A. Smith & Scammon, 1987.

76. Chassin et al., 1981; Engels, Knibbe, & de Haan, 1997; McCaul et al., 1982.

77. D. R. Black, Tobler, & Sciacca, 1998; Botvin & Eng, 1982; Hermann & McWhirter, 1997. For reviews of the studies in this vein, see Flay, 1987; Gerstein & Green, 1993, pp. 76–117.

78. Parcel, 1976; Sobel & Hornbacher, 1973. See, for example, the 22 skills contributing to self-management ability in children and adolescents outlined by Thoresen & Kirmil-Gray, 1983. Some applications of PRECEDE in developing skills include Daltroy et al., 1993; Fireman, Friday, Gira, Vierthaler, & Michaels, 1981; Hubbal, 1996; Lomas, 1993; Mann & Putnam, 1989, 1990; Mann, Putnam, Lindsay, & Davis, 1990; McKell, 1996; Nguyen et al., 1995; Schumann & Mosley, 1994; Taggart et al., 1991; M. L. Wong, Chan, Koh, & Wong, 1994–95, 1996.

79. See Chapters 6, 8, and 9 for more on these social-action skills.

80. Milio, 1976, p. 436. See also Milio, 1983.

81. D. G. Simons-Morton, Parcel, Brink, Harvey, & Tiernan, 1991. This and the other CDC Handbooks listed in subsequent citations each applies the Precede model to the assessment of needs and the planning of interventions for selected health problems and target populations. They provide detailed procedural guidelines on collecting and analyzing the data necessary to arrive at efficient judgments about the behavioral determinants and the predisposing, enabling, and reinforcing factors for behavioral change. Other applications of PRECEDE-PROCEED in assessing enabling factors in tobacco control include C. Boyd, 1993; Fawcett et al., 1997; Glenn, 1994; Hofford & Spelman, 1996; Lipnickey, 1986; Paradis et al., 1995; Parcel et al., 1989, 1995; Polcyn, Price, Jurs, & Roberts, 1991; Pucci & Haglund, 1994; Sanders-Phillips, 1996; Sun & Sun, 1995; Zhang & Qiu, 1993.

82. B. G. Simons-Morton, Brink, Parcel, et al., 1989. Other applications of PRECEDE-PROCEED in assessing enabling factors and other determinants of alcohol-related behavior include Donovan, 1991; Higgins & MacDonald, 1992; Hunnicutt, Newman, Davis, & Crawford, 1993; Kraft, 1988; Newman, Martin, & Weppner, 1982; B. G. Simons-Morton, Brink, Simons-Morton, et al., 1989; Stivers, 1994; Vertinsky & Mangham, 1991; Villas, Cardenas, & Jameson, 1994.

83. Mowatt, Isaly, & Thayer, 1985.

84. D. G. Simons-Morton et al., 1988.

85. Botvin & Eng, 1982; Ellickson & Bell, 1990a; N. Gordon, 1986.

86. D. G. Simons-Morton et al., 1988.

87. M. I. Harrison, 1987; Huberman & Miles, 1984; Kaluzny, Schenck, & Ricketts, 1986; Kantor, 1983; Lippitt, Langseth, & Mossop, 1985; Porras & Hoffer, 1986.

88. Burt & Peterson, 1998; M. A. Clark, Kviz, & Warnecke, 1998; Sargent, Mott, & Stevens, 1998; Segall & Wynd, 1990.

89. Casswell, Stewart, & Duignan, 1989; Pucci, Joseph, & Siegel, 1998; C. Smith, Roberts, & Pendleton, 1988; Stoddard, Johnson, & Boley-Cruz, 1998; Wallack, 1983; Warner, 1986.

90. Godin & Shephard, 1990; Green, Cargo, & Ottoson, 1994; Rejeski, Brawley, & Thompson, 1997.

91. S. L. Bailey & Hubbard, 1990; Chassin, Mann, & Sher, 1988; Drellishak, 1997; Lindsey, 1997.

92. Best et al., 1988; Males, 1995; Sigelman, Goldenberg, & Dwyer, 1998.

93. Chassin, Corty, et al., 1984; Gerstein & Green, 1993.

94. Arkin, 1989; Gilmore & Campbell, 1996.

95. Arkin, 1989; Basch, 1987; Gilmore & Campbell, 1996. See Chapter 2 for more detail on focus-group methods and applications. For recent examples, see Manfredi, Lacey, & Balch, 1997; Moreno, Alvarado, & Forrest, 1997; Mwanga, Mugashe, & Aagaard-Hansen, 1998; Rafferty & Radosh, 1997.

96. Faden, 1987; McLeroy, Gottlieb, & Burdine, 1987.

97. Green, 1986b, 1994a.

98. Some authors refer to this level of needs assessment as *behavioral diagnosis* (the term we used for the previous phase of PRECEDE), but their intent is the same—to identify factors that influence behavior. See, for example, Arsham, 1980; Bartlett, 1982; Jenkins, 1979; Kanfer & Saslow, 1969.

99. For examples of analyses of behavioral determinants specific to ethnic and other demographic groups, see Epstein, Botvin, & Diaz, 1998; N. H. Gottlieb & Green, 1987; O'Loughlin, Paradis, & Gray-Donald, 1998; Winkleby, Kraemer, & Varady, 1998.

100. Zapka & Mamon, 1982.

101. Green & Lewis, 1986; see esp. Chapter 6 for inventories and references on instrument selection and development, and Appendix C (pp. 331–341) for a questionnaire developed for the National Survey of Personal Health Practices and Consequences and adapted for community-level application. A Canadian national survey, also based on the Precede factors, is described in Rootman, 1988. Other measures and exemplary survey instruments are found in Lorig et al., 1996. See also, Louis Harris and Associates, 1996; Lovato & Allensworth, 1989.

102. Phillips, Morrison, & Aday, 1998; Vissandjee, Barlow, & Fraser, 1997. Such local sources of data can be most illuminating when contrasted with state or national data. A review of national data sources for the United States, organized according to the Precede model factors influencing behavior, is provided by R. W. Wilson & Iverson, 1982.

103. See, for example, Brink, Simons-Morton, Parcel, & Tiernan, 1988.

104. Rokeach, 1970.

105. E. M. Rogers, 1995. More refined analyses of the rates of change and diffusion for the successive stages of change and for different innovations are suggested in Crow et al., 1986; Green, 1975.

Chapter 6

Administrative and Policy Assessment: Turning the Corner from PRECEDE to PROCEED

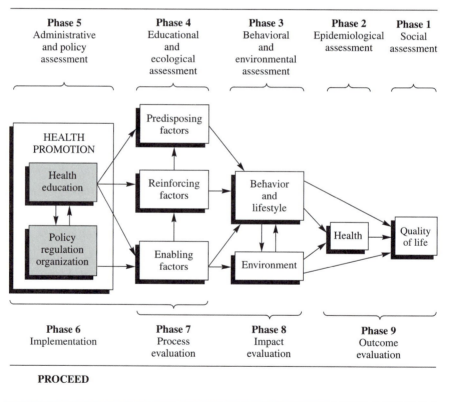

Phase 5	Phase 4	Phase 3	Phase 2	Phase 1
Administrative and policy assessment	Educational and ecological assessment	Behavioral and environmental assessment	Epidemiological assessment	Social assessment

Phase 6	Phase 7	Phase 8	Phase 9
Implementation	Process evaluation	Impact evaluation	Outcome evaluation

PROCEED

Once you have identified your program priorities, targets, and objectives, you stand on the threshold of converting these assessment results into program action. The success of implementation is greatly enhanced when organizational and policy supports of, as well as barriers to a proposed program, have been clearly identified and appropriately addressed. Some of the barriers will be internal structures in the implementing organization (or several organizations if the planning has involved a coalition). New policies, regulations, or administrative orders can overcome these barriers by reorganizing or reassigning responsibility within organizations. Other barriers may lie in the behavior or operating procedures of the implementing organization or other organizations whose cooperation is required. Here, the implementation of health promotion might gain cooperation through educating decision makers or negotiating exchange agreements. In some instances, enforcement of existing agreements, rules and laws, or advocacy and promotion of new regulatory legislation may be required at the local, state, or provincial level.

The primary purpose of this chapter[1] is to help you over that threshold by calling your attention to some key administrative and policy factors, specifically:

- The resources needed and available to launch and sustain your program
- The organizational barriers and facilitators that can effect program implementation
- The policies you can use to support your program or that need to be changed to enable the program to proceed

The insight you gain from this phase of the assessment process will help you put the final touches on your formal plan with a timetable, an assignment of resources and responsibilities, and a budget. With these final touches, you turn the corner from PRECEDE to PROCEED. In this phase, you also identify the specific **settings** in which health promotion activities must take place. The implementing organization may itself provide a setting for implementing the population focus of the program. The setting dictates the specific methods, materials, and other intervention components. We shall discuss the considerations for selecting appropriate methods to match the setting and the targets of change (predisposing, enabling, and reinforcing factors) in Chapters 8–12.

With a complete plan in hand, you PROCEED to implementation and evaluation, which draws immediately on the findings from the administrative assessment. Even though evaluation is an inherent, built-in aspect of the entire Precede-Proceed planning framework, an evaluation plan (see Chapter 7) also needs to be implemented and will require some level of similar policy, regulatory, and organizational support. *Policy, regulatory,* and *organizational* assessments (the "PRO" in PROCEED) are designed to reveal the enabling constructs for educational and ecological development (the "CEED" in PROCEED).

SOME DEFINITIONS

Before reviewing the key elements for the administrative assessment, we should consider some definitions. **Administrative assessment** refers here to an analysis of the policies, resources, and circumstances in an organizational setting that either facilitate or hinder the development of the health promotion program. **Policy** refers to the set of objectives and rules guiding the activities of an organization or an administration. **Regulation** refers to the act of enforcing policies, rules, or laws. It applies in health promotion particularly where existing policies are not being enforced to protect the health of some from the illegal behavior of others, such as in community actions against selling cigarettes to minors or drunk driving. It overlaps with **health protection,** but in health promotion it usually has more to do with behavior or the social environment than with the physical environment. **Organization** refers in this chapter to the act of marshaling and coordinating the resources necessary to implement a program. In Chapter 8, **community organization** will refer to the set of procedures and processes by which a population and its institutions mobilize to solve a common problem or pursue a common goal. **Implementation** refers here to the act of converting program objectives into actions through policy changes, regulation, and organization.

THE ADMINISTRATIVE ASSESSMENT

Having outlined methods on identifying educational and ecological determinants in Chapter 5, we shall turn now to the process of assessing the resources available to change those determinants. One begins at this stage and in later ones by matching the determinants of behavioral and environmental change to educational and organizational strategies and then budgeting the time and material resources to implement the methods and strategies. The detailed considerations of selecting or developing and implementing the methods and strategies will be addressed in the setting-specific chapters, because it is the setting or channel through which one will reach the population that dictates which methods and strategies are most appropriate. A comprehensive program may involve several settings, possibly all of the settings analyzed in Chapters 8–12. Representatives of those settings would ideally have been included in the planning processes leading up to this point; however, at times it only becomes clear at this point that a setting not previously involved needs to be a channel for the program. Involvement in this phase of planning can insure developers will address the resource requirements of such a setting.

STEP 1: ASSESSMENT OF RESOURCES NEEDED

The first step in administrative assessment is to review the resources required to implement the proposed educational methods and strategies. This entails an examination of the time frames for accomplishing the objectives and of the types and numbers of people needed to carry out the program.

Time. Because it is nonrenewable, the first and most critical resource is time. Once expended, time cannot be recovered. It is inflexible in its supply, and it affects the availability and cost of all other resources. Time required is estimated at several levels of PRECEDE with the formulation of realistic objectives. Each objective states the time (date) by which that objective needs to be accomplished in order for the next higher level objective to be accomplished. Thus, certain educational and organizational objectives must be accomplished before certain behavioral and environmental objectives can be expected to materialize, and these in turn must precede any palpable change in health or quality-of-life outcomes. For example, suppose you have established the following predisposing educational objectives:

> Within the first four months of a measles immunization program, parents in the target population will (1) show a 60% increase in their knowledge that a measles vaccine is available and (2) show a 50% increase in their belief that their children are susceptible to measles.

Your enabling objectives might include a 4-month target of dispatching 60 mobilized immunization stations, one in each school and shopping center in the community, and a 3-month target of obtaining commitments from 50 school principals and 10 shopping center managers. All these objectives must be accomplished within the time frames stated to achieve a behavioral objective of a 4% increase in schoolchildren receiving measles immunization (from 90% previously immunized to 94%) at the end of 6 months. (Because this is a onetime behavior, you need not bother with an objective for reinforcing factors.)

These objectives would clearly limit your time frame for implementing specific aspects of the program plan. A timetable or **Gantt chart** can be laid out as in Figure 6-1 to show graphically the start and finish dates for each activity. It also shows the sequence and overlap of activities in time, as well as the number of different activities that will be proceeding simultaneously during each period.[2]

From the Gantt chart in Figure 6-1, you could explicitly state the time requirements for each activity and compare them with those of every other activity. This allows an analysis not only of time requirements for each activity but also, reading down a column, of activity requirements for each period. Some activities are discrete events or actions that span less than a month. Others, such as the first and the last two in Figure 6-1, span a period of two or more units of time (the chart may be drawn in units of days, weeks, months, quarters, or years).

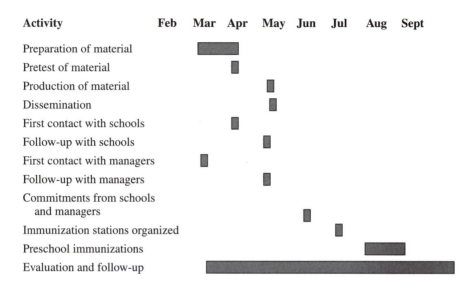

FIGURE 6-1

Time requirements can be graphed in the form of a Gantt chart to identify the specific periods when activities must be implemented, shown here for a school-entry immunization program.

This takes the administrative assessment of resources required to the second resource, personnel.

Personnel. Staffing requirements take precedence over other budgetary considerations in the resource analysis, because the personnel category generally constitutes the largest and most restricted line item in most budgets. People cost more than most resources and are more difficult to put in place than most equipment and material resources. Civil service and affirmative action hiring policies, union contracts, and due process in moving personnel all limit the flexibility and discretion with which you could mold this resource to your program needs. The personnel analysis is further complicated by the subtle considerations of talent, skills, personalities, and personal preferences and attitudes toward particular types of work to be done. The human resource frame for analysis of the interplay between an organization and its people emphasizes the skills, insights, ideas, energy, and commitment of people as the most important assets of an organization.[3]

A Gantt chart displaying your time analysis (Figure 6-1) can provide the basis for the first cut in analyzing personnel requirements. For example, the talents and skills of different personnel will quite likely be required at different times. You could define these in your situation by using the names of existing personnel; however, you would more properly define them by their function or

TABLE 6-1

Personnel loading can be charted for the example of the 6-month immunization program by attaching estimated hours for each category of worker to the tasks shown in Figure 6-1

	Week										Total
Person	1	2	3	4	5	6	7	8	9 ... 24		Hours
Administrator	20	20	20	20	20	20	20	20	20	...	480
Health educator	40	40	40	40	40	40	40	40	40	...	960
Medical consultant	8	8	8	4	4					30	62
Graphic artist	8		8								16
Nurses										800	800
Secretary	20	20	20	20	20	20	20	20	20	...	480

the professional, technical, administrative, or clerical skills required. Here it is often useful to break the Gantt chart into smaller units of time, say weeks, days, or even hours, depending on the overall duration and scope of the program. The quantitative analysis of personnel requirements then might take the form shown in Table 6-1.

Each activity in Figure 6-1 contains several subtasks, which are performed by different types of personnel. To move from a Gantt chart to a more specific understanding of the types of personnel and other costs required, you would consider the specific tasks or steps inherent in each activity.

For example, preparing material might require the following tasks or steps:

Research content of materials
Interview experts
Develop first draft
Review first draft
Prepare final draft

Pretesting—the next activity—might require some different tasks, such as:

Arrange pretest logistics—space, time, and so forth
Contact pretest participants
Document pretest reactions
Revise draft materials

Final production would require meeting with printers, reviewing final copy, and so on.

The estimate of personnel hours required each week enables planners to make a cost analysis of personnel, as well as a time allocation (loading) analysis that permits the administrator at the next higher level to consider where and when existing personnel might be reassigned to support the program without hiring new personnel. The personnel loading chart documents two sets of assumptions critical to effective project administration: (1) What types of staff members are needed? and (2) How many hours (or days) of each member's time are required to successfully complete each task and activity? In the example shown in Table 6-1, the personnel requirements include a half-time administrator and a full-time health education specialist throughout the program. The administrator might be a health education specialist with a master's degree and community experience. The other health educator, assigned to the communication and dissemination responsibilities, might hold a baccalaureate degree and have less experience. This kind of personnel analysis must be based on a matching of personnel with administrative, educational, technical, and organizational requirements dictated by the process objectives outlined in the previous chapter.

Budget. You can easily convert the time and personnel requirements into cost estimates by multiplying each line in the personnel loading chart by an average hourly wage or salary estimate for each category of worker. You might hire these personnel, borrow them from another program within the same organization, or contract for their services as consultants (e.g., the medical consultant and graphic artist, during the developmental phase, the two full-time nurses during the final 10 weeks). Whatever the method of payment, the hourly costs should be recorded in the budget requirement at this stage because these are real requirements and therefore real costs to be anticipated. If they prove too much for the organization, you can explore options for transfer of personnel, borrowing of personnel, recruitment of volunteers, donated services from other agencies, and other possibilities. If some of these can be contributed or volunteered hours in the final negotiation and allocation of responsibilities, they can be credited to the project as "in-kind" contributions mobilized by the organization or the community coalition. The more in-kind resources the proposed program can show it has raised, the more convincing the proposal will be as a community initiative to which organizations have a real commitment.

The other budgetary requirements will include personnel *benefits* for salaried workers (usually 20–25% of salaries for professional workers), plus materials or supplies, printing costs, postage, photocopying, telephone costs, equipment, data processing, and travel. In addition, most organizations have a fixed overhead or indirect cost rate such as 20% or 50%. This is an average maintenance rate they add to any direct cost estimate to provide for the administrative services of the front office, the rental and upkeep of the building and offices, utilities, and sometimes local telephone or other fixed costs of the offices in which special projects will be housed. For example, if the direct cost of a program is estimated at $10,000 in personnel time and materials, the budget might be $12,000 to cover the usual 20-percent overhead the agency has established as necessary from experience. See Table 6-2 for an example of a preliminary budget.

TABLE 6-2

Initial budget spreadsheets can be based on the foregoing analysis of requirements, estimated here based on 1998 costs or rates

Initial budget estimates based on analysis of resource requirements before assessment of resources available

Budget Items	Hours	Rate	Totals
Personnel			
Administrator	480	$29	$ 13,920
Health educator	960	23	22,080
Nurses	800	20	16,000
Secretary	480	14	6,720
Subtotal			$ 58,720
Personnel benefits (fringe) @20%			$ 11,744
Total personnel costs			**$ 70,464**
Supplies			
Printing brochure			$ 2,000
Postage (20,000 × .32)			6,400
Office supplies			300
Vaccination supplies (800 × $3)			2,400
Total supplies			**$ 11,100**
Services			
Telephone			$ 500
Photocopying			400
Consultants			
Data processing	25	$12	$ 300
Medical consultant	62	75	4,650
Graphic artist	16	25	400
Total services			**$ 6,250**
Travel			
Local (400 mi. @ .31)			$ 124
State conference ($650 air; $150 per diem)			800
Total travel			**$ 924**
Total Direct Costs			**$ 88,738**
Indirect Costs (20% of direct costs)			**$ 17,748**
Total Budget Estimate			**$ 106,486**

Attention to Detail. Whether preparing a budget for their organization or for an external grant application to support their program, planners must pay close attention to the requirements of the funding organization. For example, some funders limit the indirect cost rate that can be charged. Some prefer to see personnel time expressed as a percentage of the individual's annual work hours (to help gauge the level of commitment to the project), instead of being expressed as a number of project hours (as in Table 6-2). Some funders may even request both versions of personnel time—percent of time and project hours by task.

One should always be prepared to back up every line item in the budget with a more detailed version and narrative justification, even if one does not submit the detailed budgets. For example, if travel costs are listed as a lump sum on a summary project budget, that sum should be derived from estimates for the component parts—such as air travel, meals, ground transportation, and hotel costs—not a "ballpark guesstimate" for the broader category. Always review a project budget from the perspective of the reader, as with any written work, and ask these questions: Do the items make sense? Are any unusual items explained? Is there back-up documentation for each estimate?

Spreadsheet programs (such as Lotus 1-2-3 or Microsoft Excel) can help one create budget estimates and manipulate them ("what-if" analyses) to gauge the budgetary impact of different scenarios (e.g., another staff member, fewer brochures, more travel). Spreadsheet programs are generally faster and more accurate than is repeatedly entering numbers by hand on a calculator, but they still require careful data entry and double-checking of each total and subtotal. As you gain project experience, compare your initial budget estimates to actual expenditures to understand which items consistently have been underestimated (or overestimated), and adjust future budgets accordingly.

STEP 2: ASSESSMENT OF AVAILABLE RESOURCES

Part of the educational assessment identifies methods or materials appropriate to some of the educational objectives. Such materials and methods might need to be developed from scratch, as implied by the budget items in Table 6-2 for the development and printing of a brochure to blanket the community with information about measles and the need to immunize children before school starts. Sometimes the material has been developed in a previous program or by a national or state agency that can make the material available at little or no cost to one's agency. The costs saved by using centrally developed educational materials or materials developed previously for another program can sometimes reduce a budget considerably, but the materials might not be tailored well to the local situation or current circumstances. Such tradeoffs between costs and the ideal arrangements for your program will arise throughout the administrative and policy assessments.

Personnel. In most health promotion programs, you may find a common assumption: Existing personnel will suffice throughout the implementation of the program. If the preceding assessments, however, have produced a program design that requires more personnel than the sponsoring organization has available at its disposal, then you may want to consider the following options:

1. Identify and seek part-time commitments from personnel from other departments or units within your organization. If they are not authorized to allocate their own time, you will need commitments from their supervisors as well. Temporary arrangements of this kind are common when separate departments share common goals, which is often the case if the other department has the kind of personnel you need.

2. Retrain personnel within your department to take on tasks outside their usual scope.

3. Explore the potential for recruitment of volunteers from the community. Short-term programs, in particular, can tap the underutilized pool of talent and energy available for volunteer effort for a worthy cause.[4]

4. Explore the potential for cooperative agreements with other agencies or organizations in the community in order to fill in the gaps in your personnel. Be sure your organization can reciprocate in the future.

5. Develop a grant proposal for funding, partial funding, or matched funding of your program by a government agency, philanthropic foundation, or corporate donor. The work you will have done in following the Precede planning process follows the logical format most granting agencies wish to see in an application. With the addition of your evaluation plan and final budget request, you will have a grant application in hand.

6. Appeal directly to the public for donations.

7. Price the service at a cost-recovery level of fees you will charge some or all users of the services. With options 6 and 7, you must be cautious that you stay within affordable limits, that you stay within range of market value for the services, and that you provide assurances that those in your priority target groups who might not be able to afford the services will still have access to them.

8. If none of the previous options seems appropriate, feasible, or sufficient, and if the program represents a permanent or long-term commitment of the organization, then you may justifiably pursue policy changes in the organization such that a more fundamental reorganization or redistribution of resources to your department or unit would be established before embarking on the program.

Other Budgetary Constraints. The foregoing options for augmenting personnel might apply to some other resources available from other departments or organizations as financial or in-kind contributions to the program.[5] They represent the main courses of action you can pursue singly or in combination to close the gap between resources required and resources available within your organization to carry out the desired program.

When you cannot find resources, the fallback position, of course, is to trim the sails on your program plan and propose more modest objectives and less powerful methods of intervention. Because this course represents a compromise of the plan, you should undertake it only with due consideration to the consequences for the integrity of the plan. Specific questions you should ask before giving up too many parts of the plan or levels of intervention with budget cuts include the following:

1. *The threshold level:* Will the reduced level of resources still allow enough intervention to reach a threshold of impact that will achieve subsequent objectives? The notion of a threshold level of resources suggests that there is a minimum level of investment below which the program will be too weak to achieve a useful result.[6] Only a few documented examples of such levels in actual programs[7] support this theoretical notion.

2. *The point of diminishing returns:* Is there a point of diminishing returns beyond which additional resources do not necessarily achieve commensurate gains in impact or outcome? If so, fewer resources might not hinder the achievement of at least some benefits. This, too, is a largely theoretical concept in health education and health promotion.[8] The same studies cited in the previous paragraph contain the limited data available on points of diminishing returns.

3. *Critical elements:* Does the program plan have a critical element without which the objectives cannot be achieved? If so, will the budget cut or shortage of resources preclude achieving that one objective or element? In a work-site program to reduce lower-back injuries in nurses, for example, one might determine that everything that can be done in the program depends on the nurses having release time from their duties to participate in the educational and exercise training program. If the hospital cannot provide such time for these nurses, the director of occupational health would be advised not to proceed with the program.

4. *Critical expectations:* Can the target levels of the objectives be lowered without jeopardizing the integrity of the program or the expectations of the constituents or sponsors of the program? If the behavioral change target of immunization can be reduced from 94% to 92% for schoolchildren without risking a major outbreak of measles, the savings in outreach resources could be considerable. This is because, as we have seen in the earlier discussions of diffusion theory, the **late adopters** are harder for a program to reach than the **late majority.** An equivalent reduction in the target levels during the early phases of a program, say from 14% to 10%, would not yield a commensurate cost savings because early adopters are easier to reach than late ones.

5. *Critical timing and cash flow:* Can the target dates for the objectives be set back to spread the program effort over a longer period? By itself, this will not save resources in the long run, but it will reduce costs in the initial year by shifting them to later periods. The initial costs could be the major budgetary barrier because of temporary fiscal circumstances. By slowing the pace of the program implementation, some outlays could be delayed in anticipation of better budgetary times. This amounts to an adjustment of "cash flow."

6. *Critical population segments:* Can the types of people selected as priority target groups be reordered to give lower priority to the hard to reach? This is too often the most tempting adjustment in underfunded programs. Those who need the program the most are often the most expensive to reach and can least afford to subsidize the program with fees for service. This sometimes leads to a decision to make the underbudgeted program available on a first-come, first-served basis. This should be a last resort in accepting a reduced budget because the integrity of the longer-term objectives, including objectives to reduce disparities and increase equity, will likely be compromised. Although they cost more to reach per unit of education or service delivered, the poorer and more isolated segments of the target population will gain more in health improvement because they have more to gain if they are effectively reached.

STEP 3: ASSESSMENT OF FACTORS INFLUENCING IMPLEMENTATION

Besides the availability of resources, a host of other factors may enhance or hinder the smooth **implementation** of your program plan. Chase, among others, has listed the key obstacles to implementation.[9] A thoughtful implementation plan is not complete without a careful assessment of those factors, including a provision that assets and barriers can be acknowledged publicly. Clearly, some barriers will be essentially attitudinal or political or reflect power relationships that you cannot politely make a matter of public record in your formal plan, but you ignore them at the peril of your program.

Staff Commitment and Attitudes. Before a plan is complete, it needs to make the rounds of comment and suggestions from those who will have a role in implementing it, especially if they have not been directly involved in formulating the plan up to this point. Staff members of the implementing agencies will be in the best position to anticipate barriers in their various roles and will welcome the opportunity to point out some of the pitfalls in your plan *before* you ask them to implement it. Though they may not have participated earlier in the planning, their involvement at this stage is essential to their commitment to the objectives and methods of the program. It does not guarantee their commitment, but without their participation in planning, their commitment and their attitude toward the program are almost certain to be undependable.

Program Goal(s). Plans that require changes in standard operating procedures place the goals and objectives of the new plans into question. If these conflict with previously accepted goals and objectives, you must resolve the conflict by clarifying priorities.[10] As Ross and Mico put it, "The goals must accord with the client system's existing policy."[11]

Rate of Change. Incremental change is easier to implement than radical, ambitious, nonincremental changes.[12] Break your program plan's implementation steps down into small, manageable pieces.[13]

Familiarity. Are the procedures and methods to be employed familiar to staff members who must implement them? Do they depart radically from standard operating procedures? Even if skills are not at issue, unfamiliar methods and procedures require careful introduction and orientation to avoid being rejected, ignored, or poorly implemented.[14]

Complexity. A change requiring multiple transactions or complex relationships and coordination will be more difficult to implement than will single-action or single-person procedures.[15]

Space. One of the most precious commodities in many organizations is office space. If your program plan proposes to use existing office space for another purpose or to move staff members from one space to another, you will likely step on someone's toes. Space should be treated as a resource to be allocated according to rules or procedures similar to those suggested earlier for personnel and other budgetary items.

Community Circumstances. Beyond your own organization, the community will respond to your proposed program at several levels. The principle of participation, emphasized throughout the previous chapters, should alert one to the need to weigh the community's assets and barriers as one moves through the planning process. Inevitably, even among those who have participated in the planning process, some people will express misgivings about how the new program will affect them and their programs. Some of these misgivings will translate into passive resistance, some into subtle efforts to minimize, discredit, or even sabotage the program. The best protection against these defensive maneuvers in the community, besides education and earlier involvement in the planning, is to invite those organizations most threatened by the program to be cosponsors or collaborators. If, for whatever reason, early engagement and involvement did not occur, it is never too late to invite others to share in the credit and the public visibility of the program in exchange for their support.

Even the most thoughtful strategic plan will probably not be able to take all assets, potential barriers, and sources of opposition into account. What then? The remaining barriers and sources of support to be assessed can be considered broader political and structural barriers. These must be addressed in the final diagnostic phase, and some of them can only be changed through external political processes because they lie beyond the direct control of one's agency.

Table 6-3 groups several variables according to four general categories: policy, the implementing organization, the political milieu, and the environment. Notice that each variable, depending upon the circumstances, can be a positive, facilitating force or a negative, hindering one.

Quality Assurance, Training, and Supervision. When you board a jetliner, you probably trust that the pilot and crew have the competence and skill to get you to your destination. Your confidence has been established because airlines have to adhere to tested standards and are committed to ongoing in-service training to assure high-quality performance in those who operate and maintain the aircraft. In the same sense, the effective implementation of a health promotion program requires competence and skill on the part of those delivering the program. Findings from the School Health Curriculum Project revealed that the teachers implemented only 34% of the teaching and learning activities in the curriculum as they were intended to be implemented.[16] This suggests the need for monitoring the implementation process as the first step in process evaluation (see Chapter 7). It also suggests that policies and programs must provide for professional discretion and options so that they can be adapted to local situations and changing circumstances. Training and supervision of personnel provide the best assurance of implementation. Each training program is an educational program in itself and deserves a similar planning process to that described by the behavioral, environmental, and educational assessments in the Precede framework. Supervision can also be approached as an educational process: Behavior change goals can be set mutually by the supervisor and supervisee. Factors predisposing, enabling, and reinforcing the intended behavior can be analyzed periodically; interventions can be planned to predispose, enable, and reinforce implementation through staff meetings, training, written materials, and rewards for high performance. Examples of PRECEDE applied to professional training and **quality assessment** in the medical care setting will be presented in Chapter 11.

POLICY ASSESSMENT

In Chapter 5, we identified various enabling factors that influence high-priority health behaviors. We also examined how to assess resources for the selected educational methods that help develop skills required to enable the behavior and some community organization methods that make resources more accessible to

TABLE 6-3

Effects of policy, organizational, and political factors on implementation are shown here as either facilitating or hindering implementation

| Variables | Effects on Implementation | |
	Positive or Facilitating	Negative or Hindering
Policy		
Theory	Solid	Unproven
Assumptions	Defined	Unclear
Goals	Stated	Nonexistent
Change		
Amount	Small	Large
Rate	Incremental	Ambitious
Familiarity	Familiar	Unfamiliar
Centrality	Central	Peripheral
Complexity	Few transactions	Many transactions
Resources	Available	Nonexistent
Specification	Some	None
Flexibility	Alternative solutions	One right answer
Impact	Early stages	Later stages
Implementing organization		
Structure		
Goal	Relevant to policy	Irrelevant to policy
Task	Suitable	Unsuitable
Scale	Small	Large
Climate	Supportive	Unsupportive
Technical capacity		
Technology	Appropriate	Inappropriate
Resources	Available	Unavailable
Employee disposition		
Approach	Problem solving	Opportunistic
Motivation	Maintained	Declines
Values	Congruent	Incongruent
Attitudes	Favorable	Unfavorable
Beliefs	Faith in policy	No faith in policy
Employee behavior	Changeable	Resistant
Political milieu		
Power		
Strength	Strong	Weak
Support	Present	Absent
Environment		
Timing	"Right"	"Wrong"
Intended beneficiaries	Needs	No needs
Other organizations	Controllable	Uncontrollable

SOURCE: Adapted from "Reconciling Concept and Context: Theory of Implementation," by J. M. Ottoson and L. W. Green, 1987, in W. B. Ward and M. H. Becker (Eds.), *Advances in Health Education and Promotion,* vol. 2, Greenwich, CT: JAI Press; used with permission of the publisher.

people whose motivation to act is frustrated by the inaccessibility of such factors. We presented still other enabling factors that direct educational efforts or appeals to the community cannot be expected to change because they involve legal, political, or environmental conditions more or less "locked in" by existing policies or regulations. These issues constitute the focus of the policy assessment.

STEP 1: ASSESSMENT OF THE ORGANIZATIONAL MISSION, POLICIES, AND REGULATIONS

Before implementing a plan, one needs to know how it fits with existing organizational mission, policies, and regulations. Some of the barriers identified in the preceding administrative assessment may also have revealed incompatibilities between organizational mandates and the plan. Be aware that most organizations operate under a blend of formal and informal mandates—most of which are not set in stone. Conflicts might arise also with the policies of a collaborating organization or group. In the face of such incompatibilities, one has three choices: (1) to adapt the proposed plan to be consistent with the organizational mission and policies, (2) to seek to change the policy or organizational mandate, or (3) some of both.

Being Informed. Before choosing a course of action, one must understand the mission and culture of the organization. If new to the organization, one would be wise to follow the tenets of "primary prevention" by taking advantage of the customary orientation sessions offered new employees. One should read the organization's annual report, examine its vision and mission statements, and take the time to visit with veteran employees who have an "institutional memory." If the plan is consistent with existing policy and organizational mandates, one can strengthen it by documenting and communicating more effectively the specific policies it serves and the ways the plan and policies can support each other. Many new program plans are announced with an opening line invoking the organizational policy that authorizes or justifies the proposed program. The preamble to most new government plans or regulations, for example, will cite the authorizing legislation or statute that makes the plan necessary or possible. This kind of preface or covering memo is often signed by the director or chief executive officer, giving the plan not only the force of legislation or policy but also the prestige or authority of the chief administrator.

Anticipating. One's plan can be in alignment with the organization's mission but *inconsistent* or at odds with a policy or position held by stakeholders or an influential organization. Health practitioners concerned with violence prevention, comprehensive school health, HIV/AIDS education, and tobacco control have learned the value of anticipating the reactions of these groups early in the planning process.

**ANTICIPATING AND OVERCOMING BARRIERS:
A PRACTICAL EXAMPLE IN MANAGED CARE**

Identifying barriers to program implementation is one thing, taking action to overcome them is another. Imagine that a handful of physicians and health workers at one of the largest HMOs in the United States wanted to develop and implement a program of health promotion services appropriate for the clinical setting. Suppose further that as they conceptualized their plan, they identified the following familiar barriers:

1. The health care system and its culture limit flexibility for physicians, and the intention to help alone is inadequate justification for change.
2. Time constraints and patient demand make the physician's job one of responding to complaints, not one of initiating preventive action.
3. Feedback from preventive care is negative or neutral (e.g., the physician does not receive feedback about whether late-stage breast cancer was averted by promoting mammography).

These are precisely the barriers identified by Thompson and his colleagues at the Group Health Cooperative (GHC) in Puget Sound, Washington. In 1995, two decades after implementing their initiative, the GHC team presented the findings from their 20 years of experience providing clinical preventive health promotion services, using the Precede-Proceed model as

Failure to address the concerns of groups with conflicting policy perspectives can have serious negative consequences, such as budget cuts or conflicts with key decision makers or legislators. Addressing such a situation after the fact is inevitably an uphill battle. By anticipating a potential conflict, planners can rely on their negotiation and communication skills, their political acumen, and the scientific and theoretical soundness of their plan to achieve support for the proposed outcome.

For example, imagine an HIV/AIDS prevention effort that includes a school health education component, planning in a region with some history of ultraconservative groups organizing campaigns to derail any school program pertaining to sexuality. Although small in number, these groups are well organized, vocal, and typically make unsubstantiated, and often false, accusations about the content and intentions of such programs. For example, they may claim that school-based HIV/AIDS programs lead to an increase in sexual activity among participating students. By anticipating such claims, program planners can, early in the planning process, educate community residents by sharing with them a well-documented the conceptual basis for their interventions at the organizational and patient level.[17] Thompson and his co-workers reported the following outcomes: late-stage breast cancer was reduced by 32%; 89% of 2-year-old children had complete immunizations; the proportion of adult smokers decreased from 25% to 17% (1985–1994); and bicycle safety helmet use among children increased from 4% to 48% (1987–1992).

According to Thompson, these outcomes were achieved only after they had assessed, and developed a strategy to overcome, the aforementioned organizational barriers. A key element in their strategy was to establish, early on in the planning process, a GHC-wide committee on prevention. One of the principal purposes of this committee, which comprised representatives from virtually every interest group within the organization, was to "foster dialogue on prevention issues and to develop guidelines and program recommendations."[18] In the face of potential organizational barriers, the successful formulation and management of the committee seemed to accomplish two things. One was increased dedication within the organization through the active participation and involvement of representatives across the GHC. The second was a legitimization of the program through the development of guidelines and standards for disease prevention and health promotion. This example highlights the practical relevance of working through an administrative assessment. It also offers another important, subtle reminder. Even in the earliest stages of planning, experienced practitioners have their antennae out—sensitive to potential barriers and ever cognizant of resource needs.

evaluation of a school-based program designed to reduce HIV infection among adolescents in New York and Chicago. Gutmacher and colleagues found that making condoms available does significantly increase the use of condoms among sexually active teens. Their data also showed that "making condoms available does not encourage students who have never had sex to become sexually active."[19] Armed with credible documentation, experienced planners can, through their continuous interaction with the community, warn residents to be on the alert for false claims by special interest groups and preempt false accusations that are likely to follow.

Flexibility. The first question one can ask about any policy that appears to be inconsistent with a program plan is, How flexible is that policy? Most good policies are flexible because it is impossible to know in advance all the problems and opportunities an implementing organization or program will face.[20] The best test of flexibility is to find a previous program implemented under the policy and to examine its deviations, if any, from the policy. This will provide one with both an indicator of flexibility and a precedent to cite in defending one's request for an exception or waiver of policy. If the previous implementation experience was uniformly or mostly positive, one may have a reason to invoke the policy in support of the program, but flexibility might still be the reason other programs flourished under the policy.

STEP 2: ASSESSING POLITICAL FORCES

How do political forces influence the planning or implementation of a health promotion program? Any time finite resources have to be allocated among several programs but the decision makers do not agree on the distribution of those finite resources, politics will likely influence ultimate decision. Specifically, decisions will be influenced by what the decision makers do or do not know about the goals and content of the competing programs and also by how their friends or constituents value the proposed program. Planners should consider the following principles as they assess the very real political forces that shape policies and, therefore, their programs.

Level of Analysis. The political milieu can be analyzed at both the intraorganizational[21] and the interorganizational level.[22] Most of the suggestions for intraorganizational analysis and change that can be considered legitimate activities of the salaried insider have been presented in the foregoing sections of this chapter. If one attempts to bring about change in another organization as an outsider, one has a greater need and justification for employing political methods, because organizations resist change from without. In health promotion, the interorganizational level of analysis is particularly important, because many of the programs and policies needed to alter lifestyles and environments are controlled by multiple organizations, some of them entirely outside the health sector.

Much of the community organization literature in health deals with the development of cooperation between organizations within the health sector.[23] In his durable definition of community organization, Ross emphasizes the cooperative element. He defines it as "a process by which a community identifies its needs or objectives, ranks these needs or objectives, develops the confidence and will to work at these objectives, finds the resources (internal and external) to do so, and in so doing, extends and develops cooperative and collaborative attitudes and practices in the community."[24] The World Health Organization's *Health for All* strategy is a classic example of a global effort to encourage cooperation while placing a strong emphasis on "intersectoral" coordination in health policies.[25] Many of the case studies of how such intersectoral action has been developed in health promotion come from nutrition programs involving public and private sector cooperation in Australia[26] and the United States.[27]

The Zero-Sum Game. Contrary to the cooperation model of community organization, the political conflict perspective assumes that multiple, *independent* actors are in conflict over goals, resources, and actions. Parochial priorities, goals, interests, stakes, and deadlines determine their perceptions.[28] The actors see the stakes as a fixed pool of resources to be divided among the political sides. This means each transaction results in a gain for someone that is won at someone else's expense—a zero-sum game with a winner and a loser.

Systems Approach. Blending a systems approach with a political perspective, the separate actors with their separate goals are seen not as independent but as *interdependent.*[29] This means that one's gain need not be another's loss, because both depend on each other's success to make the community or system function effectively. Indeed, anyone's loss is everyone's loss, with perhaps a few exceptions. One exception occurs where two or more individuals or organizations have identical goals and depend on the same limited resources to pursue them. If both seek to maximize their goal without consideration for the other and exhaust the finite resources on which both depend, then the other must suffer. Such is the purely competitive marketplace. Such is the circumstance of a fitness center in competition with another center in a neighborhood with a limited number of people who can afford to pay the membership or user fees. Their options are for one center to move to another neighborhood, for both to recruit from a wider service area beyond the neighborhood, or for both to compete more aggressively through cost cutting, price cutting, and recruitment within the neighborhood. When one loses its competitive edge, the other might buy the weaker one and be done with the competition.

True, the competitive market model helps produce innovation and efficiencies. It sometimes misses the mark, however, in social and health services because the "market" tends to be defined by those who can afford to pay for the services rather than those who need them the most. When the availability of resources for the service are limited and when the health of people may suffer for lack of the service, publicly supported (tax-based) services may be required to fill gaps in a private-sector–dominated, market-driven service economy. A systems approach, democratically planned and cooperatively negotiated *with* the government, helps guard against the depletion of finite resources by a few.[30] It seeks to allocate resources in the most equitable and efficient way, to expand the market or service area, to provide for specialization within the market or service area, and to minimize duplication.

Those who enter the political arena do so because they have a stake in policy and must engage conflict, or sometimes even create it, to pursue their policy agenda.[31] One's purpose in assessing the politics of policy is to anticipate the political sides, the political actors, and the power relationships that will line up for and against the policies one must promote to bring about the enabling support, regulation, and organizational or environmental changes required for a given program. With the sides, actors, and relationships identified, the remaining task is to propose a set of exchanges that will enable each of the sides or actors to gain something in a "win-win" rather than "win-lose" transaction.

Exchange Theory. One theory of organizational and political behavior is that people cooperate when the organization or policy allows each of them to pursue their individual goals and supports each of them in some way. Under those circumstances, they are willing to give up something in order to gain the stability and predictability of the organization or policy that serves them in some way. The key to a practical political analysis, following the systems and exchange approach, is to find the "something" that each can gain in exchange for organizational or policy change.[32]

Power Equalization Approach. Unfortunately, the gains and sacrifices of exchange theory are not equally distributed in a complex community or system. Some have less to gain and more to sacrifice than others. Some have more to gain, but the gain seems trivial relative to the sacrifice they would make. At this point in political analysis, one must stand back from the attempt to make everyone happy and ask, "What is the common good?" This raises the utilitarian ideal of John Stuart Mill, who sought a political philosophy that would assure "the most good for the most people." Because power is unequally distributed in the community, the majority of people sometimes must make sacrifices or at least forgo their potential gains in favor of a few. Garrett Hardin's classic "Tragedy of the Commons" illustrated this in relation to population and the environment.[33] Where those sacrifices are basic human needs such as health, communities have the obligation to consider curtailment of the freedoms of the few to exploit or harm others. This is done through legal and regulatory means when a protective law exists, or by political means when the political will is strong enough to equalize the distribution of power long enough to get a new law or policy passed.

Power Educative Approach. The preferred means of bringing about policy and organizational changes, under the circumstances just described, is to educate community or organizational leaders, including those whose behavior jeopardizes the health of others. This approach seeks to enlighten them to the harm that is being done and to appeal to their humanity and long-term interest in maintaining the community or system.[34] Implicit in this approach is the possibility of confrontation with legal action or political action if the situation is not corrected. Also implicit is the risk of bad publicity and sweeping legislative or regulatory reforms if their behavior does not change voluntarily.

Conflict Approach. Failing the educative approach, the only avenue sometimes left to equalize or tilt the balance of power on a political issue is organized confrontation and conflict in the form of strikes, petitions, consumer boycotts, pickets, referenda, or legal action to bring about policy, regulatory, or organizational change. Similar effects on policy can be initiated through lobbying, organization of public interest groups to promote social action or to elect sympathetic candidates, and demonstrations or publicity to arouse public awareness and sentiment on the issue. This can become a program in itself, with a separate plan, or a part of a broader health promotion strategy.

Advocacy and Educating the Electorate. Recent years have seen the growth of health promotion literature on advocacy toward overcoming the lobbying power of industry or other special interest groups, especially regarding tobacco, alcohol, and environmental issues.[35] Further, much literature describes general strategies and approaches taken by health educators and other professionals in policy advocacy.[36] Specific approaches, guidelines, resources, and strategies have been proposed for health educators and other professionals to use the media and to engage the political process more directly and more effectively on behalf of specific populations and health promotion issues. Examples include health promotion policy initiatives for minorities,[37] the elderly,[38] increasing access to health services,[39] AIDS,[40] and the environment.[41]

One cannot build a strong and sustained advocacy for public health on a foundation of neutral or negative perceptions. A 1994 study found that neither the general citizenry nor decision makers in the United States had a very sound understanding of the scope or value of public health—confirming that public health is indeed the silent miracle.[42] Focus-group results from the same study, however, also demonstrated that public appreciation for the role and value of public health could be readily stimulated once a concerted effort was made to point out its benefits. This kind of information can provide a sound building block for policy supportive to public health. As Carr-Gregg has observed, government policies are typically adopted only when the public is adequately informed and ready.[43]

Empowerment Education and Community Development. A specific variation on the advocacy and **education-of-the-electorate** approaches represents a convergence of the self-care movement and the traditional community development approach in which the community takes much more of the initiative. In the advocacy approach, a politically skilled organization takes on the advocacy tasks on behalf of the community or interest group. In the educated electorate approach, either the organization or a small group within it sets out to educate people to bring about political action to change the organization or its policies. The **empowerment education** approach encourages people *within* the community to assume control over the entire process of educating themselves, defining their own problems, setting their own priorities, developing their own self-help programs, and, if necessary, challenging the power structure to remove hazards or to make resources available.[44]

Freudenberg's book *Not in Our Backyards!* presents case histories of chemical pollution and discusses coalition building, actions taken by public groups and communities to protect themselves, and various educational, legal, and legislative strategies groups have used on their own behalf.[45] A case study of a West Virginia experience describes a 6-year community self-help program that approximates the empowerment education approach.[46] The focus on a medical self-care model in this case study might have limited its clear reflection of the community organization and empowerment education approach, but the power of the participatory process in this community is thoroughly documented.[47] The following box presents a more recent case example.

AN URBAN CASE EXAMPLE

A case study analyzing the effectiveness of planning and policy making to counter the reemergence of tuberculosis in two urban settings provides an appropriate summary for the main points highlighted in the section on policy assessment. Anne Dievler studied the contrasting experiences in planning specifically as it facilitated effective policy making to support tuberculosis (TB) control in Washington, D.C., and New York City.[48] Dievler's analysis suggested that significantly different declines in TB case rates from 1992 to 1996 favoring New York occurred at least in part because planners there acknowledged the political and bureaucratic aspects of planning. Based on the findings from her comparative case study, Dievler offered the following suggestions; note how they overlap with the key elements we have mentioned regarding policy assessment.

CONSENSUS BUILDING:

It is important to be able to identify and agree on the scope and magnitude of the problem. In the District, the problem seemed to break over whether there was an epidemic, a potential for one, or no problem at all. In contrast, in NYC, the government clearly defined and delineated the problem and achieved a greater internal and external consensus on the magnitude of the problem. (p. 180)

FORMULATE STRATEGIES:

Planning processes need to address the inevitable politics of strategy formulation. In the District, higher level government officials pursued strategies based on their own goals and interests and reacted to pressure from the outside. In NYC, the leadership, in conjunction with program managers and staff, took a more proactive role in promoting scientifically sound strategies, as well as more controversial strategies.[49]

OVERCOMING IMPLEMENTATION OBSTACLES:

Dievler documented that the District plan was "widely criticized as having inappropriate issues, vague tasks, and no means of implementation" (p. 175). Further,

> One might argue that the District's unique political status . . . contributed to some of the implementation failure observed. . . . However, since the bulk of the funding for TB control was coming from the federal government and not District coffers, and since most of the policy decisions concerning TB were not subject to review by Congress . . . the kinds and extent of political and bureaucratic obstacles in the District were similar to other large metropolitan areas. In the District, the planning process did little to address these obstacles, but in New York City, some of the most critical bureaucratic obstacles were overcome. Resulting plans were also very specific in NYC, with activities, responsibilities, and time schedules for implementation outlined. (pp. 181–182)

IMPLEMENTATION: ASSURING QUALITY

Imagine how your predecessors in the mid-1940s must have felt when they came across the following passage from a book by the noted public health physician, H. S. Mustard:

> A new "profession," known as "health educators," is arising. Too often these workers are without the restraint that comes from scientific training and are not well grounded in the factual material relating to health and disease. They do, however, possess a stimulating enthusiasm and, in varying degrees, competence in catching the public interest.[50]

At about the same time Mustard was making his less-than-flattering observation, formal efforts were already underway in the United States to improve the quality of graduate training for health educators.[51] Since then, thanks to the vision and tenacity of early health education pioneers, the quality and depth of the science, theory, and practice of health education has improved steadily. Concurrently, largely through collaborative efforts among national professional health education and health promotion societies and organizations, substantial progress has been made toward improving the quality of health promotion and health education practice in the areas of teacher preparation,[52] graduate training,[53] and credentialing.[54] This kind of progress enables health education and health promotion professionals to focus systematically on quality assurance.

Within the context of *implementing* a health promotion program or its elements, we define **quality assurance** as the systematic application of audits, checks, and corrections to ensure that the strategies and methods applied, relative to program objectives, reflect the highest quality feasible. This definition makes several assumptions. First, it assumes that "quality" strategies, techniques, and methods for implementation exist. Based on a rich literature demonstrating effective applications in a variety of settings, planners can often identify strategies and practices demonstrated to be effective. A second assumption is that the protocols or procedures for performing these strategies, techniques, or methods have been established. *The Standards for the Preparation of Graduate-Level Health Educators*[55] provides an example of leadership by professional organizations in delineating standards for specific responsibilities and competencies for quality health education performance. Finally, a third assumption is that some process or system is in place to enable the assessment of quality implementation. The administrative and policy assessment phase of the Precede-Proceed model represents such a process.

For example, as was demonstrated earlier in this chapter, the administrative and policy assessment inevitably prompts an important question related to human resources: "Do we have, or can we get, the personnel necessary to implement the program as planned?" But this question leads to another, equally important question: "Assuming we have or can obtain the people needed, will they have the competencies and skills necessary to effectively implement the program?" This latter question highlights a universal reality—that targeted, high-quality training and attentive supervision of personnel are essential to ensuring effective program implementation. Thus, the assessment of training needs is quite an important aspect of administrative and policy assessment.[56]

As planners work through the first four phases of the Precede-Proceed process, their assessments will uncover areas of content and/or skill likely to be good candidates for in-service training. The steps in doing the assessment of training needs, consistent with earlier assessment tasks, will be familiar: (1) to identify the discrepancies between the current skills among the staff and those required in the proposed program, (2) to come to some consensus about which gaps matter most, and (3) given time and resource constraints, to determine which gaps are most modifiable through training.

Because training programs are by definition educational programs, they deserve a similar planning process to that described by the behavioral, environmental, and educational assessments in the Precede framework. Supervision can also be approached as an educational process: behavior change goals can be set mutually by the supervisor and employee. Factors predisposing, enabling, and reinforcing the intended behavior can be analyzed periodically. One can also plan interventions to predispose, enable, and reinforce implementation through staff meetings, training, written materials, and rewards for high performance. Examples of PRECEDE applied to professional training in the medical care setting will be presented in Chapter 11. New technologies applied to training, such as the EMPOWER (Enabling Methods of Planning and Organizing Within Everyone's Reach) software, will be presented in Chapter 12.

In the final analysis, textbooks can offer little on implementation that will improve on a well-thought-out plan, an adequate budget, solid organizational and policy support, constructive training and supervision of staff, and careful monitoring in the process evaluation stage (to be discussed in Chapter 7). The keys to successful implementation beyond these five ingredients are experience, sensitivity to people's needs, flexibility in the face of changing circumstances, keeping an eye on long-term goals, and a sense of humor.

Most of these ingredients come with time and the opportunity to start small and build on success. The only shortcut to some of the required experience might come through a critical reading of the literature, focusing particularly on readings that feature explanations of program applications. For example, one can read about effective outreach to the elderly,[57] a community organization project to stop herbicide spraying in Massachusetts,[58] issues encountered in developing health promotion coalitions and consortia,[59] a health education program about AIDS among seropositive blood donors in New York,[60] and another about AIDS education in a minority high-risk community in Detroit.[61] Good examples can also be gleaned from descriptions of health education and health promotion case studies,[62] and more recently, people have innovatively used case stories to illustrate the effective application of community-based health promotion strategies and **tactics**.[63]

With the Internet, access to the best and most recent information about all aspects of the health promotion planning process, including implementation, lies virtually within everyone's reach. Of the following organizations, most have web sites: government, philanthropic, and voluntary health agencies at the national, state/provincial, and local level; private-sector health and medical care organizations; almost all colleges and universities; and the majority of professional health promotion organizations and societies. The resources available from these various sites include, among other things, health status databases, program descriptions, guidelines and criteria for grant applications, evaluation reports, and technical assistance sources. For example, when planners use the web site at the Institute for Health Promotion Research at the University of British Columbia (http://www.ihpr.ubc.ca), they will be able to access and search—by author, setting, population, or health problem—over 750 published applications of the Precede-Proceed model, as well as download updated bibliographies and news keyed to this book, and guidelines for participatory research.

SUMMARY

The administrative assessment entails the analysis of resources required by a given program, the resources available in the organization or community, and the barriers to implementation of the program. The policy assessment then asks what political, regulatory, and organizational supports and barriers one can change to facilitate the program and to enable the development of educational and environmental supports for community action. These steps take one from Precede planning to Proceed implementation. Evaluation, then, becomes part of both the plan and of the implementation process.

Planning and policy in health education and health promotion can provide a clear purpose, resources, and protection for the programs they produce, but administrators cannot mark every step on the path of implementation without retarding the very growth and development of the people they intend to help. Plans and policies must leave room to adapt to changing local circumstances, personalities, opportunities, and feedback from evaluation.

PRECEDE assures that a program will be *appropriate* to a person's or population's needs and circumstances. PROCEED assures that the program will be *available, accessible, acceptable,* and *accountable.* Only an appropriate program is worth implementing, but even the most appropriate program will fail to reach those who need it if the program is unavailable, inaccessible, or unacceptable to them. PROCEED assesses the resources required to assure a program's *availability,* organizational changes required to assure its *accessibility,* and political and regulatory changes required to assure its *acceptability.* Finally, quality assurance through evaluation and training assures that the program will be *accountable* to the policy makers, administrators, consumers, clients, and any other stakeholders who need to know whether the program met their standards of acceptability.

Training and supervision of personnel combined with evaluation are the keys to accountability and provide the best assurance of implementation. In this context, *training needs* refers to specific in-service content or skill development as demanded by the role staff would be asked to fulfill in the specific program being planned. Each training program deserves a full planning process similar to that in the Precede framework. Supervision can also be approached as an educational process for both supervisor and supervisee. Factors predisposing, enabling, and reinforcing the intended behavior can be analyzed periodically; interventions can be planned to predispose, enable, and reinforce implementation.

Implementation relies on a well-thought-out plan, an adequate budget, solid organizational and policy support, constructive training and supervision of staff, and careful monitoring in the process evaluation stage. Beyond this, successful implementation depends on experience, sensitivity to people's needs, flexibility in the face of changing circumstances, maintaining a long-term perspective, and a sense of humor.

EXERCISES

1. Propose the essential features of a program with at least one intervention, directed at each high priority predisposing, enabling, and reinforcing factors.

2. Identify the resources required for your program with a specific budget and timetable or Gantt chart.
3. Analyze how your program would affect and be affected by other programs and units within the sponsoring or implementing organization, and propose the organizational and policy changes required to support your program.
4. Describe the interorganizational and intersectoral coordination that would be required to implement your program.
5. Describe the approaches your program might take to ensure its sustainability beyond the initial funding cycle.

NOTES AND CITATIONS

1. Susan Brink, Dr.P.H., contributed to the previous edition of this chapter. We are indebted to Judith Ottoson, M.P.H., Ed.D., for her research on implementation and training, which provided a basis for parts of this chapter.

2. Software programs for microcomputer construction of Gantt charts and other tools for planning the flow of program activities are readily available. See Chapter 12 and, for a specific example in PRECEDE-PROCEED, Gold, Green, & Kreuter, 1997.

3. Bolman & Deal, 1991. This matches the "capacity-building" perspective of health promotion applied to notions of institutionalizing programs and developing communities; see R. M. Goodman et al., 1998, which, however, unnecessarily polarized the subject with the suggestion that "community capacity should stand in contrast to other popular approaches to community health and development, such as health risk factor and needs assessments" (p. 259). See Green, 1989, for a health promotion perspective that seeks to build capacity of people through community and organizational development, not instead of successful needs assessment and control of risk factors.

4. DePree, 1997; DePue, Wells, Lasater, & Carleton, 1990; Rimer, Keintz, Glassman, & Kinman, 1986; Seiden & Blonna, 1983; Silverfine, Brieger, & Churchill, 1990.

5. Butterfoss, Goodman, & Wandersman, 1993; Feighery & Rogers, 1990; Green, 1990; J. R. Miller, 1984; P. Mullen, Kukowski, & Mazelis, 1979; Stachenko, 1996; Wandersman, Goodman, & Butterfoss, 1997.

6. Green, 1977.

7. R. Bertera & Green, 1979; Chwalow, Green, Levine, & Deeds, 1978; Connell, Turner, & Mason, 1985; Cucherat & Boissel, 1998; Green, Wang, & Ephross, 1974; Hatcher, Green, Levine, & Flagle, 1986; Risser, Hoffman, Bellah, & Green, 1985.

8. Fielding, 1982a; Green, 1974, 1977; Green, Wang, & Ephross, 1974; Wang, Ephross & Green, 1975.

9. Chase, 1979. Chase's extensive list has been updated and adapted to health promotion in Ottoson and Green, 1987; for specific case analyses, see also, Ward et al., 1982; J. R. Weiss, Wallerstein, & MacLean, 1995; Wickizer, Wagner, & Perrin, 1998.

10. Conway, Hu, & Harrington, 1997; Lillquist, Haenlein, & Mettlin, 1996; Milewa, 1997; Neugebauer, 1996; Van Meter & Van Horn, 1975.

11. H. S. Ross & Mico, 1980, p. 222.

12. T. Smith, 1973.

13. Schaeffer, 1985.

14. N. H. Gottlieb, Lovato, Weinstein, Green, & Eriksen, 1992; Gustafson, 1979.

15. P. Berman & McLaughlin, 1976; Chase, 1979; W. L. Miller, Crabtree, & Stange, 1988.

16. Basch et al., 1985. See also Blaine, Forster, & Pham, 1997; Hausman, Ruzek, & Burt, 1995; Kingery, 1995; D. Levin & Coronel, 1997; Perry, Sellers, & Cook, 1997; Probart, McDonnell, & Anger, 1997; Renaud et al., 1997; Scheirer, Shediac, & Cassady, 1995; Wickizer, Wagner, & Perrin, 1998; Wojtowicz, 1990. For an application of PRECEDE-PROCEED in assessing the problems of implementation, see P. H. Smith, Danis, & Helmick, 1998.

17. R. S. Thompson, Talpin, McAfee, Mandelson, & Smith, 1995.

18. Ibid., p. 1113.

19. Guttmacher et al., 1997, p. 1433.

20. Rein & Rabinovitz, 1997.

21. Bolman & Deal, 1991. For examples of intraorganizational adaptations to facilitate the implementation of health-related innovations and policies, including "reinvention" of the innovation or policy, see Dearing, Larson, Randall, & Pope, 1988; Kottke, Brekke, & Marquez, 1997; Schriger, Baraff, & Cretin, 1997; Stine & Ellefson, 1997; S. Woodruff, Candelaria, & Zaslow, 1996.

22. Bardach, 1977; Fawcett et al., 1997; Hargrove, 1975; Rutten, 1995.

23. Bracht, 1990; Breckon, Harvey, & Lancaster, 1998; Fawcett, Paine, Francisco, & Vliet, 1993; Minkler, 1997; Minkler, Patton, & Cissell, 1989.

24. M. Ross & Lappin, 1967, p. 14.

25. *Targets for Health for All,* 1986.

26. Chapman, 1990.

27. Fawcett et al., 1997; Samuels, 1990.

28. Alinsky, 1972.

29. Butterfoss, Goodman, & Wandersman, 1993; Elder, Schmid, Dower, & Hedlund, 1993; Quirk & Seymour, 1991.

30. S. Levine, White, & Scotch, 1963.

31. Chapman & Lupton, 1995; Freudenberg, 1984b; Wallack, Dorfman, Jernigan, & Themba, 1993.

32. Yukl, 1994.

33. Hardin, 1968.

34. Cataldo & Coates, 1986, esp. pp. 399–419; Lovato, Green, & Stainbrook, 1993.

35. For general approaches to media advocacy, see endnote 31 and DeJong, 1996; A. Russell, Voas, & Chaloupka, 1995; Scholer, Sunder, & Flora, 1996; Wallack, 1994; Wallack & Dorfman, 1996; K. Woodruff, 1996. For other examples, see R. Blum & Samuels, 1990; Casswell, Stewart, & Duignan, 1989; Farrant & Taft, 1988; Wallack, 1983.

36. Collin, 1982–1983; Freudenberg, 1978; L. M. Hoffman, 1989; Howze & Redman, 1992; Mahaffey & Hanks, 1982; Steckler & Dawson, 1982; Steckler, Dawson, Goodman, & Epstein, 1987.

37. See, for example, Braithwaite & Lythcott, 1989; Liburd & Bowie, 1989; S. B. Thomas, 1990.

38. Minkler, 1997; Minkler & Checkoway, 1988.

39. Geiger, 1984.

40. Krieger & Lashof, 1988; McKinney, 1993; Rundall & Phillips, 1990.

41. Dietz, Stern, & Rycroft, 1989; Freudenberg, 1984b; Green, Richard, & Potvin, 1996.

42. *Marketing Core Functions,* 1994.

43. Carr-Gregg, 1993.

44. Green, 1983b; Minkler, 1985; Pilisuk, Parks, Kelly, & Turner, 1982; Shor & Freire, 1987; Tjerandsen, 1980; Wallerstein & Bernstein, 1988, 1996.

45. Freudenberg, 1984b.

46. Schiller, Steckler, Dawson, & Patton, 1987.

47. Wallerstein, 1990.

48. Dievler, 1997.

49. An example of "scientifically sound strategies" would be a process such as "Directly Observed Therapy" (DOT) where health professionals or trained outreach workers directly observe a patient's oral intake of medicine. A "controversial strategy" might be restraining non-compliant patients.

50. Mustard, 1945, p. 176.

51. Gielen, McDonald, & Auld, 1997.

52. American Association for Health, Physical Education and Recreation, 1969, 1974; American School Health Association, 1976.

53. American Public Health Association, Committee on Professional Education, 1969; Bensley & Pope, 1992; Caswell, 1981; Society for Public Health Education, Ad Hoc Task Force on Professional Preparation and Practice of Health Education, 1977.

54. Cleary, 1995; National Task Force on the Preparation and Practice of Health Educators, 1985; U.S. Department of Health and Human Services, 1980.

55. *Standards for the Preparation of Graduate-Level Health Educators,* 1997.

56. In this context, "training needs" refer to specific in-service content or skill development as demanded by the role staff would be asked to fulfill in the specific program being planned.

57. Kemper, 1986; Minkler, 1985, 1997 (see Chap. 15).

58. Winder, 1985.

59. M. F. Davis & Iverson, 1984; DeFrank & Levenson, 1987; Kegler, Steckler, & McLeroy, 1998; Pelletier, Klehr, & McPhee, 1988.

60. P. D. Cleary et al., 1986.

61. L. S. Williams, 1986.

62. Carlaw, 1982; H. P. Cleary, Kichen, & Ensor, 1985. See also compilations by various resource centers and clearinghouses such as the American Hospital Association, the American Public Health Association, the CDC Center for Chronic Disease Control and Health Promotion, the U.S. Office of Substance Abuse Prevention, the Stanford Health Promotion Resource Center, the National Health Information Clearinghouse, and the Combined Health Education Data Base accessible through Medline.

63. Kreuter, Lezin, Kreuter, & Green, 1998.

Chapter 7

Evaluation and the Accountable Practitioner

A single chapter can scarcely scratch the surface of program evaluation in health education, much less in the broader arena of health promotion. For each of the health problems and settings for health promotion, entire textbooks[1] and specific review articles have been published to address the scientific and technical issues of evaluation in this field.[2] Recent national and international conferences have been dedicated to the state of the art and the epistemological issues in evaluation.[3] The World Health Organization has issued numerous manuals to guide evaluation at global, national, regional, and local levels.[4] This chapter limits its scope to the essential tasks of evaluation as they are developed and carried out within the realities of program planning and management in health promotion practice.

TEN QUESTIONS

Evaluation poses some or all of ten questions. These include the embarrassing questions a critical scientist, supervisor, agency head, board member, or legislator might ask. They include the tough questions often posed by grant review panels. They also include the innocent but penetrating questions a lay member of a planning committee or a program recipient might ask, or questions raised by colleagues when one formally presents the findings of a health promotion program. Responses to these questions illuminate pathways that practitioners can follow when faced with the challenges and complexities—sometimes big, sometimes small—that inevitably accompany the evaluation of a program. The good news is, having attended to the assessment steps of PRECEDE and PROCEED, you will already have in hand most of the essential information you need for an evaluation and the answers to most of these questions.

1. WHY EVALUATE? THE VIEWS OF DIFFERENT STAKEHOLDERS

Depending on the perspective of the user or consumer of evaluative information, the reasons given for evaluating differ. Where one stands on evaluation depends on how one regards policy and program.

- The elected official needs evaluation results to demonstrate that a given program reached and served his or her constituents and met the requirements of a legislative mandate or administrative policy.
- The program manager uses information from evaluations to guide program decisions.
- The evaluation research specialist, behavioral scientist, or epidemiologist uses evaluation data to determine whether improvements in health outcomes were causally linked to a given program, intervention, or behavioral change.[5]

As different as these reasons may appear, a common thread binds them: the need to know what works. The products of evaluation can helpfully inform each of these parties and other stakeholders. Their enlightenment, in turn, can provide support for continuing and improving useful programs and for discontinuing and reallocating resources from unproductive programs.[6]

2. IS EVALUATION REALLY NECESSARY?

Some stakeholders may see evaluation of some programs as a nuisance at best, an obstruction to urgent program action at worst. The politician and the public will be most interested in evaluations of costly programs and controversial ones. They might view evaluation of routine, well-established programs as a waste of resources. The wider professional and scientific community will be most interested in evaluation of the most innovative programs. Though the program manager will share these interests, he or she will recognize the need for at least some minimal level of evaluation of *every* program. Because the responsible practitioner needs to have something to show for the time and effort expended, he or she will seek some form of feedback on performance or impact. Nevertheless, program managers and practitioners might view some kinds of evaluation as threatening.

The accountable practitioner or program manager approaches each new population and program combination as an experiment.[7] The Precede assessment results supply the hypotheses and the Proceed implementation and evaluation test that hypotheses. Whether the evaluation is elaborate, extensive, and thorough or simple, limited, and superficial will depend on its cost, controversy, and innovativeness; in every case, though, *some* evaluation will be essential for keeping program managers and practitioners accountable. If a given Precede planning process required few assumptions because there was plenty of prior research and certainty linking each cause with each effect in the causal chain, then the only evaluation necessary is the minimum required by the program manager to account for the expenditure of resources. If the linkages within PRECEDE were tenuous, requiring some guesswork about causal relationships, then a more elaborate evaluation may be in order to confirm or disconfirm the assumptions. The assumptions derived from educated guesswork represent hypotheses needing to be tested.

3. WHAT IS EVALUATION, REALLY?

Definition. Dictionaries generally define *evaluation* in two ways: to ascertain or judge the worth of something, and to examine carefully. The primary tasks for the evaluator are "carefully examining" and "judging the worth" of methods, personnel, materials, or programs. In the context of health education and health promotion, we have defined *evaluation* simply as "the *comparison* of an *object of interest* against a *standard of acceptability.*"[8]

Objects of Interest. Objects of interest include any or all of the factors that one takes into account in applying the Precede-Proceed framework. The objects may be measures of quality of life; health status indicators; behavioral and environmental factors; predisposing, enabling, and reinforcing factors; intervention activities; methods of delivery; changes in policies, regulations, or organizations; level of staff expertise; and quality of performance and educational materials. Any or all may be the objects of interest for evaluation. The interest in *program* evaluation per se lies in some *change* in the object that one can associate with some change in program activity or input.

Order of Interest. Each of the inputs, intermediate effects, and ultimate outcomes of health promotion programs can be objects of interest in an evaluation. In a systematic search for determinants, root causes, and primary-prevention solutions, previous chapters have worked from right to left (against the arrows) along the causal chain implied by the Precede model. Evaluation applies the same logic and model except that one moves from left to right—from immediate policies, activities, resources, and implementation, to intermediate effects, to ultimate health outcomes and social benefits. The objects of interest remain the same; the order of their examination and judgment is reversed.

Objectives. Goals and targets, or **objectives,** identify the objects of interest in a well-developed plan. The term *objectives* is derived from the word *object*. A hierarchy of objectives—from ultimate social and health objectives to intermediate behavioral and environmental objectives to more immediate educational, organi-

zational, regulatory, and policy objectives—presents the objects of interest in reverse order of immediacy. Recall that objectives state *who* is expected to experience *how much* of *what change* by *when* (see Chapter 4). The objects of interest center on "who" and "what change." We regard the development of quantitative objectives for health promotion, as well as their translation into policy-guiding programs and allocation of resources, as having helped break the poverty cycle of health education, shown in Figure 7-1.

The advent of health promotion in policy as a way of widening the focus of health education to encompass both educational or behavioral and broader social and environmental determinants of health helped break the poverty cycle in several ways, as in Figure 7-2. It strengthened the analysis of evaluations (1) so those broader determinants of health were taken into consideration as causes (2). This produced stronger theory and models of planning, such as PRECEDE-PROCEED, which led to improved planning (3). With better plans and more credible, evidence-based planning, one could declare objectives, obtain greater policy support, and be accountable for more concrete, quantified objectives within specified periods (4). The U.S. and Australian objectives in disease prevention and health promotion have provided notable examples of how this process of policy support for health promotion evolved.[9] The consensus that went into the formulation of objectives also provided a foundation for health-impact assessment of the policies of other sectors.[10]

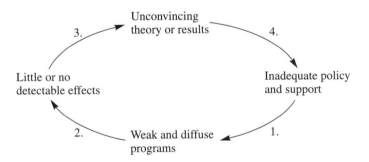

FIGURE 7-1

The cycle of poverty that plagued health education for many decades related to the inability to get adequate allocations from policy makers to support strong health education programs, resulting in (1) weak and diffuse programs. These produced (2) limited or undetectable results, which led in turn to poor evaluations and (3) little advancement of theory. The cycle persisted because, with weak theory and evidence, health education could not convince policy makers to allocate more resources to health education.

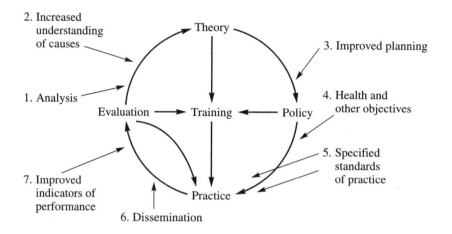

FIGURE 7-2

Building on stronger evaluation of programs that had a wider range of objects of interest than health education seemed to have, health promotion helped break the cycle of poverty at several levels.

4. WHAT ARE YOUR STANDARDS OF ACCEPTABILITY?

Standards of acceptability were specified in the "how much" and "when" estimates in the objectives developed during the planning process. Standards state how an object of interest is expected to measure up. They also serve as targets, which, when attained or exceeded, signal success, improvement, or growth.[11] For health promotion programs, the standards will be the expected *level* of improvement in the social, economic, health, environmental, behavioral, educational, organizational, or policy conditions stated in the objectives.[12] They may also apply, as the field matures, to specified standards of practice for judging the quality of work by professionals in the field (5 in Figure 7-2), the dissemination of those standards through credentialing and accreditation mechanisms (6), and ultimately the development, validation, and refinement of performance indicators (7).[13]

Now come the embarrassing questions if the objectives were not explicit and specific enough about "how much" and "by when." Legislators, directors, board members, and other policy makers and funding sources become impatient for results. They want to believe they made good investments in a program, but they need evidence to justify continuing the investment. Other priorities emerge over time, causing some of the policy makers to look for unproductive investments from which resources can be siphoned to fund new programs. Invariably they will expect more than their level of investment and the elapsed time should warrant, but one can fall back on the standards they accepted when they first funded the program if those standards are realistically and explicitly stated in the program objectives. Standards can be set in several ways.

Arbitrary Standards. Program managers or policy makers can simply declare that they want to see a given change, for example, a 50% rate of participation in program X by all employees. Such a seemingly arbitrary standard must come from somewhere. The apparent fiat probably has some historical precedent or vague rationale in the mind of its promoter. The first task of the evaluator sometimes must be to decipher or trace the origin or rationale of an apparently arbitrary standard of acceptability.

Scientific Standards ("Best Practices"). At the opposite extreme from arbitrary standards lie the standards based on evidence as reflected by the latest published evaluations or randomized trials. Evidence-based standards deem acceptable those levels of outcome achieved in scientifically controlled studies. Such standards are usually based on a systematic review of the literature to obtain averages from the best studies. For example, a practitioner charged with establishing a standard for a smoking-cessation program consults the data such as those presented in Table 7-1 summarizing the quit rates for a variety of smoking-cessation strategies at a 6-month follow-up.[14] The objectives for a program applying one or more of these

TABLE 7-1

This summary of smoking-cessation success rates at 6 months following first quitting, with rates based on large numbers of controlled studies, show a wide range of acceptable scientific standards for the efficacy of different classes of methods. When they are further multiplied by the potential of estimated reach of each class of methods, the objectives for a nation or a state or province can be estimated, as shown for the United States (US) and for British Columbia (BC), Canada

Intervention	Effectiveness %	Reach	Impact US	Impact BC
None (unaided)	3	22,800,000	684,000	7,600
Rx NRT	14	2,500,000	280,000	3,111
OTC NRT	14	6,300,000	560,000	6,222
Behavioral	24	395,000	94,800	1,053
Inpatient Rx	32	500	160	2

SOURCE: Efficacy and reach data from "Tobacco Dependence Treatment: Review and Prospects," by S. Shiffman, K. M. Mason, and J. E. Henningfield, 1998, *Annual Review of Public Health, 19,* pp. 335–358. Reach data (number of people reached by the method) for US from same source; reach data for BC based on extrapolation to BC population. With permission, from the *Annual Review of Public Health* Volume 19, © 1998, by Annual Reviews.

methods might use these figures as the basis for estimating "how much" by "when." Standards based on previous research evidence might more accurately be called "theoretical standards" insofar as programs can only partially replicate the formally tested methods in a review like that in Table 7-1. Use the figures in the "Effectiveness" and "Reach" columns to estimate how much impact a program could have on the United States or on the province of British Columbia (last two columns). The best evidence comes from a "real" program. The scientific or theoretical standard says, in effect, "If everything in our program goes just as it did in the formal experiments with this method, here is the smoking-cessation rate we should expect to achieve at 6 months and at 1 year following the program."

Evidence enters the equation at several levels of the population-based planning and evaluation cycle, as recalled from Chapter 1 in the version shown in Figure 7-3. Here, the use of evidence applies to (A) assessing the needs of the population, (B) assessing the causes of those needs based on previous research, (C) assessing the evidence for effective strategies to affect those causes from previous evaluations, and (D) assessing the current program from the prospective evaluation. In the case of D, the focus of this chapter, the current program plan can be viewed as a hypothesis and the implementation of the program itself as an experiment.

Historical Standards. Administrators usually set objectives for programs based on last year's performance in the same program. This might be an extension of the temporal trend of outcomes in the program if it has gone on for a long period. This method applies most readily to outcome objectives one can easily measure, such as birth rates, mortality rates, or attendance at clinics or other services where head counts are made routinely.

Normative Standards. By setting objectives on the basis of what other such programs have achieved in similar organizations or communities, one applies a normative standard. Normative and historical standards can be readily constructed for program objectives and evaluation purposes when the object of interest is an outcome measured in routinely collected data. These might include such data as vital events (births, marriages, deaths), hospital discharges, school attendance, communicable disease morbidity, ambient air quality, automobile crashes, and drug- or alcohol-related arrests. The most common standard for many community health promotion programs is the state average; for many state- or provincewide health promotion programs, the national average.

Compromise Standards. Standards frequently emerge from a consensus based on the informed opinions of experienced administrators, researchers, and practitioners, as well as endorsement by recognized professional organizations or societies.[15]

Case Example. Consider the *Healthy People 2000* and *Healthy People 2010* objectives for the United States in disease prevention and health promotion.[16] They developed first as *scientific* standards based on extensive reviews of the literature

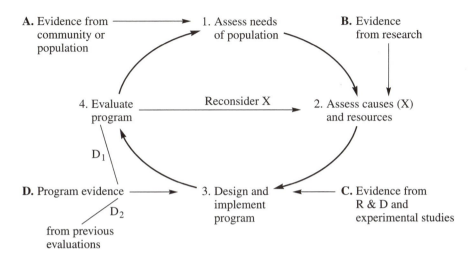

FIGURE 7-3

"Evidence-based practice" should refer not only to the evidence from previous research (B and C) but also to the evidence from the population (A) and evidence from the prospective evaluation of the current program. Each type of evidence is directed at a different part of the population-based planning cycle introduced in Chapter 1.

carried out by federal government staff with the assistance of consultants.[17] For many of the objectives, few formal evaluations and few baseline measures could be generalized to the whole nation. *Historical* trends for some of these indicated a steady rise or fall in the rates up through the late 1980s. These trend lines could be extrapolated or projected to estimate where the nation might land in the year 2000 if nothing were done to change the rate, and where the country might be if program performance improved. Some *normative* objectives could be set on the basis of what other Western nations had accomplished, especially European countries whose infant mortality rates, for example, were generally better than those of the United States.

   In the end, these scientific, historical, and normative standards were submitted to a group of experts at a national consensus conference to hammer out agreements on the most appropriate standards. A draft of the objectives for the nation was first distributed to several thousand organizations around the country for review and comment following the first. The feedback was reconciled back at the federal Office of Disease Prevention and Health Promotion. The final product was a set of 226 objectives reflecting a compromise of scientific, historical, and normative standards of acceptability. A similar process has been followed in formulating the U.S. objectives for the nation in disease prevention and health promotion for the year 2000, with greater involvement of minority groups and state and local people at an earlier stage in the process. The structure and logical

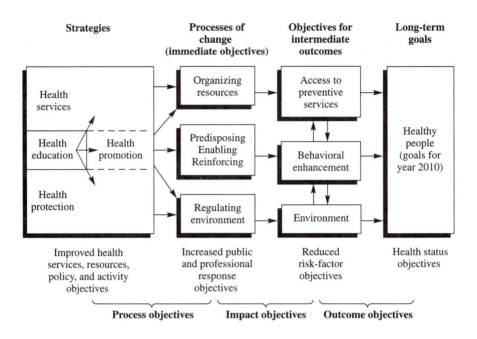

| Strategies | Processes of change (immediate objectives) | Objectives for intermediate outcomes | Long-term goals |

FIGURE 7-4

The U.S. Healthy People 1990, 2000, and 2010 objectives follow a logic of approximate relationships among the objects of interest corresponding to the Precede-Proceed model, as shown here.

relationships of the 1990, 2000, and 2010 objectives for the nation can be seen in relation to the Precede-Proceed model shown in Figure 7-4.

Besides illustrating the various sources of standards of acceptability for objectives, the U.S. goal-setting experience brought home some other lessons for evaluation. One was that many goals had to be set in the absence of adequate data, because some of the most pressing problems for disease prevention and health promotion for the nation had no data system in place.[18] Program managers and practitioners must not be bullied by evaluators to limit the scope and objectives of their programs to those things that are measurable, especially those things for which measurement systems are in place. This would trivialize most programs. Some of the most important and emergent problems, needs, and aspirations of a population will become measurable only when policy and programs give them enough attention to draw scientists and data-collection agencies into the action arena. Within five years of the publication of the first U.S. objectives for the nation, most of the previously unmeasured objectives in health promotion had become covered by National Health Interview surveys.[19]

A second lesson learned in the development of these objectives was the need to tailor them to special populations, particularly minorities, the elderly, and regional or local populations for whom the averages for the nation are the least relevant. Despite the best efforts to put the 1990 objectives through a consensus development process, the special populations still had to be consulted independently and their special needs addressed apart from the objectives and priorities for the majority.[20] This lesson has been applied in the Year 2000 and 2010 objective-setting process.

Both of these lessons pertain equally to standards and objectives for local programs. Data will follow priorities. The statistics on minority populations, if they exist at all, simply get lost when lumped with the majority, and it is often the minorities whose needs for health promotion deserve the highest priority.

As emphasized throughout this book, participation is the linchpin of effective community programs. All participants and stakeholders in a program should have their views represented in the earliest planning activities, in the establishment of objectives, and in the implementation and evaluation of health promotion programs. Such views are essential to the collaborative dialogue needed if plausible, "acceptable" standards are to be set and respected.

Model Standards. The relationship of objectives to standards, as well as the importance of collaborative input in establishing standards, is vividly illustrated in *Healthy Communities 2000: Model Standards.*[21] Collaborators from major organizations representing local, state, and national public health interests undertook this work. They hoped the project would lead eventually to a norm by which local health authorities would use quantified measures of health and program processes to define the objectives and assess the impact of programs. An evaluation of a state-local negotiation process to implement the model standards in 18 local health agencies over a 2-year period in California concludes that "the use of Model Standards appeared to contribute to establishing program priorities, emphasizing the measurement of outcomes, improving the data management systems, and evaluating the current performance of programs."[22]

These standards, expressed either as program process or as risk-factor or health outcome objectives, were originally put forth as "models" for 34 prevention program areas. Tables 7-2 and 7-3 provide examples of the model standards for health education and chronic disease control, respectively. Note that the standards are expressed as process or outcome objectives, an important distinction for program evaluation that we shall discuss in detail later.

In establishing the model standards, the original work group followed a flexible conceptual framework, an approach policy makers and practitioners should emulate:

> Standards must be significantly flexible to accommodate differences in the mix of preventable diseases and conditions facing communities. . . . Because of this variation

TABLE 7-2

These model standards for health education represent a consensus of several professional associations concerned with quality assurance in community health promotion programs

Goal: Community residents will have the necessary knowledge, skills, capacity, and opportunity to improve and maintain individual, family, and community health; use preventive health services, practices, and facilities appropriately; understand and participate, where feasible, in decision making concerning their health care; understand and carry out prescribed medical instructions; and participate in community health decision making.

Focus	Process Objectives	Indicators
Integration of health education services	**P-1.** By 20___ all community prevention programs will have an identifiable strategy for the use of health education, including at a minimum: a. Specification of population clusters with identifiable health problems or risks b. Assessment of behavior related to those problems c. Statement of educational objectives d. Educational methods to be employed with each target group e. Timelines for implementation f. Periodic evaluation of educational effectiveness *Note:* Health education programs to be effective must influence health practices in a positive direction, and the statement of educational objectives should be based on the cause-and-effect relationship between behaviors and health.	a. Existence and utilization of strategy b. Percentage of programs having identifiable strategy
Promotion of individual health maintenance	**P-2.** By 20___ the health education component of all community prevention programs will be conducted to provide the necessary knowledge, skills, and capacity to ensure that indivuduals can do the following: a: Assume greater personal responsibility for improving and maintaining optimal health for themselves, their families, and their community: e.g., smoking cessation b. Use preventive services, practices, and facilities appropriately: e.g., well-baby care c. Participate in community health decision making d. Understand the nature of their work and related health risks	a. Percentage of prevention programs that emphasize (as relevant) increased individual responsibility for health b. Evidence of citizen participation in community-health decision making c. Evidence of methods used for public education and information d. Documentation of individuals within the community participating in health promotion activities e. Existence of worker right-to-know legislation and programs

TABLE 7-3

The model standards for chronic disease control show greater emphasis on impact and outcome indicators than do the health education standards in Table 7-2. Health promotion has held itself to increasingly rigorous impact and outcome standards of acceptability as it has taken responsibility for other aspects of chronic disease control beyond the health education component

Goal: The community will experience a minimum of preventable illness, disability, and premature death; medical service utilization and attendant costs attributable to chronic diseases and conditions will be reduced.

Focus	Outcome Objectives	Indicators
	O-1. By 20___ deaths due to _____ will be reduced to _____ among _____ .	Cause-specific death rates
	O-2. By 20___ the prevalence of _____ will be reduced to _____ among _____ .	Prevalence of specific condition or risk factor
	Note: Specific conditions or risk factors include the following: a. Smoking b. Uncontrolled hypertension c. Problem drinking d. Drinking and driving e. Nonuse of seat belts f. Poor nutrition: e.g., undernutrition and obesity g. Hypercholesterolemia h. Lack of physical fitness i. Occupational and environmental exposures	
	O-3. By 20___ the indicence of _____ will be reduced to _____ among _____ .	Incidence
	O-4. By 20___ preventable complications associated with _____ will be reduced to _____ among _____ .	a. Hospital admissions rate associated with specific preventable complication
	Note: Specific chronic diseases or conditions include the following: a. Atherosclerotic, hypertensive, and other cardiovascular disease: e.g., coronary artery disease, rheumatic heart disease, stroke, myocardial infarction b. Bone and joint disease: e.g., arthritis, osteoporosis c. Cancer, specific sites: e.g., lung, breast, bladder, gastrointestinal tract, cervix, oral cavity d. Chronic obstructive lung disease e. Cirrhosis f. Congenital anomalies g. Diabetes and other metabolic diseases h. Hearing impairment	b. Hospital days of stay associated with specific preventable complication c. Disability days and restricted activity days associated with specific preventable complication d. Incidence or prevalence of specific preventable complication

in problems and service availability, it is neither useful or feasible to propose rigid, quantified national objectives for every community. Rather, a framework is presented that permits the quantification of objectives in every community irrespective of size, locale, nature of preventable problem, and present availability of preventive services.[23]

5. WHY IS EVALUATION SO THREATENING? OR, " WHY ME?"

For some, the mere mention of the word *evaluation* brings discomfort. Perhaps it trumpets the possible detection of something gone awry, or it sounds a warning that scarce program resources may be diverted. Whatever triggers the anxiety, it can be considerably diminished by attending to a systematic planning process that precedes the implementation and evaluation of the program. Carol Weiss offered this insight:

> The sins of the program are often visited on the evaluation. When programs are well-conceptualized, and developed, with clearly defined and consistent methods of work, the lot of evaluation is relatively easy. But when programs are disorganized, beset with disruptions, ineffectively designed, or poorly managed, the evaluation falls heir to the problems of the setting.[24]

The first antidote to evaluation anxiety, then, is good planning. One of the benefits gained by working through the Precede and Proceed processes is that baseline data and objectives (or at least explicit assumptions about cause-and-effect relationships), so essential to carrying out a program evaluation, are built into the process. The care given to using valid and reliable measurement techniques in the assessment phases proves valuable in evaluation as well. A fully developed Precede plan, with realistic social, health, behavioral, environmental, and educational objectives and with program activities and methods that are sound and targeted to those objectives, should lend itself easily to an evaluation that will detect the changes implicit in the objectives.

Anxiety also springs up when evaluation provokes defensiveness in the program managers and practitioners. This can occur especially in evaluations conducted by outsiders. It applies not only to social and health services, but to business evaluations as well.[25] With good integration of evaluation planning with program planning, one can prevent or overcome such defensiveness. Application of the assessment processes in PRECEDE helps practitioners cultivate an attitude and spirit of inquiry, a key principle for the educational philosopher John Dewey.[26] Dewey's description of "inquiry" captures the essence of evaluation as an integral part of professional practice: an ongoing, self-corrective process through which we gradually gain a richer understanding of those things that shape our judgments. He felt that we must continually submit our judgments and claims to a "community of inquirers," because an effective democracy depends on a community of free and open-minded inquirers.

A third source of evaluation anxiety is the understanding that a program is too complex to be comprehended by evaluation, and the problems it seeks to change too complex to be affected by this program alone. Health promotion programs tend to grapple with problems that are at once biological and political, environmental and behavioral, individual and collective. Such complexity becomes even more intense when geographic and population differences are taken into account. These circumstances demand that practitioners make adjustments based on the differences inherent in the application of health promotion programs. The purpose of evaluation in health promotion must not be seen as finding the perfect program that can be packaged and parachuted into every community. The first purpose evaluation should serve is to help improve and adapt the program to the circumstances at hand.

Schlesinger emphasizes the need for knowledge of local circumstances and flexibility of programs to adapt to such circumstances; he cautions decision makers to avoid the illusion that programs can be perfected prior to implementation and, once in place, left to run on automatic pilot.

> Indeed, perhaps the most important legacy of the Great Society programs of the 1960s was not that they were ill-conceived, but that even relatively well-designed programs must be adapted to changing conditions and needs of their beneficiaries. For much of the two decades after their enactment, we allowed these programs to languish, and their effectiveness suffered as a result. In designing future programs, we must be sensitive to the need for flexibility and change based on program experience.[27]

Accountable practitioners actively share observations with others and understand that feedback generates information essential for program improvement. For them, part of the job is to ask questions like these: Is this program working toward achieving its objectives? Why is it working the way it is? How can we do it better, more efficiently, and perhaps at less cost? Or with less inconvenience to our clients? Evaluation that provides for this interactive, learning-oriented rather than judgmental approach to new data will not only gain the support of practitioners and the affected public, but also feed back more quickly and thoroughly into program improvements and policy changes.[28] This view approaches the "fourth generation evaluation" described by Guba and Lincoln, where the first generation was measurement oriented; the second, description oriented; and the third, judgment oriented.[29]

6. WHAT TYPE OF OUTCOME IS APPROPRIATE AND SUFFICIENT TO INDICATE SUCCESS?

A health promotion program can be evaluated at one or more of three levels: process, impact, and outcome. The indicators and methodologies for detecting and comparing these indicators will vary at each level (Figure 7-5).

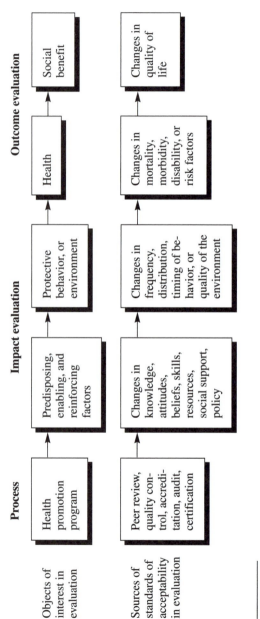

FIGURE 7-5

Three levels of evaluation for accountability suggest the objects of interest and the sources of standards of acceptability for each.

Process Evaluation. The first level is designated **process evaluation** because the observations on the *process* of the program are the first to be available. The early detection of problems of training and implementation will enable the program manager to make adjustments before the problems get out of hand. This is the time to experiment with methods, to "pilot" untried program components, and to examine new material for its readability, cultural sensitivity, and acceptability to the audience.[30]

Consider the following case. A rural cardiovascular prevention program had orchestrated multiple activities targeted at reducing selected cardiovascular disease risk factors, including several related to hypertension. To take advantage of a national campaign effort, "May is National Hypertension Month," special efforts were made to promote community participation in the various public information, screening, and counseling activities that accompany the campaign. At a weekly program meeting early in May, intervention workers in the field reported that a sizable number of residents seemed to be misinterpreting the slogan: "May is Hypertension Month." They saw it to mean that May is the month you are at highest risk to get hypertension, just as January and February are the months you are mostly likely to come down with the flu![31] It is quite possible that persons with that perception might indeed attend to risk-reduction recommendations only in the month of May, mistakenly believing that such vigilance is unnecessary during the rest of the year.

In this example, staff members were alerted to an unanticipated program effect by means of the weekly meetings designed to provide routine monitoring of the "program processes." Had there been no commitment to review program process, the unanticipated reaction to the campaign could have led to behaviors directly opposite those intended.

In process evaluation, the potential objects of interest include all program inputs, implementation activities, and stakeholder reactions. Inputs may include the policy or theoretical tenets of the program, the plausibility and specificity of program goals and objectives, and the resources (funds, personnel, space) allocated or expended. Implementation activities include staff performance, methods of data collection, regulatory and organizational activity, media distributed or broadcast, and events sponsored. Stakeholder reactions include the reviews of the program plans by board members, focus-group reactions of the intended recipients to the program materials, the level of participation among program recipients, and the response of collaborating organizations and recipients to the program. The line between input and implementation is vague and, in the final analysis, probably unimportant for practical purposes.

The quality of the process can be determined by various methods: quantitatively, by periodic surveys, audits, and counts of services rendered; qualitatively, by internal administrative surveillance of bookkeeping, contracts, and personnel or by peer review, accreditation, certification, consumer reports, and other "external" or independent testing and observational methods.[32] The critical product from process evaluation is a clear, descriptive picture of the quality of the program elements being put in place and what is taking place as the program proceeds. Numerous practical examples of innovative applications of process evaluation—also referred to as **formative evaluation**—can be found in the health promotion literature.[33]

Evaluation of implementation becomes all the more important when one is required to judge whether the program could be exported to other sites or to judge the soundness of the theory or policy underlying the program.[34] Such judgments generally assume that the program has been implemented as prescribed by policy or theory and has reached the intended clients as designed. If that assumption is wrong—and it probably should be, considering what was said earlier about the need for flexibility and adaptation of programs—then the evaluation will commit the *Type III error*.[35] The Type III error refers to concluding that the program was ineffective though in fact the program was never really implemented as designed. Process evaluation can help discern where the program's implementation has strayed from the policy, theory, or protocol, so that any generalization from the subsequent impact or outcome results can be interpreted in the light of known deviations from the intended program.

Impact Evaluation. The second level, **impact evaluation,** assesses the immediate effect the program (or some aspect of it) has on target behaviors and their predisposing, enabling, and reinforcing antecedents or on influential environmental factors.[36] The clarity, specificity, and plausibility of the behavioral and educational objectives generated in phases three and four of the Precede planning process provide the foundation for evaluating program impact.[37] A full-scale health promotion program should expect to find some impact on behavior, but components of the program, such as mass media, might not yield palpable behavioral impact if evaluated in isolation.[38]

Outcome Evaluation. At the third level, **outcome evaluation,** the objects of interest are those health status and quality-of-life indicators that have been crafted in the earliest stages of the planning process. They are typically referenced in terms of mortality, disease, or disability rates for a given portion of the population. Social indicators such as hunger, unemployment, homelessness, or elderly people living independently are often expressed as a percentage of the population. Examples of outcome evaluations that have applied the Precede-Proceed model can be found in recent published reports.[39]

The ability to detect changes in impact or outcome variables depends heavily on the specificity of the standards, the precision of their measurement, the size of the effect, and the size of the population or sample on which the measures are taken. These issues will be developed further in this chapter under Question 9, "How much is enough?"

7. HOW MUCH PRECISION AND CONTROL DO YOU NEED?

In the Precede-Proceed process, one begins by identifying a priority health or quality-of-life problem and then conducts a systematic search for the root causes holding the greatest promise of yielding social and health benefits. One *assumes* that health promotion activity and resources can be mobilized and deployed to change those root causes. The justification for that assumption—that selected health promotion activities can have the desired effect—is usually based on a combination of the practitioner's vision and experience and on relevant findings from previously published studies. Impact and outcome evaluation studies should be considered when there exists limited scientific evidence on the association between the desired outcome and the intervention selected.

The decision-making process in program planning and evaluation parallels the routine evaluations we make every day of our lives. When faced with a problem, we informally pose questions related to that problem, generate some options we might take to solve it, weigh the options, and act. The specific course of action we take frequently depends on the resources and time available, as well as the demands we feel of accountability to others for our actions.

Suppose you have an urgent need to haul some trash over a fair distance to a dump site. From among the following vehicles, you need to select one to haul the trash: a rental moving van, a small and sometimes unreliable pickup truck, a wheelbarrow, and a 1955 Corvette you are keeping for a friend. You rule out the wheelbarrow—it is too small and the distance too far; assuming you want to keep your friend, you rule out the use of the Corvette. This leaves the rental moving van and the small pickup truck. Although both will do the job, you note the van will be more efficient in that it can do the job in only one trip; you estimate three trips if you use the pickup. The rental van will cost you more. Thus, the decision depends on factors such as time and the availability of resources, as well as accountability to others.

The most pertinent question an evaluator can ask is "What do I and other stakeholders need to know, as a result of this evaluation?" The answer to this question enables the evaluator to determine, from the range of evaluation strategies available, which approaches will be acceptable and which not. Furthermore, among the approaches deemed "acceptable," some will be more appropriate than others, some more expensive, and some more time consuming; some will yield more data than necessary. One can err on the side of too little evaluation to satisfy the needs of stakeholders, and one can err on the side of wasting resources and time on unnecessary data and misplaced precision.

Consider two scenarios. In scenario A, a federal public health agency awards a sizeable grant to a university with the intent of finding out whether a health promotion program consisting of a public education campaign and a physician education component leads to specific outcomes. These include (1) an increase in the number of women who undergo mammographic screening, (2) an increase in the detection of early breast cancer, and (3) a decrease over time in breast cancer mortality within the population exposed to the intervention.

In scenario B, a state or provincial health department makes some modest resources available to interested local health jurisdictions to determine if local health agencies could effectively implement some selected community-based primary prevention strategies already shown, through previous community trials, to be effective in delaying the onset of smoking in children age 10–14.

The program planning process should be the same for both cases: the delineation of the health problem, the sound assessment of the salient behavioral and environmental factors and the probable precursors of those factors, the identification of specific program objectives at several levels, and the selection or development of intervention strategies targeted at those objectives. Even though the program planning activities will be quite similar, the evaluation questions posed in A and B are different and tasks needed to carry out the respective evaluations will differ markedly in several ways.

When Outcome Is the Focus. In scenario A, among the many possible process and impact evaluation questions likely to be posited, one outcome question is ultimate: "Does exposure to this program result in reductions in breast cancer mortality?" This is an evaluation *research* question. The information needed to formulate a confident answer requires considerable effort, as Figure 1-5 attests.

Attributing changes in a population to a given program, or program component, requires evidence. The strength of that evidence will depend on the evaluation methods used. The methods must be able to take into account the size of the sample studied, the validity and reliability of the measurements used, and the study design. *Study design* refers to the method employed to control for the variety of factors that could be alternative explanations for the effects in question.

The selection of evaluation methods depends on a variety of complex factors and circumstances. Consider a few of the questions that the evaluation researcher must address:

- What does the funding agency want?
- Is the timeline realistic? How soon will impact or outcomes be measurable, relative to how soon they are expected?
- How accessible is the population to be studied?
- Will the participants in the study be represented in the planning?
- Is it feasible to assign people randomly to the intervention to provide for an experimental study design? If not, what are the plausible alternatives?
- What are the clearance and approval procedures for studies using human subjects?
- Are standardized measurement instruments available to detect intermediate outcomes of interest or will new ones have to be developed and field tested?

- What are the requirements for data collection (sample size, interviewing, record reviews, etc.), data analysis, and approvals (institutional review boards and informed consent)?
- Are the financial and staff resources adequate to carry out this study as intended?

It is impossible to contemplate these questions seriously without getting a feeling for the magnitude of effort demanded by such an undertaking. Without substantial technical and economic support, it is unrealistic and inappropriate to expect community programs, with modest resources and limited staff, to undertake such evaluation research tasks.

When Process Is the Focus. Scenario B poses a different question. The state or provincial health officials want to determine if selected health promotion methods and protocols, previously demonstrated to be appropriate and effective in epidemiological, clinical, and evaluation research studies, could be implemented within the context of the routine services found in a local health department.

As in scenario A, one could generate a long list of interesting process and impact evaluation questions for the situation in B. For example, *impact* evaluation might ask whether the intended school-age population were being reached and, if so, could the desired *impact* on their motivation or behavior be detected? A *process* evaluation might seek to identify characteristics that tend to differentiate teachers who faithfully employ the recommended methods from those who do not. A process variable that researchers increasingly include in program evaluations is the extent to which a practitioner applies a method as it has been previously applied and found effective in controlled studies.

The practitioners' fidelity to educational protocols and methods accounts for differences in impact in several studies of health education.[40] Although fidelity may matter, program directors and practitioners need to take care not to demand it slavishly and interpret it literally. Striving to deliver the methods and protocols of the program *exactly* as prescribed in conclusions drawn from a model research project results in perfunctory practice.[41] The assumption too often in promoting "best practices" literally from research evidence is that previous research on a given population, in a specific place and time, under the direction of research investigators, can justify the precise intervention that should be implemented in *all* populations and situations. This assumption reduces the professional practitioner of health promotion to a technician or even an automaton. Armed with diagnostic planning skills and the theoretical knowledge to interpret *why* a given method worked, the inquiring practitioner will have the competence and confidence needed to make the procedural *adaptations* required with each new population or situation.

As in other levels of evaluation, to answer process evaluation questions, one must compare "objects of interest" with "standards of acceptability." Relevant objects of interest might include qualifications of staff, intensity and duration of instruction, access to and appropriateness of facilities, channels of communication, cultural sensitivity of instructional materials, the extent to which family and peer involvement is encouraged, the number of inspections made to enforce a nonsmoking regulation, and competence in applying appropriate community organization methods. The attainment of "standards of acceptability" could be assessed by the combined application of quantitative and qualitative methods.

Quantitative methods might include a record of the number and duration of the sessions conducted, the number of school-age children reached, and a record of the type and times mass media messages were actually delivered. Among qualitative methods, one might include a description of the professional preparation, experience, and general qualifications of teachers and program staff who interact with program participants; recipients' reactions to the program either by observation or self-report; and observation of the program delivery.[42] Examples of qualitative and quantitative standards of acceptability for sexually transmitted disease (STD) prevention programs are shown in Table 7-4 at each of the three levels and for various target populations.

The complexities of sampling and research design demanded in scenario A do not apply in B, but the professional commitment to rigor does. Both approaches require attention to detail, consistency and care in documentation, and objectivity in analysis and reporting. One reason for the poor reception of qualitative and process evaluation results in that they too often have been collected or reported with less rigor and objectivity than quantitative data, which are harder to mask with cosmetic prose.

8. WHAT DO EVALUATION DESIGNS ENABLE US TO DO?

One can think of the *design* as the framework the evaluator uses to provide a basis for *comparing* the object of interest with a standard of acceptability. Comparisons can be over time or between groups, or both.

An important purpose in selecting a study design is to reduce the possibility of errors in the interpretation of the results. This is accomplished by maximizing the reliability and validity of the information collected in the evaluation. A *reliable* measurement is consistent and stable. If we apply a measurement once, then repeat it a second time, or another interviewer or observer applies it again, reliability measures the certainty with which we can expect the results to be the same (assuming that little has happened between the two data points to alter the response). A measurement is *valid* when it yields an accurate or "true" measure of what it is supposed to measure; as such, valid measures are also reliable.

The following scene takes place in the year 2000: You ask a person her age and she responds, "30." Two weeks later you ask her what her date of birth is and she replies, "June 1, 1970," which confirms her self-reported age. These two

TABLE 7-4

This matrix illustrates the types of objectives for each of three levels of evaluation: process, impact, and outcome, for sexually transmitted disease (STD) control

Health Promotion's Target Population	Process Objectives and Measurements	Impact Objectives and Measures	Outcome Objectives and Measures
Adolescent students	Provision of accurate education about STDs to all junior and senior high school students by 1990 (nat.); implementation of school-based STD educational programs for all junior and senior high school students in the school district (local)	What percentage of students are able to recognize STDs, know how to protect against infection, and express intentions to use preventive measures.	Improve health status: By 2000, reported gonorrhea incidence should be reduced to a rate of 280 cases per 100,000.
High-risk groups in the community	Identification of and establishment of contact with all high-risk goups (e.g., gays, adolescents) in the community through hotlines and other outreach programs.	Increase in self-referrals and referral of sexual contacts for STD screening and treatment at an earlier stage; increase in general knowledge and practice of behaviors that decrease risk of STD contact.	By 2000, reported incidence of pelvic inflammatory disease should be reduced to a rate of 60 cases per 100,000 women.
General knowledge: subgroups within total populations	Provision of government funds for and assistance for demonstration projects of community based STD prevention.	Data on what types of STD education approaches are most effective for particular organizational settings.	By 2000, reported incidence of primary and secondary syphilis should be reduced to a rate of 7 cases per 100,000 population per year, with a reduction in congenital syphilis to 1.5 cases per 100,000 children less than 1 year of age.
Health care professionals	Completion of the development and distribution, and assistance in the implementation, of the Quality Assurance Guidelines for STD Clinical Care; provision of statewide continuing education workshops for health care professionals on how to identify high-risk individuals and how to educate patients for STD prevention (local).	By 1985, at least 95% of health care providers seeing suspected cases of STD should be capable of diagnosing and treating all recognized STDs. Increase in early referrals among private patients; increase in knowledge of STD prevention measures.	

SOURCE: Adapted from "Productive Research Designs for Health Education Investigations," by L. W. Green and N. Gordon, 1982, *Health Education, 13*, pp. 4–10. Used with permission of the publisher.

reports are consistent over time, and may be correctly judged to be reliable. If later you discover that her birth certificate indicates that the actual date of birth was June 1, 1969, you know that the reliable verbal reports were not valid.

Practitioners benefit by cultivating a working knowledge of this notion of validity, because, among other things, it is paramount in choosing among research designs. Consider this conversation between a program manager (PM), who coordinates a work-site health promotion program for a company called "New Directions," and the Chief Executive Officer (CEO) of the company.

> CEO: My advisors have read the health promotion evaluation report. Good work.
>
> PM: Thank you.
>
> CEO: What do you think are the most important findings?
>
> PM: We think there are two. First, 24% of the those who signed up for the smoking cessation program are still not smoking after 2 months. Next, of the 900 employees in the company, 250 turned out for at least one of the physical activity programs. Of those, 125 (50%) remain involved in regular aerobic activities.
>
> CEO: Impressive. I'm considering the implementation the program in the four regional offices of New Directions. However, the senior management staff have raised two questions I can't answer; I hope you can. First, how do we know that the smoking-cessation rates and the increases in physical activity are not the result of recent national campaigns and extensive local news reports? And second, if the evidence does show that our programs really do account for the differences noted, how do we know these programs will work in our various regional offices?

In the parlance of evaluation research, the CEO's staff was concerned about two basic "threats to validity." By wondering if other events (national campaigns and news reports) might explain the outcomes, they were questioning the **internal validity** of the claim that the positive changes in smoking and physical activity really stemmed from the program. The concern over whether similar results could be expected if the program is implemented in other New Directions sites raised the question of **external validity.** That is, how generalizable is the program? How confident can the CEO be about achieving similar results in the other regions?

Here follow brief descriptions of six evaluation designs ranging from the simple but often neglected collection of routine data to the collection of data in highly rigorous, highly controlled experimental settings. At the two extremes lies the historical record-keeping approach, which is the least complex and is applicable to most programs, and the controlled experimental approach, usually impractical. Each has its own utility. Practitioners will base their selections on their evaluation questions and the data required to answer them. All designs can be implemented in two or three steps.

Design A: The Historical Record-Keeping Approach. The record-keeping approach is the minimum expected of any professional health promotion practitioner at any time. It yields tables, charts, or graphs that provide an ongoing account of what is occurring in a program. The procedure is manageable even under the most adverse operational circumstances. For example, it may be sufficient merely to count the number of people served each day and then add up the daily figures to tabulate or chart the weekly, monthly, or yearly trends.

The first step is to construct a graph showing the expected relationship between inputs and outcomes. The second step is to set up a record-keeping procedure to accumulate the data. The last step is to calculate and chart the data periodically, plotting the direction and magnitude of change taking place over time. How often should one tabulate and chart the data? That depends on the number of times the events being tabulated occur and how often one needs to report trends to stakeholders. An example of a design-A graph is given in Figure 7-7.

Figure 7-6 demonstrates the sequential benefits of different educational and policy changes during three phases of a program conducted by a clinic for sexually transmitted diseases over a 2-year-plus period. You can see the impact of each educational strategy both in changes in the absolute number of patients appearing at the clinic and in the composition of the patient population. The change in interviewing policy (C) was a change from asking patients to identify their sexual contacts to encouraging them to take the responsibility for seeing that their sexual partners received treatment. The behavioral impact in terms of the male:female ratio of patients at this point was most notable.[43] The ratios (looked at in combination with the graph) show increases in women and whites using the clinic until the numbers were closer to equal. Other examples of this simplest of designs for evaluation are listed in the bibliography.[44]

A similar evaluation of a VD hotline in New Jersey permitted a cost-benefit analysis of the program. Records were kept of the number of calls handled by hotline operators during one year (process) and the number of clinic and emergency room visits for STD screening and treatment for 6 months following start of hotline operation (impact). Results showed that emergency room and clinic visits for STD care were 53% greater during the period when the hotline was operating than during the same time period of the year before the hotline's existence. The cost per call in operating the hotline was calculated (process measure). Unfortunately, the cost-benefit evaluation was hampered by an absence of information about financial and person-hour costs for hotline publicity and by poor data on additional cost that resulted from the clinic and emergency room handling of STD patients.[45] This case illustrates the importance of including interagency cooperation for coordinated record keeping in an evaluation plan to assure the availability of data needed.

Design B: The Periodic Inventory Approach. The inventory approach requires making a special effort periodically (rather than continuously) to collect data. Sometimes

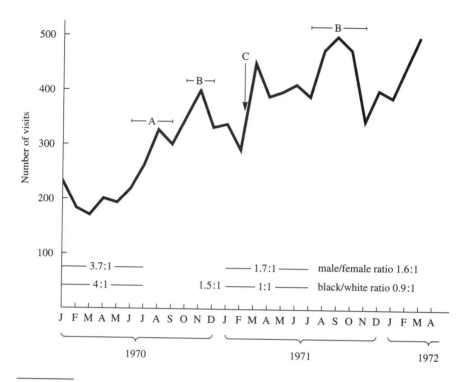

FIGURE 7-6

This graph, produced simply from recording the number of people visiting a clinic, their gender, and their color, provides a clear evaluation of the relative impact of different methods used to recruit patients with sexually transmitted diseases. A = contacting street groups, B = radio announcements, C = change in interviewing policy, encouraging patients to refer their sexual contacts to come to the clinic.

SOURCE: "Adapting the Venereal Disease to Today's Problem," by J. B. Atwater, 1974, *American Journal of Public Health, 64,* pp. 433–437; reprinted with permission of the American Public Health Association.

the prevailing record-keeping system does not incorporate the data required, and changing the system, perhaps expanding it, would disrupt the service program too much. Rather than accumulating the data on an ongoing basis, as is done with design A, one can obtain the data by conducting special surveys.

First the evaluator sets target dates for the assessments. Then, he or she identifies the expected target levels. Finally, he or she takes the surveys as a way of estimating the levels achieved at the selected points in time.[46]

Comparisons in this design are historical in the sense that success is defined in relation to a prior period of performance in the same program or population.

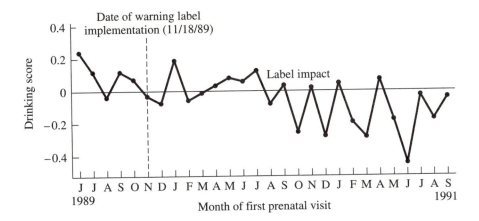

FIGURE 7-7

This graph, applying design B, required questionnaires to be administered to inner-city, low-income African-American women in Detroit who initiated prenatal care at a hospital clinic each month from 5 months before a national alcohol-labeling program began to nearly 2 years after it was in force. The graph provides a clear picture of how warning labels affected alcohol consumption during pregnancy.

SOURCE: "FAS Prevention Strategies: Passive and Active Measures," by J. R. Hankin, 1994, *Alcohol Health and Research World, 18,* pp. 62–66.

Often referred to as the "before-and-after design," the "pre-postest design," or the "historical time-series approach," the inventory approach can be much more than just two measures taken before the start and after the completion of the program. It is frequently used to take tests of knowledge gain or attitude and behavior changes during a program in school and clinical settings.[47]

A variation on the periodic inventory approach is the *interrupted* time-series design. In this variation, the program may be systematically stopped and started to see whether the impact or outcome measures (records or interviews) show corresponding changes.

Figure 7-7 illustrates this method from an evaluation of the U.S. alcohol labeling law that warns pregnant women that drinking alcohol during pregnancy could cause birth defects.[48]

For some kinds of programs, such as smoking-cessation programs, the critical points for measuring behavior are highly standardized.[49] Reviews of the literature reveal the times people are likeliest to drop out or relapse in programs dealing with such matters as smoking, hypertension treatment, antibiotic therapy, and oral contraceptive use.[50]

Design C: The Comparative, "Benchmarking" Approach. Evaluation by means of the comparative approach is an extension of the inventory or record-keeping approach. The same procedures are followed, except that data from sources external to the program are obtained for comparison. One can usually find similar data on programs in other places; one can borrow or copy the record forms used in these programs or join with other programs or services in a common, standardized format for collecting such data. One would then periodically compare the programs on the same basis as design A or B.

Various kinds of state or national data can be used for comparison. For example, the National Health Discharge Survey provides data derived from standardized questionnaires that can be compared with data collected in local programs. National norms suggest what health educators can expect in relation to breast examination, Pap smears, smoking cessation, and other health behaviors.[51] Comparability is an essential feature of cumulative evaluation. For this reason, it is better to use standardized formats for collecting data than to develop original questionnaires except where data requirements are unique. Many examples of the comparative or normative approach can be found in the literature.[52]

Design D: The Controlled-Comparison, Quasi-Experimental Approach. In the controlled-comparison approach, an evaluator first identifies a community or population similar demographically to the target population, but one *not* receiving the intervention program. He or she then applies design A or B in the intervention *and* comparison populations and periodically collects relevant data to enable comparisons. One might want to compare the effects of various kinds of interventions in similar populations—in schools, for example, or in communities.

The Stanford, Minnesota, North Karelia, Texas, Kentucky, COMMIT, and CARP community studies are the most notable contemporary examples of the community application.[53] At Stanford, for example, the original three communities studied in the cardiovascular risk-reduction project included one in which an intensive educational effort had been made, another in which only a mass media effort was made, and another in which neither effort was made, although there were comparable resources and facilities. The effectiveness of the strategies used in each of the three experimental communities and their various subpopulations was compared using impact and outcome data from surveys. Other examples of this approach can be found in the literature.[54]

The Rotterdam evaluation of the STD media/hotline campaign compared trends in new visits to the STD clinic during the intervention for civilians with those of seamen who were not likely to have been exposed to the campaigns and were thus a "control" group (see Figure 7-8).[55] This example points out the importance of controlling for seasonal fluctuations or possible changes in the demographics of the population sampled when analyzing patterns of incidence and prevalence over long periods.

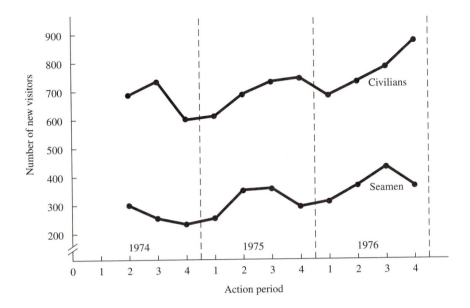

FIGURE 7-8

Though similar to Figures 7-7 (design A) and 7-8 (design B), this graph used design D to compare visit rates to an STD clinic in Rotterdam before and after the civilian population was exposed to media recruitment efforts. The seaman were less exposed to the media campaign because they tended to be off at sea. As such, they provided a natural quasi-control group, which is difficult to find in mass media evaluations.

Design E: The Controlled-Experimental Approach. The controlled-experimental approach is comparable to the clinical trial in medical studies. It requires a formal procedure for random assignment of individuals within the target population to two (or sometimes more) groups. If two, one group will receive the program (experimental group) and one will not (control group). In this approach, it must be possible and ethical to deny certain people the treatment. The control group typically receives "usual treatment" rather than nothing. Once the groups are set up but before the program is underway, the evaluator applies design A or B for both the experimental and the control groups. Often, baseline data are collected on all groups, but this is not essential and depends on the kinds of change one hopes to detect. Records, observations, or survey data over time are then graphed to see how the groups compare at various points in the treatment.[56] Smoking-cessation and weight-control programs are often evaluated according to design E.

Design F: The Evaluative Research Project. The most complex of the evaluation designs, what might be described as a full-scale evaluative research project, is unlikely to be feasible in most community programs. Procedures resemble those for design E, the controlled-experimental approach, except that multiple groups are randomized in factorial designs, and multiple measures are obtained on intermediate variables such as changes in knowledge, attitudes, and skills as well as on outcomes and impact variables such as behavior and health. Group tendencies are compared, as are intragroup effects. The design can accommodate numerous refinements. For example, one can use it to detect the independent effects of the components of a program on selected impact and outcome variables. The program components in question would have to be well defined and the sample would have to be large enough to enable the detection of changes in the randomized subgroups that were systematically exposed to the program components independently and in combination.[57]

Such a design was used to demonstrate how the application of the Precede model could produce changes not only in behavior, but also in the mortality rates of low-income, urban African-American patients with high blood pressure.[58] This project provided much of the data on which the Precede model was first tested formally. Experimental evaluation research studies of this nature are needed to continue to advance the knowledge base of health education and health promotion. However, because they require the application of complex, costly research designs, they are inappropriate undertakings for most community programs, where the mission is service delivery.

Somewhere between the simplicity of design A, with its inconclusive but suggestive findings, and the expense and complexity of design F lies a level of evaluation with the appropriate degree of feasibility, practicability, and rigor for a given program. The problem with complicated designs is that they usually have to be carried out under highly controlled conditions, which makes the behavioral circumstances unusual or unnatural.[59] Often, one must remove people from their social milieu, the ordinary context for their behavior. It is seldom easy to find willing participants for controlled, randomized experiments. Further, such designs require informed consent for those in the control as well as those in the experimental group. This usually requires health education for both groups, which means the control group does not truly lack a planned intervention.

In short, what one gains in internal validity through the more rigorous randomized procedures one may sacrifice in feasibility and in generalizability of findings. Can findings from highly controlled classroom, clinical, or community trials be generalized to private practice and community-based programs?[60] Certainly, one obvious factor is the extent to which the population or community exposed to the program resembles the one in the study; the closer the match, the greater the likelihood of a generalizable effect. However, the most powerful predictor of success in replicating the result is the ability of the practitioner(s) to make the program adjustments and refinements required as a function of the unique needs of their own target population. Thus, even when interventions have been found effective in rigorously controlled studies, the practitioner considering their use in a new population or situation still needs PRECEDE or some similar assessment of needs and determinants to appropriately adjust the interventions.

9. HOW MUCH IS ENOUGH?

Even when practitioners have the best of intentions, evaluation can be disruptive. Further, no element of evaluation has more potential for disruption than the collection of data. Program participants, nonparticipants, and staff may resent being asked or required to complete questionnaires (in person or by telephone); program and clerical staff are frequently asked to carry an increased workload; some may interpret the costs of collecting *and* coding as a drain on scarce resources that could have gone to the program; and staff may perceive that the only beneficiary of the evaluation will be those academic professors and doctoral students who secure their promotion, tenure, or degrees as a result of the publications generated by the data collected by the program staff.

These problems cannot be completely eliminated; they will emerge, more or less, even under the best of circumstances. Nonetheless, by developing, with input from program staff and key stakeholders, a strategic plan for the evaluation, evaluators can minimize the potential for disruption. Here are some elements key to developing such a plan:

1. If possible, designate a staff member with responsibility for coordination of data collection.
2. Based on the measurable objectives delineated in the first four phases of PRECEDE, specify
   a. The hypotheses, derived from the objectives
   b. A list of those objects of interest representing independent variables or intervention strategies, methods, or materials
   c. A list of those objects of interest representing the dependent variables (anticipated impact or outcomes)
3. Construct several "dummy" tables or charts to help you visualize how the data may be organized and eventually summarized. Table 7-5 gives an example of a dummy table. Insert hypothetical numbers, percentages, or rates reflecting the standards of acceptability.
4. Make a list of the information you need.
5. Develop a timeline or work schedule for the remaining steps in the planning and execution of the evaluation, such as shown in Figure 7-9.
6. Identify the data collection techniques that are appropriate and feasible for the information you need.
7. Identify
   a. sources of existing data that may be used
   b. existing data gathering instruments
   c. instruments that need to be developed

TABLE 7-5

This matrix lays out the essential data required for an analysis of change in smoking status among a group of people assessed at baseline and at 1 year following exposure to a cessation recruitment effort or 1 year following enrollment in a smoking-cessation program

	Year 1 Smoking Status		
Baseline Smoking Status	Never Smoked	Former Smoker	Current Smoker
Never smoked			
Former smoker			
Current smoker			

8. Establish a data-collection plan including details on what data will be collected when and by whom.
9. Develop a plan for the reporting phase including formal presentations of results, a final report, publication of papers, and general dissemination plan.

Evaluators must be able to find the appropriate middle ground between undesirable extremes: falling prey to the temptation of data collection "overkill" and choosing methods and measures of minimal burden that render minimal information. As usual, the best advice is to use common sense: Keep focused on the purpose of the evaluation.

10. HOW SHOULD PROCESS, IMPACT, AND OUTCOME MEASURES BE CALCULATED AND PRESENTED?[61]

Analysis of results produces the rewards for one's labor in designing and implementing a program evaluation. It provides for responsible disclosure to the relevant public: program participants, administrators, and health education staff. Our purpose here is to offer a cumulative series of calculations that lead from estimates of need to cost-effectiveness and cost-benefit estimates. Such estimates allow decisions to be made about the relative advantages or disadvantages of implementing and sustaining a health promotion program. Such decisions are best informed if the estimates are derived from widely accepted and standardized procedures and expressed in common terms in both the research and the evaluation report.

Although practitioners and philosophers might argue that the benefits of health promotion go far beyond what can be reflected in numbers, these calculations are often necessary to gain policy and administrative support.[62] The

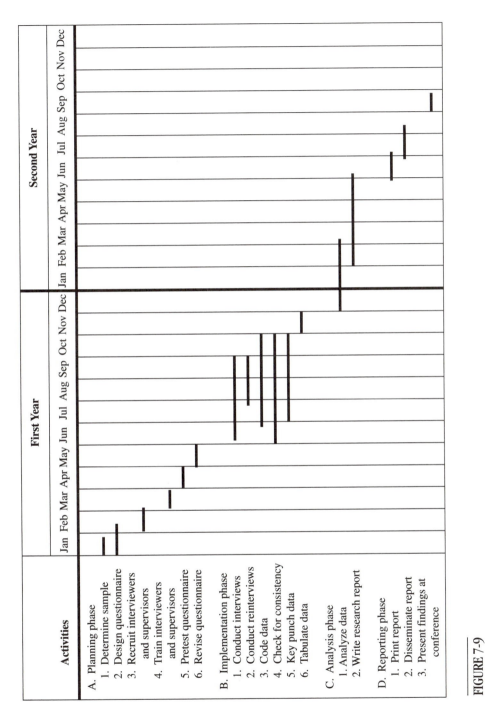

FIGURE 7-9

This timeline or Gantt chart identifies the typical tasks, their order, and their duration, within an evaluation involving user or population surveys.

allocation of scarce resources often demands evidence of outcomes or economic benefits. Health education, no less than other service disciplines, is asked to account for its products and outcomes.[63]

CALCULATING THE INPUTS AND OUTPUTS OF HEALTH EDUCATION

Table 7-6 summarizes 17 calculations that provide a comprehensive analysis of needs, inputs, and outputs of a health promotion program. The table summarizes the calculations for two separate health promotion programs. Both hypothetical programs involve smoking cessation. The first smoking-cessation program targets 1,000 classroom teachers; the second targets 100 school principals or head teachers.

The calculations summarized in Table 7-6 relate to 17 concepts relevant to health promotion assessment: need, **reach,** coverage, impact, **efficacy,** effectiveness, program cost, **efficiency,** cost-effectiveness, benefits, cost-benefit, income, net gain or loss, start-up cost, operating cost, operating cost-effectiveness, and operating cost-benefit. We shall define each of these concepts in terms of its standard calculations. In the analyses, the evaluator wants answers to the following questions:

- Which of the two programs will provide the best coverage of the 100 schools?
- Which program will achieve a greater adoption of health behaviors associated with the intervention?
- What are the relative costs and cost-effectiveness of the two programs?
- What are the relative benefits and cost-benefit ratios of the two programs?
- If the programs generate revenue, what will be their net proceeds or costs?
- What will it take to maintain the preferred program for future offerings?
- What will be the ongoing cost-effectiveness and cost-benefit ratios after the program is running routinely?

POPULATION CONCERNS

A. Need. Need refers to the population in need or the population eligible for the program. In Table 7-6, these are the 10,000 classroom teachers affiliated with the 100 schools in Program 1 or the 100 school principals for these same 100 schools for Program 2. Ideally, we would like to define need in terms of the number of participants who might benefit from the smoking-prevention program, such as the students who might not take up smoking if they were influenced by nonsmoking

TABLE 7-6

The comparative calculations for each of two programs show the trade-offs between population estimates of need, reach, coverage, impact, efficacy, and on through various measures of effectiveness, efficiency, and benefits

Type of Calculation	Program 1 (teachers)	Program 2 (principals)
A. Need (estimated population eligible)	10,000	100
B. Reach (attendance)	1,000	50
C. Coverage [(B/A) × 100]	10%	50%
D. Impact (immediate effects)	100	40
E. Efficacy [(D/B)100]	10%	80%
F. Effectiveness [(D/A) × 100]	1%	40%
G. Program cost	$10,000	$200
H. Efficiency (G/B)	$10/teacher	$4/principal
I. Cost-effectiveness (G/D)	$100/effect	$5/effect
J. Benefits (D × value)	$100,000	$4,000
K. Cost-benefit (J/G as ratio)	10/1	20/1
L. Income	$6,000	0
M. Net gain (or loss) (L − G)	(−$4,000)	(−$200)
N. Start-up costs	$1,000	$100
O. Operating cost (G − L − N)	$3,000	$100
P. Operating cost-effectiveness (O/D)	$30/effect	$2.50/effect
Q. Operating cost-benefit (J/D)	$33/$1	$40/$1

SOURCE: *Measurement and Evaluation in Health Education and Health Promotion,* by L. W. Green & F. Marcus Lewis, 1986, Palo Alto, CA: Mayfield; reprinted with permission of Mayfield Publishing Co.

teachers as role models, but this quantity is unknown and potentially infinite. Therefore, we define need in terms of the population eligible to receive the alternative programs.

The population in need is usually estimated from census data or from previous estimates of the target population. Any of these estimates must often be qualified by screening or exclusion criteria. For example, in Table 7-6 the target teachers and the target principals may be only those who currently smoke two or more packs of cigarettes a day. Estimates of need are interpolated from local, regional, or national data. The estimate is then a synthesized estimate based on available data and screening criteria.

The need estimate becomes the denominator for subsequent calculations for the proportion of the population reached by the program and the overall effectiveness of the program.

B. Reach. The second number or statistic we need is the count of the eligible population who would be or were actually exposed to the program being evaluated: This is the program's *reach*. Sometimes this figure is estimated from previous experience with such programs, from the rules that might be invoked to get people into the program, or from market analysis. If the analysis is completed after the program is implemented, reach is merely a count of the number of individuals who participated in the program during a period such as a month or a year. If the program is a mass media program, reach is much more difficult to estimate.

In Table 7-6, the reach for Program 1 is expected or observed to be 1,000 classroom teachers. Program 2 reaches 50 school principals.

C. Coverage. Coverage is the percentage reached of the number in need. Program 1 has a 10% coverage (1,000/10,000) and Program 2 has a 50% coverage (50/100). Coverage standardizes the absolute numbers of reach and need and allows us to compare the coverage of Program 1 with that of Program 2. By standardizing the figures, we can also compare the coverage of programs in the current fiscal or academic period with those offered in the past.

D. Impact. Impact refers to the immediate, short-term, or intermediate effects of the health promotion program. The evaluator includes the impact variables because they are available within the time frame of most evaluations and, in the absence of data on expected final outcomes, they provide some evidence of progress. Often, these impact variables are measures of health behaviors because they provide more convincing evidence of the effects of the program than do measures of enabling, predisposing, or reinforcing variables.

Table 7-6 shows the impact of the two proposed programs: In Program 1, 100 of the 1,000 school teachers were still not smoking 6 months after the program stopped. In contrast, 40 of the 50 school principals were still not smoking at 6 months after the program.

E. Efficacy. Efficacy refers to the impact of the program for those people who actually attended it. To obtain an estimate of program efficacy, we merely divide the impact number by the number reached (D/B) and multiply that amount by 100 to convert the proportion to a percentage.

From Table 7-6, we see that Program 1 produced the intended impact on more teachers than Program 2 did on school principals, but the efficacy of Program 2 was 80% for 50 school principals reached, compared with only 10% for the school teachers reached by Program 1.

Efficacy considers the relative impact of the program only on those who received it. What about the people who did not participate in the program but who were part of the target population?

F. Effectiveness. Effectiveness is the proportion of people intended to receive the program who successfully changed as intended. In public health programs, one is particularly interested in the level of change for those who were initially intended to receive the program, not just in the change for those who actually participated in it.

Seldom is the distinction between efficacy and effectiveness maintained in evaluation reports. People tend to evaluate the effects of programs on captive audiences. We hold that such reports are evaluations of the program's efficacy, not its effectiveness. The figures on effectiveness in Table 7-6 suggest that Program 2 is more effective (it successfully changed a higher proportion of people eligible to receive it) than Program 1. Program 1 had a 1% rate of effectiveness; Program 2, 40%.

ECONOMIC MEASURES

Eventually we shall want to assure ourselves and others that we achieved the impact, both efficacy and effectiveness, at a reasonable cost.[64] To do this, we next consider measures of cost, efficiency, cost-effectiveness, and cost relative to benefits.

G. Program Cost. Cost is an estimate of the program expenditures outside of the evaluation cost. Cost estimates, therefore, should not include data collection or other evaluation functions. The availability of cost data is often sufficient to advise policy on the preferred program alternative, especially when two or more competing programs appear equally effective in the impact analyses.[65]

Record-keeping practices should be included as part of the cost estimates only if they are essential to the ongoing implementation and integrity of the program. If pre- and posttests are viewed as part of the total program experience and not just as evaluation strategies, their costs should be included. To obtain unbiased estimates of program cost, ledgers should be initiated at the beginning of the program to keep accurate track of actual expenditures. Staff salary, including support staff, should be prorated and included in the cost estimate. In Table 7-6, Program 1 costs $10,000 and Program 2 costs $200.[66]

H. Efficiency. Efficiency is the proportion of program cost to reach; or, the unit cost of each person who actually attended the program. From Table 7-6 we see that the efficiency of Program 1 was $10 for each teacher who attended ($10,000/1,000) compared with $4 for each school principal who attended in Program 2.

Efficiency calculations convert the numbers expressing the reach and the raw cost of the program into a relatively comparable single expression of the cost per person attending or reached by the program. Note that Program 1 at $10,000 was 50 times more expensive than Program 2, but the efficiency measure reveals that Program 1 was actually only 2.5 times more expensive per professional reached than was Program 2.

I. Cost-Effectiveness. Cost-effectiveness is the cost per unit of observed impact or effect; the measure standardizes cost relative to a specific effect. Results are expressed as a ratio of dollar cost per unit of impact. From Table 7-6 we see a ratio of $10,000/100 or $100 for every school teacher in Program 1 who quit smoking and $200/40 or $5 for every school principal who quit smoking in Program 2. It appears that we can obtain the same effect 20 times cheaper with school principals than we can with school teachers. These estimates might run counter to the initial first impressions from lines A, B, and D in Table 7-6, which we could use to argue for Program 1 over Program 2.

J. Benefits. Benefits are the ultimate gains to a society, organization, or sponsor from the program's effects. Not limited to efficiency and cost-effectiveness data, benefit calculations interest primarily taxpayers and others who fund social programs. Such people want to know the program's profound effects, basic to society's quality of life—not merely the efficient transfer of resources into programs or the transfer of programs into behavioral impact.

How can analyses go beyond the measures of efficiency and cost-effectiveness to capture adequately the ultimate value of health education programs? Unfortunately, economists, legislators, the public, and health educators tend not to agree on a common yardstick. We use an approach that bases benefits on one or on a few tangible outcomes that go beyond the strictly medical outcomes but not beyond the measurable and near-future outcomes for which actual dollars can be tracked.[67] With regard to modeling healthy behavior for the students in the schools, we assume that each teacher in Program 1 who changes his or her smoking practice will have greater influence on the students' smoking prevention and smoking-cessation behavior than will the school principals in Program 2. We make this assumption on the basis of the school teacher's more frequent personal contact with the students both during school and at after-school events. In addition, the classroom teacher often can tangibly affect the classroom environment and educational milieu in ways that directly support nonsmoking behavior.

With any previous research or with a set of informed conservative estimates, we can translate these relative advantages into monetary values for the changes in the school teachers' and the principals' behavior. Applying the most conservative assumptions, which is advisable in cost-benefit analyses, we assume the following:

1. Each school teacher in Program 1 will directly affect smoking cessation or smoking prevention behavior in 10 students per year, at an average value of $100 per year of smoking averted, for a total of $1,000 gained in nonsmoking students for every year of nonsmoking teacher.
2. Each principal in Program 2 will directly affect smoking prevention or smoking cessation behavior in 1 student per year. The annual value in smoking averted in students by preventing smoking in principals can be placed at $100, using this outcome as the value.

Multiplying the number of teachers (100) and principals (40) on whom the program had an impact (D) by the value attached to each teacher's effects on the students ($1,000) and each principal's effects on the students ($100), we obtain the benefits in Table 7-6.

K. Cost-Benefit. Cost-benefit is the ratio of the benefits to the program cost. By convention, this is typically expressed in terms of the benefits expected for every unit of currency invested in the program. From Table 7-6 we see that the calculations for cost-benefit suggest that we must recommend in favor of Program 2 over Program 1; we can predict two times as much return in the program for the school principals as in the other. Qualifications are in order, however.

A comparison between programs may ask, "Which of the two programs gives us the best benefit-to-cost ratio?" But a choice between programs may not always be necessary. Rather, one may want to get the best combination of results by taking into account the political and administrative realities, including access to health education resources.

Based on a criterion rather than a normative reference perspective, evidence from Table 7-6 shows that Program 1 produces a substantial return on the dollar investment. A 10-to-1 benefit-to-cost ratio is analogous to a 1,000% return in interest on savings or a 10-fold increase on the value of stocks. Such returns are noteworthy and provide evidence of the importance of Program 1 independent of its comparison with Program 2.

L. Income. Income calculations are estimates of the revenue-generating potential of a program. Such calculations are particularly important when one must consider whether one can operate the program. It is one thing to know that a program is a sure winner; it is another to have the resources available to make the investment. Sources of revenue include grants, donations, recurring or zero-based budgets from a parent organization, and fees for services rendered; however, most of these sources of revenue are unstable. The agency must often ask if the program could support itself or generate revenue.

In Table 7-6, we posit that each school teacher will pay $6 to attend the smoking-cessation program. The school principals, on the other hand, will most likely decline to pay anything. This represents a $6,000 income for Program 1 with no equivalent for Program 2.

M. Net Gain. Net gain or loss is the computed difference between the generated income and the program's cost. Note that net gain or loss does not include the speculative future gains implied by the cost-benefit ratios in line K. If those benefits are expected, one can add them to future income. For example, if the $100,000 benefit from Program 1 with the classroom teachers is expected to be actual savings to the agency, the agency's net gain at the end of one year would be

$96,000 ($100,000 − $4,000) rather than a loss of $4,000. Most likely, some part of the savings reflected in the cost-benefit analysis would accrue to the agency, not all of it.

EXTRAPOLATING TO FUTURE PROGRAMS

How will the program play in other sites, in new settings, with new populations, and under new circumstances? We now turn to a final set of calculations related to start-up and operations.

N. Start-Up Costs. Start-up costs are the initial expenditures not typically repeated. They often involve the costs of planning, software development or review, and capital outlays for such items as equipment and program materials.

O. Operating Cost. Operating cost is the recurring cost required to continue and maintain a program, excluding start-up costs. Often, planners use the operating cost to decide whether or not to continue a program. The operating cost is calculated by adding the original cost estimate (Table 7-6, line G) with the income or net gain or loss (lines L and M) and then subtracting the start-up costs (line N). Any research costs embedded in the original budget should be removed.

P. Operating Cost-Effectiveness. Operating cost-effectiveness is the cost-effectiveness estimate for maintaining the program. It considers the operating cost, not the previously used estimate of total program cost. Because it includes the initial start-up costs, total program cost overestimates of the cost of operating the program. Calculations for operating cost-effectiveness use the operating cost of the program in the numerator (O/D). From Table 7-6 we see that the agency needs to spend $30.00 per participant to sustain Program 1 to obtain the desired effect; Program 2 requires $2.50 per person for the same effect.

Q. Operating Cost-Benefit. Similarly, the ongoing benefit-to-cost ratio partitions start-up and developmental expenditures out of the cost estimate in the denominator, leaving only the program maintenance costs. The numerator, as in the earlier cost-benefit ratio, is the monetized estimate of value gained from the program. For *operating cost-benefit,* the ratio is expressed as money gained per unit of currency spent on maintaining the program for a given period, usually a year.

SUMMARY

This chapter has highlighted some concepts and approaches to evaluation particularly relevant for the health promotion practitioner or manager. Program evaluation is defined, with emphasis given to standards of acceptability. Professional commitment to accountability is best served by an inquiring practitioner who approaches the planning and implementation of each health promotion program as a social experiment. The Precede-Proceed model produces a series of hypotheses about presumed relationships between interventions and outcomes. Evaluation provides the "test" of those hypotheses. Evaluation design provides the experimental or quasi-experimental conditions for the test.

In the absence of a planned evaluation design that facilitates the collection and analysis of valid information, the processes and effects of a program are likely to go undetected. If accidentally detected, they tend to be over- or understated. In this chapter, we presented descriptions and examples of process, impact, and outcome levels and emphasized their practical application for the practitioner in the field. Several designs for evaluation were described in simple steps, with examples listed in the reference notes for each design. By concluding the Precede-Proceed process with the results of an evaluation, practitioners, program managers, and policy makers prepare themselves to approach the next population or health problem armed with a better understanding of health promotion needs and effective ways to address them.

Data flow sometimes uncontrollably, sometimes controllably, from health promotion projects or programs. Control of the flow of data depends on having an analysis plan—ways to accumulate the data systematically so they provide meaningful sums, divided by meaningful denominators, with quotients related to relevant yardsticks or social values. Because social values are so difficult to measure, "bottom-line" valuation is most often expressed in monetary terms.

We have proposed a series of quantitative definitions that seem to capture the most widespread, consistent, and logical uses of the terms *need, reach, coverage, impact, efficacy, effectiveness, program cost, efficiency, cost-effectiveness, benefits, cost-benefits, income, net gain, start-up costs, operating costs, operating cost-effectiveness, and operating cost-benefit*. These quantitative definitions, illustrated with two examples in Table 7-6, could help one improve the consistency of reporting and understanding of evaluation results.

EXERCISES

1. Retrieve your program objective from Chapter 3, your behavioral and environmental objectives from Chapter 4, and three educational objectives from Chapter 5. For *each* objective, identify *two* different "standards of acceptability"; explain the strengths and weaknesses of each standard.
2. Using the circumstances described in the smoking and physical activity program offered at the company called New Directions (see section on evaluation designs), explain how you would answer the two questions posed by the CEO if you had employed (a) Design A, (b) Design C, (c) Design D.

3. Propose an evaluation plan for your program, indicating the data to be collected, the procedures for collection, and the comparisons you intend to make. Use charts or graphs with hypothetical data. As a part of the plan, include *two* design options, one that you would apply if research support is reasonable and the other if the resources are minimal.

NOTES AND CITATIONS

1. Dignan, 1995; Fetterman, Kaftarian, & Wandersman, 1996; Green & Lewis, 1986; Hawe, Degeling, & Hall, 1990; Kar, 1989; Lorig et al., 1996; McDowell & Newell, 1996; Rossi & Freeman, 1993; Sarvela & McDermott, 1993; Temmreck, 1998; Wholey, Hatry, & Newcomer, 1994; Windsor, Baranowski, Clark, & Cutter, 1994.

2. Specific problems and examples of health promotion evaluations can be found in many of the publications cited in other chapters. For more general discussions of evaluation issues and techniques applicable to health promotion, see Abelin, Brzezinski, & Carstairs, 1987; Bjaras, Haglund, & Rifkin, 1991; Flay, 1986a; Lorig et al., 1996; McCuan & Green, 1991; Nutbeam, Smith, & Catford, 1990; Rychetnik, Nutbeam, & Hawe, 1997; Speller, Evans, & Head, 1997; Wagner & Guild, 1989.

3. Lowe, 1992; Maclean & Eakin, 1992.

4. Cholat-Traquet, 1996; Creese & D. Parker, 1994; Global Programme on AIDS, 1994; *Guidance for Conducting Policy and Programme Evaluation in WHO,* 1997.

5. Green, 1992a.

6. Altman, 1995; Green, 1987c; M. Q. Patton, 1997.

7. D. T. Campbell, 1969.

8. For various elaborations of this definition, see Green, 1974, 1977, 1986a; Green & Figa-Talamanca, 1974; Green & Lewis, 1986; Kreuter & Green, 1978.

9. Chomik, 1998; Green, 1991, 1995; McGinnis, Harrell, Artz, Files, & Maiese, 1996; Nutbeam & Harris, 1995; Nutbeam & Wise, 1996; Nutbeam, Wise, Bauman, Harris, & Leeder, 1993; Richmond & Kotelchuck, 1991.

10. Ratner, Green, Frankish, Chomik, & Larsen, 1997.

11. The most common type of evaluation is goal oriented, but this is not the only kind. Some have taken exception to it. See, for example, P. D. Mullen & Iverson, 1982; Scriven, 1972. An emerging "realist theory" of evaluation practice responds to postmodern criticism of positivist assumptions in conventional evaluation methods. See Mark, Henry, & Julnes, 1998. The continuing development in health promotion of empowerment evaluation (Fetterman, 1994; Fetterman, Kafterian, & Wandersman, 1996), participatory evaluation approaches (Green, George, et al., 1995; Israel, Schulz, Parker, & Becker, 1998; P. Park, Brydon-Miller, Hall, & Jackson, 1993), and "portfolio approaches" (Shiell & Hawe, 1995) call into question the assumptions of "accountability to whom" in evaluation.

12. Setting standards for evaluation or "program audit" or "health impact assessment" from program objectives has a growing literature of its own. See, for example, Guild, 1990; Harris & Wise, 1996; Nutbeam, Wise, Bauman, Harris, & Leeder, 1993; Ratner, Green, Frankish, Chomik, & Larsen, 1997.

13. H. P. Cleary, 1995; M. J. Cleary & Neiger, 1998; Doyle, Woods, & Deming, 1995; C. E. Lewis, 1998a; Livingood, Woodhouse, & Waring, 1995; Pollack & Middleton, 1994.

14. Shiffman, Mason, & Henningfield, 1998. For an older but more extensive review and more detailed tabulation of methods, see Schwartz, 1987.

15. One must cast standards of acceptability in historical perspective in any case. "The history of public health might well be written as a persistent redefinition of the unacceptable," according to Vickers, 1958. Examples of "standards of acceptability" proffered by groups of professionals include M. Franz et al., 1986; World Health Organization, 1981; the series of six handbooks by IOX Assessment Associates, 1988; Handbook for Evaluating Drug Abuse and Alcohol Prevention Programs, 1987. The most sweeping consensus-development procedures resulting in national objectives made up of compromise standards of acceptability are the U.S objectives for the nation discussed in the next section.

16. *Healthy People 2000,* 1991. Drafts of the 2010 objectives were available for public comment as this book went to press.

17. Green, 1980b; McGinnis, 1982.

18. Green, R. W. Wilson, & Bauer, 1983.

19. Andersen & Mullner, 1990; Green, Blakenbaker, et al., 1987; National Center for Health Statistics, 1990; U.S. Department of Health and Human Services, 1986.

20. U.S. Department of Health and Human Services, 1981b. See also Secretary's Task Force on Black and Minority Health, 1985; and commentary on the report by Nickens, 1990, esp. pp. 133–134. The year 2000 objectives process incorporated the focused attention to minority issues; see Mason, 1990, esp. pp. 27–28.

21. See *Model Standards,* 1985, and its later edition, *Healthy Communities 2000,* 1991.

22. Spain, Eastman, & Kizer, 1989, p. 969.

23. *Model Standards,* 1985, p. 5.

24. C. H. Weiss, 1973, p. 54.

25. O. W. Cummings et al., 1988.

26. Dewey, 1938. See also Dewey, 1909.

27. Schlesinger, 1988, p. 902.

28. Fetterman, Kaftarian, & Wandersman, 1996; Green, George, et al., 1995.

29. Guba &. Lincoln, 1989.

30. Brindis, Hughes, & Newacheck, 1998; Delaney & Adams, 1997; Doyle, Smith, & Hosokawa, 1989; R. M. Goodman, Steckler, & Alciati, 1997; Viadro, Earp, & Altpeter, 1997; Wickizer, Wagner, & Perrin, 1998.

31. Kotchen et al., 1986. See also endnote 13.

32. Andrzejeswski & Lagua, 1997; Bausell, 1983; Bernier, 1996; Colton, 1997; Green & Brooks-Bertram, 1978; Henderson, 1987; Kernaghan & Giloth, 1988; D. Levin & Coronel, 1997; G. Macdonald, 1997a, 1997b; Mark & Pines, 1995; Mullen & Zapka, 1989; Neufeld & Norman, 1985; Pincus, 1996; Rootman, 1997; Saan, 1997; Salzer, Nixon, & Bickman, 1997; Speller, Evans, & Head, 1997; Terris, 1998; Van Den Broucke & Lenders, 1997; Zapka, 1985; Ziglio, 1997.

33. The following references provide a variety of methodological approaches to the evaluation of program process: Basch, 1987; Blake et al., 1987; Brunk & Goeppinger, 1990; Finnegan, Murray, Kurth, & McCarthy, 1989. Examples where the Precede model was applied include W. B. Brown, Williamson, & Carlaw, 1988; Contento, Kell, Keiley, & Corcoran, 1992; Dignan, Michielutte, Sharp, Young, & Daniels, 1991; Graff, Pearson, LeVan, & Sofian, 1987; Knox, Mandel, & Lazarowicz, 1981; Macaulay et al., 1997; Mahloch, Taylor, Taplin, & Urban, 1993; McAlister et al., 1982; Michielutte & Beal, 1990; Steckler, Orville, Eng, & Dawson, 1989, 1992; Taggart, Bush, Zuckerman, & Theiss, 1990; van Assema, Steenbakkers, & Kok, 1994; Vasse, Nijhuis, Kok, & Kroodsma, 1997; Worden et al., 1988.

34. Basch et al., 1985; Botelho & Richmond, 1996; Candeias, 1991; DePue, Wells, Lasater, & Carleton, 1990; Dodek & Ottoson, 1996; N. H. Gottlieb, Lovato, Weinstein, Green, & Eriksen, 1992; Helmer, Dunn, & Lubritz, 1995; Hendrickson, Wood, & Parcel, 1996; Hubbard & Ottoson, 1997; Laitakari, 1998; Ottoson & Green, 1987; Pucci & Haglund, 1994; Pulley, McAlister,

& O'Reilly, 1996; Spivak, Prothrow-Smith, & Hausman, 1995. An extensive application of the Precede-Proceed model in guiding and evaluating implementation in a large HMO is reported by R. S. Thompson, Taplin, McAfee, Mandelson, & Smith, 1995. See also endnotes 16, 21, 22, and 57 in Chapter 6.

35. Basch et al., 1985; Dobson & Cook, 1980; Rezmovic, 1982. In medical and health services research and evaluation, the Type III error is usually counted as an ineffective program, because in these fields a distinction is made between efficacy and effectiveness. *Efficacy* here refers to the achievement of intended results under ideal "laboratory" conditions. *Effectiveness* refers to the achievement of intended results in the field, where the program is in the hands of practitioners who will implement it with their own twist, adapting it to suit local circumstances. See Flay, 1986a.

36. Again, the line between the audience reactions in process evaluation and the antecedents to behavior in impact evaluation is fuzzy. Classification of an evaluation as process or impact within these overlapping spheres has little meaning or importance to anyone except a few evaluation experts. In the field, process evaluation and impact evaluations will tend to blend in their timing and methods. See Leviton & Valdiserri, 1990; Ramirez & McAlister, 1989.

37. Examples of impact evaluations where the Precede model was used include Brink, B. Simons-Morton, & Zane, 1989; Bush et al., 1989; Pentz, MacKinnon, et al., 1989; Vickery et al., 1983; Walter & Wynder, 1989; B. L. Wells, DePue, Lasater, & Carleton, 1988; Windsor, 1984.

38. Flay & Cook, 1981; Redman, Spencer, & Sanson-Fisher, 1990; Wallack, 1981. When the campaign's objective is to influence policy through increased public awareness, then one can appropriately measure media success by tracking the number of news stories on the issue, legislative acts proposed and passed, or other political outcomes. See DeJong & Winsten, 1990; Wallack, 1980.

39. D. M. Levine et al., 1979; Maiman, Green, Gibson, & Mackenzie, 1979; Mann & Sullivan, 1987; McGowan & Green, 1995; Morisky et al., 1983; Terry et al., 1981; Walter, 1989.

40. A lament often heard from researchers conducting school and work-site health promotion studies, explaining the sometimes disappointing results of their evaluations, is that the curriculum or program was not implemented as intended. "Fidelity" was often identified as the factor influencing outcomes in "The School Health Education Evaluation Study," 1985. See also Basch, 1984; McCaul & Glasgow, 1985; Walker, 1992.

41. This is one of several dilemmas of evaluation in health education described in Green, 1977. This problem of fidelity was discussed earlier in this chapter in relation to the Type III error in evaluation. More recent evaluations and reviews have given greater play to the need for adaptation in effective implementation, e.g., Gerstein & Green, 1993; R. M. Goodman, Tenney, Smith, & Steckler, 1992; MacDonald & Green, 1994; McCormick, Steckler, & McLeroy, 1995; Parcel, Eriksen, et al., 1989; Parcel et al., 1991; Parham, Goodman, Steckler, Schmid, & Koch, 1993; Pentz & Trebow, 1991.

42. A pioneering text in qualitative evaluation is M. Q. Patton, 1990. See also R. M. Goodman & Steckler, 1989b; Steckler, 1989.

43. Atwater, 1974.

44. Drazen, Nevid, Pace, & O'Brien, 1982; Fawcett et al., 1997; Spiegel & Lindaman, 1977; Taggart, Bush, Zuckerman, & Theiss, 1990; Warner, 1977.

45. Bryant, Stender, Frist, & Somers, 1976.

46. Here are examples of the inventory approach: Bertera, Oehl, & Telepchak, 1990; K. F. Dennison, Galante, & Golaszewski, 1996; A. J. Hill, 1996; Taggart et al., 1991; U.S. Department of Health and Human Services, 1986; Worrall, Hickson, Barnett, & Yiu, 1998; Zabora, Morrison, Olsen, & Ashley, 1997.

47. This is usually referred to as *formative evaluation* when the purpose is to make adjustments in the program as it is developing. See for example Basch, 1989; Basch et al., 1985; Mendelsohn, 1973.

48. Hankin, 1994.

49. U.S. Department of Health and Human Services, 1990. See also D. B. Black & Cameron, 1997; DiClemente & Prochaska, 1982; Glynn, Gruder, & Jerski, 1986; Leupker, Pallonen, Murray, & Pirie, 1989; D. M. Murray & Perry, 1987; Pechacek, Fox, Murray, & Leupker, 1984; Windsor & Orleans, 1986.

50. J. Allen, Lowman, & Miller, 1996; Connors, Maisto, & Donovan, 1996; Eddy, Fitzhugh, & Wang, 1997; Green & Krotki, 1968; Lando, Pirie, & Schmid, 1996; Law & Tang, 1995; Longabaugh, Rubin, & Lowman, 1996; Lowe, Windsor, & Woodby, 1997; Marlatt & Gordon, 1985; Secker-Walker, Solomon, & Mead, 1995; Wang, Ephross, & Green, 1975.

51. R. W. Wilson & Iverson, 1982.

52. For example, Douglas, Wertley, & Chaffee, 1970; Wang et al., 1979; Windsor, 1984.

53. Blackburn, 1987; Farquhar, 1978; Farquhar et al., 1990; Fortmann et al., 1981; Kotchen et al., 1986; Nutbeam & Catford, 1987; Ramirez & McAlister, 1989. For summary discussions and reviews of the evaluation designs of the cardiovascular disease prevention projects at Stanford, Minnesota, Pawtucket, North Karelia, and Wales, see Blackburn, 1987; a series of descriptions in Matarazzo et al., 1984; Nutbeam, Smith, & Catford, 1990; Shea & Basch, 1990; Tudor-Smith, Nutbeam, Moore, & Catford, 1998.

54. Farquhar, Maccoby, & Wood, 1977; Macauley et al., 1997; Maccoby, Farquhar, & Wood, 1977.

55. Schuurman & de Haes, 1980.

56. Dershewitz & Williamson, 1977; Roter, 1977; Sayegh & Green, 1976.

57. Bailey & Zambrano, 1974; Elwood, Ericson, & Lieberman, 1978.

58. Green, Levine, & Deeds, 1975; Green, Levine, Wolle, & Deeds, 1979; Hatcher, Green, Levine, & Flagle, 1986; D. M. Levine et al., 1979; Morisky et al., 1983.

59. Green, 1977; Green & Lewis, 1986; Windsor, Baranowski, Clark, & Cutter, 1994.

60. Bertram & Brooks-Bertram, 1977; Figa-Talamanca, 1975; Kreuter & Green, 1978; Stuart, 1969.

61. This section is based on Chapter 12 in Green & Lewis, 1986. See this book for a more extensive discussion of the measures and application to a different example.

62. Banta & Luce, 1983.

63. Batey & Lewis, 1982; Lewis & Batey, 1982; C. E. Smith, Kleinbeck, Fernengel, & Mayer, 1997; Steckler & Dawson, 1982.

64. Porter, 1981.

65. Lovato, Green, & Stainbrook, 1993.

66. For examples of costing programs in school health, see Risser, Hoffman, Bellah, & Green, 1985. In smoking cessation, see Cromwell, Bartosch, & Baker, 1997; Curry, Grothaus, & Pabiniak, 1998; Green, Rimer, & Bertera, 1978; Law & Tang, 1995. In family planning, see Bertera & Green, 1979; Trussell, Koenig, & Stewart, 1997. In hypertension education, see Cantor et al., 1985; Crowley, Dunt, & Day, 1995; O'Neill, Normand, & McKnight, 1996.

67. Green & Lewis, 1986.

Chapter 8

Applications
in Community Settings

PRECEDE asks and helps answer what, who, and why questions. What are the quality-of-life, health, behavioral, and environmental problems or aspirations? Who has those problems or aspirations? Why do they have them (what are their causes or determinants)? What assets can be built on? PROCEED asks what resources, barriers, policies, regulations, and organizational factors need to be adjusted so one can make a program work and can set up an implementation and evaluation design. The overall process is ecological because, from the social assessment through to implementation and evaluation, the program's future context and circumstances directly influence planning decisions. The next five chapters discuss the application of the Precede-Proceed model in five settings or contexts: community, work site, school, medical or health care, and new information and communication technologies.

This chapter addresses some issues planners need to consider when applying the Precede-Proceed model in the community setting. It is divided into three sections. The first begins with an expanded definition of the word *community* and follows with a description of the subtle differences between *community interventions* and *interventions in communities*. It also discusses the realities and limitations of *participation*. The second section examines the complexities inherent in establishing, managing, and maintaining community coalitions. The third section illustrates how the application of Precede-Proceed principles in the community setting leads to multiple intervention tactics that constitute a comprehensive health promotion strategy. Practical tools to help planners identify and apply multiple intervention tactics are reviewed, with special emphasis on mass media applications.

COMMUNITY: A MEDIUM FOR CHANGE AND A CHANGING MEDIUM

DEFINING COMMUNITY

The term *community* is easily understood in common parlance. When it is used in the context of health practice or research, though, its varied meanings force the use of an operational definition. Operational definitions of community are sure to bring simultaneous cries of "too restricting" and "lacks precision." This chapter uses the term *community* to refer to two characteristics—the first structural, the second functional. Structurally, a community is an area with geographic and often political boundaries demarcated as a district, county, metropolitan area, city, township, or neighborhood.[1] Functionally, a community is a place where "members have a sense of identity and belonging, shared values, norms, communication, and helping patterns."[2] Effective community workers understand the dynamic social characteristics and the less dynamic cultural traditions of a community, and they plan interventions with sensitivity to them.

The structural aspect of the definition limits activity to a local focus, leaving the larger national, provincial, and state endeavors for consideration elsewhere.[3] Even so, this definition leaves room to roam. For instance, political nuances that can influence program planning and implementation will vary according to the cultural context of a given community or neighborhood. In some instances, *informal* political forces exert more influence on policy formulation and program implementation than do the *formal* political structures usually associated with official boundaries.[4] For example, it would be foolhardy to launch a health promotion program in Harlem simply on the grounds that the mayor of New York City endorsed it, just as it would be in London's Lewisham area with merely the blessing of that city's lord mayor. On the other hand, proceeding without such political support could be equally foolhardy. For instance, attempts to organize Nigerian villagers to control malaria or guinea worm disease outbreaks would be impossible without the overt approval and support of the village chief. Ultimately, the geopolitical scope of a program must be left to the prudent judgment and sensitive action of those working with the program. It must be guided by the local people who know the culture and traditions of the community and by Proceed analyses of the resources available from the community and other levels (state, provincial, or national) to support the program.[5]

Grounded in the principles of participatory democracy and social justice, community-based programs hold considerable potential for making population changes. They accomplish such changes primarily as a result of reaching larger numbers of people through mass media and multiple channels of communication, building widespread normative, economic, and political support for the changes and possibly stimulating change in a community's social fabric. The justification for community-based approaches is by no means limited to passionate rhetoric. Numerous studies[6] support and justify the theoretical and philosophical tenets underlying community-based approaches, and research findings from community interventions constitute some of public health's most significant success stories.[7]

COMMUNITY INTERVENTIONS AND INTERVENTIONS IN COMMUNITIES

The following terms sound alike, but they are different. *Community interventions* seek small but pervasive changes that apply to the majority of the population; the approach is community-wide. *Interventions in a community* seek more intensive or profound change in a subpopulation, usually within or from a specific community site such as a workplace, hospital or clinic, nursing home, or school; this approach is targeted.

Most population-wide approaches are designed to produce small changes across an entire population. The social arithmetic of this idea is that the net effect of influencing a small percentage change in an entire population will yield more profound public health benefits than will those strategies aimed exclusively at the 10% of the population deemed to be at highest risk. Demonstration programs reported in the international literature, beginning with the large-scale family planning and immunization programs reported in the 1960s and early 1970s, have fueled enthusiasm for the community-based approach to health promotion.[8] This trend gained ground through reports on a series of cardiovascular and cancer community-intervention trials initiated in the late 1970s and early 1980s,[9] and it continued with descriptions of a wide variety of community applications supported by government[10] and philanthropy[11] in the 1990s. The environmental movement has sought a similar level of community-wide activation around issues such as recycling, toxic waste disposal, water conservation, and carpooling.[12] The AIDS epidemic and HIV infections revived a parallel and converging interest in community approaches to health education.[13]

While numerous public health analysts[14] have offered epidemiological and sociological justifications for supporting these population approaches, others have wisely cautioned that either-or approaches can be counterproductive. Both approaches aim at promoting health and reducing preventable health problems and disability, and both have independent and additive effects.[15] The benefits of creating a balance between community interventions and interventions in communities become especially compelling when their complementary merits are examined from different perspectives.

The Epidemiological Case for the Community Approach. By the numbers alone, the community-wide approach appears irresistibly advantageous to the point that some would argue to transfer resources from high-risk approaches. In North

Karelia, only 2% of the target population lost weight in the initial years, but this amounted to 60,000 persons, far more than could have been reached through doctors' offices.[16] The Australian "Quit. For Life" media campaign produced what might seem a measly 2.8% reduction in smoking prevalence,[17] which would be considered a failure by targeted smoking-cessation program standards,[18] but it amounted to 83,000 fewer smokers in Sydney. A television and community organization effort to support smokers' quitting in Canada yielded a 2.9% reduction in smoking prevalence, which translated to 8,800 fewer smokers than expected from extrapolated trends in Canada.[19] The scattered but relentless antismoking efforts in the United States between 1964 and 1978 produced a net annual smoking prevalence reduction of only 1%. But this produced in turn an estimated 200,000 fewer premature smoking-related deaths, with many more expected to be avoided as former smokers age through the 1980s and 1990s.[20]

These epidemiological examples of the extensive, though proportionately small, benefits of community-wide or population interventions relative to the more effective but limited range of targeted, institutionally-based interventions argue for a place at the health promotion table for community approaches.

The Social-Psychological Case for the Community Approach. From their review of the decades of work on sexually transmitted disease control, Solomon and DeJong conclude, "More than any other recommendation, we urge that AIDS risk-reduction strategies focus on establishing a social climate in which people feel that it is the norm and not the exception to adopt AIDS risk-reduction behavior."[21] This concept of building a social norm for behavior conducive to health lies at the heart of the social psychological justification for community approaches to health promotion.[22] Clearly the antismoking policy initiatives have succeeded in doing just that. Designated drivers rather than drinking and driving appears to be making similar strides in becoming a norm. Low-fat eating has begun to take on the markings of a social norm, at least in more affluent communities and their upscale restaurants.[23] To assure that health-promoting norms touch the *entire* community, however, efforts to reach high-risk subpopulations must continue. Research studies suggest that computers and video games, when appropriately targeted, can reach segments of a community missed by traditional communication strategies.[24]

The social psychological case does not argue for a choice between community-wide and targeted approaches. It argues for a combination of them. As every social marketing and classroom experience demonstrates, targeting or "market segmentation" effectively produces tailored, relevant, and effective teaching and persuasive messages that reach individuals.[25] But individual change can be powerfully *predisposed* by the individual's own perception that others have made the change successfully (role models) and with satisfaction (vicarious reinforcement). Furthermore, the individual process of making the change can be *enabled,* by imitation or modeling and by help from friends, and *reinforced,* by the approval of significant others. These processes of social support and influence are facilitated if enough social change is taking place around the individual—that is, if other people and environmental circumstances support the change in the same period. This is the fundamental thesis of reciprocal determinism in cognitive learning theory.[26]

The combination of targeted and community approaches reconciles the debate between individualized and system approaches, which some have characterized as a debate between health education and health promotion or between educational and environmental approaches.[27] Community approaches count on individual innovators to blaze the trail for social change, but such approaches must reinforce their changes and increase their reach by building greater environmental and normative supports for the changes. Ordinances to control smoking in public places, for example, support those who have quit smoking and protect them from exposure to others' smoking while encouraging still others to quit.[28]

Community programs strive to provide the general environmental and social supports for change through policies and mass media; they also try to bring about the institutional interventions to strengthen psychological readiness through families, schools, work sites, and health care settings, where relatively individualized communications can be organized. In the long run, policies and mass media also help shape psychological readiness. Institutional settings provide ideal opportunities for social and environmental supports for change. The combination of interventions at multiple levels achieves the community diffusion effect necessary to reach those who cannot be reached personally.

The Economic Case for the Community Approach. The Ottawa Charter on Health Promotion and virtually all policy declarations related to the enhancement of health and quality of life acknowledge the reality that the major determinants of health, for both populations and individuals, are directly linked to social, cultural, and economic factors.[29] As Frank has observed, "One's immediate social and economic environment and the way this environment interacts with one's psychological resources and coping skills, has much more to do with the determination of health status than was recognized in early epidemiological studies of chronic disease etiology."[30] For example, trends in market economies over the past two decades suggest that the initial demand for healthful food and fitness products tended to be driven by the consumer preferences of the more upscale and middle majority segments of the population and less so by the poorer, typically late-adopter segments. In this innovative stage, the consumption of healthful products was profitable to producers to the extent that prices, typically set for those in higher income brackets, were met. Those same prices were usually prohibitive to those with modest economic means. Over time, congruent with the principles of diffusion theory,[31] the interest in and demand for healthful products have spread beyond the middle majority segments of the population. This demand constitutes an economic incentive motivating producers and distributors to find ways to

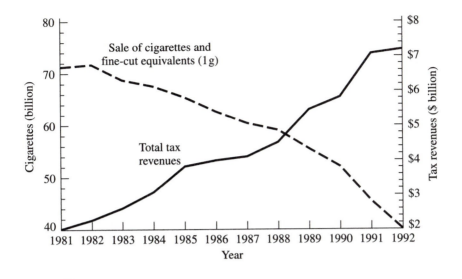

FIGURE 8-1

Domestic sales of cigarettes inversely mirrored domestic tobacco taxes in Canada between 1981 and 1992.

SOURCE: Non-Smokers' Rights Association, Ottawa, Ontario, Canada.

make these products accessible to larger portions of society. Such was the case when low-fat alternatives were introduced into the marketplace. Over time, healthful alternatives have gradually become more accessible, even through fast food restaurants and convenience grocery stores, where the poorer segments obtain much of their food.[32]

The pricing of tobacco products represents a compelling flip side to this discussion—an example of a health benefit resulting from *higher* prices. Figure 8-1 shows that increases in the tobacco tax from 1981 to 1992 in Canada were inversely related to decreases in tobacco consumption in those same years. Following the tax increase, as shown in Figure 8-2, the prevalence of smoking among teens, a lower income, hard-to-reach population, declined by over 50%. The Canadian experience with taxes on cigarettes as an effective means of controlling consumption among teenagers also needs to be seen in the context of the controls on media exposure as a result of laws passed in Canada that restrict advertising more severely than in the United States.

Figure 8-3 shows a similar trend from 1977 to 1997 among high-school seniors in the United States. In that figure, note that the percent of high-school seniors who smoke goes up between 1993 and 1997, even though the price per pack of cigarettes remains the same. While price does strongly influence the consumption of tobacco, it is not the only force. Experts remind us that during that

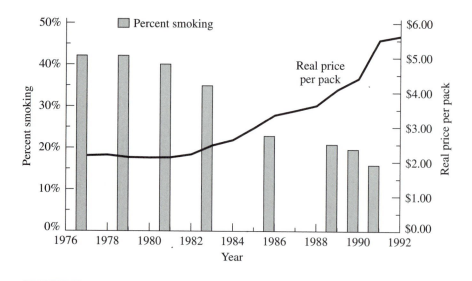

FIGURE 8-2

The percentage of Canadians 15 to 19 years old smoking daily between 1977 and 1992 followed the trend in real prices of cigarettes (adjusted for inflation).

SOURCES: National Clearinghouse on Tobacco and Health; Statistics Canada.

same period, the tobacco industry in the United States carried out extensive advertising campaigns aimed at young smokers.[33]

As in all other aspects of life, economic measures are powerful health policy tools, with both positive and negative consequences for large segments of the population. Accordingly, those planning community-based health promotion programs should pay heed to the economic context of the population they plan to serve. Some jurisdictions have sought alternatives to taxation on products like alcohol and tobacco as a way of controlling consumption and paying for the damage of these products, viewing such taxes as regressive. British Columbia, for example, has initiated legal action against the tobacco industry to collect a tax directly from them for health damages paid by the province; the terms specifically forbid the tobacco manufacturers from passing this tax on to the consumers.

The Political Case for the Community Approach. The strength of numbers makes the epidemiological case, the strength of social norms makes the sociological case and the strengths of purchasing power and taxes make the economic case for community-wide strategies in health promotion; the combination of these makes the political case. Policy changes needed to support behavior in some health promotion programs will tend to favor numbers, norms, and money. The political power of the middle majority lies in the number of votes this segment of the

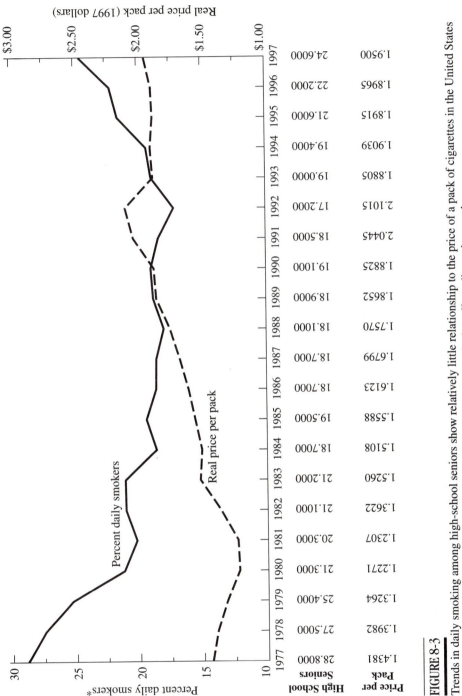

High School Seniors	Price per Pack	Year
28.8000	1.4381	1977
27.5000	1.3982	1978
25.4000	1.3264	1979
21.3000	1.2271	1980
20.3000	1.2307	1981
21.1000	1.3622	1982
21.2000	1.5260	1983
18.7000	1.5108	1984
19.5000	1.5588	1985
18.7000	1.6123	1986
18.7000	1.6799	1987
18.1000	1.7570	1988
18.9000	1.8652	1989
19.1000	1.8825	1990
18.5000	2.0445	1991
17.2000	2.1015	1992
19.0000	1.8805	1993
19.4000	1.9039	1994
21.6000	1.8915	1995
22.2000	1.8965	1996
24.6000	1.9500	1997

Percent daily smokers

Real price per pack

Real price per pack (1997 dollars)

Percent daily smokers*

FIGURE 8-3

Trends in daily smoking among high-school seniors show relatively little relationship to the price of a pack of cigarettes in the United States between 1977 and 1997 because of the tobacco industry's intensive marketing efforts directed at youth.

SOURCES: General Accounting Office; Institute for Social Research, University of Michigan, Monitoring the Future Project; The Tobacco Institute.

population represents. The political power of social norms lies in the voter sentiments and public opinion reflected by broadly accepted norms. The political
power of money lies in contributions to campaign funding and lobbying. The
numbers and norms clearly give the middle majority of the population an advantage in democratic policy making.

Economic influence on politics might seem to favor the most affluent minority, but increasingly politicians feel pressures to diversify their sources of campaign funding and prefer many small donations from the mainstream to few large
donations from the rich special-interest groups. Gaining or holding elected office
on the strength of a few large campaign donations leaves a politician with limited
options and tainted integrity. Similarly, the lowest-income minority of the population commands little political influence, having neither money nor numbers.
Health promotion strategies that increase broad public awareness, interest, and
commitment therefore stand a much greater chance of gaining political support
than do those directed exclusively at either high- or low-income populations.

Programs and policy issues related exclusively to the needs of the poor,
minorities, and other politically marginal groups gain less support in Congress,
Parliament, and state or provincial legislatures than do issues framed as affecting
everyone. As Wilson concluded from his analysis of policy in the United States,

> In the final analysis, the question of reform is a political one. Accordingly, if the
> issues are couched in terms of promoting economic security for all Americans, if the
> essential political message underscores the need for economic and social reform that
> benefits all groups in society, not just poor minorities, a basis for generating a broad-
> based political coalition to achieve such reform would be created. Minority leaders
> could play an important role in this coalition once they fully recognize the need to
> shift or expand their definition of racial problems in America and to broaden the
> scope of suggested policy programs to address them.[34]

THE DEMONSTRATION AND "MULTIPLIER" VALUE OF SMALLER PROGRAMS

In relation to intervention methods, two fundamental differences between community interventions and interventions in communities exist. One is the comparative magnitude of the undertaking, which is determined by the size of the group
or population for whom the program is intended. The other is the number of organizations as well as the levels of organization needed to be involved. Consequently, the quantitative aspects of the intervention process should vary mainly as
a function of the size and scope of the program, but the added complexities of
organizing and managing a community-wide program make the qualitative
aspects quite different for the two types of interventions.

A commitment to a community intervention is a big commitment, but big is
not always better. Health workers using interventions in a community can take

advantage of the strong reinforcement that group dynamics within institutions, support systems, and interpersonal channels of communication bring to a program. Such interpersonal and small-group interventions are more common, more manageable, and probably better understood than are community-wide programs, as subsequent chapters will show. Institution-based programs lend themselves better to systematic, controlled research, hence their stronger research base. In addition, site- or area-specific interventions carried out within communities offer great potential for long-term, positive social change. When these smaller intervention efforts are sensitively carried out within the envelope of the community, they tend to become focal points for attention. At first they may be viewed merely as curious experiments. Over time, though, curiosity gives way to genuine interest and imitation. As more people begin to sense that respectable individuals and organizations think the undertaking is good, more people agree to it.[35] As more organizations adopt or extend components of the program, they produce a multiplier effect.[36]

A classic example of this effect concerns three forces that accounted for health improvements in Mississippi from 1956 to 1981, especially among African Americans. The first was the passage of federal laws providing for new human service entitlement for food stamps, Head Start programs, medicare and medicaid, and housing improvements. The second and third forces reveal the multiplier effect.

> A second force was the establishment of a variety of health services and health undertakings, originally by concerned external groups such as the Medical Commission on Human Rights and later by Mississippians themselves. These indigenous efforts were, in part, responses to innovations of outside origin, e.g., in maternal and child care. Overall, while some health projects like the Tufts University's Mound Bayou Health Center were well funded, long lasting, and capable of providing a variety of services to a defined Black population in the Delta, many projects were very small, ephemeral, and maintained on shoestrings. Nevertheless, the health projects of the 1960's and the early 1970's introduced new concerns for health standards, often improved methods, and involvements of communities in the improvement of health. The third force arose out of the first two. It was the growth of valid health information among both races. This led to an awareness of health needs, enhanced capacities for self-help, and greater demands for quality from health services providers.[37]

A contemporary extension of this multiplier effect is evident in the analysis reported by Schooler and her colleagues.[38] They document how technology and methods learned from the early cardiovascular-disease prevention trials begun in the 1970s have been translated into specific applications worldwide. Table 8-1 presents a partial listing of these applications.

The theoretical underpinnings of the health promotion methods and the application of those methods will vary little between community interventions and interventions in communities. The differences will lie largely in their magnitude and complexity.

TABLE 8-1

Examples of community-based interventions shown here are modeled after the cardiovascular disease community prevention trials from the 1970s through the early 1990s

Description	Units and Population Size	Intervention Years	Intervention Activities	Population-Wide Risk Factor Results
The Martignacco Project (Italy)	2 towns: 1 treatment; 1 reference (N = 12,910)	1977–1983	Newpaper, other print, direct education, events	Cholesterol (men only), blood pressure, CHD risk, CVD events
North Coast Healthy Lifestyle Programme (Australia)	3 towns: 2 treatments; 1 reference (N = 61,560)	1978–1980	TV, radio, newspaper, other print, direct education, events	Smoking
Swiss National Research Programme	4 towns: 2 treatments; 2 references (N = 56,000)	1978–1980	TV, radio, newspaper, other print, direct education, events, environment	Smoking, blood pressure, obesity
Coronary Risk Factor Study (South Africa)	3 towns: 2 treatments; 1 reference (N = 17,750)	1979–1983	Other print, direct education, events	Smoking, blood pressure, composite CHD risk
German Cardiovascular Prevention Study	4 cities, 2 towns, 1 rural community; former West Germany reference (N = 1,228,400)	1985–1991	Newspaper, other print, direct education, events, environment	Blood pressure, smoking (men only), cholesterol
Norsjö study (Sweden)	3 areas: 1 municipality treatment; 2 counties reference (N = 5,300)	1985–1995	TV, radio, newspaper, direct education, events	Cholesterol
Heart-to-Heart Project (South Carolina)	2 towns: 1 treatment; 1 reference (N = 107,254)	1987–1991	TV, radio, other print, direct education, events, environment	Smoking, cholesterol
Slangerup "Heart Area" Project (Denmark)	2 rural/small towns: 1 treatment; 1 reference (N = 8,000)	1989–1990	TV, radio, other print, direct education, events, environment	

SOURCE: Adapted from "Synthesis and Issues from Community Prevention Trials," by C. Schooler, J. W. Farquhar, S. P. Fortmann, and J. A. Flora, 1997, *Annals of Epidemiology*, 7 (Suppl.), S57, S59. With permission.

COMMUNITY PARTICIPATION

One thing that should not differ between community interventions and interventions in the community is the importance of engaging community participation, highlighted in Chapter 2. Early involvement of community members in identifying their own needs, setting their own priorities, and planning their own programs is, in itself, a form of intervention. It provides the opportunity for ownership. This can lead to a sense of empowerment and self-determination—those difficult-to-measure intangibles that can make the difference between long-term success and failure.

Is It Real or Symbolic? As health promotion practitioners take steps to create and nurture community participation, they must repeatedly ask themselves, "Am I fostering participation that is real or symbolic?" Consider just two of many factors that typically surface in community-based work. First, by definition, communities are made up of a variety of stakeholders who tend to hold very different views and expectations. Second, many community-based programs are driven or supported by outside funding, either in response to opportunities (in the form of grants from outside funders) or threats (which they must unite against to survive). Both of these factors—diversity in stakeholders and economic support—are certainly assets. Ironically, these same assets, if mismanaged, can become a source of mistrust that in turn leads to the perception that participation is actually "tokenism."

The Dilemma of External Funding. To some extent, this mismanagement occurred in efforts to elicit broad-based community participation for federally funded, large-scale research and demonstration efforts. These large scientific studies were conceived and, for the most part, planned by public health officials at the federal level and by the professors who received the grants. In some instances, efforts to engage the community typically occurred after the initial planning had started. A national peer review panel approved the protocol and the grant was approved by a federal agency. Thus, the active participation of the community came only after the grant was in hand. Asking communities and organizations to implement programs planned elsewhere and evaluated on someone else's terms might gain some followers, but often with commitments only "as long as the money lasts."

Academics working on large community interventions are faced with a dilemma. Public health workers cry out for the resources needed to bring prevention to the community. Though taken by the idea, decision makers want proof that it will make a difference. Guidelines for scientific trials and rigorously evaluated demonstrations are delineated by the federal government. Academics design proposals. "Participation" begins when key influencers in the target communities are informed of the university's intent to apply for the grant and their willingness to cooperate is secured. If the community is invited to participate in the implementation but not the policy and planning stages, they may feel they are being used as free labor or a laboratory for university-initiated projects. This dilemma reflects an inability to design unbiased scientific tests of community interventions without damaging the variable (active community participation) that is most likely to account for successful community structural and cultural change, as well as behavioral change in individuals.[39] Early activation of the community in these instances may falsely raise community hopes and expectations should funding not be secured. Nevertheless, some communities take this aborted effort as a nudge to develop their own programs without external funding. Alternately, some of the communities that receive research grant funding fail to carry on the programs initiated under these or other grants.[40]

The scientific benefits of the early community studies may have justified their restraints on the early and active participation of community members. Even so, the compelling evidence pointing to the benefits of community participation now demands a continuing search for funding mechanisms between levels of government and procedures of grant making that provide for greater community involvement.[41]

Two Points of View. A study of changes in the organization of local community services centers in Quebec provides a clear illustration of how differing perceptions of authority, and consequently power, can lead to problems and disagreements. The defenders of local autonomy opposed central government programming on the grounds that it would result in low-level adaptation to local needs, bureaucratization of services, and the discouragement of local participation. In response to these concerns, the Canadian health policy analyst Bozzini commented:

> This danger is real, but the analysis should be freed from ideological preconceptions. First, nobody should, *a priori* be scandalized because the state offers, over the whole Quebec territory, a homogeneous set of services addressing the most prevalent needs of the citizens. Furthermore, centralized programming does not mean a lack of local autonomy in the ways of doing things; against this anti-institutional rhetoric, the present situation shows that this autonomy is quite large including locally determined styles of community organization.[42]

All of this suggests the need for practitioners to be clear in their understanding of what community participation means. Having several influential community authorities on a steering committee is politically wise and undoubtedly will strengthen a program's chances for support, but it does not constitute "community participation." In reviewing the ethical issues inherent in fostering such participation, Minkler and Pies[43] pose this important question:

> When our agencies or funders propose what is really only symbolic or lip-service community participation, how do we formulate effective value based arguments to reinforce the importance of not only bringing community members to the table but also hearing their concerns and ensuring that their input is heavily reflected in the final product?

One way planners can begin to address this pithy question is to incorporate the principles of participatory research into both planning and evaluation. An essential feature of participatory research is that the people affected by an issue are involved in identifying the research questions about it and in interpreting the results for the purposes of policy or other action in relation to it. Involving them early in the planning assures that they have a say in the research assessment of needs and assets, which is part of the planning during PRECEDE. Maintaining their involvement through the evaluation phases of PROCEED will ensure that the results will be interpreted and translated into actions relevant to their further needs.

COALITIONS: GROUPS TO BE RECKONED WITH

Whether meeting basic needs in Nigeria,[44] influencing policy action to prevent childhood lead poisoning in New York City,[45] trying to strengthen collaboration in a minority neighborhood,[46] establish healthy public policy in an impoverished inner-city area of London,[47] or working to create health services for the rural homeless,[48] community coalitions emerge as an essential part of any community-based intervention program.

Coalition refers to a grouping of varied organizations in which the collective interests converge on a central, shared objective but whose member organizations have separate agendas and interests of their own. Thus, coalition members will bring their own organization's perspectives and resources to the table, but they also are expected to work toward achieving goals set by the coalition as a whole.

Coalitions operate at different points on what Wandersman has described as a "continuum of decision-making," ranging from an advisory role to full control over resources.[49] Coalitions often tackle multiple planning and financial oversight. In the planning realm, they are responsible for conducting needs assessments, setting priorities, and choosing interventions. At the financial end of the spectrum, coalitions and consortia may be responsible for disbursing and monitoring funds awarded to others in the community. In both cases, a coalition's capacity and skill in undertaking these managerial functions can drastically affect its survival.[50] It is precisely in such complex situations that applications of the Precede-Proceed model will help keep planners on track.

COALITIONS IN CONTEXT: SOCIAL CAPITAL

Another important feature of community-based consortia and coalitions is the community context in which they operate. In their alternating roles as leaders, facilitators, convenors, and participants in community life, coalition members find that the social norms and histories of their communities influence collaborative efforts.[51] For example, if a planner is trying to establish a health promotion coalition in an area where there is a legacy of mistrust or failed attempts, the coalition's formation may occur in an atmosphere of suspicion or hostility. No matter how well its members go about the tasks of forming and implementing collaborative activities, a history of strained relationships can only be overcome through the rebuilding of trust, and this requires more time than some program planning and implementation schedules permit. Goodman notes that a community's readiness and capacity are demonstrated through the ability to "mobilize, structure, initiate, refine, and sustain an organized response," but that community development efforts are often sacrificed in an effort to move quickly to interventions and results.[52] Ironically, lack of attention to these underlying factors may be exactly what jeopardizes the intervention.

Emerging research on the theory of social capital explores the extent to which a community's history and its underlying structures, beliefs, and levels of trust may mediate the success or failure of collaborative efforts. We define *social capital* as the processes and conditions among people and organizations that lead to accomplishing a goal of mutual social benefit. In theory, those processes and conditions are manifested by four interrelated constructs: trust, cooperation, civic engagement, and reciprocity.

Beyond theory, research provides evidence not only that the constructs of social capital can be measured but also that they tend to predict positive outcomes when detected in high levels. For example, Kawachi[53] and his colleagues have demonstrated that low levels of social capital (as measured by mistrust) are linked to increased mortality; they employed a two-dimensional measure of social capital (social trust and group membership). Sampson, Raudenbush, and Earls studied the relationship between what they call "collective efficacy" (self-reported measures of the willingness of adults in a community intervene when they observe deviant behaviors by youth) and evidence of violence in an inner-city Chicago neighborhood.[54] Higher levels of collective efficacy in a neighborhood, a manifestation of mutual trust and solidarity, were associated with lower levels of violence in that same neighborhood. In a study of over 600 children 2–5 years of age and their caregivers (all of whom participated in a longitudinal child abuse and neglect study), Runyan and his co-workers[55] found that only 13% of the children were classified as "doing well," based on standard developmental measures. Their analysis revealed that measures of social capital, specifically "social support" and "support within the neighborhood," were the indicators that best discriminated children who "did well" and those who did not.

The capacity to assess levels of social capital in a community could have important methodological and policy implications for community health promotion. Currently, in spite of the extensive literature pointing to the social, economic, and political determinants of contemporary health problems, very few government or philanthropic resources are earmarked for building or strengthening the community capacity needed to maintain coalitions or the complex community interventions those coalitions support. If valid measurement can show that social capital or some aspect of community capacity is clearly linked to the effective application of community-based public health programs, funders will have to reexamine their present policies. Specifically, funders will be able to make more-informed decisions about the most productive ways to contribute infusions of health-related funding to a given community—either to bolster the capacity required for successful interventions or to move directly to the interventions themselves.

THE POLITICS OF COALITIONS AND COMMUNITY POWER

The following scenario takes place quite often in public health. Decision makers receive several program initiatives requiring support. All the options have merit, but the available resources cannot support all the options. In spite of what seems to be compelling data and information to some, decision makers do not agree on how the resources should be disbursed. Under these circumstances, political factors enter the decision-making process. In this context, public perceptions, or the perceived needs of special interest groups, tend to carry extraordinary weight. Political decision making is not inherently good or bad—it is just real. Communities are political. Over the years, academics[56] and political commentators[57] alike have used *game* as a metaphor to describe politics. Virtually all social systems have informal rules for the exchange of ideas and for negotiations. Those who want to initiate activities in a community need to be mindful of such rules. Here are some practical principles that will give you a feel for the game and its rules.

1. *There are never enough resources to cover all the demands for them.*
   A program is, figuratively speaking, in a competitive market. Thus, not only does a program have to meet the professional practice standards the planner sets for it, it must also have attributes that appeal to decision makers and a large segment of their constituents.
2. *Often, the ultimate decision as to what resources will be allocated to what demand are made by those who are not expert in the issues.* Therefore, special efforts need to be made to insure that decision makers are informed by credible experts as to the value of a project, and that the same information is reinforced through the decision makers' constituents or allies.
3. *Although decisions are sometimes influenced by the sheer weight of popular clamor, they are often influenced by the effective penetration of the decision makers' inner circle.* Therefore, program advocates need to know how to gain access to that inner circle.
4. *The conventional wisdom that "people tend to support what they 'own' is well supported in the literature."*[58] Therefore, because personal commitment follows ownership, one should make special efforts to help local leaders feel that the initiative or program in question is "theirs."

Even the entry-level practitioner quickly realizes that failure to pay attention to these and other political issues could prevent the best of programs from getting off the ground or, once initiated, from being sustained. Most health workers, however, especially those employed by official or government agencies, are discouraged, if not forbidden, from taking what might be construed as political action. Often they are informed that their program activities should remain independent of politics. Legally, this means campaigning for a political candidate or lobbying for legislation is prohibited during work time or in the name of one's organization. Practically, it means avoiding any appearance of using public funds to influence legislative or electoral decisions. These important principles by no means prohibit government health workers from using one of their most powerful tools, education, to keep decision makers and the general public informed about the progress of health promotion programs and the benefits they yield.

COALITIONS: SOME BASIC PRINCIPLES

In culling the literature in search of the indispensable rules that guide health promotion planners in the process of coalition building, one finds but a few.[59] More plentiful are examples of coalition efforts, each crafted to address the unique needs and sensitivities of a given community.[60]

To augment a review of the literature on the effectiveness of community coalitions for the Health Resources and Services Administration, Kreuter and Lezin[61] incorporated a telephone survey of health professionals[62] known to have extensive research or practical field experience with community health coalitions. The purpose of the survey was to elicit their expert views on what constitutes realistic expectations for community health coalitions. The results, summarized in Table 8-2, highlight the value of establishing a clear purpose, realistic expectations, and a reasonable time frame for a coalition.

BASIC STEPS TO KEEP IN MIND

Borrowing from the information in Table 8-2 and our own experiences, we offer the following as practical steps to consider when establishing and nurturing a community health promotion coalition.

1. Establish the Agenda. A small steering or planning committee, composed of colleagues dedicated to addressing the same health priority, is usually the first step in forming a coalition.[63] The steering committee can begin the work of the coalition by defining the purpose, proposing potential members, and organizing the first meeting. If the smaller group's deliberations lead to the formation of a broad-based coalition, the steering committee members may turn the leadership over to

TABLE 8-2
Expert panel opinions are shown here on realistic
expectations for community coalitions

Goals judged to be realistic
- Exchange information among coalition members
- Achieve a common goal among coalition members
- Promote collaboration among coalition members
- Legitimize the issue or focus of coalition

Goals judged to be realistic with reservations
- Program planning
- Influence policy
- Influence resource allocation for a given problem or issue

Goals judged to be generally unrealistic
- Program implementation
- Create organizational or systems change in a community
- Directly influence health outcomes

Key expectations for a coalition in the first year
- Get organized
- Establish a clear vision and mission—a common purpose
- Clarify mode of operations
- Formalize process, procedures; as necessary, establish subcommittees around agreed-on objectives
- Establish trust
- Develop an unambiguous plan of action
- Ascertain the group skills required to manage the coalition effectively

What factors predict the effectiveness of a coalition?
- Having a well-defined, specific issue on which to direct energies
- Having an agreed-on vision and goal
- Coalition members acknowledging that, given a problem or issue they are trying to address, they are more likely to succeed as part of an alliance rather than individually
- Having an adversary (e.g., health problem or an organizational or environmental threat to quality of life) that is clear and unambiguous
- A coalition taking a leadership, not a management, role—remaining focused on the vision, not getting bogged down in minute details

SOURCE: *"Are Consortia/Collaboratives Effective in Changing Health Status and Health Systems? A Critical Review of the Literature,"* by M. W. Kreuter and N. Lezin, prepared for the Office of Planning, Evaluation and Legislation (OPEL), Health Resources and Services Administration, June 19, 1998. With permission.

other members of the coalition or may retain a major management and support or staffing role.

Because many of the people capable of making a difference at the community level are already committed to other community projects, the aim of the coalition and its agenda must be compelling and appeal to the interests of these busy leaders. It must elicit in the prospective coalition member sentiments like "This is really important" or "This agenda ties in with our mission" or "I've heard Dr. Martha Francis, an influential community leader, challenge us to tackle this issue." In general, the more concrete and specific the coalition's goal, the better. Of course, if the goal is too specific, it discourages the formation of a broad constituency. Nevertheless, given the choice between a vague, motherhood-and-apple-pie goal and a precise, well-understood goal, one is better off negotiating the expansion of a specific goal than starting with a more general agenda that runs the risk of having universal but lukewarm appeal.[64]

2. Seek Broad Representation. Clarifying the key role(s) of the coalition will provide insight to the planners on the matter of recruiting the most effective coalition members. Nix's list of the types of leaders who typically influence community health programs offers a good point of departure:[65] (1) top-level community influentials who "legitimize" the program, (2) subarea (neighborhood) leaders if the program includes more than one area, (3) key health leaders, (4) leaders of the most influential organizations or companies, (5) leaders of factions and those who can act as "go-betweens" or links to several groups, (6) leaders of the target population (opinion leaders who represent the underserved, minority groups and those at high risk), (7) specialists with skills and knowledge relevant to the goals of the program, and (8) officials who control or support health programs (mayor, health director, commissioner, etc.).

We would add to this list two other influential groups: the media and the faith community. A formative evaluation of CDC's Planned Approach to Community Health (PATCH) program found that the most successful applications had media representation in the core group (coalition).[66] In addition to the obvious advantage of direct contact with a principal communication channel within the community and the political support that can bring, media representatives frequently bring invaluable skills in conducting market research. They also can articulate the health messages of the coalition to different audiences and reach out to other members of the media. Researchers have also demonstrated the influential role that the faith community can have on establishing community health promotion programs.[67]

As coalition members are recruited, keep in mind that close collaboration and cooperation are not always the automatic by-products of joining a coalition. Even with the shared goal of improving quality of life, public, private, and voluntary health organizations do compete with one another. For example, although the voluntary cancer, heart, lung, diabetes, and other health organizations may share prevention goals, they also compete with one another for donations from the community. If representatives of such competing organizations are a part of the same coalition, planners must maintain their sensitivity to the subtle, but very real, differences among those groups.[68]

One caveat for enthusiastic, entry-level practitioners is this: Be wary of giving community members the impression that the effort they are undertaking is a brand-new idea that will be the answer to their prayers. The fact is that most communities are already organized and have probably been down this road before; some likely serve on other community groups that also have a health agenda. By demonstrating interest and respect for prior experience, the practitioner can capitalize on the experience of coalition members.

3. Pay Attention to Details. Establishing a strong, representative coalition with a common agenda is one thing, managing that coalition is another. When you enter a room full of the community's most influential people, will you be ready?

    a. *Do your homework.* Generally, work goes better and faster when you know and understand the people you work with. Prior to your first meeting, find out about coalition members' interests and hobbies as well as their professional background and health concerns. If you have data describing the health issue(s) to be addressed, make certain that the coalition members have received it in advance and in a format and language they can easily understand.

    b. *Be hospitable.* Because active community leaders usually have more requests for their participation than they can honor, they may sometimes look for a reason to say "no." By creating a focused agenda and a hospitable environment for your coalition meetings, you increase the likelihood that people will participate. If at all possible, schedule meetings at the same location and a time most convenient for the majority of the group. The meeting room should be arranged to encourage discussion, and the chairs comfortable. Be prepared for the meeting with easy-to-read name tags, plenty of typed agendas and handouts, and any audiovisual equipment that you think might be needed during the meeting. Depending on the norms of the group, provide refreshments or food as appropriate.

4. The Crucial First Meeting. The first meeting is the most important one. It sets the tone for the coalition and establishes a model for the meetings to follow. Consider the following steps for the first meeting.

First, frame the agenda by asking the question, "What do we want the coalition members to leave the meeting with?" At a minimum, participants should leave the first meeting (1) with an understanding of the key issues or problems the coalitions will be addressing, (2) aware of the potential to address those issues and problems, (3) believing that the work of the coalition could be a worthy priority for their organization and for the community at large, (4) knowing other members of the coalition and understanding what they and the organizations they represent can and cannot contribute to the work of the coalition, and (5) knowing that the coalition is well staffed and organized.

Second, begin the meeting with a round-robin of self-introductions limited to name, title, organization or group representation, and perhaps why they came. Keep it short—opportunities will arise for more detailed discussion at two points later in the meeting. Following the brief introductions, a presentation about the proposal should be given by a respected person in the community, one who is articulate and has been well briefed on the details of the program to date. The presentation should include both a clear statement of the problem or goal the program will be addressing and local data to document its importance. An effective strategy is to describe the likely long-term health, social, and economic effects on the community if no action is taken on the problem. Even better, paint a vision of community well-being if action is taken. Keep this introductory presentation short, no more than 15 minutes. If visuals are used, make certain that they are clear, uncomplicated, and easy to grasp. Pretest all audiovisual equipment.

Third, provide time immediately following the presentation for questions and discussion. Have program staff ready to assist with the question and discussion period if necessary. Do not merely remain open for new ideas and criticism—ask for them.

Fourth, after the discussion, invite coalition members to share their responses to the following questions:

a. What is the primary mission of my agency, organization, or group?
b. What is it about this problem or program that is linked to our mission or interests?
c. With regard to the problem or the program envisioned, what kinds of activities would be appropriate for my agency or organization?
d. What *can't* my agency or organization do?
e. Do you know of others who ought to be part of this coalition?

Fifth, the final task will be defined in part by the extent to which the coalition reaches agreement on the overall coalition agenda or program goal. If the tone of the meeting reflects such a general consensus, the next step will be to begin a systematic process to delineate the major tasks that need attention and to identify coalition members willing to take on those tasks. If people still disagree on particular aspects of the coalition agenda, those disagreements will need to be clarified and resolved before moving on.

CREATING AN ORGANIZATIONAL FRAMEWORK

Although well worn, the aphorism "a picture is worth a thousand words" aptly describes the organizational chart for a community-based program for the prevention of drug abuse in Kansas City[69] presented in Figure 8-4. This chart merits attention for several reasons. First, it reflects the continuity and the flow of relationships in the program, starting with the community assessment at the top and concluding with clearly cited health and social benefits at the bottom. Second, the flow of activities that stem from the box labeled "Training of program implementors" provides a practical illustration of the various types of activities typically found in a community health promotion program. Third, the chart paints a coherent picture of what is envisioned—busy coalition members and stakeholders appreciate such coherence. Finally, note how the training activity highlighted in Figure 8-4 reinforces the point made in Chapter 6: Assessing and strengthening community capacity, readiness, confidence and skills are part of "Proceeding" from the planning process to the organizing and implementation process. Murray Ross, generally regarded as the father of postwar community organization practice, considered increased community competence or problem-solving ability to be a defining characteristic of a community organization process.[70]

APPLICATIONS IN COMMUNITIES

The assessment processes described in Chapters 3, 4, and 5 reveal critical insight into the multiple factors that influence health and quality of life for a given target population. These assessment processes have been applied in community settings across numerous health problems, including domestic violence,[71] smoking among women,[72] prevention of child pedestrian injuries,[73] cervical cancer screening and follow-up,[74] breast cancer screening among African-American women,[75] and maternal nutrition, specifically enhancing the consumption of food rich in vitamin A by women in Mali.[76] When carefully examined in the light of sound behavioral, social, and educational theory, information generated by these assessments will help uncover the most effective combination of educational, organizational, and policy approaches.

A KENTUCKY CASE STUDY

A well-known community intervention study illustrates how these principles of selection and rationale for multiple intervention strategies have been put into action with beneficial results. Kentucky is a rural state with high rates of mortality from cardiovascular disease and hypertension. As elsewhere, those with the lowest incomes and standards of living bear a disproportionate burden of those preventable deaths. In an attempt to address this public health problem, Kotchen and her colleagues[77] carried out a community-based study in two adjacent, sparsely populated, rural Kentucky counties. The combined population of the two intervention counties was approximately 32,000; many of those residents lived in relative isolation. The population was predominantly white, with adults having

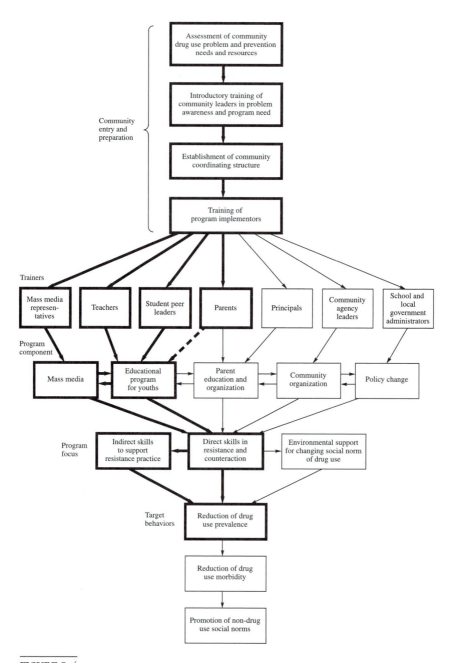

FIGURE 8-4

In this organizational framework for a community program for primary prevention of adolescent drug abuse, training and program components progress from left to right over a 6-year period.

SOURCE: M. A. Pentz et al., "A Multicommunity Trial for Primary Prevention of Drug Abuse," 1989, *Journal of the American Medical Association, 261*(22), 3259–3266. With permission.

completed an average of 8 years of schooling. Coal mining was the major industry, but 20% of the men were unemployed, disabled, or retired.

Results. After five years, comparisons of blood pressure outcomes of the intervention counties with those in a demographically similar control county revealed significant decreases in both systolic and diastolic blood pressure in both men and women in the two intervention counties. These decreases occurred despite 5-year increases in age; increased age tends to correlate with increased blood pressure. Results showed that the intervention influenced improved medication compliance and, therefore, control over hypertensive disease. The most striking outcome was the evidence linking the intervention effort to measurable declines in mortality. The 3-year moving averages for cardiovascular death rates, showing declines in the two intervention counties and no change in the control county, are presented in Figure 8-5.

Strategy: Multiple Tactics. What strategy did Kotchen and her co-workers use to achieve such a dramatic public health success? First, they hired a full-time coordinator who was enthusiastic and energetic and who knew the community and was respected by them. Then, using insights gained from a community assessment, the implementers gradually began to implement a comprehensive strategy that included the following:

1. Establishing a "Community High Blood Pressure Control Program Council" with the charge to provide direction to community-wide activities directed at controlling high blood pressure. Council membership included representatives from public schools, the Cooperative Agriculture Extension Service, local health departments, the local medical society, businesses, and interested citizens.
2. Using existing resources and organizations to play a major role in the delivery and promotion of the program.
3. Expanding an existing hypertension registry within the health department to include those people in the intervention counties identified as having high blood pressure. These individuals received periodic mailings of information on high blood pressure control and risk reduction, as well as descriptions of various community resources and activities of possible interest to them.
4. Using the local Cooperative Extension Service Nutrition Aide Program, already established in the community, as the channel to provide cardiovascular risk reduction assistance to those identified by their physicians as being in greatest need.
5. Developing a 4-H Club cardiovascular-risk-reduction program in which teenagers used peer teaching techniques to present educational lessons to fifth graders.
6. Introducing a school blood pressure screening program into two high schools to identify adolescents with high blood pressure.

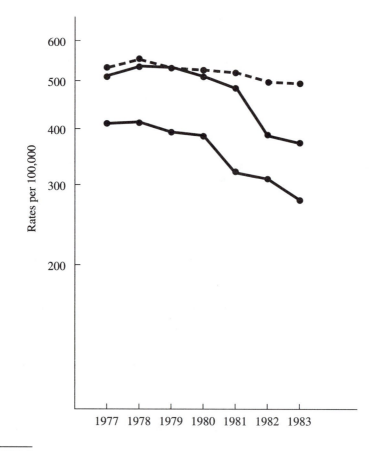

FIGURE 8-5

Three-year moving averages for cardiovascular disease death rates by year for two intervention counties and one control county, shown here for the Kentucky case study (1983
rates are based on 2-year moving averages). Control county, • • • ; intervention counties,
—. Significant decline in mortality is shown for each of the intervention counties
(P < .0004). Mortality trend coefficient for the intervention counties is significantly
different from that of the control county (P < .04).

SOURCE: "Impact of a Rural High Blood Pressure Control Program on Hypertension Control and
Cardiovascular Disease Mortality," by J. M. Kotchen, H. E. McKean, S. Jackson-Thayer, et al., 1986,
Journal of the American Medical Association, 255, 2177–2182, with permission of the American
Medical Association.

7. Creating a volunteer blood pressure screening and monitoring network
in the smaller churches and in businesses in the area. This network provided outreach to individuals within these organizations and to the residents in close proximity.

8. Adding a work-site high blood pressure screening program to an existing screening program provided by local health departments.

9. Securing the support of the local newspapers and radio stations as a means to reach the community as a whole with information about cardiovascular disease risk factors, benefits, and the feasibility of reducing those risks. While the project did purchase some air time, most of the media coverage was either aired as news or donated.

10. Implementing continuing education programs for nurses.

11. Providing health education programs to community clubs, homemaker groups, county fairs, health fairs, and large family reunions—a tradition in rural Kentucky.

The strategy taken in the Kentucky experience provides yet another reminder that the application of multiple intervention tactics is a hallmark of an effective community health promotion program.

Implications for Practitioners. The principal variable the program planners wanted to affect was the blood pressure level of those at highest risk. Yet, as evidenced by the list of activities, the program covered many other facets of the entire community, with special elements strategically aimed at those who were at high risk. How did they arrive at choosing that particular combination of strategies? The expansion and activation of the health department hypertension registry was an especially strategic method because it provided a channel through which direct contact could be made with those at highest risk.

One of the main reasons planners need to be thorough in the behavioral and educational/organizational assessment phases of PRECEDE is that such thoroughness increases the chances for detecting the critical targets for change. In the Kentucky case, the target behavior and its benefits are obvious; keeping blood pressure under control prevents strokes and saves lives. The predisposing, enabling, and reinforcing factors that influence behavior conducive to blood pressure control become the factors that shape the program.

Recall from Chapter 4 the discussion of the broken-appointment cycle (Figure 4-2). The broken appointment ultimately resulted in a specific, problematic behavior: not taking medications. By retracing the loops in the cycle, we see a combination of affective, environmental, and behavioral barriers that would stop most of us in our tracks. The registry provided a means to make contact with, encourage, and reinforce known hypertensives in using their medications and practicing risk-reduction behaviors, including coming into the health department or going to their physicians for blood pressure checks. Social support for their behavior came at three levels: (1) positive reinforcement from the nurses in the health department and from their physician; (2) the social norm endorsing risk reduction manifested by media, church activities, the cooperative extension service, school programs, community fairs, and family gatherings; and (3) messages in direct mail. Other community intervention projects have also found that mailings offer an inexpensive and effective follow-up method for high blood pressure screening programs.[78]

Implementation Lesson.   Well-planned and grounded in sound theory, the Kentucky plan also gave thoughtful consideration to the practical implementation questions asked in PROCEED. This program had no "high-tech," expensive program components.[79] Although there were direct costs (materials, special training, travel) and indirect costs (volunteer time, participant time at screens), the costs for the intervention components were quite modest. This is not to suggest that they could be easily replicated—good planning and intervention are anything but easy—but cost should not be a prohibitive factor for replication of this kind of program in rural areas.

The Kentucky team also observed a change in the community physicians' perception that hypertension was indeed an important health problem. They also suspected that this change in physicians' perception was a precursor to the subsequent support of the program by the community physicians.[80] The project, and its multiple activities, apparently heightened physicians' attention to this modifiable public health problem. This, in turn, resulted in rather undramatic but critical changes in their interactions with patients regarding hypertension and cardiovascular disease risk factors.

THE NORTH KARELIA PROJECT

Those who plan comprehensive community health education and health promotion programs should find comfort in the fact that there were strong similarities between the Kentucky demonstration and one of the most thoroughly researched and well-documented community-based intervention programs: the North Karelia, Finland Project. The study was designed to determine whether well-known coronary heart disease risk factors (smoking, serum cholesterol, and elevated blood pressure) could be reduced by multiple community-based interventions. The project began in 1972 as an intervention trial comparing two provinces with populations over 200,000 each. North Karelia was the intervention community and Kuopio was the reference or comparison.

The Design. Figure 8-6 presents a schema of the North Karelia model described as follows:

> The external input from the project affects the community both through mass media communication to the population at large (where its effect is mediated through interpersonal communication) and even more so through formal and informal opinion leaders acting as change agents to influence various aspects of community organization. This two-pronged approach is aimed at increasing knowledge, at persuasion, at

COMMUNITY

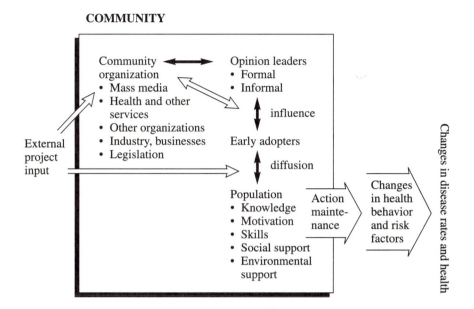

FIGURE 8-6

This model of community intervention in North Karelia reflects the 25 years of monitoring that has followed the initial program.

SOURCE: "The Community-Based Strategy to Prevent Coronary Heart Disease: Conclusions From the 10 Years of the North Karelia Project," by P. Puska, A. Nissinen, J. Tuomilehto, et al., 1985, *Annual Reviews of Public Health, 6,* 147–193. With permission, from the *Annual Reviews of Public Health* Volume 6, © 1985, by Annual Reviews.

teaching practical skills, and at providing the necessary social skills in the population. The acquisition and maintenance of new behaviors ultimately leads to a more favorable risk factor profile, reduced disease rates and improved health.[81]

The Impact.   Twenty-year results (1972–1992) reveal a decrease in coronary mortality of 52% in men and 68% in women for all of Finland.[82] The general trends in the risk factors between the intervention and comparison provinces over that same 20-year period are as follows. During the first five years, serum cholesterol and blood pressure levels fell more in North Karelia than in Kuopio; thereafter, both declined at a similar rate. Smoking declined more dramatically in North Karelia over the first decade. During the next 10 years, a small decline was noted in both areas. Figures 8-7 and 8-8 provide compelling evidence that the dramatic declines in risk factors from 1972 to 1992 were causally associated with the observed decline in mortality in Finland during that same 20-year period.

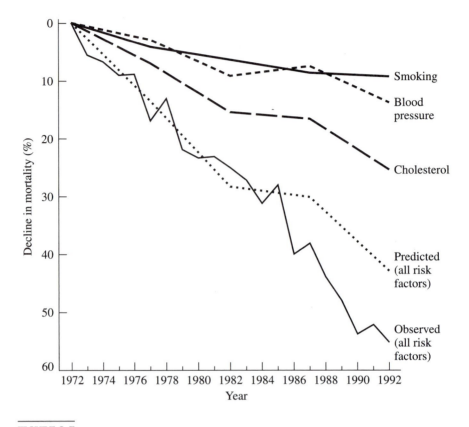

FIGURE 8-7

Observed and predicted decline in mortality from ischemic heart disease in men age 35–64 in Finland reflects the impact of the program.

SOURCE: Reprinted from "Changes in Risk Factors Explain Changes in Mortality from Ischemic Heart Disease in Finland," by E. Vartiainen et al., 1994, *British Medical Journal, 309,* p. 25. With permission of BMJ Publishing Group.

Diffusion. Initially undertaken as a community intervention research trial comparing two provinces within Finland, the intervention rapidly began to spread to the entire country. While we may never be able to account for all the forces that influence community change, the North Karelia experience offers health promotion planners some important lessons that we believe are generalizable. Early on in the project, research findings provided evidence that declines were occurring in risk factors within the North Karelia intervention population.[83] These findings generated a wide variety of national initiatives to promote heart health, including cholesterol guidelines endorsed by both the Finnish Cardiac Society and Internists'

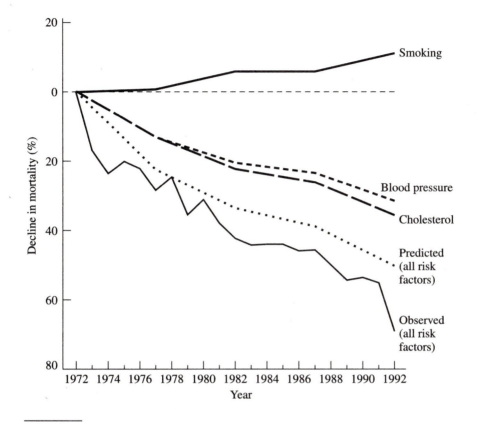

FIGURE 8-8

Observed and predicted decline in mortality from ischemic heart disease in women age 35–64 in Finland.

SOURCE: Reprinted from "Changes in Risk Factors Explain Changes in Mortality from Ischemic Heart Disease in Finland," by E. Vartiainen et al., 1994, *British Medical Journal, 309*, p. 25. With permission of BMJ Publishing Group.

Association. This was followed by national communication campaigns recommending screening and promoting public awareness of what constitutes a normal, healthy level of blood cholesterol. Interestingly, these health promotion efforts prompted a countercampaign by the dairy industry against the cholesterol hypothesis. The ensuing public debate elevated the national conversation about heart health and resulted in greater public awareness and interest in healthful nutrition. A marked decline in the consumption of milk fat and a corresponding increase in the consumption of vegetable oil followed this series of events.[84] Notice how these events follow the principles of diffusion theory discussed in Chapter 5.

When asked how he would explain the apparent success of the North Karelia Project, Pekka Puska, the project's director, said:

> Our philosophy was to get out into the community to meet and work with the people. We made special efforts to have meaningful discussions with representatives of businesses, the dairy industry, teachers, the media, and our colleagues in the health field. Our efforts went much deeper than television ads and posters. Although it was difficult work, everyone involved with the project followed this "boots deep in the mud" approach.[85]

Penetrate the Community. Although on opposite sides of the world and working with markedly different cultures and political systems, the Kentucky and North Karelia projects used similar approaches to planning and organizing. Both actively engaged the community, used sound data assessment to frame their respective intervention strategies, and sought to strengthen environmental supports thorough organizational change and policies. These actions, inherent in PRECEDE-PROCEED, provided a sound foundation that led to dramatic public health benefits in both examples. In reviewing these two as well as other successful community projects documented in the literature, one finds that the capacity and ability to penetrate the community sufficiently to yield an outcome must accompany sound planning. In the Kentucky example, recall that they hired a full-time coordinator with energy and strong community ties. Recall as well Puska's description of working in the community "boots deep in the mud" with efforts that "went much deeper than television ads and posters."

One of the hallmarks of effective community health promotion interventions seems to be that they do more than scratch the surface of a community. The Bootheel Heart Health Project, a community-based cardiovascular risk-reduction project, targets a rural area in southeastern Missouri characterized by high rates of poverty and illiteracy, low education, high unemployment, and medical underservice. Five-year results indicate that the Bootheel intervention strategies have been responsible for favorable changes in levels of cholesterol, physical activity, and obesity.[86] Key to the success of the intervention was the formation and maintenance of county-wide heart health coalitions. In a detailed account of how these coalitions sustained their functions over 5 years, Brownson and colleagues[87] provide added support for the view that undertakings are not only demanding but have to be taken slowly: "Each county had its own distinct character and infrastructure. Project staff found that our planned approach to development of these coalitions had to be tailored to the unique needs and interests of each group. Our 'plan' became more of an evolving process based on what we learned along the way." The level of effort and commitment implicit in these examples requires both skill and capacity: the technical, organizational, and interpersonal skills needed to communicate, listen, and negotiate with multiple stakeholders and interest groups and the capacity or resources to penetrate below the surface of the community and sustain the effort long enough to make an impact.

Never Promise Too Much Too Soon. But how long is "long enough to make an impact?" In Kentucky, Missouri, and North Karelia, some results were detected within 5 years—some would say this is "quick" by health promotion standards. In North Karelia, however, the most dramatic effects accumulated over a 20-year period. These time frames suggest that in addition to skill and capacity, one needs patience to stay the course of a well-planned intervention. In our enthusiasm, we sometimes run the risk of promising too much, too soon. As PRECEDE-PROCEED illustrates, however, there are few direct, simple paths to lasting change—whether this change is to occur in individual behavior or in larger political and social systems.

We join with Mittelmark,[88] Hancock,[89] and others reporting on the effectiveness of community-wide intervention approaches in urging planners to make every effort to ensure that they establish achievable outcome goals within realistic time frames. Figure 8-9 provides a graphic reminder of this counsel. It shows the conceptual planning framework for the Kaiser Family Foundation Community Health Promotion Grant Program,[90] which was based on PRECEDE-PROCEED. First, note how examples of educational, organizational, and policy tactics are strategically matched to benchmarks positioned between the health goals identified in the far right box and the box to left labeled "health promotion builds." Note also how the multiple methods, expressed in terms of short-term, intermediate, and long-term objectives, have been bracketed into reasonable projected time frames. Encouraging results from many community studies offer a clear lesson: To achieve sustainable programs, we must be willing to get "boots deep in the mud" while keeping a realistic eye on the distant horizon, be that 5 or 25 years.

SELECTING MULTIPLE STRATEGIES

Since the mid-1980s, many have tried to translate the intervention ideas developed in scientific, university-led community trials into practical, community-led applications in the field. Many of those translation efforts generated practical tools to help planners identify and apply multiple strategies for intervention. A few are reviewed here.

Ideas From PATCH. In 1983, the Centers for Disease Control (CDC) developed a program called the Planned Approach to Community Health (PATCH).[91] PATCH is grounded in the assessment planning principles of PRECEDE and is designed to translate the complex methods of community intervention to communities via the state health agency. All PATCH training goes on at the community level, in vivo, and involves the collaborative efforts of health promotion staff from the local and state health departments and CDC, as well as local community participants. Within this partnership context, methods in community mobilization,

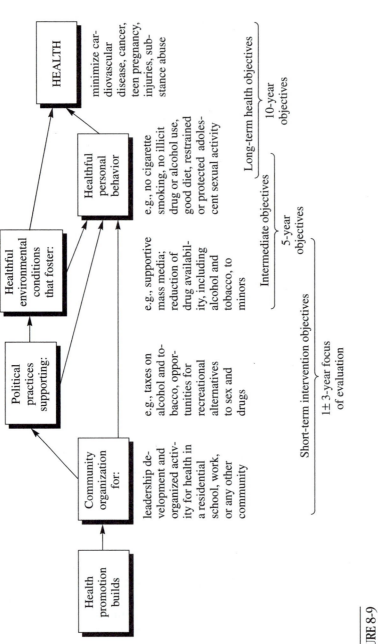

FIGURE 8-9

The sequence of relationships from community health promotion to health outcomes was reflected in the model for a national community health promotion grant program.

SOURCE: Adapted for Kaiser Family Foundation, *Strategic Plan for Health Promotion Program* (Menlo Park, CA: Henry J. Kaiser Family Foundation, 1989) from "The Future of Public Health: Prospects in the United States for the 1990s," by L. Breslow, 1990, *Annual Review of Public Health, 11,* 20. With permission, from the *Annual Review of Public Health* Volume 11, © 1989, by Annual Reviews.

assessment, and intervention are covered in considerable detail. It takes about a year and a half for a PATCH community to move from the community mobilization and assessment process to the point of the first intervention. Based on a 1992–1993 survey of local health departments in the United States conducted by the National Association of City and County Health Officers (NACCHO),[92] 239 local health agencies (12% of those responding) have used or applied the planning principles of the PATCH program. In the PATCH training process, the concept of multiple strategies is introduced by using the framework shown in Figure 8-10.

This technique was refined by public health specialists at the Center for Health Promotion Research and Development, University of Texas Health Science Center at Houston.[93] The health department is identified in the box to the left. Within the system of public health in the United States, local health agencies have a responsibility to stimulate community health promotion activity.[94] The diagram focuses the planner's attention on three levels of strategic action: (1) governmental, (2) organizational, and (3) individual.

Example: Auto Fatalities. Suppose the health outcome of interest was a specific reduction in the number of automobile fatalities by a given time. Planners would first turn their attention to the column of boxes under "Actions for intervention" and would translate those general activities into concrete examples taking into account the circumstances of their locality. For example, if the community was part of a state or province that required seat belt use but the law was not enforced, a strategy to promote enforcement would be a logical activity to specify in the box labeled "Governmental change." Establishing a responsible beverage service training program or a designated driver program for those establishments that serve alcoholic beverages would fall under "Organizational change"; actions under "Environmental and personal conditions" might include having the participating establishments adopt designated driver policies, providing incentives for adoption, and providing their employees with responsible beverage service training programs. Working through this framework is a simple but effective way to help planners think not only in terms of multiple strategies but also in terms of the multiple levels of governmental and organizational systems that can either facilitate or impede implementation.

Intervention Matrix. Once planners are comfortable with the concept of three levels of change, they can gain valuable insight by applying another planning tool, the intervention matrix (Table 8-3). The three levels of change (government, organizational, and individual) are positioned on the vertical axis; the settings in which various strategies are likely to reach specific target populations are identified along the horizontal axis. The matrix was designed as a means to identify both existing resources and gaps in prospective health promotion programs.

Schools, work sites, health care institutions, and the community appear as the general settings in Table 8-3. After identifying these settings more specifically

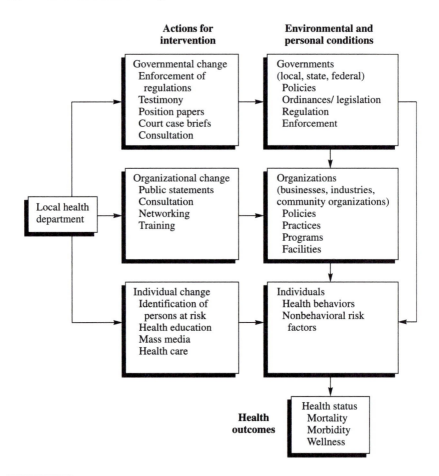

FIGURE 8-10

Local health departments play a central role in community-based risk reduction.

SOURCES: Centers for Disease Control; University of Texas Center for Health Promotion Research and Development.

(which schools, work sites, clinics, hospitals), planners might expand the variety of settings, depending on the problem in question. For example, in many areas, exercise facilities,[95] religious institutions,[96] health fairs,[97] bars and restaurants,[98] and grocery stores[99] can be critical settings for health promotion activity. In rural areas, outreach to the home may be necessary.[100]

To see the relationships between the earlier planning principles of PRECEDE and PROCEED and the selection of intervention strategies, planners can work through an exercise that leads to an integrated summary chart similar to the one characterized in Table 8-4. In this example, the PATCH community chose the

TABLE 8-3

The intervention planning matrix shown here was used in the community intervention handbooks and in the PATCH program sponsored by the U.S. Centers for Disease Control and Prevention

| Target | Setting | | | |
	School	Worksite	Health-Care Institution	Community
Individuals	Students' health behaviors	Employees' health behaviors	Patients' behaviors	Community residents' health behaviors
Organizations	School policies, programs, practices, and facilities to foster healthful behaviors by students	Worksite policies, programs, practices, and facilities to foster healthful behaviors by employees	Institution policies, programs, practices, and facilities to foster healthful behaviors by patients	Policies, programs, practices, and facilities of community-serving organizations, and institutions to foster healthful behaviors by community residents
Governments	Legislation, regulation, services, and resources affecting schools to foster healthful behaviors by students	Legislation, regulation, services, and resources affecting worksites to foster healthful behaviors by employees	Legislation, regulation, services, and resources affecting institutions to foster healthful behaviors by patients	Legislation, regulation, services, and resources affecting community sites to foster healthful behaviors by community residents.

SOURCE: "Community Intervention Handbooks for Comprehensive Health Promotion Programming," by S. G. Brink, D. Simons-Morton, G. Parcel, and K. Tiernan, 1988, *Family and Community Health, 11,* 28–35.

reduction of motor vehicle fatalities as the health problem and seat belt nonuse and driving under the influence of alcohol or drugs as the primary behaviors; poorly marked and lighted streets and seat belt laws that were unenforced were the primary environmental problems. Table 8-4 combines the intervention variables of site and actions for interventions with diagnostic information generated from the Precede process and from theory—in this case, the theory of stages of change.[101]

Matrix techniques have several uses. They can help one to take an inventory of existing resources or to set priorities for new strategies or for fund-raising

TABLE 8-4

Summary matrix for planning community health promotion programs

Health Problem: To reduce motor vehicle fatalities
Behavioral Problems: Driving under the influence
                    Not using seat belts
Environmental Problems: Poorly marked and poorly lighted streets
                        Poorly enforced seat belt law

| | Intervention Factors | | Diagnostic Factors | |
Strategies	Site	Action for Intervention	Contributing Factors	Adoption Stage
BEHAVIORAL PROBLEMS				
Driving under the influence				
Lobby concerning state liquor laws	C	LR	E	Sk
Substance-free high-school graduation party	S	En	P/E/R	Aw/Sk/R
Poster contest in middle schools	S	Ed	P/R	Aw/R
Bartender education	W	Ed	E	Sk
Substance-free events for teens	C/S	En	P/E/R	R/Mn
Education and community work assignments for those convicted of driving under the influence	H/C	Ed	E/R	Sk/Mn
News media events	C	Ed	P/E	Aw/Mn
Not using seat belts				
Poster contest in elementary school	S	Ed	P/R	Aw/R
Seat belt use required in company car	W	LR	E	Sk
Buckle-up contest in high school	S	Ed	P/R	Mo/Mn
Buckle-up signs on major roads	C	Ed		Aw/R
Seat belts in school buses	C	En	E	Sk
Installation Saturday (to install seat belts on cars lacking them)	C	En	E	Sk
News media events	C	Ed	P/E	Aw/Mn
ENVIRONMENTAL PROBLEMS				
Conduct and publicize findings from study of hazards in areas of high fatality	C	En/Ed	E	Aw
Lobby local activities for improved markings and lighting	C	LR/Ed	E	Mn/Sk
Pressure local authorities to enforce seat belt law	C	LR/Ed	E	Mn/Sk

SOURCE: Letters denote the following. *Site:* C = community, H = health care, W = work site, S = school. *Action for intervention:* Ed = educational, En = environmental, LR = legislative/regulatory. *Contributing factors:* E = enabling, P = predisposing, R = reinforcing. *Adoption stage:* Aw = awareness, Mn = Maintenance, Mo = motivation, Sk = skills.

where resources are lacking. They can serve as heuristic devices to expand the perspective of planners with limited experience in community work. Often, a talented practitioner hired to coordinate a community health promotion program brings mostly experience gained in a given setting, perhaps in schools or working with clinic patients. Working through and understanding the rationale of intervention matrices can help call attention to the need for regulatory or media approaches that otherwise may not have come to mind. Another useful application of the matrix approach is to apply or test other theoretical assumptions (where adoption appears in Figure 8-11).[102] Such an exercise of theory application can give the planner insight to determine what the proposed intervention should include. Consider the example in the following section.

Stages of Change: Applying Theory. Prochaska and DiClemente's stages of change model operates on the assumption that people do not change chronic behaviors discretely; that is, smokers do not just stop smoking, nor do sedentary persons suddenly become active. Rather, change in habitual behavior occurs continuously through four stages: (1) *precontemplation,* a condition in which people have expressed no interest in or are not thinking about change; (2) *contemplation,* the period in which serious thought is given to change; (3) *action,* the 6-month period after an overt effort to change has been made, and (4) *maintenance,* the period from 6 months after a behavior change until the behavioral problem in question is completely terminated. By incorporating this model in the intervention matrix exercise, the practitioner is sensitized to the idea that change strategies differ according to the stage people are in. According to Prochaska, the vast majority of prevention programs are designed for the small minority of the people in the ready-for-action stage. Using national survey data, he estimated that among those who were smokers in 1985, their 1986 stages were as follows:

> 4% were in the maintenance stage, 12% were in action, 15% were ready for action, 34% in contemplation and 35% in the precontemplation stage. Even with a health behavior that has received the most publicity, has the greatest consensus about its deleterious consequences, and has 10,000,000 served by the National Cancer Institute intervention projects alone, nearly 70% of the smokers are not ready to take action on their own.[103]

Another way to view the stages in the psychological process of change is in relation to the major forces operating on or within the individual at the time. Diffusion and adoption theory, discussed in previous chapters, divides the process of individual change into four phases: awareness, interest, trial, and adoption. These can be further refined to six phases, shown in Table 8-5, along with features of the community that can be developed or mobilized to support the individual at each phase.

Assuming the validity of the stages of change and stages of adoption models, what are the implications for the practitioner who is unaware that a substantial portion of the target population is *not* ready for action? One would be the

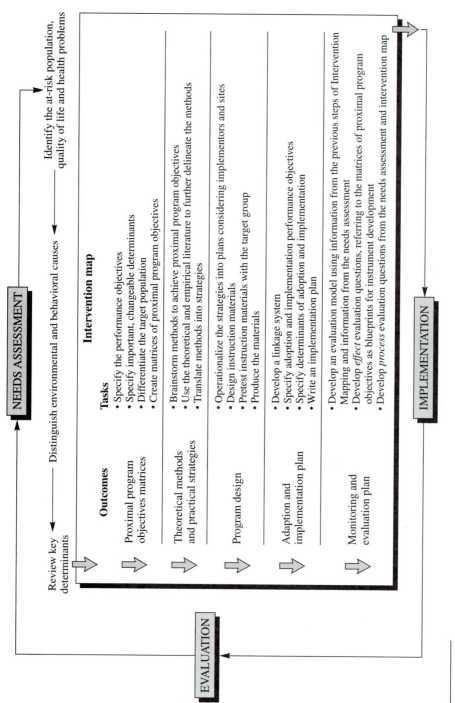

FIGURE 8-11

Overview schema of intervention mapping process.

SOURCE: "Intervention Mapping: A Process for Developing Theory-Based Health Education Programs," by L. K. Bartholomew, G. S. Parcel, and G. Kok, 1999, *Health Education and Behavior.* Reprinted with permission.

TABLE 8-5

Features of the community supporting each phase of the psychological process of change are shown here (contrast with Table 8-9)

Phase in Psychological Process of Change		Supporting Features of the Community
1 Exposure	←	Social setting with access to media
↓		
2 Attention	←	Interest of family, peers, and other significant people
↓		
3 Comprehension	←	Group discussion and feedback, question-and-answer sessions
↓		
4 Belief	←	Direct persuasion and social influence, actions of informal leaders
↓		
5 Decision	←	Group decision making, public commitments, repeated encouragements that build self-confidence
↓		
6 Learning	←	Demonstration and guided practice with feedback and continued confidence, advice, and directed assistance

SOURCE: "Macro-Intervention to Support Health Behavior," by L. W. Green and A. M. McAlister, 1984, *Health Education Quarterly, 11,* 322–339.

tendency to overestimate what could realistically be achieved, especially if the interventions are directed at the stages that involve the fewest people at the time of the program. Program failure can result from misapplication of relevant theory just as surely as from improper execution or inappropriate measurement.[104]

Intervention Mapping. In their conceptualization of intervention mapping, Bartholomew, Parcel, and Kok have expanded on the matrix approach.[105] The process is designed to help fill a gap they have observed in health promotion practice: specific guidance in helping planners translate the findings from their social, behavioral, environmental, organizational, and policy assessments into theoretically sound and appropriate interventions. Intervention mapping is analogous to geographic mapping in that once planners locate where they are going (program objectives), they are guided by clear signposts in the form of instructive diagrams and matrices that incorporate the outputs of the assessment process with sound theory. Figure 8-11 illustrates how intervention mapping is integrated into the overall process that includes needs assessment, evaluation, and implementation. It begins in the upper right hand corner of the figure with "needs assessment" steps consistent with the early phases of the Precede-Proceed model. The five steps of intervention mapping are listed under "Outcomes" and the tasks required to effectively carry out each step are listed in bullet points to the right.

The matrices used in the process provide planners with a specificity they will find most useful. For example, Table 8-6 provides a hypothetical example that focuses on the role of the parents who have children with asthma. This is the kind of matrix that would be created under the fourth bullet point for the first step in the mapping process in Figure 8-11.

Just as planners must take care not to establish unrealistic time and outcome expectations, neither should they view intervention mapping as a quick and easy way to identify interventions. As Bartholomew and her colleagues point out,

---

TABLE 8-6

This sample Matrix of Proximal Program Objectives at the Individual Level applies to parents of children with asthma

Parent Performance Objectives	Determinants	
	Behavioral Capability	Self-Efficacy
1. Monitors environment and circumstances to anticipate risk of asthma attack	Recognizes signs of impending attack, including environmental triggers	Feels confident in recognizing signs and environmental triggers that could trigger child's asthma
2. Effective communication with health care provider	Enters health care provider's office with a goal and technique to promote discourse and information gathering	Feels confident in developing goals for gathering information

Parent Performance Objectives	Determinants	
	Outcome Expectancy	Rewards
1. Monitors environment and circumstances to anticipate risk of asthma attack	Expects that recognizing signs and environmental triggers will lead to better asthma management	Parent sees that child is able to participate in wider range of activities due to better asthma management
2. Effective communication with health care provider	Expects that having a communication goal will increase effectiveness of interactions with health care provider	Health care provider comments on increased effectiveness of interactions Parent feels they have better information about child's asthma

SOURCE: Adapted from "Intervention Mapping: A Process for Developing Theory-Based Health Education Programs," by L. K. Bartholomew, G. S. Parcel, and G. Kok, in press, *Health Education and Behavior.* With permission.

unlike a road map, intervention mapping is an iterative process where "the planner is expected to return to early planning steps as insights are gained, and as the effects of early decisions on subsequent steps are experienced."[106]

REACHING THE MASSES

It is almost impossible to find a community intervention program devoid of one or a combination of the following mass media strategies: Internet, television, radio, newspapers, magazines, outdoor advertising, transit advertising, direct mail, telemarketing, and special promotional events. The application of mass media techniques is second only to the activation of community participation through community organization and coalition building as a critical element in community intervention. The literature is abundant with detailed accounts of (1) large-scale national or regional public health applications,[107] (2) applications at the community level,[108] and (3) the theoretical rationale for planning and implementing mass media strategies.[109]

This explosion of interest in mass media techniques by health promotion practitioners is an international phenomenon that in part confirms Manoff's assumptions about the power and utility of mass media in health promotion. He has identified seven beneficial characteristics of mass media:[110]

1. *Mass media carry special authority:* That which is seen in the cinema or on television, heard on the radio, or read in the paper has special impact.
2. *Mass media assure control over the message:* Since the content and tone of the health messages is critical, the most desirable means of communication is the one that guarantees that whatever it is, whenever it is communicated, and from whomever it comes, the message will stay the same.
3. *Media lend cumulative impact to the message:* The whole program is more than the arithmetic sum of the parts; mass media create a communications synergism.
4. *Mass media reach the masses.*
5. *Mass media telescope time:* They have maximum further-faster capacity.
6. *Mass media influence other major audiences in important ways while directing a message to the target audience:* Even though a seat belt message may be targeted at middle-aged men, others exposed to the message (women, children, co-workers) can serve to reinforce the message or may themselves be influenced to consider action.
7. *The mass media campaign enhances all other methods employed in health education:* It provides an umbrella for attention to the issue.

Segmenting. Acknowledging the importance of coordinating multiple intervention strategies, Preston, Baranowski, and Higginbotham[111] have devised a practical scheme to aid practitioners in the selection of those strategies. Using diffusion and adoption of innovations as their primary theoretical base, they begin by identifying eight generic points of community intervention. Table 8-7 illustrates the eight points of intervention in the context of a dietary change example. These points move from methods employed primarily for heightening awareness, through those that can transmit messages about reasons for change, to potential early adopters and eventually to skills enhancement and changes in community standards.

Major media (1) are newspapers, radio, and television intended to reach large audiences. Minor media (2) includes newsletters, bulletins, and other notices targeted at specific audiences because of their membership in a group. Institutional interventions (3) are efforts to focus interventions on the institution in which a behavior is likely to take place, such as a restaurant for eating, a tavern or pub for drinking alcohol, or a grocery store for buying food. Special events (4) are those designed to create heightened public awareness and attention to a problem or program and often involve celebrities or prizes. Formal social networks (5) include community organizations such as churches, fraternal groups, work sites, and schools. Informal social networks (6) are those characterized by informal but frequent neighborhood or friendship gatherings. Center-based points of intervention (7) are those in which professional staff provide services or programs, as in universities, clinics, or fitness centers. Created social networks (8) could be e-mail listserv groups, self-help groups, or mutual-aid groups created by the program on an ad hoc basis. They may or may not outlive the program.

The different points of intervention will have varying effects on persons at different stages of the community adoption process. Attention also must be paid to the sequencing and timing of those points of intervention. In the Proceed process highlighted in previous chapters, time was a critical element in assessing the barriers to and facilitators of program implementation. The multiple interventions of a program do not explode onto the scene at once. Based on a variety of factors, including the theoretical underpinnings of the program, the various intervention components need to be timed to address the strategic objectives of the program.

In Table 8-8, Preston and her colleagues present a timeline for the implementation of interventions, again using dietary change as the example.

The timing of the intervention strategy, therefore, takes into consideration four general purposes for the program: public awareness, the introduction of information and reasons for change into the established social system for earlier adopters, the enhancement of skills needed to make desired changes, and the modeling of new behaviors for later adopters.[112]

Note how staging intervention components in terms of their timing for intervention addresses the central concern raised in DiClemente and Prochaska's stages of change model. Working with individuals in one-to-one counseling or teaching relationships makes such staging relatively easy, because the readiness of the learner can be readily detected or inferred. But in community health

TABLE 8-7

Types of intervention and segments of the community likely to be reached

Types of Community Intervention	Early Adopters	Early Majority	Late Majority
1. Major media			
Newspaper	X	X	
Radio	X	X	
Cablevision and television	X	X	X
2. Minor media			
Church newsletters	X	X	X
Employer newsletters	X	X	
Customer bill inserts	X	X	
3. Institutional intervention (supermarkets, grocery stores, restaurants, fast food stores)			
Point of purchase information	X	X	X
Making more food available	X	X	X
Grocery bag inserts	X	X	X
Taste testing	X	X	X
4. Special events			
Health screening events in churches, grocery stores	X	X	X
Cooking contests	X	X	
5. Existing formal social structures and networks			
Occupation-based programs	X	X	
Churches	X	X	
Community, fraternities, sororities			X
Medical care delivery	X		
Schools	X	X	X
6. Existing informal social networks			
Living room sessions (education and taste testing) with family-invited participants (Tupperware Party concept)		X	X
Events in service centers, beauty and barber shops, neighborhood action committees		X	X
Training community lay health advisors		X	X
7. Center-based programs			
Test kitchen taste testing of new versions of recipes	X	X	X
8. Created social networks			
Developing a ward or block system		X	X

SOURCE: "Orchestrating the Points of Community Intervention," By M. A. Preston, T. Baranowski, and J. C. Higginbotham, 1988–1989, *International Quarterly of Community Health Education, 9,* 11–34. Reprinted with permission.

TABLE 8-8
Timeline for intervention strategy

Type of Intervention	Six Months Prior to Intervention						Six Months of Intervention					
	1	2	3	4	5	6	1	2	3	4	5	6
Center based												
Test kitchen	P	P	P	P	P	P						
Ongoing behavior, grocery stores												
Food purchasing		P	P	P	E	E	E	E	E	E	E	
Shelf labeling					P	P	I	I	I	I	I	I
Food tasting	P	P	P	P	P	P	I	I	I	I	I	I
Ongoing behavior, restaurants												
Additional menu selections	P	P	P	P	P	E	E	E	E	E	E	E
Menu labeling						I	I	I	I	I	I	I
Major media												
Newspaper						P	A	N	N	N	N	N
Radio						P	A	N	N	N	N	N
Television						P	A	N	N	N	N	N
Minor media												
Paycheck inserts						P	A	A	A			
Newsletter notices						P	A	N	N	N	N	N
Screening handouts						P	A	A				
Grocery bag stuffers						P	A	A	A	A	A	A
Special events												
Cooking contests						P	A	A				
Public health screenings						P	A	A				
Formal structures												
Group intervention	P	P	P	P	P	P	B	B	B	B		
Informal structures												
Group network intervention	P	P	P	P	P	P				B	B	B

NOTE: P = preparation, A = public awareness (media), N = notification (media), I = information dissemination, E = enabling behavior changes, B = behavior change (educational sessions).

SOURCE: "Orchestrating the Points of Community Intervention," by M. A. Preston, T. Baranowski, and J. C. Higginbotham, 1988–1989, *International Quarterly of Community Health Education, 9,* 11–34. Reprinted with permission.

promotion, generalizations must be made about where the population lies on the continuum or, more accurately, how the population distributes over the stages of change at a given time in the course of the program.

A Su Salud. *A Su Salud* (To Your Health) was designed as a mass media health promotion program to reduce selected chronic disease risk factors among Mexican Americans in southwest Texas.[113] The smoking-cessation element of this program provides an excellent example of how one can use theory and data in the planning process. Data generated from formative evaluation methods, especially focus groups, were combined with two theories: (1) Bandura's conceptualization of social modeling and social support[114] and (2) the previously cited stages of change theory.

In developing the community organization components of the program, planners mobilized the community supports (see Table 8-5) by actively involving community groups and institutions. As to the media components of *A Su Salud,* the supporting features of communications associated with each stage were developed, as shown in Table 8-9.

Table 8-10 summarizes the three general stages of change applied specifically to smoking cessation; it also offers examples of role model messages for each stage as developed in the mass media component of *A Su Salud.* Developers recruited Mexican Americans enrolled in smoking-cessation programs and had them present messages in their own words. Then, scripts were developed for narrators to highlight these messages.

Social Marketing: Square One for a Campaign. Most definitions of *social marketing* characterize it as a system or process, using both qualitative and quantitative data and information about a given population, to bring about the adoption or acceptability of ideas or practices in that population. Lefebvre and Flora[115] add specificity to this general description when they describe the social marketing process in terms of eight specific components.

1. *Consumer orientation:* A focus on the needs and interests of the target population
2. *Voluntary exchanges:* The assumption that adoption of new ideas or practices involves the voluntary exchange of some resource (money, services, time) for a perceived benefit
3. *Audience analysis and segmentation:* The application of qualitative research methods to obtain information on the needs and special characteristics of the target population that has been segmented to permit a more specific message
4. *Formative research:* Message design and pretesting of materials to be used in the campaign

TABLE 8-9

Features of communications supporting each phase of individual response to mass media

Phase in Psychological Process of Change		Supporting Features of the Community
1 Exposure $\downarrow$	←	Use of most popular media of communication, program repetition
2 Attention $\downarrow$	←	Message relevance, attractiveness, novelty, drama, humor, and suspense
3 Comprehension $\downarrow$	←	Use of simple concepts with illustration and analogy
4 Belief $\downarrow$	←	Expert and trustworthy sources, counterarguments refuted
5 Decision $\downarrow$	←	Display of incentives and values of different consequences of action, message enhancing self-confidence
6 Learning	←	Step-by-step demonstrations, guides for practice and feedback, repetition

SOURCE: "Macro-Intervention to Support Health Behavior," by L. W. Green and A. L. McAlister, 1984, *Health Education Quarterly, 11,* 322–339. Reprinted with permission.

5. *Channel analysis:* The identification of the various channels of communication, including media outlets, community organizations, businesses, and "life path points"
6. *Marketing mix:* The process of identifying the product, price, place, and promotional characteristics of intervention planning and implementation
7. *Process tracking:* A system to track the delivery of the program and to assess trends in the use of services, resources, facilities, or information sources provided, promoted, or subsidized by the program; a critical evaluation tool
8. *Management:* A commitment to a coordinated management system to assure quality of planning, implementation, and feedback.

Quantitative health data, so essential in measuring the severity of a problem and in assessing the effects of a program, are rarely available to give the planner insights into why a target population resists the adoption of certain actions. It is the consumer-oriented aspect of the social marketing process that makes it so complementary to epidemiological data and, therefore, so relevant for planning an intervention.

Take It Outside. An interesting and population-wide health promotion media campaign was carried out by the Kansas Health Foundation (KHF).[116] In 1997, the foundation's board approved a campaign taking a stand against secondhand

TABLE 8-10

Broad categories of the stages of change and the corresponding examples of media messages provided by role models on television in the *A Su Salud* project in southwest Texas

Three Stages of Smoking Cessation	Examples Provided by Role Models
I. Preparation Information about smoking: decisional balance Dissatisfaction with dependence on cigarettes	"I decided to quit because I was pregnant. It's OK to risk my own life, but not my unborn child." "I wanted to be here [living] to see my children grown."
II. Taking action Positive efficacy expectations Social support and reinforcement for nonsmoking Reevaluation of self	"My husband supported my decision and he joined me in the decision to stop smoking." "I physically feel better, less fatigued, less tense. I feel better."
III. Maintenance Increased efficacy expectations for specific situtations Avoiding stimuli associated with smoking Acquisition of new coping responses General social support for stress-coping	"In social situations, I would review the reasons why I quit smoking . . ." "When nervous due to not smoking, I would talk to someone or eat a piece of candy."

SOURCE: "Mass Media Campaign: *A Su Salud*," by A. G. Ramirez and A. L. McAlister, 1988, *Preventive Medicine, 17,* 608–621. Reprinted with permission.

smoke. In Sedgwick County, where the city of Wichita and the foundation head-quarters are located, surveys showed that 40% of smokers had children living at home. These data, coupled with a desire to bring new information into the tobacco control debate, led the foundation, in cooperation with multiple local stakeholder groups, to focus the campaign on the dangers of secondhand smoke for children.

Focus-group data on smokers, combined with information gained through visiting Internet chat rooms, revealed that smokers had heard antismoking messages so often that the messages did not register. In response, the campaign specifically avoided asking smokers to quit, to avoid angering them. Instead, the specific call to action was "If you choose to smoke, *take it outside.*" This was a deliberate attempt to emphasize the smokers' choice and control over their behavior and to make the requested action easier to accept and implement. The campaign ran a gauntlet of both anticipated and unanticipated difficulties before its launch date. The latter included negative reactions from focus groups, which led to the creation of new ads within a month of the launch date. Among the anticipated problems was a series of attacks from the tobacco industry, which targeted not only the foundation but many of its grantees.

To preempt controversy, the foundation reached out to key leaders in the community before the official launch date. The Governor of Kansas not only joined a news conference with foundation staff but also participated by appearing in one of the later television spots. In a stroke of good fortune, a news conference to announce the campaign and emphasize children's health coincided with news of the impending tobacco settlements in states throughout the county. Materials were also mailed to child-care providers and a second news conference was held at a day-care center.

The campaign included television and radio ads as well as billboards throughout Wichita. The goal was to reach 99% of the market with a frequency of 36 exposures in 6 months. In addition, nontraditional media—Internet banners and the sides of buses—helped spread the message. Each ad featured a toll-free number; callers received packets with brochures and resources on smoking cessation. These calls averaged 40 per week, for a total of 1,492. After the pilot, surveys demonstrated that awareness of secondhand smoke as harmful had increased 14%, and 18% more smokers agreed that it was not too much trouble to "take it outside." In terms of smoking behaviors, surveys had consistently shown that 25% of Wichita's population were smokers. At the campaign's midpoint, 19% said they were smokers. To substantiate this drop, another survey with a larger sample was conducted—it showed the same percentage. At the end of the campaign, 17% of respondents said they were smokers. Even if these respondents were not being truthful about their smoking behavior, the survey may at least have documented that the ads had helped create an environment in which people considered smoking as unacceptable.

Physical Activity. Smith and Scammon conducted a market segment analysis to examine the beliefs and perceptions that may influence adults' exercise behavior. They found that (1) people were generally misinformed about the frequency, intensity, and duration of activity needed to obtain a cardiovascular benefit; (2) people thought that their own doctor was the "most important" source of information regarding exercise; and (3) subjects did not consider the health benefits of exercise to be as critical as the psychological or emotional benefits of exercise.[117] These findings obviously have much to contribute to health promotion programs seeking to increase physical activity in the population.

Examples from Developing Countries. Considerable attention has been paid to the creative use of social marketing methods in the major cardiovascular community intervention trials. The effective application of social marketing to health promotion is by no means limited to affluent "media markets," however. Brieger,

Ramakrishna, and Adeniyi[118] applied social marketing research in an especially creative way. In their health promotion program, aimed at controlling dracunculiasis (guinea worm) in Idere, Nigeria, they combined key principles of community participation with social marketing strategies in an attempt to increase the use of filters as a means of protection against this infection. They took steps to include in the planning process people from the participating towns and hamlets. Based on results from qualitative research efforts, including focus groups, a program was established wherein local tailors made the cloth used to filter the water, other community members helped debate the price, and still others became salespeople. Figure 8-12 illustrates their model of integrating community involvement with the application of social marketing principles.

We can also point to many other examples of social marketing strategies effectively applied in developing countries. A University of South Carolina team together with Ivory Coast collaborators[119] used focus groups as a cost-effective way to obtain rich and valid information that led to improvements in controlling childhood diarrhea and malaria in sub-Saharan Africa. Another group[120] used social marketing research to increase contraceptive use in Bangladesh. Gordon[121] showed that the coordination of a national media campaign with a well-planned community intervention effort effectively addressed the problem of dengue fever in the Dominican Republic.

Irrespective of where they are on the globe, public health workers will need to become more skilled in the methods and techniques of health communications, mass media, and social marketing. Developing a trusting contact with those whose culture, language, or beliefs differ from one's own is a complex task that takes resources: time, money, and skill. Planners must argue and budget for the first two; they must *possess* the third. Practitioners with competence in the application of social marketing research methods gain special insight into precise program planning and implementation.

Yet, there remain large gaps in practitioners' ability to reach individuals at high risk, who greatly need preventive services and education. Even when implementers do reach such a population, their methods of communications prove ineffective. For the most part, these gaps continue not because of a lack of practitioners' desire and efforts to close them. They continue because of glaring deficiencies in communication and education training, cultural sensitivity, and resources available to health organizations.

As always, the literature is the primary means for responsible practitioners to stay abreast of innovations. Yet, the multidimensional complexity of health promotion does not lend itself to easy communication through the written word. Even the most artful wordsmith cannot capture all of the subtleties that "make a difference." Those government and private-sector institutions responsible for public health training have not kept pace with the methodological demands of the practitioner. Accessible training systems that work with trainees in the community are needed to facilitate the rapid translation of new methods, including social marketing, to those who need it most: frontline health practitioners.

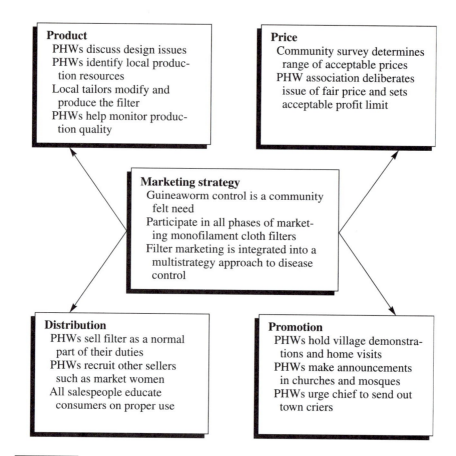

FIGURE 8-12

Community involvement in social marketing of monofilament nylon-cloth water filters for guineaworm control in Idere, Nigeria.

SOURCE: "Community Involvement in Social Marketing: Guineaworm Control," by W. R. Brieger, J. Ramakrishna, and J. D. Adeniyi, 1987–1988, *International Quarterly of Community Health Education, 8,* 297–316. Reprinted with permission.

SUMMARY

Practitioners who base their community intervention planning on the Precede-Proceed model (1) build from a base of community ownership of the problems and the solutions; (2) base program decisions on sound theory, meaningful data, and local experience; (3) have an evaluation plan in place to monitor program progress and detect program effects; (4) know what types of interventions work best for specific populations and circumstances; and (5) have an organizational and advocacy plan to orchestrate multiple intervention strategies into a complementary, cohesive program. This chapter has emphasized community participation and has distinguished between interventions in communities and community interventions. Some guidelines were offered for engaging the realities of community politics, including practical suggestions for the formation, implementation, and maintenance of community coalitions. The importance of applying multiple strategies was highlighted in a review of well-documented, community-based health promotion programs with a caveat: Don't underestimate the magnitude of the task and fall prey to setting unrealistic outcomes and time frames. Finally, practical guidelines for selecting multiple intervention tactics were offered, followed by examples of successful media applications in communities.

EXERCISES

1. What is the difference between community intervention and interventions in a community? Why is it important to make that distinction?
2. Based on your interpretation of the forces of change in Mississippi, what should planners look for over the long term as a result of well-planned community-based interventions?
3. What is the paradox that major university-based community intervention trials have faced?
4. Consider any one of the following problems as the focus of a planned program effort: alcohol-related injuries and death, dracunculiasis, smoking, or AIDS. Name two political issues that planners might face if they were to try a community intervention in *your home town*. Explain how you would keep those issues from becoming a problem.
5. In terms of relevant theory, explain why the Kentucky program worked, in terms of social learning theory.
6. Apply the social marketing steps and the intervention matrix to your own program plan.
7. Suppose someone said to you, "Marketing is Madison Avenue glitz, great for selling cars and beer, but there's no place for it in health science. Besides, it just focuses on the individual, which is victim blaming!" How would you respond?

NOTES AND CITATIONS

1. Green & Ottoson, 1999, pp. 40–41.
2. Israel, 1985, p. 72. *Sense of community* is defined and developed more fully in J. Allen & Allen, 1990; Brodsky, 1996; Chavis, Hogge, McMillan, & Wandersman, 1986; Chavis & Wandersman,

1990; W. Davidson & Cotter, 1993; Lorion & Newbrough, 1996; McMillan, 1996; Plas & Lewis, 1996.

3. Even though we have consciously separated community-based approaches from those carried out at the national, provincial, or state levels, the positive, complementary effect that national and regional policies and campaigns have on local efforts should not be minimized. In fact, where appropriate and feasible, community-based programs should try to time their interventions to coordinate with larger population campaigns to obtain the media benefits as well as other resources that support the campaign. See, for example, Comino, Bauman, & Hardy, 1995; Glantz, 1997; Goldman & Glantz, 1998; R. M. Goodman, Wheeler, & Lee, 1995; Green, 1997b; Popham et al., 1993, 1994. Most of the principles and methods that apply to community health promotion can be applied with adaptation at the state-provincial or national level. See Arkin, 1990. For synthesis of PRECEDE-PROCEED with other models in guiding media campaigns, see Flynn et al., 1992; Green & McAlister, 1984; Winnett, Altman, & King, 1990; Worden, Flynn, & Carpenter, 1996; Worden, Flynn, Solomon et al., 1996.

4. E. R. Brown, 1984. Brown's phases of development in community health care policy were later applied in the development of indicators of community action to promote "social health." See Rothman & Brown, 1989.

5. Another dimension of *community* important to the national and international development of health promotion is the community of interest. National advocacy organizations such as Public Voice for Food Policy, the Smoking Control Advocacy Resource Center, Americans for Non-smokers' Rights, Mothers Against Drunk Driving, and others all relate to a constituency of concerned citizens scattered around a country. Voluntary health associations and professional associations, similarly, advocate and develop health promotion initiatives through their networks of members and chapters distributed around the country. Each of these represents a community in every sense except for the locality criterion applied in this chapter. Some can support local initiatives. Much of the discussion in this chapter, however, can be applied to organizing through these interest groups on a state, national, or international scale. For more on national advocacy groups and their methods, see Paehlke, 1989; Pertschuk & Erikson, 1987; Pertschuk & Schaetzel, 1989; Wallack & Dorfman, 1996; Wallack, Dorfman, Jernigan, & Themba, 1993.

6. Berkman & Syme, 1979; Marmot, Kogevinas, & Elston, 1987; Orth-Gomer, Rosingren, & Wilhelmsen, 1993; G. D. Smith, Shipley, & Rose, 1990.

7. Fortmann et al., 1995; Puska, Tuomilehto, Korhonen, & Vartianinen, 1995.

8. Cuca & Pierce, 1977; Green & McAlister, 1984.

9. See note 46 in Chapter 7; and esp. Farquhar et al., 1990; Farquhar, Fortmann, Wood, & Haskell, 1983; Lasater et al., 1984; Luepker et al., 1994; Nutbeam & Catford, 1987.

10. COMMIT Research Group, 1995; Kegler, Steckler, & McLeroy, 1998; Nutbeam, Smith, Murphy, & Catford, 1993; Plough & Olafson, 1994.

11. Kaiser Family Foundation, 1987; Kellogg Foundation, 1997; Louis Harris and Associates, 1997; Neuhauser, Schwab, Syme, Bieber, & Obarski, 1998; Potapchuk, Crocker, & Schechter, 1997; Schorr & Kubisch, 1995; Wickizer, Wagner, & Perrin, 1998.

12. Berger, 1997; Daneshvary, Daneshvary, & Schwer, 1988; Freudenberg, 1984b; Paehlke, 1989.

13. Aday, Pounds, Marconi, & Bowen, 1994; Becker & Joseph, 1988; Coates, Stall, & Hoff, 1988; Leviton & Valdiser, 1990; Markland & Vincent, 1990; McKinney, 1993. Ostrow, 1989; Patton, 1985; L. S. Williams, 1986; For more specific applications of PRECEDE-PROCEED to community action on HIV/AIDS, see Bolan, 1986; Freudenberg, 1989; Kroger, 1991; Mantell, DiVittis, & Auerbach, 1997, esp. pp. 199–203; Meredith, O'Reilly, & Schulz, 1989; Trussler & Marchand, 1997; U.S. Department of Health and Human Services, 1988a, esp. Section D.

14. *Integration of Risk Factor Interventions*, 1986; Kottke et al., 1985; Rose, 1992.

15. B. Lewis, Mann, & Mancini, 1986. For a case illustration of the systematic integration of community-wide and high-risk strategies using PRECEDE-PROCEED, see Daniel & Green, 1995. For further reflections on balancing these two perspectives in the context of health care and community, see Chapter 11 and Green, Costagliola, & Chwalow, 1991; Green, Lewis, & Levine, 1980.

16. Puska, McAlister, Pekkola, & Koskela, 1981.

17. Dwyer, Pierce, Hannam, & Burke, 1986; Pierce, Macaskill, & Hill, 1990.

18. Lando, Loken, Howard-Pitney, & Pechacek, 1990; Lando, McGovern, Barrios, & Etringer, 1990.

19. Millar & Naegele, 1987.

20. Warner & Murt, 1983.

21. Solomon & DeJong, 1986, p. 314.

22. Dwore & Kreuter, 1980; Green, 1970a, 1970b; Green & McAlister, 1984. For applications of the concept of norms within PRECEDE-PROCEED planning or evaluation efforts, see Farley, 1997; N. H. Gottlieb et al., 1990; Kristal et al., 1995; Maxwell, Bastani, & Warda, 1998; Newman & Martin, 1982; M. W. Ross & Rosser, 1989; Schumann & Mosley, 1994; Secker-Walker, Flynn, & Solomon, 1996; B. G. Simons-Morton, Brink, & Simons-Morton et al., 1989; Sleet, 1987; Sloane & Zimmer, 1992.

23. Block, Rosenberger, & Patterson, 1988; National Restaurant Association, 1989; Popkin, Haines, & Reidy, 1989; Samuels, 1990; *Trends,* 1989.

24. Boberg, Gustafson, Hawkins, & Chan, 1995; Bosworth, Gustafson, & Hawkins, 1994; Hawkins et al., 1987; Thomas, Cahill, & Santilli, 1997.

25. Ashford, 1998; Campbell et al., 1994; Kreuter, Vehige, & McGuire, 1996; G. Sorensen, Emmons, Hunt, & Johnston, 1998; Zabora, Morrison, Olsen, & Ashley, 1997.

26. Bandura, 1986; N. M. Clark, 1987; Parcel & Baranowski, 1981.

27. For critical reviews of such debates, see Green, 1994a; Green & Raeburn, 1988; Minkler, 1989; Rimer, 1990; D. G. Simons-Morton, Simons-Morton, Parcel, & Bunker, 1988.

28. Biener & Siegel, 1997; Borland, Owen, Hill, & Schofield, 1991; Willemsen, deVries, van Breukelen, & Oldenburg, 1996.

29. J. W. Frank & Mustard, 1994; Mackenback, 1991; Romer & Kim, 1995.

30. J. W. Frank, 1995, p. 162.

31. Diffusion theory is described in considerable detail in Chapter 5 and later in this chapter.

32. R. M. Goodman, Wheeler, & Lee, 1995; Green & Ottoson, 1999; Green & McAlister, 1984; Samuels, 1990. We are cognizant, however, of the limitations of this argument as it relates to the poorest segments, the unemployed and welfare-dependent; see W. J. Wilson, 1987.

33. Personal conversation with Gary Giovino, Chief of the Epidemiology Branch, Office on Smoking and Health, National Center for Chronic Disease Prevention and Health Promotion, National Centers for Disease Control, Atlanta, GA, June 13, 1998. See also Green, 1997b; Lewit, Hyland, Kerrebrock, & Cummings, 1997.

34. W. J. Wilson, 1987, p. 124. See also Gerstein & Green, 1993.

35. Carlaw, Mittlemark, Bracht, & Luepker, 1984; Green, Gottlieb, & Parcel, 1991. An alternative view of organizational adoption of innovations sees the process as largely internal and rational or responsive to consumer demands rather than imitative or interorganizational. See for example R. M. Goodman, Steckler, & Kegler, 1997; Schiller, Steckler, Dawson, & Patton, 1987.

36. Hawe, Noort, King, & Jordens, 1997; Kreuter, Christenson, & DiVincenzo, 1982.

37. Shimkin, 1986–1987, pp. 154–155.

38. Schooler, Farquhar, Fortmann, & Flora, 1997.

39. Green, 1977, 1986f; McGowan & Green, 1995.

40. Altman, 1995; R. M. Goodman & Steckler, 1989b; Shediac-Rizkallah & Bone, 1998.

41. Green, 1986f. For a journalistic description of a grantmaking strategy designed to apply this model of early participation and to stimulate support to communities from the state level, see R. M. Williams, 1990.

42. Bozzini, 1988, p. 369.

43. Minkler & Pies, 1997, p. 134.

44. Brieger, Onyido, & Ekanem, 1996; Okafor, 1985. For a specific Precede-Proceed application in Nigeria, see Adenyanju, 1987–1988.

45. Kass & Freudenberg, 1997.

46. E. B. Fisher et al., 1992; R. M. Goodman & Steckler, 1987–1988, 1989a, 1989b; Green, 1989; Shediac-Rizkallah & Bone, 1998.

47. Farrant & Taft, 1988. Cf. Wharf Higgins & Green, 1994.

48. Dahl, Gustafson, & McCullagh, 1993.

49. Wandersman, 1981.

50. Altman et al., 1991; Green & Ottoson, 1999.

51. Altman, 1995.

52. R. M. Goodman et al., 1996, p. 36.

53. Kawachi, Kennedy, Lochner, & Prothro-Stith, 1997.

54. Sampson, Raudenbush, & Earls, 1997.

55. Runyan et al., 1998.

56. Bardoch, 1977; J. M. Clark, 1939.

57. H. Smith, 1988.

58. Flynn, 1995; B. Thompson & Kinne, 1990.

59. Allensworth, 1987; American Medical Association Auxiliary, 1987; T. Black, 1983; C. Brown, 1984; Butterfoss, Goodman, & Wandersman, 1993; Feighery & Rogers, 1990; S. Miller, 1983; Mulford & Klonglan, 1982; Pertschuk & Erikson, 1987; Wandersman, Goodman, & Butterfoss, 1997.

60. Bibeau, Howell, Rife, & Taylor, 1996; DeFrank & Levenson, 1987; Freudenberg & Golub, 1987; S. Gottlieb, 1986, Kumpfer, Turner, Hopkins, Librett, 1993; Lefebvre et al., 1986; R. K. Lewis et al., 1996; McKinney, 1993; I. Miller, 1987; Orthoefer, Bain, Empereur, & Nesbit, 1988.

61. Kreuter & Lezin, 1997.

62. The researchers and practitioners who participated in this survey include David Altman, Bowman Gray School of Medicine, Wake Forest, NC; William Beery, Group Health Cooperative of Puget Sound, Seattle, WA; James Frankish, Institute of Health Promotion Research, University of British Columbia; Robert Goodman, School of Public Health, Tulane School of Public Health and Tropical Medicine, New Orleans, LA; Brick Lancaster, National Center for Chronic Disease Prevention and Health Promotion (NCCDPHP), Centers for Disease Control and Prevention (CDC), Atlanta, GA; Katherine Marconi, Bureau of Health Resources and Development, HRSA, Rockville, MD; Martha McKinney, Community Health Solutions, Inc.; Dearell Niemeyer, NCCDPHP, CDC; Randy Schwartz, Division of Health Promotion and Education, Maine Bureau of Health; and Nancy Watkins, NCCDPHP, CDC. The survey was conducted by telephone during April 1997.

63. Endres, 1990.

64. Specificity of objectives has been addressed in previous chapters as an issue in planning and evaluation. The issue here is with specificity as a facilitator of interorganizational understanding, commitment and cooperation in implementing a policy or common objective. See Elmore, 1976; Pressman & Wildavsky, 1973; Van Meter & Van Horn, 1975.

65. Nix, 1977, pp. 90–91. For software, see Gold, Green, & Kreuter, 1997.

66. Steckler, Orville, Eng, & Dawson, 1989.

67. Eng, Hatch, & Callan, 1985; Hatch & Jackson, 1981; Vincent, Clearie, & Johnson, 1988; Vincent, Clearie, & Schluchter, 1987; B. L. Wells, DePue, Lasater, & Carleton, 1988.

68. For a taxonomy of community-based organizations, see Cuoto, 1990. For "caveats on coalitions" that relate to the issue of natural competition among organizational members of a coalition, as well as our "Noah's Ark principle of partnering," which acknowledges the limits of

trying to micromanage the implementation of programs by a coalition, see Green & Ottoson, 1999, pp. 52–53, as well as p. 598, which lists web sites concerning coalitions.

69. Pentz, Dwyer, et al., 1989.

70. M. Ross, 1955, cited in Minkler, 1990, p. 257.

71. Ashley, 1993; Sanders-Phillips, 1996; P. H. Smith, Danis, & Helmick, 1998.

72. Secker-Walker, Flynn, Solomon, 1996.

73. Stevenson, Jones, Cross, Howat, & Hall, 1996.

74. Dignan, Michielutte, Wells, & Bahnson, 1994; Michielutte, Dignan, Bahnson, & Wells, 1994.

75. Danigelis et al., 1995.

76. Parvanta, Cottert, Anthony, & Parlato, 1997.

77. Kotchen et al., 1986.

78. D. M. Murray et al., 1988. For examples of direct mail strategies applied to other issues in health promotion, see also Byles, Redman, & Boyle, 1995; Cardinal & Sachs, 1995; Wewers & Ahijevych, 1995.

79. There was no need for more expensive communication efforts (such as a paid media campaign) given the efficiency of existing informal communications networks and the ready cooperation of the local radio and newspaper. We hasten to point out, however, that more expensive campaigns may be cost-effective when indicated by geographic, demographic, and media characteristics.

80. Personal communication, Jane Kotchen, August 25, 1989.

81. P. Puska et al., 1985, pp. 162–163.

82. Puska, Tuomilehto, Nissinen, & Vartiainen, 1995.

83. Salonen, Puska, & Mustaniemi, 1979.

84. See discussion on page 503 in Vartiainen et al., 1994.

85. Personal conversation between Marshall Kreuter and Pekka Puska in Budapest, May 31, 1996 [audiotaped].

86. R. C. Brownson et al., 1996.

87. C. A. Brownson, Dean, Dabney, & Brownson, 1998, p. 161.

88. Mittelmark, Hunt, Heath, & Schmid, 1993.

89. Hancock et al., 1997.

90. Kaiser Family Foundation, 1989.

91. Kreuter, 1992; Green & Kreuter, 1992; C. F. Nelson, Kreuter, & Watkins, 1986; C. F. Nelson, Kreuter, Watkins, & Stoddard, 1986, Chap. 47.

92. National Association of County and City Health Officials and the Centers for Disease Control and Prevention, 1995, p. 60.

93. Brink, Simons-Morton, Parcel, & Tiernan, 1988; Green & Kreuter, 1992.

94. As of September 1990, there were 50 PATCH sites in 17 U.S. states. According to a 1992–1993 survey of local health departments in the United States conducted by The National Association of City and County Health Officials (NACCHA), 239 local health agencies (12% of those responding) use PATCH and/or some PATCH-like organizational planning strategy; see National Association of County and City Health Officials and the Centers for Disease Control and Prevention, 1995, p. 60.

95. Sallis et al., 1990.

96. DePue, Wells, Lasater, & Carleton, 1990; Eng, Hatch, & Callan, 1985; Markland & Vincent, 1990; Ransdell & Rehling, 1996; S. Thomas, Quinn, Billingsley, & Caldwell, 1994.

97. Clayman, Chamberlain, & Hong, 1995; Office of Disease Prevention and Health Promotion, 1981; Spoon, Benedict, & Buonamici, 1997.

98. Biener & Siegel, 1997; R. L. Miller, Klotz, & Eckholdt, 1998; Mosher, 1990; O'Donnell, 1985; Saltz, 1987.

99. Cheadle et al., 1990; Ernst et al., 1986; Hunt et al., 1990; Kristal, Goldenhar, & Morton, 1997; Mayer, Dubbert, & Elder, 1989; Mullis et al., 1987; Paine-Andrews, Fancisco, & Coen, 1996; Pennington, Wisniowski, & Logan, 1988.

100. A program that thoroughly applied the Precede model to planning for the prevention of a veterinary health problem required direct outreach to individual dairy farmers: W. B. Brown, Williamson, & Carlaw, 1988. Results of the program are reported in N. B. Williamson et al., 1988. See also Soubhi & Potvin, 1999.

101. Prochaska & DiClemente, 1983; Prochaska, DiClemente, & Norcross, 1992.

102. See for example Green, 1976a; Green, Gottlieb, & Parcel, 1991; Nutbeam, 1996; Sanderson et al., 1996.

103. Prochaska, 1989, p. 6.

104. C. H. Wiess, 1972.

105. This description of intervention mapping is based on an original manuscript and used with the permission of the authors: K. Bartholomew, Parcel, & Kok, in press.

106. Ibid., ms. p. 4. Cf. Bartlett & Green, 1980, for an earlier mapping approach.

107. The entire issue of each of several journals has been devoted to mass media applications. See for example R. Blum & Samuels, 1990; Green, Mullen, & Maloney, 1984.

108. For example, Alcalay et al., 1987–1988; Farquhar et al., 1990; Lefebvre et al., 1986; H. V. McCoy, Dodds, & Nolan, 1990. For examples of mass media applied within Precede-Proceed planning processes, see Ashley, 1993; Bakdash, 1983; Bakdash, Lange, & McMillan, 1983; Bartlett & Green, 1980; Centers for Disease Control, 1987; Dignan et al., 1991; Flynn et al., 1992; Ramirez & McAlister, 1989; Worden et al., 1990, 1996.

109. General references include Glanz & Rimer, 1995; Kotler, 1989; Lefebvre & Rochlin, 1997; Leviton, Mrazek, & Stoto, 1996; Manoff, 1985; K. Tones, 1994; Walsh, Rudd, Moeykens, & Maloney, 1993. For applications related to health education planning, see also Bonaguro & Miaoulis, 1983, which specifically integrates social marketing with the Precede model; De Pietro, 1987; Kotler & Roberto, 1989, esp. pp. 285–294, which describes Project LEAN as a case study of planning a national social marketing program for dietary fat consumption; Miaoulis & Bonaguro, 1980–1981; Novelli, 1990; Romer & Kim, 1995.

110. Manoff, 1985, pp. 76–77.

111. Preston, Baranowski, & Higginbotham, 1988–1989.

112. Ibid., p. 31. Note parallel with predisposing, enabling, and reinforcing.

113. Ramirez & McAlister, 1989.

114. Bandura, 1977b. Se also R. I. Evans et al., 1981; Parcel & Baranowski, 1981.

115. Lefebvre & Flora, 1988.

116. Direct telephone communication with Tammi Bradley, Vice President for Communications, Kansas Health Foundation, Wichita, July 8, 1998; "Let's Take It Outside," 1998.

117. J. A. Smith & Scammon, 1987. This was an application of PRECEDE-PROCEED.

118. Brieger, Ramakrishna, & Adeniyi, 1986–1987.

119. Glik et al., 1987–1988.

120. Schellstede & Ciszewski, 1984.

121. A. J. Gordon, 1988.

Chapter 9

Applications
in Occupational Settings[1]

We have characterized PRECEDE-PROCEED as a "robust" model, referring to its adaptability and broad utility in various settings. Since the first publication of the Precede model in 1974[2] the health promotion the literature has provided numerous examples of its application in planning and evaluating programs for various populations in diverse settings within communities.[3] This chapter examines some of the unique challenges of promoting health in the work site; and it also explores how the application and adaptation of Precede and Proceed can make that task more efficient and effective.[4] We might also refer to the model as a *minimalist* theory of health promotion, insofar as it offers the "simplest possible description or conceptualization of a field . . . [and] states some fundamental principles as part of or in addition to integrating the phenomena via new concepts."[5] The same Precede-Proceed principles stated in previous chapters—participation, assessing quality-of-life outcomes beyond health, and combining behavioral and environmental perspectives in working back to the determinants of health—apply to the workplace. These all apply, whether the work-site initiative comes from a community health agency,[6] from the workers themselves,[7] or from employers.[8]

THE ECOLOGICAL CONTEXT OF WORKPLACE HEALTH PROMOTION[9]

The 1980s and early 1990s saw the rapid diffusion, expanding roles, and changing contexts of work-site programs. This initial review reconstructs the paths that health promotion in the workplace has followed. It places experience from past programs in their historical, legislative, demographic, epidemiological, economic, technological, and scientific contexts. It also examines the changing ecological context of work-site health promotion as a convergence of developments in three related workplace developments: economic and demographic changes, occupational health and safety, and employee assistance programs. Though some of these changes have spurred developments in workplace health promotion over the last two decades, others of them threaten to undermine the development as the new century dawns.

The historical path is not marked neatly by progressive milestones. Evidence from evaluations and reputations of occupational health and safety, ergonomics, employee assistance, and work-site wellness and health promotion programs suggest overall progress, achieved by way of converging paths. The ecological context of today's workplace health promotion can be seen in the historical evolution of these paths, as shown in Figure 9-1, out of the demographic, the economic, the regulatory or legislative, and the substance abuse contexts. This flowchart of the converging paths provides a map to the first part of this chapter.

These paths bring us to a crossroads at the turn of the century. The point of convergence ahead confronts the workplace health promotion field with uncertainties about where it will lie in future organizational charts. Will the medical or engineering models of occupational health and safety and of ergonomics dominate? Or will the mental health models of employee assistance programs come forward? Will the behavioral science or the holistic health models of work site wellness emerge as the main paradigm? Or will the new public health model of health promotion prevail? This chapter traces the converging paths to discern how the context of health promotion in the workplace has changed and how the blending of these models will define the future of health promotion in the workplace.

Three other paths emerge in our tracings of the ecological context for health promotion in the workplace. One path defines the degree to which academic research and government policies have stimulated innovations in the workplace. Another defines the direction of influence from innovative business and professional leaders whose vision and initiative in workplace health promotion have stimulated research and policy. The third path emerges from unions and worker initiative in both stimulating health protection reforms in the workplace and resisting health promotion. To guard against bias and confusion of cause and effect in our presentation of issues and developments, we base this chapter on a combination of academic, business, and government sources from at least two countries—the United States and Canada. Though some differences exist between these sources, we find them generally consistent in their implications for the future of workplace health promotion.

HISTORICAL CONTEXT OF HEALTH IN THE WORKPLACE

A new era concerned with employee health unfolded in response to several factors influencing standards for the workplace environment. Occupational health services developed originally to treat and later to prevent job-related injuries and illnesses. **Employee Assistance Programs** (EAPs) later grew out of the targeting of alcohol as a major determinant of industrial injuries, decreased productivity, and psychosocial problems. Workplace health promotion then emerged from

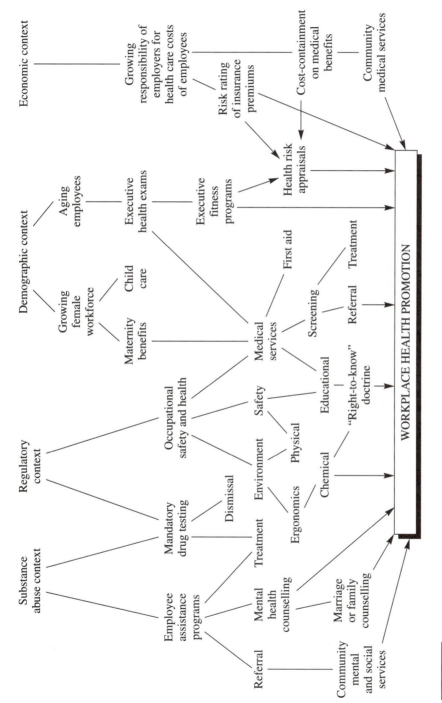

FIGURE 9-1

The ecological context of workplace health promotion can be understood in part from the historical convergence of pathways by which employers have adapted to earlier contexts of changing demography, economics, government regulation, and substance abuse by employees.

SOURCE: "The Changing Context of Health Promotion in the Workplace," by L. W. Green and M. Cargo, 1994, in M. P. O'Donnell and J. S. Harris (Eds.), Albany, NY: Delmar. Reprinted with permission of Delmar Publishers, Inc.

myriad converging trends, the most influential of which in the United States, where workplace health promotion has seen its greatest push, was the increased burden placed on employers by escalating health care costs for illnesses that were not necessarily or entirely job related. These three program areas have evolved independently, with the common (though seldom shared) goal of improving employee health. They also goaded and facilitated the development and implementation of occupational health, employee assistance programs, and health promotion by business and industry. We have sought to identify the common social, economic, and scientific forces behind these three movements and to assess their collective potential to facilitate change in employee health.

Four phenomena have influenced the growth of work-site health promotion in postindustrial nations. One is the changing demographic profiles in most workplaces, especially with the aging of the workforce and the increase in female participation. Second is the economic context, with growing concern for the burden on industry of rising medical care costs, health insurance premiums, and cost of lost productivity in unhealthy workers. Whether employers pay this cost directly, as in the United States, or indirectly through corporate and employer taxes, as in most countries, it represents a burden on industry that makes them less competitive than they might be. The third trend is the growing recognition of the influence of the behavioral and environmental determinants of health, absenteeism, and productivity, which has led to the regulatory and substance abuse context. The fourth is the mounting evidence that health education and health promotion strategies have been effective in altering the behavioral and environmental determinants of health.

DEMOGRAPHIC CONTEXT

Willie "The Actor" Sutton, the infamous American bankrobber was once asked, "Why do you rob banks?" He allegedly answered, "Because that's where the money is!" Health promotion tends to be organized around schools for children and work-sites for adults because that's where the people are. Work sites are to many adults what schools are to children and youth—places where most of the daylight hours are spent, where friendships are made, where many of the rewards that make one feel worthy are dealt, and where one can be reinforced by peers and significant others. They are also places where one feels pressures to perform and deliver.

About three-fourths of the adult men (16 years and over) and nearly 60% of the adult women in the United States were in the labor force as of 1996.[10] Of the married working men, 60% had working wives.[11] Figure 9-2 shows the rates of participation in the U.S labor force for men and women. From 1970 to 1985, the increase in the female workforce participation rate, especially working mothers, reshaped the attitudes of employers toward employee benefits and working conditions.[12] The workplace has replaced the neighborhood as the community of

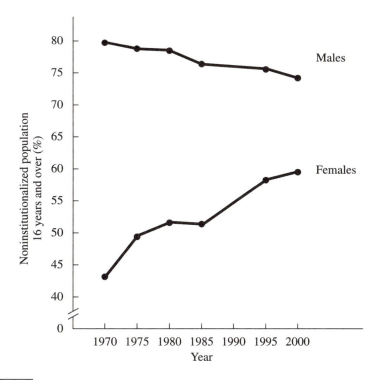

FIGURE 9-2

Civilian labor force participation rates for the U.S. population age 16 years and older, 1970–2000, show the striking increase in female employment.

SOURCE: *Monthly Labor Review,* by U.S. Department of Labor, Bureau of Labor Statistics, 1998; *Statistical Abstract of the United States, 1999,* by U.S. Bureau of the Census, 1998, Washington, DC: U.S. Government Printing Office.

reference and social identity for many urban and suburban North Americans and Europeans.[13] These demographic and social trends, combined with the pervasive influence of occupational environments on adult health, quality of life, behavior, and lifestyle, make them logical if not ideal settings for health promotion programs.

REGULATORY CONTEXT: OCCUPATIONAL HEALTH AND SAFETY LEGISLATION

Industrial hygiene and the occupational health and safety movement focused on protecting health through the control of potential hazards in the work environment. The field emerged from (1) the recognition that employees are strongly influenced by their work environment and (2) the realization that many illnesses related to the work environment could be controlled, some even eliminated.

Legislative Initiatives. The passage in 1970 of the Occupational Safety and Health Act (OSHA) in the United States[14] and similar legislation in the United Kingdom (1974),[15] Canada (1970s),[16] Australia (1972, 1977, 1985),[17] France (1946, revised 1976, 1982),[18] West Germany (1974),[19] and Sweden (1978)[20] led to the rise of occupational health and safety education activities. Standards were established to protect the worker's health. These standards had the support of the international labor movement and the advantage of the international codes that were developing during this period. In this context, health promotion found a natural ally in the workplace and a potentially favorable climate.

The Problem of Coordination. The U.S. Occupational Safety and Health Act of 1970 placed the responsibility for and enforcement of occupational health and safety in one federal agency, the Occupational Health and Safety Administration, and its counterpart state agencies. Reactions to the act have led to increasing polarization between labor and management. The polarization and fragmentation does not end there. The legislation for Employee Assistance Programs (EAPs) and health promotion programs emerged from different congressional committees and are governed by different federal and state agencies. The National Institute of Alcoholism and Alcohol Abuse and the National Institute of Drug Abuse in the Department of Health and Human Services (DHHS) administer EAPs. The Department of Labor and the National Institute of Occupational Safety and Health (NIOSH) administer OSHA. NIOSH is located in the Centers for Disease Control, which is part of DHHS. The lack of horizontal integration among these governing legislative committees and administrative agencies has constrained the development of a more comprehensive approach to program implementation in policies and regulations. The Office of Disease Prevention and Health Promotion under the Assistant Secretary of Health and its *Healthy People* objectives for the nation in disease prevention and health promotion, however, has provided a coordinating mechanism for these agencies and sectors to work together toward more comprehensive workplace health programs.

In Canada, labor legislation is under provincial jurisdiction, with each province and territory having its own occupational health and safety legislation. The federal government has laws for its own employees and for employees of industries under its jurisdiction. Occupational health and safety laws were passed in the 1970s for most provinces. In Britain, implementation of the Health and Safety Work Act is the responsibility of the Health and Safety Executive.[21] As in most countries other than the United States, British employers have not experienced great economic pressures to prevent disease and promote health in their employees. This changed somewhat with the advent of the employer's responsibility for statutory sick pay under the 1986 Social Security Act. Britain's enlight-

ened occupational health policies, though, had never been entirely motivated by either economic or health concerns. Rather, they originated from benevolent employers in the 18th and 19th centuries seeking to protect workers from occupational disease and injury.

Problems Requiring Regulatory Intervention. Many people work in an environment containing a host of potential hazards such as harmful physical agents (e.g., heat, vibrations, noise), toxic chemicals, stressful routines, or dangerous equipment. Exposure to the hazardous elements in the workplace takes its toll in the form of employee illness, disability, and death. In 1993, work-related injuries in the United States cost $121 billion in medical care, lost productivity, and wages; these increased from the 1983–1987 average of 7.7 injuries per 100 workers to 8.4 in 1994. This occurred while injury deaths and work-related injury deaths were declining in general.[22] Some three-fourths of new cases of occupational illness in private industry occur in manufacturing. The service industry accounts for about one-eighth of the cases. Occupational illnesses associated with repeated trauma or conditions caused by repeated motion, pressure, or vibration constitute just over 50% of the reported cases, marking a significant increase in number and percentage of total illnesses reported. Industries with the highest accident frequency rates (disabling injuries per 100,000 work hours) also have the highest severity rates (days lost per 1 million work hours). By their very nature, certain industries such as agriculture, mining, marine transportation, quarrying, and construction tend to post the greatest hazard. Motor vehicle injuries account for the greatest proportion of all work-related fatalities.[23]

Environmental Protections Versus Health Promotion. The occupational health and safety acts in many countries resulted in strategies to protect employees from the biological, physical, chemical and environmental hazards of the workplace. The emphasis of employer responsibility for environmental protection began as early as 1912, with workmen's compensation laws. Many trade unions have consistently viewed worker health as the employer's responsibility. As a result, unions initially resisted the introduction of health promotion, which they viewed as a smokescreen to mask failed environmental reforms and to shift the blame for worker illness and injury onto the behavior of workers. This was of great concern for those workers exposed to potentially health-threatening working conditions such as chemicals.

The work environment was the first target of employee health concerns and has persisted as the primary concern of labor unions and reform-minded health professionals. As health promotion moves closer to occupational health and safety, attention to the environment will increase in health promotion planning as well.

Protection of Women. A decision by the U.S. Supreme Court in 1991 changed the occupational safety and health policy as it affects the working conditions of women. The court decision ruled against the Johnston Controls, which was originally legislated to protect women from exposure to potential reproductive hazards such as lead and which prevented women from being hired into positions that would place them at reproductive risk. The new legislation shifts the focus from hiring restrictions to environmental reforms, requiring hazard-free workplaces for high-risk employees to ensure their equal work opportunity.

Since World War II, women have moved increasingly into occupations previously designed for men, including heavy manual labor. The increase in the percentage of working mothers has reshaped the attitudes of employers toward working conditions and family matters such as day care, flexible working hours, job sharing, and childbirth leave for both parents.

Educational Protections. Legislative action introduced the "right to know" doctrine, assuring workers information about workplace health hazards. Prior to the OSHA, employers were not required to inform workers of chemical or other workplace hazards that could cause adverse health effects. Passage of the act was an attempt to remedy occupational injury and disease through primary prevention. This approach involved establishing safety standards and placing limits on exposures to hazardous substances. It then became the responsibility of the employers to comply with these standards or incur fines.

The act has been criticized for being paternalistic, because it assumes that workplace health risks can be eliminated, an approach that leaves minimal opportunity for worker participation or decision making.[24] The High-Risk Occupational Disease Notification and Prevention Bill of 1987 was a further effort to remedy the deficiencies of the OHSA by establishing a system for identifying, notifying, and assisting workers at high risk for occupational disease.[25]

One could argue that educational methods directed at the behavior or the **informed consent** of workers, when combined with management and environmental reforms to improve the working conditions, gained greater participation and action because employers and employees were meeting each other halfway. Another advantage of the combined educational and environmental approach was that some of the work-site hazards affected worker behavior. Some were synergistic in their effects, such as smoking and exposure to asbestos, solvents, and other air pollutants. Some had concomitant effects on the same health problems, such as alcohol and injury exposure. Some potentially affected worker productivity and health concomitantly but independently, such as stressful working conditions, being overweight, or being sedentary and lacking physical fitness. All of these interacting relationships called for intervention directed at (1) protecting the worker against hazardous and stressful working conditions and (2) promoting healthful practices such as exercise, nutritional eating, and self-examination for cancer signs and symptoms.[26]

The educational and right-to-know context of occupational health provided an additional wedge for health promotion approaches that informed workers more generally about health risks, among which lifestyle and behavioral risks could be shown to account for an even larger proportion of premature mortality and years of life lost than did the workplace environment.

Medical Surveillance. Medical surveillance was first incorporated into the occupational health field as a weapon to prevent occupational disease and injury through preplacement examinations and periodic checkups. The pamphlet *Health Education in Industry,* published by the Metropolitan Life Insurance Company around 1963, characterizes the typical workplace health program as follows:

> Today, an employee health program generally starts with a pre-placement examination. This helps to determine a person's suitability for a specific job—his technical as well as his physical and emotional fitness. It follows through with regular check-ups, and concerns itself with the employee's general well-being as well as with the specific job hazards and work environment.

Medical surveillance now covers a range of services: medical screening, medical and biological monitoring, primary and secondary prevention strategies, drug testing.[27] Medical surveillance activities systematically evaluate employees at risk for exposure to workplace hazards. When blood pressure screening was added to the battery of tests in occupational surveillance programs, issues began to arise about whether to attribute the cause of detected hypertension to the job or to other lifestyle risks.[28] The surveillance systems complemented the hazard control strategies, but they also raised ethical issues of privacy, confidentiality, and labeling, especially with the specter of HIV/AIDS testing and drug testing.[29] These have spilled into the health promotion arena with the advent of health risk appraisal questionnaires, some of which include medical screening items and questions of private behavior.[30] The possibility of genetic testing to identify risks makes the threat to privacy and the possibility of discrimination even more ominous, underscoring the urgent need for regulation.[31]

Risk Assessment. Testing for the presence of alcohol, tobacco, and illegal drugs in the employee's blood or urine has become more prevalent among employers, who sometimes used the results to dichotomize present or potential employees into users and nonusers in order to identify those with undesirable lifestyles.[32] Employers tend to implement drug testing and fitness testing to reduce the number of work-related injuries[33] and to improve productivity and product integrity, although there is little evidence to warrant this practice.[34] Most corporations have taken remedial action through the provision of EAPs, but some companies routinely fire employees with or without provisions for counseling or treatment.

Workplace medical surveillance has evolved over the decades. Its primary role today is to enhance and assess the overall effect of the health examinations, drug-testing, and health promotion aspects of a comprehensive occupational health program.[35] As we progress into the 21st century, we may expect to see a further blurring of the boundaries between work and private life, especially with increasing provisions for work at home.

Psychosocial Factors. The occupational safety and health movement concerned itself with reducing work-related health problems resulting from exposure to hazards external to the control of employees.[36] Employers, however, tended to give greater consideration to the role of behavioral, motivational, and psychological factors in job health and safety.[37] The psychosocial aspects of job demand such as pace, monotony, and degree of controls represent sources of stress that researchers have focused on to test additional ways to protect health and prevent safety risks to employees.[38] Noise was targeted in the U.S. objectives for the nation as an environmental work condition with implications for mental and physical health, as shown in Figure 9-3. The attention given to individual psychosocial factors in job health and safety served as a stimulus for the appearance of the workplace mental health movement[39] and may represent a common historical linchpin of occupational health and safety, EAP, and workplace health promotion.

Recent Trends. In reviewing the profile of occupational safety and health, one can observe significant progress in hazard control strategies, medical surveillance, and psychosocial factors in safety and health. Since the passage of the OSHA, considerable headway has been made in the prevention of occupational disease as recorded in U.S. statistics. Some of the most serious workplace hazards have disappeared or declined in prevalence. Stringent regulatory controls and standards have replaced looser guidelines, requirements have replaced recommendations, and secrecy is less common.[40] The effectiveness of safety programs is attested to by the drop in the injury frequency rate for companies reporting to the National Safety Council. Occupational injury deaths per 100,000 workers dropped 71% between 1912 to 1980. This remarkable accomplishment was matched by an additional 23% reduction from 1980 to 1986 but offset by an increase between 1987 and 1994.[41]

Even with these signs of progress, success as measured by the reduction and -elimination of work-related morbidity and mortality remains uneven. Although asbestos is used less frequently today than in the past, an estimated 10,000 deaths attributable to asbestos exposure are expected to occur in the U.S. annually until the year 2020. The progress on occupational safety and health toward the year 2000 objectives has also been uneven, as shown in Figure 9-4.[42] The deregulatory emphases of recent federal policies in the United States and other nations, to favor their industries in the intensified global competition, have loosened some of the controls on workplace hazards.

Current Limitations. The preventability of work-related illness depends on the simultaneous control and further study of the interactions among environmental, behavioral, social, and economic factors that contribute to the persistence of occupational disease in the United States. We still know relatively little about

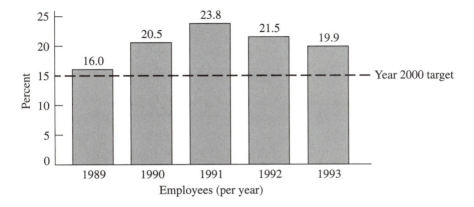

FIGURE 9-3

Progress toward the U.S. objective for reducing the average daily exposure of employees to noise levels that exceed 85 decibels by the year 2000 has been uneven, reflecting the combined forces of regulation, economics, education, and technology.

SOURCE: *Healthy People 2000 Review, 1995–96,* (p. 96), by National Center for Health Statistics, 1996, Hyattsville, MD: Public Health Service.

many synthetic chemicals, despite increases in public, regulatory, and scientific awareness and investigation. The capacity of physicians is limited to the extent that they are not trained to infer work as a potential cause of disease. Physicians also receive little training in occupational medicine. Workers exposed to hazardous substances in many cases are not notified of exposure. Medical surveillance programs are "fragmented, unreliable and outdated," underestimating the actual number of cases of occupational-related illnesses.[43]

In addition to the regulatory roles of the Occupational Health and Safety Administration already discussed, the National Institute for Occupational Safety and Health (NIOSH) is responsible for investigating the presence of hazardous working conditions. The budget of NIOSH was cut by over 50% during the 1980s and has not made up that deficit in the 1990s, limiting workplace inspections to a few high-risk industries. Uprooted from its base in Washington, D.C., where it had good exposure to political forces, NIOSH was moved to the Centers for Disease Control in Atlanta, Georgia. These factors have impeded some attempts to address workplace hazards contributing to the incidence and prevalence of occupational-related illnesses.

In summary, the environmental and medical orientation of occupational safety and health has made it compatible with and hospitable to some health promotion concepts emphasizing primary prevention. On the whole, however, the professionals and the workers (especially unions) invested in occupational health and safety have ranged from competitive to hostile in their attitude toward health promotion programs as they have been developed in many workplaces. The ascendancy of

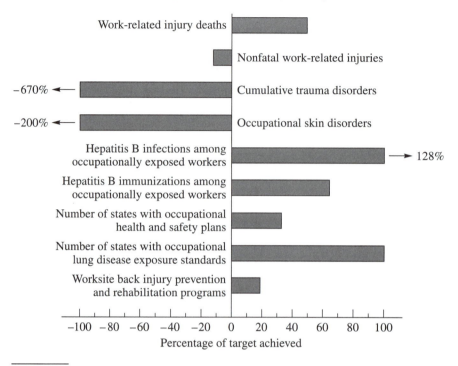

Status of occupational safety and health objectives

FIGURE 9-4

The mid-decade progress toward achievement of selected occupational safety and health objectives revealed lost ground on nonfatal work-related injuries, cumulative trauma disorders such as carpal tunnel syndrome, and occupational skin disorders.

SOURCE: *Healthy People 2000: Midcourse Review and 1995 Revisions,* (p. 73), by U.S. Department of Health and Human Services, 1996, Sudbury, MA: Jones and Bartlett.

health promotion in government policy at the same time that OSHA and NIOSH faced cutbacks in their budgets, their regulatory powers, and their influence in Washington made many occupational safety and health workers unreceptive if not antagonistic toward the advancement of workplace health promotion.

ECONOMIC CONTEXT

The other way to understand Willie Sutton's answer to why he robbed banks—"Because that's where the money is!"—would be to consider the costs and benefits of health promotion in the workplace. In 1994, U.S. employers paid about a

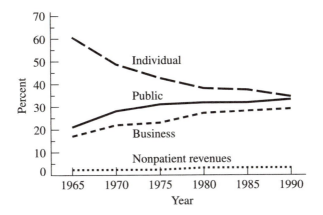

FIGURE 9-5

The business sector's and government's percentage of expenditures for health services in the United States has continued to increase since 1965, while personal expenditures have decreased.

SOURCE: Health Care Financing Administration and National Center for Health Statistics, *Healthy People 2000 Review, 1995–96,* by National Center for Health Statistics, 1996, Hyattsville, MD: Public Health Service, DHHS-PHS-96-1256.

third of the $900 billion in medical care costs through employment-linked health insurance, workers' compensation, and other payment mechanisms.[44] This continued the prior 25 years of increase in the business proportion of total health care expenditures since 1965, shown in Figure 9-5.

Containing Health Care Costs. U.S. business and industry took a fresh look at health promotion and disease prevention in the late 1970s as they faced alarming increases in the cost of medical care and insurance premiums for their employees.[45] The increase in spending on health care fell more heavily on industry than on individuals (Figure 9-5),[46] with business and government picking up a larger share of the continuing increase.

Corporate interest in health promotion was generated in large part in response to escalating health care costs. In 1988, occupational deaths and injuries cost employers and workers an estimated $47.1 billion. For each work-related injury, occupational injuries resulting in disability cost the U.S. $16,500 in lost wages, medical expenses, and insurance fees, increasing to $23,000 in 1990. By 1994, the work-related injuries alone cost $121 billion in medical care, lost productivity, and wages.[47]

Canada has not seen the same explosive growth of workplace health promotion programs or interest among employers in such programs, because its companies do not shoulder as much of the direct cost for its sick and injured employees.

Total medical care expenditures in the United States have grown at an exponential rate—from \$38.2 billion in 1965, to \$124.7 billion in 1975, to \$407.2 billion in 1985, and to \$643.4 billion in 1990.[48] The cost of health care coverage provided by employers increased over threefold from 1980 to 1990—from \$64.8 billion to \$186.2 billion. As shown in Figure 9-5, in 1990 business accounted for 29% of expenditures for health services and supplies, government 33%, and households 33%. Besides incurring a smaller proportion of their employee's health care costs, Canadian employers have seen a slower escalation of costs. The increased U.S. and Canadian interest in workplace health promotion was also influenced by changing demographic profiles, with older workers bringing more chronic conditions. Finally, both countries and others have recognized the influences of behavior and environment on health, as well as the converging evidence of the effectiveness of health education and health promotion strategies in altering the determinants of health.

The imperative of OSHA legislation forced employers to implement environmental strategies to reduce the risk of disease, disability, and premature death among employees. Health promotion was enlisted as a strategy for containing health care costs, to increase productivity, and to provide personal benefit to employees, but it did not have the regulatory teeth that occupational hazard control and safety had in OSHA-type legislation. With the advent of smoke-free workplace legislation at the state, provincial, and local levels, a new era of regulatory support for health promotion was born.[49]

Econometric Evaluation. Cost containment remains a primary motivating factor in the implementation of health promotion programs. In the early 1980s, to address the lack of cost-effectiveness and cost-benefit data to support health promotion programs, researchers estimated the cost-effectiveness and cost-benefit of existing programs.[50] There was some concern that health promotion programs were subjected to greater economic scrutiny intervention and to more stringent criteria and requirements of acceptability, including evidence of effectiveness and cost savings, than was medical care intervention. Further, some worried that cost-benefit arguments might be oversold.[51] The continued growth of health promotion programs in the 1980s in the absence of evidence for cost-effectiveness suggests the importance of other factors, such as concern for employee health and well-being or quality of work life. The diverging views regarding the profitability of health promotion may reflect employers' various rationales for program adoption. Some employers place greater weight on cost-effectiveness or cost-benefit as measured by reduced absences or increased productivity, whereas other employers emphasize the health benefits derived by employees. There appears to be at least some consensus that cost-benefit impact on the corporate bottom line by reducing health care costs, absenteeism, and other employment-related costs is probable, but it cannot be the sole basis for program implementation.[52]

The concern for cost-effectiveness and cost-benefit data encouraged an increasing number of evaluations of single modality and comprehensive programs.

Given the methodological limitations of the data, the combined evidence suggests that health promotion programs can support both health and cost-effectiveness. The majority of evaluations have focused on single modality programs such as smoking cessation, stress management, weight loss, and hypertension.

Tobacco Control. Smoking-cessation and -control programs have taken varied forms in workplaces, ranging from clinical and self-help models to organizational, regulatory, and legal reforms of smoking policies. Meta-analyses and systematic reviews of long-term quit rates from controlled smoking cessation studies in workplaces reveal a modest but significant overall effect.[53] Generally, short-term quit rates are high and diminish over time, highlighting the problem with maintaining behavior change. Quit rates are influenced by whether the company has a restrictive smoking policy and provides smoking-cessation programs; and these policies depend in part on company size.[54] This clearly demonstrates the importance of the ecological context and the need for ecological interventions to support individual changes.

The most compelling of the cost-benefit analyses of the health and economic implications of a work-site smoking-cessation program is a simulation by Warner and his colleagues. They used long-term flow of costs and benefits, based on conservative estimates from previous studies. They also factored in employee turnover, which showed that approximately half of the considerable health and economic benefits generated by a work-site smoking-cessation program accrue to the community rather than to the employer who sponsored the program. Nevertheless, the simulation shows that smoking cessation is a "very sound economic investment for the firm, and is particularly profitable when long-term benefits are included, with an eventual benefit-cost ratio of 8.75."[55] The analysis also highlights, however, that these benefits should not be overstated as to their solution to the smoking problem for the workplace and that the intervention successfully addresses only a small fraction of the costs that the firm incurs from smoking employees.

Stress Management and Nutrition. The findings from stress management studies suggest that well-designed programs oriented toward individual behavior change lead to short-term changes in various physiological variables, the most important factor being lower blood pressure, but comprehensive or combined individual and environmental programs are more effective.[56] Stress management often accompanies smoking-cessation and weight control programs. Few studies have demonstrated the cost-effectiveness of workplace nutrition programs. Low participation rates have plagued the evaluation of stress and nutrition programs, as it has others.[57]

A key study found that the program costs for a campaign strategy for weight loss amounted to $0.81 spent per pound lost.[58] Compared with other approaches, work-site competitions have been found to be highly cost-effective in recruiting participants without compromising outcome efficacy.[59] Because weight gain is such a major concern of some smokers in deciding whether to quit smoking, the linkage to smoking makes weight control and stress management a natural grouping of programs for an economically justified comprehensive set of programs.

Hypertension. Evidence suggests that by reducing absenteeism, hypertension control programs have a favorable cost-benefit ratio.[60] One study calculated the program cost at $150 per employee per year, which was considered a cost-saving investment in relation to the $10,000 incurred in medical costs when an employee has a heart attack.[61]

Comprehensive Programs. As reviewed by Pelletier, there is sufficient evidence to support the cost-effectiveness of comprehensive programs.[62] Evaluation of the Johnson & Johnson Live For Life Program is an excellent example of a cost-effectiveness evaluation using existing data along the lines of design C in Chapter 7. Experimental groups had lower increases in inpatient costs, hospital days, and admissions than did control groups.[63] Because the study design has inherent methodological limitations, this support should be viewed cautiously. Besides methodological limitations, some have called into question how well even the "comprehensive corporate health promotion programs" meet the ecological demands of a systems model of health.[64]

Limitations of Evaluation. Despite the growing body of evaluation literature supporting the cost-effectiveness of health promotion programs, researchers continue to identify the need for well-designed, methodologically sound studies. Yet, professionals in the field identify rigorous scientific standards as a barrier to evaluation.[65] Work sites viewed as laboratories pose difficulties in incorporating and maintaining the integrity of a control group. With the difficulties in implementing randomized evaluation designs, researchers may need to settle on better analyses of quasi-experimental designs that statistically control for variables they cannot control by random assignment of large numbers of workers.

Employee Dependents. Health promotion in the workplace is primarily concerned with supporting healthful lifestyle practices, but lifestyle has come to be seen as more than just behavior. The workplace has long been seen as a venue in which health promotion professionals could give greater attention to social factors influencing health.[66] This expanding focus is similar to EAP taking on family and emotional difficulties and financial problems associated with alcohol misuse. Some corporations have not limited health promotion to employees but have extended the efforts to family and retirees. Some employers recognize that these groups influence the firm's health care costs. An estimated 50% to 70% of health care costs accrue from the spouses and dependents of employees.[67] In a 1993 survey of 20 companies, dependents and retirees accounted for more health care dollars than did employees in 18 of the 20 work sites.[68] Others saw the importance of family influence on the employee and the need to make health promotion a family endeavor.

Large companies such as Du Pont (starting in 1994) and Johnson & Johnson have extended their health promotion efforts to dependents and retirees.[69] Programs directed at maternal health are a new addition to dependent care. One unhealthy baby can cost a company over $1 million, including impact on absenteeism and productivity.[70] The Baby Benefits Program and March of Dimes prenatal programs were found to impart significant cost savings to employers. The former program is consumer oriented and encourages the mother to attend the prenatal program in the first trimester. Breast-feeding programs have been found successful in assisting the mother in the transition back to work after maternity leave.[71] Pennsylvania Public Employees Health and Welfare concluded from an 18-month study that prevention programs for dependent children of employees provide effective protection of family health and reduce costs of medical care for preventable illnesses.[72] The difficulty of changing the lifestyle of adults was given as another reason for the focus on children.

SUBSTANCE ABUSE CONTEXT: EMPLOYEE ASSISTANCE PROGRAMS

The U.S. Organizational Context. In the United States, EAPs have no direct mandate from any federal legislation. Indirectly supported by the U.S. federal Drug-Free Work Act and the National Drug Control Strategy, EAPs leave private business and health professionals responsible for the development, implementation, and operation of EAPs. In the late 1970s, the Employee Assistance Program Association (EAPA), formerly known as ALMACA, released program standards that provided cursory rationalizations for the functions of EAPs.[73] As EAPs changed in scope during the 1980s, the standards were perceived as having conceptual and pragmatic deficiencies. A new set of standards released in 1990 addressed the design, implementation, and evaluation of EAPs. The new standards seek to clarify misconceptions among researchers and others about the elements of comprehensive EAPs. A managed care monograph entitled "Maximizing Behavioral Health Benefit Value through EAP Integration" was released along with the new standards. This document conveyed the message that management uses EAPs to save health care dollars with the added benefit of keeping employees healthy and on the job. In a pragmatic way, it assists businesses in applying EAP standards to the workplace, acknowledging the economic context, as in the preceding section of this chapter, but also seeking to adapt to the organizational culture.

The Canadian Organizational Context. In Canada, EAPs function differently than in the United States. The Canadian federal and provincial governments provide a broader network of assessment and treatment services, with lesser emphasis on private facilities and private consultants. Companies therefore have less concern for cost barriers when they refer troubled employees to community resources. There is greater union involvement in and commitment to EAPs in Canada than in the United States. Some Canadian unions have successfully negotiated EAPs into the collective agreement, an issue of great contention in the United States. The Canadian Labor Congress (CLC) Employee Recovery Program assists union members in establishing EAPs in their workplace. EAPs appear to be developing in other countries, the international interest and growth spurred by governments and multinational companies.

The Diffusion of EAPs. The rise and proliferation of EAPs in the United States, Canada, and other countries underscores the role of alcohol as a major determinant in industrial injuries, psychosocial problems, and decreased productivity, the costs of which are borne largely by employers. Estimates from national surveys indicate that 10% of employees in North America experience serious alcohol problems.[74] Alcohol abuse is related to several serious problems that influence the health and welfare of employees, families, and employers. In addition, up to 57% of all industrial injuries are associated with alcohol, with as many as 75% of those involved in two or more industrial accidents having alcohol problems. Many non-work-related injuries are linked to alcohol, with approximately one-half of all motor vehicle injuries involving it. Alcohol is also implicated in the high costs of psychosocial disturbances[75] and domestic violence that accrue to industry. Decreased productivity is another result of alcohol abuse of particular interest to employers. Bertera estimated annual costs per employee at $389.[76]

From Medical Model to Constructive Confrontation. Occupational alcoholism rehabilitation represents the forerunner of EAPs. Responsibility fell initially on occupational medicine departments to carry out these activities. These programs focused on tertiary care, or referral and treatment services to employees whose use of alcohol interfered with work performance.[77] Physicians treated the interference of alcohol with job performance as they would other diseases, by trying to eliminate the use of alcohol without addressing the underlying motivations for its use. It became evident that the medical model offered little help to the drinking employee. Alcohol consumption does not always manifest itself in physical illness, but rather represents behaviors requiring lifestyle modification rather than medical treatment.[78] The encounter between physician and patient was often antagonistic rather than cooperative, as patients did not voluntarily seek help for their problem but viewed it as forced on them. With federal support in the form of grant funds from the National Institute of Alcohol and Alcoholism, occupational alcoholism policies and programs incorporated a strategy referred to as constructive-confrontation.[79] This strategy, based on the identification by supervisors of workers experiencing alcohol-related problems, guided the formation and implementation of occupational alcoholism programs. Further development of this strategy—namely, the adoption of formal written policies by companies to guide the managerial actions—and the protection of employees' rights led to the outgrowth of EAPs from occupational alcoholism programs. The ideological shift away from the disease orientation of alcoholism coincided with the expanded focus of EAPs to include other drug use and eventually other family or personal problems.

Evidence of program success and incentives provided by the National Institute of Alcoholism and Alcohol Abuse led to a dramatic increase of programs in the 1970s.[80] Fewer than 100 programs were in operation in the 1960s. By 1980, an estimated 12% of the nation's workforce had access to occupational alcoholism programs.

From Treatment to Secondary Prevention. The limited focus on tertiary care inspired some EAP administrators to expand the program to include secondary prevention activities to identify and intervene with high-risk employees, including dependents and retirees. EAP professionals began to acknowledge the importance of and the need for primary prevention.[81] One review, however, found no evidence of primary prevention having taken root in any EAP as of 1987.[82]

From Screening to Self-Referral. Among other consequences, the movement from tertiary to secondary prevention has increased employers' emphasis on personal responsibility for health and well-being. Based on the training of supervisors to detect deterioration in employee job performance and on the referral of troubled employees to counseling, the EAP model has shifted toward the promotion of employee self-awareness and voluntary self-referrals.[83]

Converging Interests of EAPs and Health Promotion. EAP professionals have expressed some concern over the potential encroachment of workplace health promotion into their domain. The issue of territoriality or boundary maintenance is manifest in an alleged struggle for shared resources.[84] Some expressed a further concern that health promotion demonstrated program efficacy and cost-effectiveness at the expense of EAPs.[85] Others suggested that the concomitant emphasis of health promotion programs on self-referrals may serve to strengthen rather than jeopardize outreach efforts of EAP services.[86] The presence of "dual clients," employees who use both EAPs and health promotion services, provides further support for a "wellness-to-EAP-to-wellness" referral pattern. High blood pressure, for example, is a common condition among alcoholics. Physical fitness programs have been used to rehabilitate employees from substance dependence or emotional problems. It was even suggested as early as 1987 that the common interest in reciprocal influences of individuals and their environments may lead to an interdependency between EAPs and health promotion.[87]

Over the years there has been a gradual reorientation of substance abuse programs—from the referral and treatment of employees with identified alcohol problems to a more basic focus on those factors that precipitate socioemotional problems. Comprehensive EAPs address the emotional and personal problems that interfere with work performance and can develop into more serious and costly psychiatric or physical health disorders. The evolution of EAPs has led some to extend their services to address family and emotional difficulties, financial crises, and problems with children and family.

Although EAPs remain at a secondary prevention level of intervention, their new comprehensive orientation is responsible for the increasing popularity of EAPs in the 1980s and 1990s. This broad focus eliminates the stigma associated with an employee being labeled as an alcoholic. In addition, removal of this stigma helps reduce the denial often experienced by troubled employees in accepting referral and treatment. With the trend of increasing self-referrals, supervisors are now trained to assess employee job performance rather than diagnose potential problems related to alcohol or drug use.

We have witnessed a shift in the strategies implemented by EAPs. The initial strategy of treating alcoholic employees identified by trained staff has given way to secondary prevention, in which workers at high risk may voluntarily use EAP services for alcohol, drug, and other family or socioemotional problems. One can view the substance abuse component of work-site health promotion as the primary prevention arm of employee assistance programs. Herein, the boundaries of EAPs overlap with health promotion. The recognition of simultaneous unhealthful lifestyle behaviors and dual-client users will continue to generate even greater concern over the issue of territoriality and boundary maintenance. This particular crossroads is marked with signs reading "yield" and "proceed with caution."

THE BLENDING OF THE THREE WORK-SITE HEALTH ECOLOGIES

A few remaining features of the workplace setting for health promotion and its evolution illustrate how the approaches to health in the regulatory, medical, and psychological traditions of occupational health and safety, employee health services, and EAPs have blended into the work of health promotion.

Health Risk Appraisals. The history of medical screening in occupational health, combined with the screening and self-referral traditions of EAPs, were expressed in work-site health promotion with an early interest in the development of the Health Risk Appraisal (HRA). In the context of the work site, HRAs are used to assess the health risks and to motivate actions to reduce the lifestyle risks for chronic diseases and injury. The HRA provides a methodology for determining the probability of risk for illness and provides employers with a tool for planning, evaluation, and cost control.

Although HRAs are useful for identifying behaviors requiring modification at the individual level, programs based on this information alone tend not to attain much success. Program developers need to consider the role of the organizational environment and its resulting impact on health behavior. R. F. Allen advocated interventions directed at the culture of organizations so that the support of groups for the behavior in question would change.[88] Increasing appreciation of the eco-logical role of organizational factors in influencing health behavior has led to the development of a risk appraisal tool for health cultures.[89] In conjunction with the standard HRA, the two data sources may lead to the development of a more eco-logically comprehensive health promotion program.

Prevention Versus Health Promotion. Early stages of occupational health emphasized the conservation of health status, while more recent efforts address the promotion of health to the optimal level, to improve quality of life and work performance. The definition of occupational disease and injury includes health problems that may be aggravated by work conditions, thus expanding the concept of occupa-tional health to include conditions such as high blood pressure, cardiovascular disease, ulcers, and a variety of psychological problems.

Work Organization, Control, and Health. Karasek's pioneering work on stress in occu-pational health, beginning in the 1970s, helped establish the relationship between work organization and health.[90] A central theme that emerged from this line of inquiry is that a person's place and degree of control in the social and work envi-ronment affect health and well-being. Researchers emphasized the central role of the social environment in determining the health of individuals, and they stressed on-the-job environment as a factor in biological and social pathology. When workers have little control over their work pace and methods, higher levels of cat-echolamines, mental strain, coronary heart disease, and other health problems result.[91] Studies of civil servants in Britain[92] and bus drivers in San Francisco[93] show similar effects of stress, work pace, isolation, and hierarchical position.

With the increase in office and service occupations, the relationship between work conditions and health is of great concern: an estimated 15 million U.S. citi-zens work at video display terminals. This type of work encourages low control, social isolation, and repetition and monotony, which may have unduly influenced the increasing number of stress-related disability claims, identified as the most rapidly growing form of occupational illness within the worker's compensation systems in the United States and Canada.[94]

Organizational Culture. Business professionals, employee unions, and researchers alike respect the view that health promotion's role is to help employers move toward optimal health in a supportive work environment. Many health promotion programs struggle, however, because they function in the absence of a supportive corporate culture.[95] This could explain the problem of fit with prepackaged well-ness programs: They would be ineffective when imposed on a corporate culture different from the one in which they were developed, especially when com-pounded by an initial mismatch between the program and employee needs. Suc-cessful implementation of health promotion programs in part depends on the systematic change of norms that support unhealthful lifestyle practices.

Allen pioneered the Normative Systems Approach to Cultural Change.[96] *Norms* are the social group's expectations concerning appropriate behavior. In the work environment, employees establish certain standards of behavior that become the norms of that group. The systematic cultural change strategies outlined by Allen's approach serve to reinforce the norms for health-enhancing behavior, for empowering employees, and for stimulating cooperation for change. In the 1970s and early 1980s, smoking in offices was the norm. Within a decade, support of restrictive smoking policies had changed the norm to nonsmoking.

Health promotion programs that are designed and implemented in a way that fits the organizational culture tend to be more effective than those that do not. Researchers find that the implementation of identical programs in different work sites yield variable results, suggesting that work-site characteristics may well have a mediating effect on the desired outcome.[97] For example, the ecological effects of organizational characteristics on compliance with nonsmoking policies were studied in 710 work sites associated with the North American COMMIT study. Compliance of workers was highest in work sites where policies were more restrictive, communication of the policy was effective, cigarette vending machines were not present, smoking-cessation programs were offered, and labor-management relations were excellent.[98] The concept of fit of a given program with the organizational culture begets more sophisticated constructs for assessment. It is important to design flexible programs that can be adapted to the employee group norms and organizational characteristics; alternatively, one could adapt selected organizational characteristics and policies to the proposed program.[99]

The economic impetus for workplace health promotion has forced it to expand its initial behavioral focus to include some of the environmental, medical, and mental health concerns of occupational health and safety and EAPs. An environmental approach to disease prevention grew out of the limitations of individual approaches to health promotion, which usually depended entirely on individual effort. Individuals can easily change their own behavior when they have the necessary knowledge, skills, resources, and incentives; however, when the behaviors are deeply embedded in lifestyle, including conditions of work over which they have little or no control, change is difficult at best. Some behaviors have an addictive or compulsive component. While short-term behavior change occurs, often through exhaustive efforts, long-term change is even more difficult to achieve. Changes do occur with comprehensive programs addressing the necessary combination of predisposing, enabling, and reinforcing factors.

In summary, health promotion has been a tumbling snowball in the workplace, accumulating layers of new ideas and old components from environmental programs. From a preoccupation with cost-effectiveness to growing interests in corporate culture and an array of outcomes from short-term to long-term intangibles, health promotion continues to evolve as it spreads to new firms and new work sites within large companies. The three spheres in Figure 9-6 illustrate the

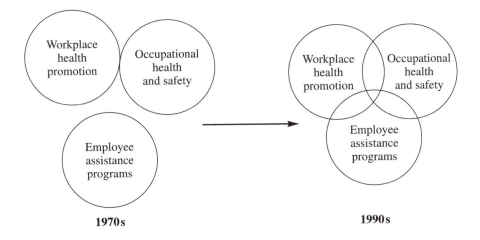

1970s   1990s

FIGURE 9-6

The three spheres of workplace health have separate histories, traditions, disciplinary attachments, ideological orientations, and legislative mandates, but they have taken on features of each other in the past decade to the point that they now overlap in their functions and activities.

convergence at the turn of the century. We might anticipate a further merging of the three spheres as the 21st century unfolds.

The Pattern of Diffusion. The trend in adoption of health promotion programs by employers parallels the diffusion curve invoked in earlier chapters. Except in a few innovative areas,[100] adopters before about 1980, often chief executive officers who had a heart attack or for other reasons were themselves true believers in a healthful lifestyle, typically installed health promotion programs for personal more than economic reasons. During the early 1980s, employers began to initiate health promotion programs because of a growing awareness of their potential health and economic benefits.[101] Through repeated exposures to health messages via myriad communications channels, the general public, including employers, began to see the relevance of the information confirming the link between health and factors they had the power to change. In Figure 9-7, these and other events, projected into the 21st century, are plotted on a diffusion curve that follows the pattern of adoption of workplace health promotion activities by employers. The fourth generation remains to unfold fully in the years ahead.

Surveys have indicated progressive increases in the variety and number of health promotion programs offered in work sites from the mid-1970s to the mid-1990s.[102] A survey of work-site health education and health promotion programs

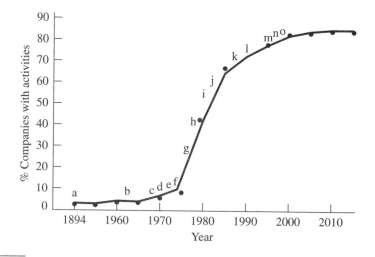

FIGURE 9-7

The diffusion curve shown here approximates the rate at which workplace health activities have spread, with the most recent acceleration resulting from the spread of health promotion. For details on the milestones, see Green & Cargo, 1994, p. 524.

sponsored by the U.S. Department of Health and Human Services in 1985 found that nearly two-thirds of all work sites with 50 or more employees had programs of some kind.[103] By 1992, this percentage had risen to 81%. Figure 9-8 compares the relative prevalence of the types of programs in 1985 and in 1992.

CAVEATS

Attention to the assessment steps of PRECEDE can help practitioners avoid two traps that could sidetrack program efforts or undermine their credibility. The first is associated with potential ethical problems, the second with the tendency to be too zealous with claims of cost containment.

ETHICAL CONCERNS

Problems may arise from (1) conflicting loyalties of health professionals, (2) focusing attention exclusively on changing the behavior of victims of work-site hazards rather than on the hazards themselves, (3) labeling and coercion of individuals, and (4) unintended consequences such as the compromising of medical

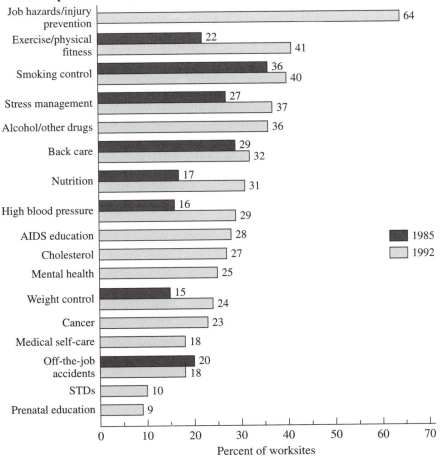

Health promotion information or activities offered by subject, 1985 and 1992

Percent of worksites

FIGURE 9-8

Percentage of work sites with 50 or more employees sponsoring each of seventeen types of health promotion information or service programs show the increase in most categories between the 1985 and 1992 surveys of private businesses in the United States.

SOURCE: *1992 National Survey of Worksite Health Promotion Activities: Summary Report,* by U.S. Department of Health and Human Services, 1993, Washington, DC: U.S. Government Printing Office.

care benefits and discrimination in hiring practices.[104] These issues point to the need for sensitivity to issues of worker participation in planning programs, justice, and privacy in the implementation of health-related programs. Attention and commitment to the principle of participation highlighted in Chapter 2 is of paramount importance in helping the practitioner recognize and effectively address these critical issues.

Perhaps no work-site health promotion issue is more sensitive than one that arises when attention to environmental problems in the workplace are ignored in favor of programs directed solely at individual responsibility for behavioral change among workers.[105] One of the greatest concerns expressed by labor groups has been the issue of "blaming the victim," particularly for people working under potentially health-threatening conditions such as exposure to chemicals. The victim-blaming trap applies equally to the neglect of environmental factors constraining or compelling behavior. For example, some stress management programs put the entire emphasis on personal coping strategies rather than on the management practices and environmental conditions that create stress.[106] The concern in both instances is that employers will use the concept of behavior change and worker responsibility for health as a smokescreen for hazards in the work environment.[107]

The health professional negotiating a work-site health promotion program must struggle with issues of allegiance or neutrality with respect to the positions of management and workers.[108] The ideal resolution is one that combines behavioral and environmental approaches to health promotion, with input from both management and workers.[109]

Through the systematic application of the Precede assessment steps, the practitioner in the work site can guard against these ethical concerns in at least two ways: (1) The social assessment can promote greater collaboration between employers and employees, assuring attention to the ultimate concerns of both. (2) The epidemiological, environmental, and behavioral assessments increase the likelihood that programs will include environmental reforms, balanced with appropriate behavioral strategies, to improve working conditions.

These assessments also help identify circumstances in which work-site hazards interact with worker behavior. As we have seen, some are synergistic in their effects, some have concomitant effects,[110] and others affect productivity and health concomitantly but independently.

Recognition of these interacting relationships between working conditions and health behavior will help health promotion planners justify the application of comprehensive approaches that provide for interventions that (1) help protect the worker against hazardous and stressful working conditions and (2) promote healthful practices such as exercise, nutritional eating, and self-examination for cancer signs or symptoms.

Employers and the white-collar workforce have responded well to the introduction and expansion of EAPs centered particularly on mental health, alcohol, and drug abuse[111] and to health promotion programs emphasizing stress management,[112] exercise facilities, and health education.[113] Blue-collar workers have shown less interest in these programs and facilities except where their introduction has been through a process of collective bargaining with attention paid to perceived problems in the work environment and in the health service benefits provided by the employer.

Caution: Do Not "Over-Sell" Economic Benefits. Earlier, the case was made that health promotion programs in the work site had considerable potential for containing the costs paid by employers for their employees' health care. While conventional wisdom may indicate that health promotion programs are good "investments" for employers, health economists and others caution practitioners to avoid exaggerating and thereby overselling the potential economic benefits to the employer's company or organization.[114]

The key to an appropriate and compelling social assessment, from the employer's perspective, is to calculate the cost per worker, or per 100 workers, of poor fitness or health outcomes and to relate these costs to the products or services central to the organization.

APPLICATION OF PRECEDE-PROCEED

PHASE 1: SOCIAL ASSESSMENT

In the work setting, as in other organizational settings, the social diagnosis and assessment of quality-of-life concerns or potential benefits to be obtained from a health promotion program produce quite different results when viewed from the distinct perspectives of workers and management.

From the Perspective of Employers. If quality of life is the bottom line for the public, then productivity or profit is the corresponding bottom line for the corporate world, where *bottom line* was coined. The term refers to the bottom of the accounting balance sheet or ledger where the assets and liabilities, or credits and debits, are totaled to get the net profit or loss, surplus or deficit. If you ask "Why?" after each reason a given employer offers for having a health promotion program for his or her employees, eventually the answer will be profit if it is a for-profit company, productivity in some other terms if a nonprofit. Certainly, employers want to have happier, healthier workers. Even so, if an employer invests in a program the only outcome of which is employee "happiness," there's a good chance that the employer won't be happy very long. The day that happier, healthier workers start missing days of work or failing to produce because they are happier or healthier is the day that employers will begin to dismantle their work-site health promotion programs. That is the bottom line.

Employers can use various criteria to set bottom-line priorities among optional programs in health promotion. Some of the most commonly used criteria are listed in Table 9-1. These reflect the orientation of employers not to health as

TABLE 9-1

Criteria used by employers in setting health promotion priorities

- Direct measures of productivity (cost-benefit analysis)
- Prior demonstration of benefits in comparable sites
- Time frame for the realization of benefits (discounting)
- Relevance of the program to health costs and risks in the company, taking the benefits package into consideration
- Employee interest in the program as an indication that having the program will help retain and recruit good employees
- Possible negative effects of the program, such as time away from work, injuries, and liability of the employer

an end in itself but to other ultimate concerns as motives to provide health promotion programs for their employees.

Two criteria, epidemiological importance and the demonstrated effectiveness of interventions, were used by the Public Health Service to establish national priorities in health promotion. These included (1) reduction of smoking, (2) reduction of alcohol and drug misuse, (3) diet and nutrition, (4) physical fitness and exercise, and (5) stress and violence control. When employers consider their own needs, resources, and potential benefits, different priorities tend to be established. For example, when immediate costs from poor employee morale, absenteeism, low productivity, and injuries are considered, alcohol abuse will be seen as the most important social problem to be addressed in the work site. Stress management and other mental health concerns might also seem paramount. If company image matters the most to management, then exercise facilities and community-oriented activities might receive highest priority.[115]

Companies have been most concerned in recent years about the increases in cost associated with their health care coverage of employees, as reflected in premium rates on group insurance, and in benefits paid on medical claims. As in most other settings, health is not an end in itself in the work site. Health is a resource that enables workers to perform more productively; it holds instrumental rather than terminal value. The social assessment, then, is something of a misnomer in the work setting as far as the employer is concerned. In its place, one would begin the Precede analysis with an assessment of the "bottom-line" concerns of productivity and profitability such as absenteeism, medical claims, sick days, worker's compensation claims, security problems, and injuries and property damage caused by smokers or by alcohol- or drug-abusing employees. Other health-related concerns affecting productivity include health insurance premiums higher than average because of poor experience rating, turnover rates requiring more frequent hiring and training, and early retirement rates. Relatively direct productivity measures (output per worker) are compared with competing companies who may or may not have health promotion programs.

These would be analyzed in Phase 1 not as indicators of the health or morbidity of the organization but as meaningful consequences of employee morbidity. They are meaningful to the employer because they cost money, time, or productivity, any of which reduces the profit margin. They add to the cost of doing business or maintaining the workforce. These costs must be passed on to the consumer or be subtracted from the services rendered or the profit taken. The first makes the company's product or service uncompetitive; the second makes it unattractive to owners or stockholders. In the end, an unhealthy workforce can make an organization untenable.

From the Perspective of Employees. The workers' perspective on quality-of-life concerns makes the social assessment for their purposes no different than for community programs. If the employers have the final say and they control the resources that will support a program in the work site, why would one bother with a social assessment of the workers? How do their social needs or their perspective matter? A community assessment carried out prior to the work-site program could serve as the social assessment from the workers' perspective, making another assessment of their quality-of-life concerns within the work site redundant. It might suffice to concentrate the social assessment of the concerns of employers, previously outlined.

A unionized shop or a highly participatory management structure in a given organization, however, makes an assessment of employee perspectives essential. Unions have opposed some behaviorally oriented health promotion programs because they saw them either as smokescreens to divert attention from environmental problems in the work site or as substitutes for other benefits in the collective bargaining package. Knowing what matters most to the workers can help a health promotion program adequately address environmental issues and appropriate other benefits. It can also serve to establish appropriate objectives and evaluation criteria for whatever programs are eventually offered. Finally, it can provide a baseline against which later concerns can be compared when the programs are evaluated.

PHASE 2: EPIDEMIOLOGICAL ASSESSMENT

While occupational health has traditionally dealt with hazards of the workplace separate from general health, the more recent movement toward integrating health promotion and occupational health has been directed toward the advancement of health to the optimal level to improve quality of life and performance. *Work-related diseases* are those that the work environment entirely or partially causes. This definition includes health problems that may be aggravated by work conditions, thus expanding the concept of occupational health to include conditions such as high blood pressure, cardiovascular disease, ulcers, and a variety of psychological problems. Epidemiological assessment is best carried out in conjunction with the behavioral and environmental assessments to include the health factors influencing the social problem (descriptive epidemiology) as well as the behavioral and environmental causes of the priority health problems (etiological epidemiology).

Table 9-2 lists the 10 leading work-related diseases identified by the National Institute of Occupational Safety and Health as the most frequent, the most severe, and of the highest priority. Both environmental and behavioral factors influence the work-related diseases and injuries cited in this table.

PHASE 3: BEHAVIORAL AND ENVIRONMENTAL ASSESSMENT

Examples of worker behavior and workplace environmental factors influencing occupational cancer are shown in Figure 9-9. Program personnel representing five labor unions identified these factors. They participated in developing interventions designed to reduce the incidence of cancer for workers at high risk of cancer because of occupational exposure.[116]

Once one has established the health problems of greatest importance (to employers and workers) in the given work site and the determinants of those health problems, the third phase of the Precede planning process is the further specification of the behavioral and environmental factors and assessment of their relative changeability. Using data on their importance (from the epidemiological

---

TABLE 9-2

The 10 leading work-related diseases and injuries identified by NIOSH for the United States

1. Occupational lung disorders
2. Musculoskeletal disorders
3. Occupational cancer
4. Fractures, amputations, traumatic deaths
5. Cardiovascular disease
6. Reproductive problems
7. Neurotoxic illness
8. Noise-induced hearing loss
9. Dermatological problems
10. Psychological disorders

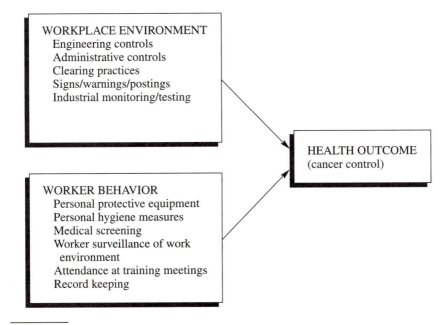

FIGURE 9-9

Behavioral and environmental assessments of cancer risks in five industries in collaboration with Painters Union representatives produced this set of relationships.

SOURCE: Consultation report to Painters Union, by C. Y. Lovato and L. W. Green, 1986.

assessment), one can rate each of the behavioral and environmental factors on importance. Among those found to be most important, some will be more amenable to change than others. Some will be related to each other, which will make change in one affect change in another. One can use these ratings and relationships to set priorities on the behavioral and environmental factors deserving primary attention in the next phase.

The number of complex factors contributing to a given health indicator usually exceeds the program resources available. It is inevitable, therefore, that some behavioral or environmental factors will receive a low priority. However, by narrowing the focus of the program at this stage of analysis and assessment of needs, one saves considerable effort in each of the subsequent steps in planning. Failing to rule out less important objectives or targets of change at this phase will mean wasteful analysis of their determinants in the next two phases, only to discover in the final phase of planning that one has insufficient resources to provide for these low-priority needs.

Because environmental factors in the work site are so much more immediate and contained than in the larger community, they deserve special attention as candidates for change in work-site health promotion planning. They also represent the factors most likely to convince workers that the commitment of the program to meaningful change is sincere. Some workers, especially those who perceive themselves at risk of environmental assaults on their health and well-being in the work site, are more likely to support and participate in the program if they see some significant attention to environmental concerns.

It seldom happens that a set of important health problems in the work site can be attributed singularly to environmental or to behavioral causes. The choice is seldom between the two; rather, it usually lies among the numerous candidates competing for attention in both the behavioral and environmental categories. DeJoy has developed an adaptation of the Precede-Proceed model that attempts to combine the occupational hygienic, ergonomical, and organizational factors and health promotion aspects of worker safety in a "comprehensive human factors model of workplace accident causation."[117]

An epidemiological assessment of the problems of sick leave, absenteeism, and accident rates in San Francisco bus drivers found hypertension, musculo-skeletal system problems, and gastrointestinal problems at excess levels in this population of workers.[118] A traditional medical approach to this assessment might have emphasized drug treatment for the hypertension, patient education on posture for the back pain, and diet for the gastrointestinal problems. By simultaneously examining the potential behavioral and environmental determinants, planners found unreasonable work schedules for the bus drivers, in combination with long shifts and social isolation. A related coping behavior was the tendency for the drivers to remain at the bus yard for several hours after their shift to "wind down" before going home. This resulted in limited time with family and friends at home, which might account for some of the hostile and impatient behavior observed in the drivers. This narrowed the focus of the behavioral and environmental assessment of coping behavior of drivers and scheduling conditions of the work site. The planners also provided for rest stops located in or near central city areas. This example, as shown in Figure 9-10, illustrates the interactions of environmental and behavioral factors that need to be examined in this phase of assessment.

The final step in these two phases of PRECEDE is to set objectives for each of these outcomes. These objectives might have to be long-range goals that will be unmeasurable or unachievable within the first year or more of the program. For example, the objective of a cancer control program designed by the Workers Institute for Safety and Health specified the following goal: to reduce the mortality of workers exposed to the bladder carcinogens used in the manufacture of textile dyes. Impossible to measure directly in the short term, mortality reductions would be inferred (projected statistically) from the increase in lead time for treatment, resulting from the program's success in reducing delay in workers' seeking diagnosis after their symptoms first appeared. Reduced mortality could also be projected from earlier treatment resulting from the program's early detection of cancer symptoms from screening.[119]

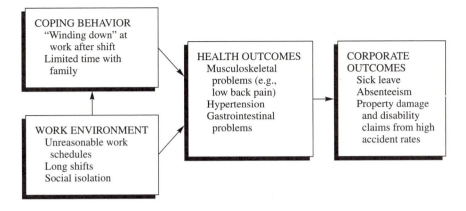

FIGURE 9-10

Behavioral and environmental assessment of work-site conditions related to health outcomes and corporate outcomes in the Municipal Transit Authority of San Francisco.

SOURCE: Based on "Strategies for Health Promotion," by L. W. Syme, 1986, *Preventive Medicine, 15,* 492–507. Reprinted with permission.

Objectives should be stated in quantitative terms so that a clear vision of the program's contribution to the organization's "bottom line" can be brought out any time the program seems to be losing its way or its support. These objectives should state how much of what health or fitness measure (e.g., a 20% reduction of medical claims for lower back pain) might be expected in which employees (e.g., in mail room workers) by when (in the second year of the program).[120]

The objectives for each of the behavioral and environmental targets of change should state how much of what factors are expected to change by when. The changes in behavior may be expressed in the behavioral objectives as percentages of employees in a given category of the workforce (e.g., an increase of 40% of mail room workers) who will adopt a new behavior or abandon a negative health practice (e.g., practicing proper lifting techniques) by when (e.g., between the first week and the twelfth week of the program).

The environmental objectives might be stated in terms of the actual installation of a new facility. For example, "Waist-high conveyor belts will be installed in the mail room next to each work station by the twelfth week of the program." Environmental objectives would often reflect the removal of an environmental hazard: "All floor level bins for mail bags will be replaced with conveyor belts."

If the objective is to be used as the program's criterion of success, one might want to specify the measurement procedure as part of the objective or as an operational definition of the behavior. For the behavioral objective in the foregoing example, this might be "as measured by an observer during a randomly selected one-hour work period each day for one week." For the environmental objectives, this might refer to a specific regulatory code or occupational health and safety standard (e.g., "in accordance with Section 1601 of the State Safety Code"), which also often provides for the inspection procedure. Alternately, it might refer the terms of a contract or the contractor to be hired for the installation or removal of the facility or hazard (e.g., "as specified in contract number AB21" or "as specified in the standard contract of company XYZ"). In the absence of codes and standards or documented specifications, the objective might need to specify the size, shape, or type of materials to be installed or removed (e.g., "constructed with ball-bearing rollers").

PHASE 4: EDUCATIONAL AND ECOLOGICAL ASSESSMENT

The task in Phase 4 is to assess the relative importance and changeability of the factors predisposing, enabling, and reinforcing the selected behavioral and environmental targets for the work-site program. These determinants of change in each of the behavioral and environmental objectives will become the immediate targets of the interventions. In a cancer-screening project for workers exposed to carcinogens, the predisposing factors determining change were identified as knowledge and awareness of the risk of bladder cancer and the advantages of early detection. Enabling factors concentrated on the development of skill in detecting symptoms and on providing cancer screening. Reinforcing factors concentrated on building social support networks through the community, co-workers, and the family.

The educational and ecological assessment is where one brings to bear most cogently the appropriate behavioral science, social, or political science and economic theories of change. Selecting which determinants might be influencing the behavioral or environmental targets is, once again, an exercise in narrowing the field from an enormous number of possible factors to a more manageable number of important and realistic targets for change.

For example, for a complex lifestyle objective such as increasing exercise or changing dietary practices to reduce fat intake, there would be dozens of component behaviors and, for each of those, dozens of possible predisposing, enabling, and reinforcing factors. The more complex the behavior, the more component parts or manifestations the behavior will have. Each component must be analyzed in Phase 4, so this phase will become too complex to be practicable unless Phase 3 has been rigorous in its priority-setting step. Critical professional judgment should eliminate the least important and least changeable behaviors from further analysis. Similarly, the environmental factors identified in Phase 3 can become too complex to analyze in Phase 4 if they have not been sufficiently delineated and reduced to the most important few deserving highest priority.

Here also, the time perspective of the previously developed objectives will dictate the pace at which change in the determinants must occur to meet the behavioral and environmental objectives. The degree of urgency, in turn, will dictate some of the selection of processes of change. To a population asked to make changes in its behavior, educational processes are slower but often more acceptable than are regulatory processes. Rules and regulations promulgated from management when the workers have not yet learned the need for the rules and have not been involved in the process of their formulation sometimes results in a backlash that offsets any gain in efficiency.[121]

The trade-offs between expediency and durability of change apply not only to the choice of emphasis between predisposing factors and enabling factors; within educational or behavioral approaches, they also apply to the "internal" (cognitive) predisposing factors and "external" reinforcing factors.[122] For example, the mobilization of incentives and rewards for behavioral change among employees through bonuses and competitions might stimulate immediate participation and change.[123] Without attendant changes in knowledge, beliefs, and attitudes, however, the behavioral changes will tend to relapse after the incentives and external rewards have stopped.

The point is that a balanced approach including both learning processes and environmental change processes is almost always advisable to ensure lasting results and changes that are both acceptable and efficient. Acceptability comes with learning and associating the proposed change with values; efficiency comes with structural or organizational facilitation and resources for change. In Phase 4, therefore, one needs to assess the predisposing and reinforcing and enabling factors determining *each* of the behavioral and environmental targets or objectives given high priority in Phase 3.

Predisposing Factors. Assessing level of commitment, then, is the first order of business in Phase 4. This predisposing factor represents the base on which all other determinants may have their effect. If the employer and worker populations have a high level of commitment or motivation for the behavioral or environmental changes identified in Phase 3, then less effort will be needed on enabling and reinforcing factors. If motivation is low, then little will happen with respect to behavioral change, no matter how much emphasis is placed on enabling and reinforcing factors. Motivation or level of commitment must be high enough to ensure participation in the program.

Studies of employee participation in work-site programs indicate that the predisposing factors with the highest correlations are (1) interest in health and (2) knowledge of the benefits of the recommended behavior.[124] Continued participation in weight control, smoking-cessation, alcohol abuse, and physical activity programs also appears to be predicted by self-efficacy.[125] High levels of perceived job stress also predict participation in exercise, weight control, and stress management programs.[126] Work stress, however, may be negatively correlated with participation in a smoking-cessation program but positively correlated with assertiveness in asking smoking co-workers not to smoke. These effects of work stress may cancel each other out.[127]

"Loss of interest or motivation" is the most frequently cited reason for dropping out of a work-site exercise program.[128] This suggests that the predisposing factors might need to be reassessed periodically to determine changes in attitudes, beliefs, or perceptions that need to be corrected to sustain the level of participation required to achieve the behavioral or environmental objectives. This brings one to the analysis of reinforcing factors, which might be thought of as boosters to reactivate fading predisposing factors.

Reinforcing Factors. Motivation is a necessary but not sufficient determinant of participation. Some of the most highly motivated workers will not continue to participate in a work-site health promotion program if they are bucking a supervisor who frowns on it or other workers who think it is silly or that it means more work for them. These social forces rewarding or punishing the proposed behavior are crucial determinants, assessed in Phase 4.

Research indicates that participant satisfaction plays a major role in continued employee participation. Satisfaction increases when employees are involved actively in planning the program.[129] Employees tend to be more satisfied with programs in which health care or health promotion personnel show warmth and personal concern in their interactions.[130] Amount of contact time and number of contacts with health care providers have been shown to relate to higher satisfaction and blood pressure control.[131]

Overall "organizational climate" has been cited frequently as a key factor in reinforcing worker participation and in ensuring supervisory support for worker participation as well.[132] Senior managers' attitudes and worker perception of their attitudes toward the program set up organizational norms encouraging participation and providing role models for behavioral change. But management-driven norms can also preclude the discussion among workers that leads to stronger self-enforcement of norms and a "subtle change in the frequency and nature of workplace interactions that may no longer discourage employee smoking," for example.[133]

Confidentiality is an important reinforcing factor for some behavioral and environmental objectives. Participation in a screening program, for example, will be quickly discouraged if workers learn that information about their health condition or family history is shared with employers, insurers, or others.[134] Recall the ethical issues of confidentiality, addressed earlier in this chapter.

Boredom with a repetitive routine discourages continued participation for some, though others may find a mindless routine comforting or liberating from work stress. Fun and variety in the health promotion program activities can reinforce participation and hold the interest of some, which might account in part for the popularity of group aerobic exercise classes and work-site competitions in weight control and other areas.[135] Incentives related to competitions or in combination with other components of a program have been found helpful in maintaining higher abstinence from smoking for 6 months.[136] Caution must be exercised, however, not to substitute token rewards for the internalization of values and beliefs necessary to sustain real behavior change over time. Token reinforcements may only yield token behavior, or deceptive claims of behavior change.[137]

Enabling Factors. Accessibility and convenience are the key enabling factors to be assessed in Phase 4. Proximity of the program to workstations, convenience of scheduling, and cost determine program accessibility; lack of access represents the largest barrier to program participation.[138] Enabling factors for environment change in the work site include cost of the environmental modifications, disruption of the flow or pace of work, and availability of space for new facilities or equipment.

An application of the Precede model analyzing the injury prevention behavior of construction workers appears in Figure 9-11, illustrating the range of factors considered in Phase 4.[139]

PHASE 5: ADMINISTRATIVE AND POLICY ASSESSMENT

Having now identified the key determinants of the behavioral and environmental objectives, one must assess the resources that could influence these determinants, as well as assess organizational or regulatory policies that will facilitate or hinder the implementation of the program. The first resource of concern is time. Release time for worker participation in health programs of any kind can be a source of considerable controversy. It adds to the cost of the program the hours of work time lost for participants. The usual solution is flexible schedules that allow workers to participate within their workshift but to make up the time during another shift.[140]

Second among resource concerns for most work-site health promotion programs is space. The main purpose of the company or organization hosting the program is not employee health but rather some other product or service production; thus, devoting space to health promotion cannot be done lightly.

Policies to support or protect employee health and health behavior have become the most hotly debated subject in work-site health promotion literature in recent years. Work-site smoking policies have been tried and evaluated in several countries with varying success.[141] Employee Assistance Programs raise similar policy issues of cost-effectiveness, ethics, employee acceptance, and civil rights.[142]

Policy, resources, and organizational support for health promotion programs in the work site relate most directly to company profit or worker productivity issues. To understand managerial attitudes toward offering new policies, programs, or facilities, one must review a company's experiences with worker

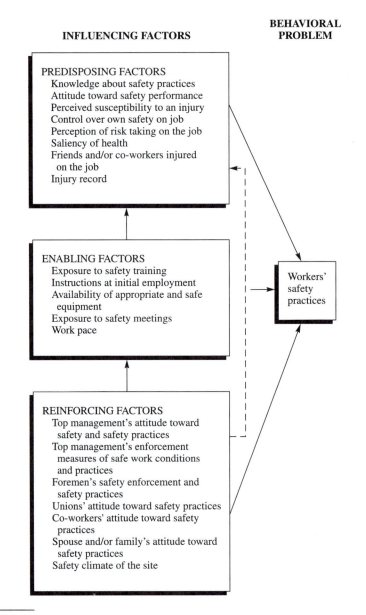

INFLUENCING FACTORS

**BEHAVIORAL
PROBLEM**

PREDISPOSING FACTORS
  Knowledge about safety practices
  Attitude toward safety performance
  Perceived susceptibility to an injury
  Control over own safety on job
  Perception of risk taking on the job
  Saliency of health
  Friends and/or co-workers injured
    on the job
  Injury record

ENABLING FACTORS
  Exposure to safety training
  Instructions at initial employment
  Availability of appropriate and safe
    equipment
  Exposure to safety meetings
  Work pace

Workers'
safety
practices

REINFORCING FACTORS
  Top management's attitude toward
    safety and safety practices
  Top management's enforcement
    measures of safe work conditions
    and practices
  Foremen's safety enforcement and
    safety practices
  Unions' attitude toward safety practices
  Co-workers' attitude toward safety
    practices
  Spouse and/or family's attitude toward
    safety practices
  Safety climate of the site

FIGURE 9-11

Predisposing, enabling, and reinforcing factors in the educational assessment of construction workers' safety practices.

SOURCE: "Safety Practices in Construction Industry," by N. Dedobbeleer & P. German, 1987, *Journal
of Occupational Medicine, 29,* 863–868. Reprinted with permission.

participation, satisfaction, and job performance in previous efforts to offer health promotion programs and so forth. Management behavior is predisposed, enabled, and reinforced just as much as everyone else's behavior. This point should lead the health promotion planner to consider applying the Precede steps to an analysis of employer behavior or to the collective bargaining behavior of workers if the obstacle to starting a program for employees lies in the motivation of management.[143]

PHASES 6–8: IMPLEMENTATION AND EVALUATION

The circumstances and politics of each work site differ, and within each work site these will change over time. No amount of planning and policy development can anticipate each new employee's and each new day's special circumstances. Implementation must therefore adapt plans and policies to changing circumstances. The organization of advisory groups during the implementation phases should help the program stay on track regarding sensitivity to managers' and workers' concerns. The provision for continuous feedback through supervisory lines of communication and anonymous suggestion boxes and questionnaires can help.

Based on experience in setting up and implementing a series of work-site health promotion programs in Lycoming County, a rural area of Pennsylvania, the County Health Improvement Program (CHIP) staff recommend the following steps in establishing and implementing programs in work sites:

1. Introduction of the program to management
2. Announcement of program to the employees
3. Recruitment and organization of a worker-management committee
4. In-house communication planning
5. Employee interest and risk-factor surveys
6. Formation of subcommittees for each risk factor
7. Exploration of community risk-factor reduction programs
8. Committee review and program selection
9. Development of a program proposal
10. Discussion of the proposal with management
11. Promotion of programs and recruitment of employees
12. Scheduling of programs
13. Program implementation-evaluation-modification-maintenance[144]

The details of these steps will vary depending on the setting, but the logic of the implementation process described in previous chapters here display their own character in the work site. The final phases of implementation-evaluation-modification-maintenance obviously represents a series of steps. They essentially recycle through the previous steps, beginning usually at Step 5 for evaluation, and possibly as early as Step 1 for program modification if the changes required are so sweeping as to require renegotiation with management. Surveys and data collection would have been done at the earliest planning stages, for purposes of assessing employee and employer perceptions of needs, or at the stage of setting objectives, when survey data were needed to establish baselines for later evaluation. Data collection might not have been possible until the evaluation phase. Whenever they might be conducted, surveys of employees follow a series of steps that can be planned and phased as suggested by Figure 9-12.

The major challenge of resource allocation arises in the implementation phase when demand exceeds resources. Sometimes this is a problem of numbers, sometimes a problem of variable needs of different types of employees. One can consider three approaches for rationing and allocating scarce program resources during the implementation phase:

- Screening or wait-listing employees on the basis of a procedure or set of criteria agreed on in the planning
- Providing self-help materials and referrals to community resources, with or without subsidies or release time
- A systematic triage and stepped program of interventions based on individualized needs assessments and tailored interventions

Screening and Wait-Listing. The most common method of rationing health promotion resources in the work site is simply limiting the eligibility. Historically, work-site health promotion programs were known as executive fitness programs, or executive health examination programs, with the obvious implication of their unavailability to many workers. Some programs screen at the other end of the hierarchy, restricting access to those with the highest risk, greatest exposure to workplace hazards, or greatest need for company subsidy or support. The use of health-risk appraisals and other screening tests to select the target groups for recruitment or admission to the program has a time-honored tradition in public health.[145]

One screening test particularly relevant to a program's effectiveness concerns level of motivation. Many workers will take up space in health promotion programs without much commitment to follow through with the behavioral change recommendations. The requirement that applicants keep a diary of their behavior for a week before starting the program has served as an effective screen in some programs.[146]

Self-Care and Community Referrals. Much of what a company can offer through personnel and facilities provided at the work site could be obtained through other organizations in the community, either in the form of self-help materials or in classes and facilities. The advantages of access and convenience at the work site are obvious, and the advantages of group support among employees can be argued. But self-help materials have a good track record for the motivated.[147]

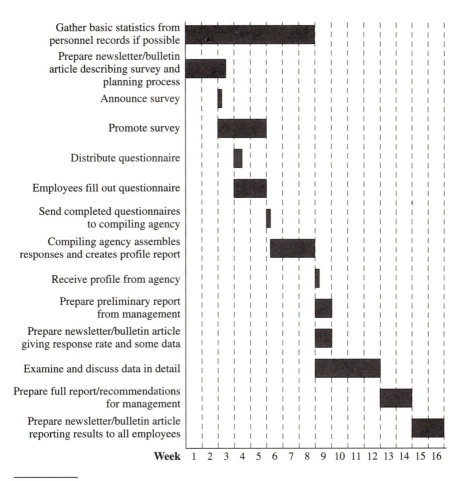

Gather basic statistics from personnel records if possible	
Prepare newsletter/bulletin article describing survey and planning process	
Announce survey	
Promote survey	
Distribute questionnaire	
Employees fill out questionnaire	
Send completed questionnaires to compiling agency	
Compiling agency assembles responses and creates profile report	
Receive profile from agency	
Prepare preliminary report from management	
Prepare newsletter/bulletin article giving response rate and some data	
Examine and discuss data in detail	
Prepare full report/recommendations for management	
Prepare newsletter/bulletin article reporting results to all employees	

Week 1 2 3 4 5 6 7 8 9 10 11 12 13 14 15 16

FIGURE 9-12

This sample Gantt chart from Health Canada suggests a series of overlapping steps in conducting a survey of employees for purposes of planning or evaluating a work-site program.
SOURCE: *Workplace Health: Discovering the Needs,* 1990, Ottawa: Health and Welfare Canada.

Subsidy of worker participation in outside programs through direct contract with the vendor or agency, through payment to the worker, or at least through release time to participate can lend credence and effectiveness to the referral process.

Triage and Stepped Program of Interventions. This third approach requires a more systematic process of assessing the needs of each employee, applicant, or participant in a program of interventions to determine which combination of interventions might be most needed and effective in achieving the program goals or

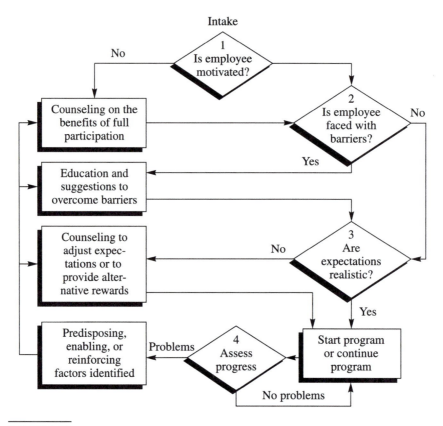

FIGURE 9-13

This algorithm follows the Precede model for the purpose of assessing potential problems of employees in initiating and maintaining a behavioral change and allocating them to actions that conserve the resources of the program for those who need specific interventions.

SOURCE: "Maintaining Employee Participation in Workplace Health Promotion Programs," by C. Y. Lovato and L. W. Green, 1990, *Health Education Quarterly, 17,* 73–88. Reprinted with permission of the publisher.

that person's goals. The Precede model can be applied in this process, especially in the educational assessment stage. Figure 9-13 offers an algorithm (flowchart) for the **triage** and **stepped approach** to assessing predisposing, enabling, and reinforcing factors in sequence and intervening to strengthen those needing more attention.[148]

Evaluation can be accomplished through program records to measure implementation and process variables, through self-tests, questionnaires, and self-monitoring reports to measure impact, and through company medical or insur-

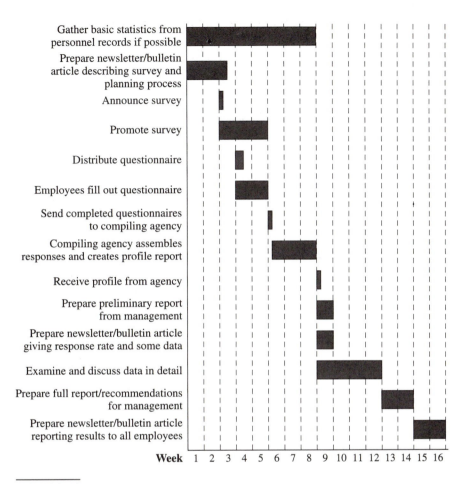

FIGURE 9-12

This sample Gantt chart from Health Canada suggests a series of overlapping steps in conducting a survey of employees for purposes of planning or evaluating a work-site program.

SOURCE: *Workplace Health: Discovering the Needs,* 1990, Ottawa: Health and Welfare Canada.

Subsidy of worker participation in outside programs through direct contract with the vendor or agency, through payment to the worker, or at least through release time to participate can lend credence and effectiveness to the referral process.

Triage and Stepped Program of Interventions. This third approach requires a more systematic process of assessing the needs of each employee, applicant, or participant in a program of interventions to determine which combination of interventions might be most needed and effective in achieving the program goals or

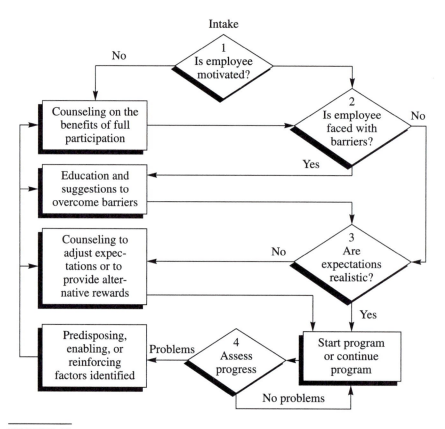

FIGURE 9-13

This algorithm follows the Precede model for the purpose of assessing potential problems of employees in initiating and maintaining a behavioral change and allocating them to actions that conserve the resources of the program for those who need specific interventions.

SOURCE: "Maintaining Employee Participation in Workplace Health Promotion Programs," by C. Y. Lovato and L. W. Green, 1990, *Health Education Quarterly, 17,* 73–88. Reprinted with permission of the publisher.

that person's goals. The Precede model can be applied in this process, especially in the educational assessment stage. Figure 9-13 offers an algorithm (flowchart) for the **triage** and **stepped approach** to assessing predisposing, enabling, and reinforcing factors in sequence and intervening to strengthen those needing more attention.[148]

Evaluation can be accomplished through program records to measure implementation and process variables, through self-tests, questionnaires, and self-monitoring reports to measure impact, and through company medical or insurance records to measure health outcomes. Absenteeism, productivity, and other company bottom-line concerns can be assessed as described in the evaluation literature cited earlier in this chapter and in Chapter 7.

A CASE STUDY: AIR QUALITY CONTROL IN A STATE AGENCY

This case[149] will illustrate issues concerning the planning process and the policy implementation and evaluation process in the work site.

SOCIAL AND EPIDEMIOLOGICAL ASSESSMENT

A large state human services agency employs about 14,000 people and has its headquarters in the state capital, with field offices organized into 10 regions. Recently, in one of the regions, 1,500 employees moved into a newly constructed facility. Shortly thereafter, employees began to experience respiratory problems and allergic reactions; they associated these reactions with the recent move. They expressed their concern about these new events and the quality of air in the environment to the building committee, who conducted an investigation of the building's ventilation system. The committee determined that, other than systematic vigorous cleaning, little could be done to improve the turnover rate of air, or the rate of replacing used with fresh air. This finding, coupled with the voice of employees who wished the new building to be smoke-free, led to a concentrated approach to improve the air quality through reducing the ambient smoke and other pollutants in the environment and encouraging employees who smoked to stop.

BEHAVIORAL AND ENVIRONMENTAL ASSESSMENT

As seen from this description, movement from the social to the behavioral and environmental assessment was as much a political process as one of professional planning. The agenda for the building committee was set by employee concerns, and no systematic effort was made to set priorities among quality-of-life concerns or health problems. The decision to change behavior and the environment through a policy reform restricting smoking was a foregone conclusion.

EDUCATIONAL AND ECOLOGICAL ASSESSMENT

The building committee, which extended its membership to include both smokers and non-smokers, did engage in an assessment process to determine its strategies for addressing the environmental issue. It forwarded responsibility for designing the smoking-cessation programs to the wellness committee, and it assessed the options for environmental and behavioral change as follows:

A. The Environment. Figure 9-14 illustrates the determinants of environmental air quality. The importance and changeability of each of the enabling factors was considered as follows:

Enabling Factors	Importance	Changeability
■ Ventilation system improvements to increase air exchange rate	++	− −
■ Cleaning ventilation system	+	++
■ Portable smoke-eaters	−	++
■ Restrictive smoking policy	++	+/−

Based on this organizational and engineering analysis, developers decided to make cleaning of the ventilation system a high priority and to reduce ambient smoke in the building by recommending that a restrictive smoking policy be established.

B. Behavior/Lifestyle. The wellness committee decided to conduct smoking-cessation programs for smoking employees in the new headquarters building. These programs were also offered to employees in some of the regional offices as part of an evaluation research project. When the executive decision was made to adopt a restrictive smoking policy, the policy was applied statewide, so smoking-cessation programs were offered statewide.

An educational and organizational assessment was conducted to help design these programs. Table 9-3 displays predisposing, reinforcing, and enabling factors for stopping smoking. This analysis flows from a behavioral perspective.

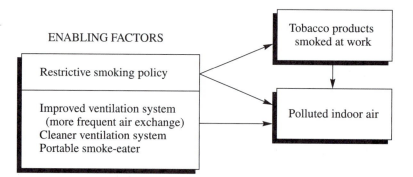

FIGURE 9-14

Enabling factors influencing air quality in an office building with central heating and air conditioning.

TABLE 9-3

Educational and organizational assessment of predisposing, reinforcing, and enabling factors related to smoking cessation

PREDISPOSING FACTORS

    Attitudes, beliefs, and values concerning the positive aspects of smoking:

        Increases concentration

        Decreases tension

        Provides a high

        Controls my weight

        Helps me fit in

    Attitudes, beliefs, and values concerning the negative aspects of smoking:

        Keeps me from fitting in

        Increases my health risk

        Increases the health risks of others

        Is not compatible with my value of health

        Costs a lot

        Makes my clothes and hair smell

        Is messy

    Belief in self-efficacy for quitting

    Habit strength: number of years smoked

    Previous cessation attempts: experience with quitting

REINFORCING FACTORS

    Social encouragement to quit and remain abstinent

        Co-worker

        Family

        Cessation group "buddy"

    Material incentives

        Financial rewards for quitting

    Restrictive policy violations

ENABLING FACTORS

    Skills for quitting

    Restrictive smoking policy

The predisposing factors are drawn primarily from the perspective of social learning theory and the Health Belief Model. They include the individuals' expectations for the positive and negative results of smoking, their self-efficacy for quitting, their intentions to quit, and their health beliefs regarding their susceptibility to and the seriousness of smoking-related diseases. Measures of an individual's smoking history—smoking frequency and duration (habit strength) and number and duration of cessation attempts—are also predisposing factors shown to predict success in quitting. The predisposing factors vary across individuals and are useful (1) in designing interventions directed to getting persons to decide to quit smoking and (2) in tailoring cessation programs to the target population.

Although the cognitive factors include a motivational component of desired outcomes from quitting, social and material incentives provide an important source of reinforcement for quitting. In addition, the restrictive policy brings negative reinforcement and punishment into play. Individuals will avoid penalties by not smoking in restricted areas, and smoking in these areas will lead to punishment. Expectation of these reinforcements is a strong source of motivation.

The possession of behavioral skills, including self-contracting, goal setting, monitoring of cigarettes, identification and management of environmental cues to smoke, self-reinforcement, and techniques for coping with urges to smoke are crucial to the individual's following through on the decision to quit. The worksite setting makes it possible to move beyond individual management of environmental cues. To reduce triggering of the smoking impulse, cues for smoking are removed from areas in which policy restricts smoking. In this way, the policy restraint on one smoker becomes a support to another smoker trying to quit.

FROM ADMINISTRATIVE AND POLICY ASSESSMENT TO IMPLEMENTATION

In our example, a smoking cessation program was devised based on the educational and organizational assessment and the resources available in the budget and in the work site. *Freedom from Smoking in Twenty Days,* a low-cost self-help program, was chosen to provide information and exercises designed to influence the predisposing factors (e.g., those identified by questions such as "Why do you smoke?" and "Why do you want to quit?") and the specific skills listed earlier as enabling factors.[150] The self-help manual includes forms for logging smoking patterns and analyzing cues or triggers for smoking, for making self-contracts, and for planning how one will cope with urges to smoke. With encouragement from the manual, smokers could select a "buddy" and find advice in the manual on how to make the most of this supportive relationship.

Additional reinforcement was mobilized at the organizational level, using two campaigns. The first was a competition between two work sites.[151] The work site with the highest proportion of smokers recruited to the program and of nonsmokers becoming "supporters" won a cold-turkey buffet the day after the Great American Smoke-Out, which is sponsored by the American Cancer Society. This mobilized social reinforcement for recruitment. A second campaign conducted later, *Winning Choices,* provided chances to win savings bonds to smokers who joined the cessation programs.[152]

The new policy restricting smoking served as an enabling factor for both the behavioral objective of smoking cessation and the environmental objective of cleaner air. As part of its work in advising the agency head on how to improve air quality, the building committee carried out a survey of employees to assess opinions on whether a more restrictive policy was needed. This survey (box C in Figure 9-15) followed the employee surveys (A and B) that had provided assessments of predisposing, enabling and reinforcing factors.

The committee also sponsored a roundtable on the smoking issue, a discussion open to all employees at the state headquarters. Based on its findings, the committee recommended that a restrictive smoking policy be adopted. The committee, however, played only an advisory role. There was concern that top administration would not act on the recommendation. A proposed Clean Air Act, which would have required smoking policies in all work sites across the state, did not pass in the state legislature that year.

At this point, an internal champion for the proposed policy emerged. A newly appointed high-level manager, who had successfully established a similar smoking policy at another agency, became an advocate for the recommended policy. The executive decision-making group developed a restrictive smoking policy for the entire agency, not just the state office.

Policy development and implementation always depend on context.[153] Two of the few generalizable principles are (1) supervisors who must implement and employees who will be affected by policy should participate in the formulation of the policy and (2) the policy should be flexible enough to cover a variety of contingencies.

A draft policy was published in the statewide employee newsletter, which invited comments. Experience in smoking policy development and implementation suggests that the mere opportunity to comment, even if employees do not avail themselves of the opportunity, goes a long way toward greater acceptance of a new policy. Sent to all employees 4 months before implementation, the final policy called for smoking to be restricted in each building, except in break rooms

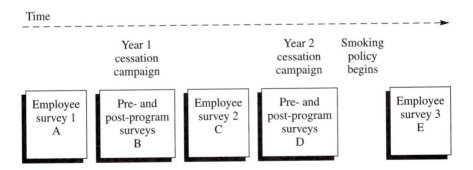

FIGURE 9-15

Quantitative data collection points in the assessment and evaluation phases of developing an educational and environmental approach to air quality in a state office building.

designated by the regional administrator. Employee meetings held at each site generated advice for the regional administrator on the preferred site of the designated break room. Had this state agency been unionized, representation of the union would have been crucial to the development and implementation of the policy.

Figure 9-16 provides an overview of key factors in policy development and implementation. The success of a smoking policy will depend on its concept or content and the process of its development (first box), on how it fits into the context of implementation (second box), and on its implementation process (third box). The careful planner will provide for employee ownership of the program through participation in its formulation and implementation. Anticipating variations in work sites helps build the necessary flexibility into the policy.

The more thorough cleaning of the ventilation system, the second environmental reform, was more easily implemented. A simple regulatory directive from the agency head to the maintenance supervisor accomplished this. Biweekly vacuuming of external vents and monthly inspections were incorporated into the job routine of maintenance personnel.

IMPLEMENTATION AND STRUCTURAL EVALUATION

The implementation and structural evaluation of the new smoking regulations was planned using the flowchart in Figure 9-15 and the model in Figure 9-16. Both qualitative and quantitative methods were used. The process of policy development was documented using internal records such as newsletter articles, memoranda, minutes of committee meetings, and interviews. A survey of a random sample of employees following policy implementation ascertained their level of involvement in policy formulation and implementation (Figure 9-15, box E). The new ventilation system maintenance was documented through memoranda and inspection reports.

An evaluation was also carried out for the implementation of the smoking-cessation program. Records were maintained of the numbers of nonsmokers volunteering as "supporters" and smokers signing up for the program, attending the orientation, and receiving the self-help manual. The percentages of smoking and nonsmoking employees in the program were calculated using prevalence estimates from an earlier baseline survey (Figure 9-15, boxes A and C, respectively). This indicated the penetration of the program into the employee population.

These process evaluation reports were completed by each regional wellness coordinator and forwarded to the state coordinator. They served as the basis for making the awards in each region for the cold-turkey buffet and savings bonds drawings in the two campaigns. In addition, all media related to the campaigns were organized by date and submitted by each region to the state office. Based on this evidence, one could determine the extent of implementation of the program within each region.

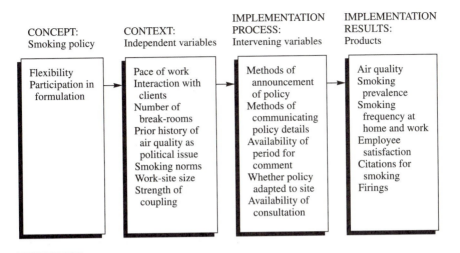

CONCEPT: Smoking policy	CONTEXT: Independent variables	IMPLEMENTATION PROCESS: Intervening variables	IMPLEMENTATION RESULTS: Products
Flexibility Participation in formulation	Pace of work Interaction with clients Number of break-rooms Prior history of air quality as political issue Smoking norms Work-site size Strength of coupling	Methods of announcement of policy Methods of communicating policy details Availability of period for comment Whether policy adapted to site Availability of consultation	Air quality Smoking prevalence Smoking frequency at home and work Employee satisfaction Citations for smoking Firings

FIGURE 9-16

Smoking policy implementation in a large state agency must reconcile the concepts of the policy with the ecological context of the setting.

PROCESS EVALUATION

Changes in predisposing factors among smokers were studied using pre- and posttest questionnaires (Figure 9-15, boxes B and D) of the beliefs and attitudes outlined in Table 9-3. Program participants were also asked what behavioral skill components in the manual they had used and, for each they had used, how helpful it had been. Items related to co-worker and family encouraging and discouraging employees' quitting working documented the extent to which co-workers and family had provided social reinforcement for the behavior change. The extent to which the new smoking policy was perceived as a factor in the processes of quitting and maintenance of cessation was also examined.

Satisfaction with the air quality in the work area and with the smoking policy was assessed. Figure 9-17 indicates the marked differences between satisfaction of smokers and nonsmokers. Most of the change occurred in the first month following implementation of the policy.

Several approaches provided for evaluation of changes in the two enabling factors related to air quality. For smoking policy, employees were surveyed regarding their satisfaction with the policy, whether employees abided by the policy, and the level of enforcement at their specific work site (Figure 9-15, box E). The evaluation team analyzed whether these factors varied by work-site context and by individuals' smoking status. Records were maintained by the state office of employee complaints about the policy, resignations related to the policy, and policy violations and associated personnel actions. The cleaning of the ventilation

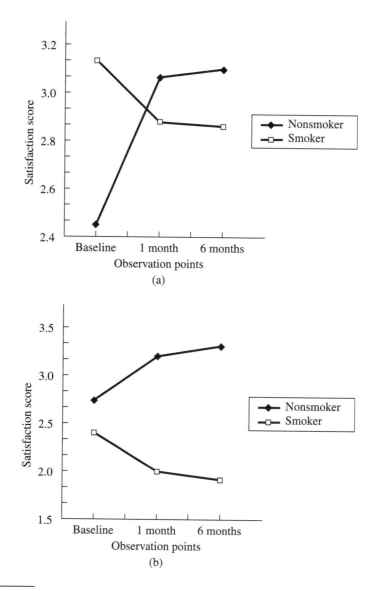

FIGURE 9-17

Satisfaction of workers with (a) air quality in their work area and (b) the smoking policy, at the time of implementation and 1 and 6 months following implementation, comparing smokers and nonsmokers.

SOURCE: "Impact of a Restrictive Work Site Smoking Policy on Smoking Behavior, Attitudes, and Norms," by N. H. Gottlieb, M. P. Eriksen, C. Y. Lovato et al., 1990, *Journal of Occupational Medicine, 32,* 16–23. Reprinted with permission.

system was monitored through regular inspection reports of dust accumulation before and after the policy was implemented.

IMPACT EVALUATION

Comparison of pre- and posttest patterns of smoking (Figure 9-15, boxes B and D) indicated whether participants had reduced the number of cigarettes they smoked or quit smoking. These self-reports of quitting were validated using biochemical analysis on a sample of employees. Besides this study of program participants, a random sample of all employees was undertaken to see if the smoking prevalence had changed across the entire workforce, not just among the employees who were in the program (Figure 9-15, boxes A, C, and E).

Comparisons were made also between smoking rates in work sites where smoking was allowed in restricted areas and those in which a complete ban was enforced within the buildings. Table 9-4 shows the results at 1 month and 6 months following implementation of the policies. Although the policies succeeded in reducing smoking in the work sites, thereby achieving the program objective of improving air quality, smokers' daily total of cigarettes might have increased with more smoking at home for those working in restricted areas.

TABLE 9-4

Smoking indicators versus time in regions with restricted smoking areas and in those with bans

	In Restricted Areas (%)			In Ban Areas (%)		
	Baseline	1 month	6 months	Baseline	1 month	6 months
	$n = 1432$	$n = 1111$	$n = 967$	$n = 279$	$n = 238$	$n = 169$
Current smokers	22.4%	21.4%	20.1%	25.1%	22.7%	16.6%
Former smokers	19.2	19.3	20.2	12.5	19.3	15.4
Never smokers	58.4	59.3	59.8	62.4	58.0	68.0
Smokers						
≥ 15 cigarettes at work	$n = 313$ 16.9	$n = 226$ 6.6	$n = 190$ 5.8	$n = 69$ 17.4	$n = 49$ 8.2	$n = 27$ 0.0
≥ 15 cigarettes daily total	$n = 314$ 48.7	$n = 232$ 40.9	$n = 194$ 52.1	$n = 69$ 63.8	$n = 51$ 53.8	$n = 28$ 60.7

SOURCE: "Impact of a Restrictive Work Site Smoking Policy on Smoking Behavior, Attitudes, and Norms," by N. H. Gottlieb, M. P. Eriksen, C. Y. Lovato et al., 1990, *Journal of Occupational Medicine, 32,* 16–23. Reprinted with permission.

Air quality was measured using self-reports of employees on pre- and post-policy surveys (Figure 9-15, boxes C and E). In addition, an environmental engineering firm conducted an analysis of air quality before and after the policy and program were implemented.

OUTCOME EVALUATION

It is not feasible within program resources to measure long-term health consequences of smoking cessation and air quality improvement in a situation such as this. The time lag for health effects is too long, the employee turnover too great, and the cost of follow-up prohibitive for most organizations. Projections of outcome, however, can be made using risk-factor equations from studies such as the Framingham Heart Study. In this case, it was possible to examine changes in self-reported respiratory symptoms before and after the program and policy were implemented. Nonsmokers in smoke-free regions reported higher satisfaction with air quality and indicated they were bothered less frequently by co-workers' smoke than were their peers in regions with a restrictive smoking policy allowing smoking in break rooms.

SUMMARY

The common mission of EAPs and workplace health promotion to improve employee health represents a point of convergence between the two philosophies, as well as a fundamental shift away from the underlying disease-and-injury-prevention philosophy of occupational health and safety. The emphasis of EAPs and health promotion on employee health and well-being rather than on work-related health problems displaced the locus of power—from determinants of health external to employees but internal to the work site to those determinants of health under greater control of employees and to those outside the work site.[154] Although conspiratorial theories abound, it appears to us that the displacement of the foci of intervention was an unconscious result of a growing interest in behavioral risk factors rather than a conscious decision to "blame the victim."[155]

Consequently, the ideologies that govern health promotion and EAPs led to an unconscious drift in responsibility for health from the environment to the individual. The tendency for many programs to emphasize behavior change at the individual level is inconsistent with our understanding of the primary determinants of health.[156] As this chapter attempted to show in its initial positioning of workplace health promotion in an ecological context, employee health and behavior are first influenced by the broader economic, technological, cultural, and structural elements of the workplace and community. The additional influence of the proximal workplace social environment that predisposes, enables, and reinforces employee health behavior is not trivial. Placing the primary burden for health on the employee without provision for supportive "healthy policy" has limited the effectiveness of many health promotion programs. Barriers to behavior change include problems with participation, retention and attrition, in addition to the maintenance of such change.

The work site presents an opportunity and a challenge for the development of health promotion. The growth of the labor force with the increased participation of women may be matched in future years with a corresponding growth in the employment of older people needing or choosing to work rather than retire. These demographic trends place new demands on employers to cope with issues of child care and employee health. Escalation of health care costs and the increasing proportion of the burden of medical costs borne by industry has brought about an explosion of alternative strategies to contain costs, with health promotion being one among many still in an experimental phase.

Whether for cost-containment or other reasons, the planning, implementation, and evaluation of work-site health promotion programs can follow the Precede and Proceed phases of the model with some adaptations. A first point of emphasis for work-place applications is in the social assessment phase, where the economic bottom-line of the employer must receive first consideration before one can expect to gain entry let alone attention to the health promotion needs of employees. Particular attention in Phase 3 to balancing the emphasis on behavioral and environmental determinants of health can serve to assure greater support from management and employees alike. Care in the implementation process to provide for continuous monitoring and feedback through advisory and communication structures will assure the continuity and sustainability of the program.

EXERCISES

1. If the counterpart of social benefits for industry are the bottom-line issues of productivity and profit, how can you express your objectives for a work-site program that will convince management to support the program?
2. Create an example in which a behavioral approach, though well-intentioned, may be construed as victim blaming. Then, using the appropriate steps in the Precede-Proceed model, illustrate how the accountable practitioner can avoid that criticism.

NOTES AND CITATIONS

1. We are indebted to Chris Y. Lovato, Nell Gottlieb, and Michael Eriksen, formerly at the University of Texas Center for Health Promotion Research and Development, and to Dave Ramsey at CDC for their contributions to this chapter in the previous edition. Margaret Cargo and C. James

Frankish at the University of British Columbia Institute of Health Promotion Research contributed to material used in this edition.

2. Green, 1974. The first worksite test of the model was R. L. Bertera, 1981.

3. See previous chapter notes for examples of broader community-wide applications and the distinction between community interventions and interventions in community settings. The next three chapters provide examples of applications in school and medical settings and in new communications and information technologies. For a continuously updated bibliography of programs based on this model of health promotion, see the Precede-Proceed web page at http://www.ubc.ihpr.ca.

4. The most extensive application of the Precede-Proceed model in a series of work-site health promotion programs, with evaluation of efficiency and effectiveness at several levels, is that by Robert Bertera for the Du Pont corporation. For his most recent publications reporting on the results of this series of programs, see R. L. Bertera, 1991, 1993, 1999. The article in which he describes how the Precede-Proceed model was applied is R. L. Bertera, 1990b.

5. Scriven, 1998, p. 62. See also Glanz & Rimer, 1995.

6. Shoveller & Langille, 1993.

7. Eakin, 1992; Green, Kreuter, Deeds & Partridge, 1980; pp. 212–224.

8. Lovato, Green, & Stainbrook, 1993.

9. This section is adapted from Green & Cargo, 1994, and Lovato, Green & Stainbrook, 1993.

10. U.S. Bureau of the Census, 1998.

11. Burden & Googins, 1987.

12. Barth, 1995.

13. Dean & Hancock, 1992; Duhl, 1986; Green, 1990; Riger & Lavrakas, 1981.

14. Wade, 1982.

15. Clutterbuck, 1980.

16. Sass, 1989. Legislation in Canada varied by province in the year of its passage.

17. Pearse & Refshauge 1987. Australian laws also varied by state in the year of their passage.

18. Cassou & Pissarro, 1988.

19. Schuckman, 1986.

20. Kleinman, 1984. Supportive environments for health: Sundovall, 1998.

21. Gevers, 1985.

22. U.S. Department of Labor, Bureau of Labor Statistics, 1995.

23. National Safety Council, 1995.

24. Brandt-Rauf & Brandt-Rauf, 1989; J. D. Miller, 1989.

25. Ringen, 1989.

26. Sloan, Gruman, & Allegrante, 1987; Walsh, Rudd, Biener, & Mangioni, 1993.

27. Ordin, 1992; Walsh, 1992.

28. R. L. Bertera, & Cuthie, 1984.

29. S. Burris, 1997.

30. Sackett & Haynes, 1976; Sloan, Gruman, & Allegrante, 1987.

31. Black, 1980; Haber, 1994.

32. Conrad & Walsh, 1992.

33. Daltroy et al, 1993.

34. S. Burris, 1997.

35. Henritze, Brammell, & McGloin, 1992; Ordin, 1992; Stonecipher & Hyner, 1993.

36. DeJoy, 1990; Eddy, Fitzhugh & Wang, 1997; Winett, King & Altman, 1989.

37. A. Cohen, Smith & Anger, 1982; Eakin, 1992.

38. Bunce, 1997; Kagan, Kagan, & Watson, 1995; Quick, Murphy, & Hurrell, 1992; Schnall, Landsbergis, & Baker, 1994. For an application of PRECEDE, see Daltroy et al., 1993.

39. Lovato, Green, & Stainbrook, 1993.

40. Landrigan, 1989.

41. U.S. Department of Labor, 1995.

42. U.S. Department of Health and Human Services, 1996, p. 73.

43. Landrigan, 1989, p. 2.

44. Kizer, Pelletier, & Fielding, 1995.

45. Collings, 1982; Lovato, Green, & Stainbrook, 1993.

46. Levit, Freeland, & Waldo, 1989.

47. National Safety Council, 1995.

48. Levit & Cowan, 1991.

49. Eriksen, 1986; Fielding, 1990a, 1991; Pucci & Hoglund, 1994.

50. Warner et al., 1988. For applications of PRECEDE, see Bertera, 1990a, 1993.

51. Warner, 1987.

52. Pelletier, 1993, 1996; Tengs et al., 1995; Warner, 1992; Warner, Smith, Smith, & Fries, 1996.

53. K. J. Fisher, Glasgow, & Terborg, 1990; Frankish & Green, 1998 (see http://www.ihpr.ubc.ca).

54. Ashley, Eakin, Bull, & Pederson, 1997; Brigham, Gross, Stitzer, & Felch, 1994; Conrad et al., 1996; Dawley et al., 1993; Flynn, Gurdon, & Secker-Walker, 1995; Frankish, Johnson, Ratner, & Lovato, 1997; Sorenson, Glasgow, Topor, & Corbett, 1997.

55. Warner et al., 1996, p. 981.

56. Leo, 1996; McLeroy, Green, Mullen, & Foshee, 1984; Pelletier & Lutz, 1998.

57. Barratt et al., 1994; Lando, Jeffery, McGovern, Forster, & Baxter, 1993; Lovato & Green, 1990.

58. D. J. Nelson et al., 1987.

59. Brownell et al., 1984; see also Matson, Lee, & Hopp, 1993.

60. H. R. Brown, Carozza, Lloyd, & Thater, 1989. See also Alderman, Green, & Flynn, 1980.

61. A. J. Brennan, 1985. For an application of PRECEDE, see Salazar, 1985.

62. Pelletier, 1993, 1996. Cf Wong, Alsagoff, & Kok, 1992.

63. Bly, Jones, & Richardson, 1986.

64. Meek, 1996; cf. Richard, Potvin, Kishchuk, Prlic, & Green, 1996.

65. Johnston, 1991.

66. House, 1981. For PRECEDE applications: Daltroy et al., 1993; Hubball, 1996.

67. Chenoweth, 1994; Sloan, 1987.

68. Chenoweth, 1993.

69. For descriptions of these and 59 other U.S. company programs, some of which are international, see Office of Disease Prevention and Health Promotion, 1993. For Canada, a similar inventory provides descriptions of 62 company health promotion programs: Health and Welfare Canada, 1992.

70. Howse, 1991.

71. Ibid. See PRECEDE analysis of breastfeeding counseling, Burglehaus et al., 1997.

72. Vass & Walsh-Allis, 1990.

73. Yandrick, 1990.

74. Des Jarlais & Hubbard, 1997.

75. Vaillant, 1983.

76. R. L. Bertera, 1991. See also Hofford & Spellman, 1996; Masi, 1984.

77. Walsh & Kelleher, 1987. See also Glenn, 1994.

78. Girdano, 1986. For PRECEDE application: Newman, Martin, & Weppner, 1982.

79. Trice & Beyer, 1984.

80. Kurtz, Googins, & Howard, 1984.

81. Ford & Ford, 1986.

82. Cook & Harrell, 1987.

83. J. B. Franz, 1987. For a European example: Vasse, Nijhuis, Kok, & Kroodsma, 1997.

84. Yandrick, 1990.

85. Ford & Ford, 1986.

86. J. B. Franz, 1987.

87. Ibid. See also Green, Richard, & Potvin, 1996.

88. R. F. Allen, 1980.

89. Frost & St. Germain, 1986.

90. Karasek & Theorell, 1990.

91. Gardell, 1982; Schechter et al., 1997; Stronks et al., 1998.

92. Marmot, Rose, Shipley, & Hamilton, 1978; Power, Hertzman, & Manor, 1997.

93. Syme, 1986.

94. J. V. Johnson & Johansson, 1991; Schechter et al., 1997.

95. Witherspoon, 1990.

96. J. Allen & Allen, 1986, 1990.

97. Emont & Cummings, 1990; Green & Cargo, 1994; Hubball, 1996.

98. Sorenson, Glasgow, Corbett, & Topor, 1992.

99. Ottoson & Green, 1987. See also Hubbard & Ottoson, 1997.

100. The innovative or bellweather states in health promotion were identified by Naisbitt, 1982; see also Naisbitt & Aburdene, 1990. For specific accounts of the early growth and diffusion of smoking-control programs in the workplace, see Eriksen, 1986; Haefele, 1990; Orleans & Shipley, 1982; Schilling, Gilchrist, & Schinke, 1985; Todaro et al., 1987; Walsh, 1984. The growth trends in other work-site health promotion activities are traced in Fielding, 1984; Fielding & Piserchia, 1989. For Europe: Tillgren, Haglund, & Romelsjo, 1996.

101. Fielding, 1982b; Fielding & Breslow, 1983; Parkinson et al., 1982.

102. Davis et al., 1984; Fielding, 1984; Fielding & Piserchia, 1989; Minnesota Department of Health, 1982; Todero, Denard, Clark et al., 1987.

103. Fielding & Piserchia, 1989.

104. Allegrante, 1986; Allegrante & Sloan, 1986; Beauchamp, 1980; M. H. Becker, 1986; Hollander & Hale, 1987; O'Rourke & Macrina, 1989; Ratcliff & Wallack, 1986.

105. McLeroy, Gottlieb, & Burdine, 1987.

106. Karasek & Theorell, 1990; McLeroy, Green, Mullen, & Foshee, 1984; Pelletier & Lutz, 1988.

107. Shipley, 1987; Sloan, Gruman, & Allegrante, 1987.

108. Eakin, 1992; Permut, 1986.

109. Vojtecky, 1986. PRECEDE example: Wong, Chan, Kok, & Wong, 1996.

110. G. S. Smith & Kraus, 1988.

111. Brody, 1988; Masi, 1984; Myers, 1985. The EAPs, however, have failed to offer primary prevention of substance abuse, just as drugs and alcohol are seldom part of health promotion programs that emphasize primary prevention. See Cook & Harrell, 1987.

112. Pelletier & Lutz, 1988; Windom, McGinnis, & Fielding, 1987.

113. Fielding & Piserchia, 1989; Hubball, 1996; Simpson & Pruitt, 1989.

114. A. Cohen & Murphy, 1989; Key & Kilian, 1983; Vojtecky, 1986; Warner, 1987, 1992.

115. Cataldo et al., 1986; Lovato, Green, & Stainbrook, 1993.

116. Lovato & Green, 1986; Lovato, Green, & Conley, 1986. For a discussion of data sources for epidemiological surveillance of occupational illness and injury in the United States, see Baker, Melius, & Millar, 1988.

117. DeJoy, 1986a, b, 1990 (quotation from p. 11); DeJoy, Murphy, & Gershon, 1995.

118. Syme, 1986.

119. Lovato & Green, 1984.

120. Chomik, 1998; A. Cohen & Murphy, 1989; Dunlop et al., 1989; Nutbeam & Harris, 1995.

121. Green, Wilson, & Lovato, 1986; Haskell & Blair, 1982; Wong & Seet, 1998.

122. Green, 1988e; Tones & Tilford, 1994.

123. Brownell & Felix, 1987; Matson, Lee, & Hopp, 1993.

124. P. Conrad, 1987; Fielding, 1984; Kristal et al., 1995; Oldridge, 1984.

125. Hubball, 1996; Sallis et al., 1986; Strecher, DeVellis, Becker, & Rosenstock, 1986.

126. K. E. Davis, Jackson, Kronenfeld, & Blair, 1987; Leo, 1996; Lovato & Green, 1990; McLeroy, Green, Mullen, & Foshee, 1984.

127. N. H. Gottlieb & Nelson, 1990.

128. Bellingham, 1994; Bjurstrom & Alexiou, 1978.

129. Alderman, Green, & Flynn, 1982; Everly & Feldman, 1985; O'Donnell & Ainsworth, 1995.

130. P. H. Bailey, Rukholm, Vanderlee, & Hyland, 1994; Feldman, 1983, 1984.

131. Alderman, Green, & Flynn, 1980.

132. Conrad, Campbell, Edington et al., 1996; Everly & Feldman, 1985; Landgreen & Baum, 1984; O'Donnell & Ainsworth, 1995; Parkinson et al., 1982.

133. N. H. Gottlieb et al., 1990, p. 22.

134. Feldman, 1984; Wong, Chan, Kok, & Wong, 1994–95, 1996.

135. Brownell & Felix, 1987; Brownell et al., 1984; Collins, Wagner, & Weissberger, 1986; Glasgow, Klesges, Mizes, & Pechacek, 1985; Matson, Lee, & Hopp, 1993.

136. Jason et al., 1990; Klesges, Vasey, & Glasgow, 1986.

137. Green, A. L. Wilson, & Lovato, 1986.

138. Bjurstrom & Alexiou, 1978; Haskell & Blair, 1982; cf., however, Kristal et al., 1995.

139. Dedobbeleer & German, 1987.

140. Lovato & Green, 1990.

141. Borland, Chapman, Owen, & Hill, 1990; Eriksen, 1986; Flynn, Gurdon, & Secker-Walker, 1995; Frankish & Green, 1994, 1998; Frankish, Johnson, Ratner, & Lovato, 1997.

142. Colantonio, 1989; Walsh & Egdahl, 1989; Walsh, Rudd, Biener, & Mangione, 1993.

143. For an application of PRECEDE to the activation of workers to bring pressure on management for a policy change regarding work-site hazards, see Appendix C-1 in previous edition: Green, Kreuter, Deeds, & Partridge, 1980, pp. 212–224.

144. Felix, Stunkard, Cohen, & Cooley, 1985.

145. Donovan, 1991; Haber, 1994; Kingery, 1995; Sloan & Gruman, 1988.

146. P. D. Mullen & Culjat, 1980.

147. Bibeau et al., 1988; A. L. Davis, Faust, & Ordentlich, 1984; Frankish & Green, 1998; T. J. Glynn, Boyd, & Gruman, 1990; Sallis et al., 1986; Windsor & Bartlett, 1984. For a meta-analysis of work-site smoking-cessation evaluations, see K. J. Fisher, Glasgow, & Terborg, 1990.

148. Lovato & Green, 1990; algorithm adapted from Green, 1993c, 1987a.

149. This case description is based on work initiated at the University of Texas Center for Health Promotion Research and Development, with support from the Texas Affiliate of the American Heart Association and grant K07-CA01286 from the National Cancer Institute. See N. H. Gottlieb et al., 1990; N. H. Gottlieb & Nelson, 1990. Some variations on the actual history of the case have been introduced for illustrative purposes. For another fully developed and evaluated case study of a work-site health promotion program based on the Precede model, see R. L. Bertera, 1990b. This project received the 1990 Program Excellence Award of the Society for Public Health Education. See also Bertera, 1990a, 1993, 1999.

150. For a description of the development and pilot testing of this American Lung Association Program, see Strecher, Rimer, & Monaco, 1989.

151. Work-site competitions have been found in several studies and reviews to have modest effectiveness in reducing smoking or weight control but substantially lower costs than classes or clinical interventions, giving them a better cost-effectiveness than other methods except self-help. See for example Altman, Flora, Fortmann, & Farquhar, 1987; Brownell & Felix, 1987. This first campaign was based particularly on the experience of Klesges, Vasey, & Glasgow, 1986.

152. The lottery contest approach to recruitment had been found in one work-site study to yield a 14% participation rate among workers in a cancer research hospital and a quit rate of 36%, higher than that reported in other studies of contests. See K. M. Cummings, Hellmann, & Emont, 1988. See also Matson, Lee, & Hopp, 1993.

153. Ottoson & Green, 1987. Also, Hubbard & Ottoson, 1997; C. H. Weiss, 1988, p. 57.

154. Roman & Blum, 1996.

155. Sorensen et al., 1997.

156. Richard, Potvin, Kishchuk, Prlic, & Green, 1996.

Chapter 10

Applications
in School Settings

We expect schools to be places of learning. We expect investments in education to yield benefits to individuals, communities, and nations. Schools are in a position to contribute to social and economic development, increased productivity, and a better quality of life for all. In many parts of the world, some schools are making significant progress. But even more could be achieved if all schools could promote the healthy development of young people as actively as they promote learning.[1]

This inspiring commentary, the opening statement in the World Health Organization's 1996 Global School Health Initiative, becomes even more compelling when we consider the demographics of schools and school-age children. In 1994, over 1 billion students were enrolled in schools around the world. In the United States, every school day sees nearly 47 million students attend elementary and secondary schools; about 6 million professional and nonprofessional workers staff those schools.[2] Thus, in the United States, schools constitute the center of work activity for nearly one fifth of the population.[3] From a public health perspective, these demographics confirm that support for health promotion in schools is a powerful and cost-effective global prevention strategy.[4]

In this chapter, we explain how the application of the Precede-Proceed model can assist school curriculum planners, administrators, parents, teachers, and advocates for children to meet the ongoing challenge of creating health-promoting schools. First, we explain how the concept of a "coordinated" school health program, widely accepted internationally as a sound organizational framework for school health, is consistent with the key principles of the Precede-Proceed model. Next, we offer examples of how findings from school health research continue to contribute to advances in school health. Then, starting with the social assessment process, we provide examples of how aspects of PRECEDE and PROCEED relate specifically to the school setting. Finally, we offer a hypothetical case applying the steps and principles to a specific school/community setting.

THE COMPONENTS OF SCHOOL HEALTH PROMOTION

The basic conceptual structure of school health programs in the United States can be traced back to 1935. In that year, a report issued by the Health Education Section of the American Physical Education Association described the school health program as consisting of three interdependent components: (1) school health services, (2) school health education, and (3) healthful school environment.[5] The simplicity and comprehensiveness of that tripartite structure has provided school health program planners with a sound and stable foundation.[6] In the late 1980s, Kolbe[7] and Allensworth and Kolbe[8] offered an expanded conceptualization of school health by adding five to the original three: (1) integrated school and community health promotion efforts, (2) school physical education, (3) school food service, (4) school counseling, and (5) school-site health promotion program for faculty and staff, as shown in Figure 10-1. Note that under the "Program components" column, the three traditional elements have been extended to include those five. The vertical arrows between the program components connote the interdependence of the program activities. The remaining arrows suggest various ways in which intermediate, short-term, and long-term outcomes can be influenced. Definitions for the eight components are listed in the glossary.

THREE ADVANTAGES

While some may suggest that the five additional components were implicitly part of the three components in the earlier characterizations of the school health program, their more explicit delineation in the expanded rendition offers three advantages. First, by giving greater visibility to integrated community and school programs, physical education, school food services, school counseling, and school-site health promotion for staff, the importance of these activities in the overall scheme of school health becomes much more salient. Salient components receive attention; they become worthy of consideration, study and support; they are viewed as essential rather than incidental, primary rather than subsidiary. Growing scientific evidence now confirms our prior assumptions about the health and human performance benefits of good nutrition[9] and prudent physical activity.[10] Activities related to school food services (including cafeteria lunches and vending machine policies) and physical education (including curriculum, facilities, and extracurricular programs) are too important not to receive the utmost attention in planning for a school health program.

The second advantage of delineating the five components is that the expanded framework suggests the need for a team approach to school health. It identifies the important players on the team—school nurses, physicians, health educators, counselors, psychologists, food service workers, physical educators,

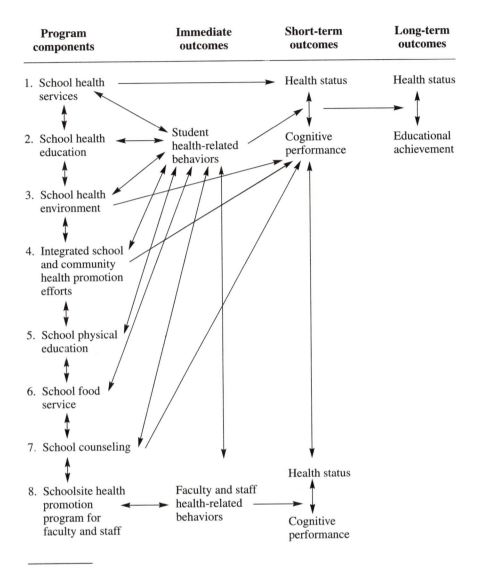

FIGURE 10-1

School health promotion components and outcomes.

SOURCE: "Increasing the Impact of School Health Promotion Programs: Emerging Research Perspectives," by L. Kolbe, 1986, *Health Education, 17*(5), 47–52.

and those responsible for the school's physical and psychosocial environment. It also acknowledges the critical supporting role played by both the family and the community and its institutions. In 1985, two distinguished U.S. public health officials offered the following call for collaboration and cooperation:

We must all maintain sensitivity to the unique educational mission of schools and the complex social and economic conditions that frequently surround them. The institutions of public health and education are complementary and, as such, they must work as partners, sharing their expertise, time, energy and resources if everyone is to realize the potential schools have in contributing to the goal of a healthier citizenry, whether that be 1990 or 2090.[11]

The third advantage of using the expanded framework is that it overtly calls attention to the fundamental mission of schools: education. In Figure 10-1, note that cognitive performance and educational achievement share equal billing with health status as short- and long-term outcome priorities. When health professionals lose sight of the school's raison d'etre, and replace it with health priorities, a collapse of interest and support from school administrators often follows.[12]

KEY CONCEPTS: "COORDINATED" AND "COMPREHENSIVE"

In *Health Is Academic: A Guide to Coordinated School Health Programs,*[13] care is taken to make a distinction between the use of the words *comprehensive* and *coordinated* in the context of school health. It is recommended that the word *coordinated* should be used in reference to the school health *program.* The rationale is that since each of the organizational entities representing eight components have independent identities and standards, they can contribute most effectively to the promotion of student health when their collective efforts are *coordinated.* For example, the component focusing on "family and community involvement in school health" directly reinforces the goal of public health professionals to engage the community, including parents, in active roles on behalf of the health of school-age children.[14]

The term *comprehensive* refers here specifically to one's approach to *health education.* Lohrmann and Wooley[15] characterize comprehensive school health education terms of these key elements:

- A developmentally and age-appropriate, planned scope and sequence of instruction from kindergarten through 12th grade, with a minimum of 50 hours of instructional time annually
- An organizing framework based on the National Health Education Standards[16] to ensure that all performance indicators are addressed at the appropriate grade level
- Health content and skills introduced in the early grades and reinforced in the later ones
- Student assessments that measure skill acquisition as well as functional knowledge

Figure 10-2 shows the relationship among National Health Education Standards, general health topics, and the six risks that constitute the leading causes of

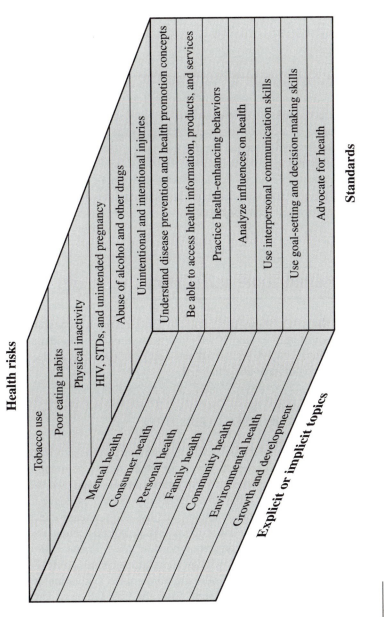

FIGURE 10-2

Standards, health risks and topics: Key elements in comprehensive school health education.

SOURCE: Reprinted by permission of the publisher from *Health Is Academic: A Guide to Coordinated School Health Problems* (p. 49), E. Marx and S. F. Wooley (eds.), 1998, New York: Teachers College Press. © 1998 by Educational Development Center, Inc. All rights reserved.

illness and death among school-age youth. When these critical dimensions are taken into account and inform the curriculum development process, the "comprehensiveness" of school health education is inevitable.

ADDRESSING COMPLEXITY

While Figure 10-1 shows the nature of coordination among the key components of a school health program, it also reflects the complexity inherent in the task of coordinating the efforts of multiple entities toward a common goal. The complexity inherent in the notion of a coordinated school health program makes a working knowledge of the Precede-Proceed model especially useful. For example, planners with an understanding of the principles of PRECEDE-PROCEED would make several helpful assumptions about the coordinated school health program approach and would conduct social assessments and administrative and policy assessments in the several stakeholder groups.

PROGRESS IN SCHOOL HEALTH RESEARCH AND POLICY

Since the printing of the first edition of this book in 1980, research on health promotion in schools has virtually exploded with new and compelling evidence on the effectiveness of comprehensive and coordinated approaches. Noteworthy policy advances in school health have also emerged.

ASSESSING THE EFFECTS OF SCHOOL HEALTH EDUCATION

After decades of defending comprehensive school health on the basis of learning principles and research evidence borrowed from other fields, contemporary school health literature is now replete with evaluations of well-designed school health education and school health programs. The most sweeping evidence to arrive in the 1980s was the nationwide evaluation of the comprehensive School Health Curriculum Project. From a handful of small-scale studies conducted before 1980 with limited controls (usually pretest-posttest designs) and with little behavioral impact measured (usually knowledge and attitude changes only),[17] the opportunity arose in 1981 to carry out a multisite randomized evaluation of this and several other health curricula with support from the U.S. Office of Disease Prevention and Health Promotion and the Centers for Disease Control.

The School Health Education Evaluation was a pioneering 3-year prospective study, involving 30,000 students in grades 4–7 from 20 states. It revealed that students who were exposed to comprehensive school health education not only

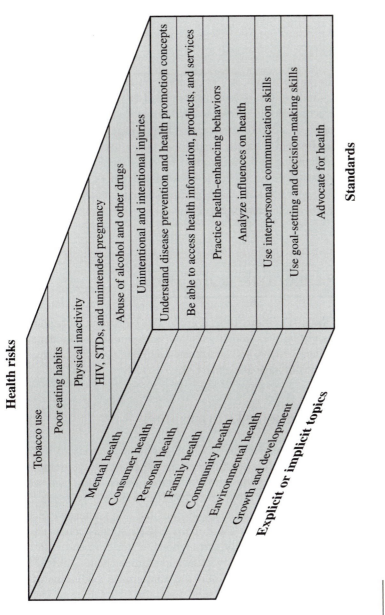

Health risks

Tobacco use

Poor eating habits

Physical inactivity

HIV, STDs, and unintended pregnancy

Abuse of alcohol and other drugs

Unintentional and intentional injuries

Standards

Understand disease prevention and health promotion concepts

Be able to access health information, products, and services

Practice health-enhancing behaviors

Analyze influences on health

Use interpersonal communication skills

Use goal-setting and decision-making skills

Advocate for health

Mental health

Consumer health

Personal health

Family health

Community health

Environmental health

Growth and development

Explicit or implicit topics

FIGURE 10-2

Standards, health risks and topics: Key elements in comprehensive school health education.

SOURCE: Reprinted by permission of the publisher from *Health Is Academic: A Guide to Coordinated School Health Problems* (p. 49), E. Marx and S. F. Wooley (eds.), 1998, New York: Teachers College Press. © 1998 by Educational Development Center, Inc. All rights reserved.

illness and death among school-age youth. When these critical dimensions are taken into account and inform the curriculum development process, the "comprehensiveness" of school health education is inevitable.

ADDRESSING COMPLEXITY

While Figure 10-1 shows the nature of coordination among the key components of a school health program, it also reflects the complexity inherent in the task of coordinating the efforts of multiple entities toward a common goal. The complexity inherent in the notion of a coordinated school health program makes a working knowledge of the Precede-Proceed model especially useful. For example, planners with an understanding of the principles of PRECEDE-PROCEED would make several helpful assumptions about the coordinated school health program approach and would conduct social assessments and administrative and policy assessments in the several stakeholder groups.

PROGRESS IN SCHOOL HEALTH RESEARCH AND POLICY

Since the printing of the first edition of this book in 1980, research on health promotion in schools has virtually exploded with new and compelling evidence on the effectiveness of comprehensive and coordinated approaches. Noteworthy policy advances in school health have also emerged.

ASSESSING THE EFFECTS OF SCHOOL HEALTH EDUCATION

After decades of defending comprehensive school health on the basis of learning principles and research evidence borrowed from other fields, contemporary school health literature is now replete with evaluations of well-designed school health education and school health programs. The most sweeping evidence to arrive in the 1980s was the nationwide evaluation of the comprehensive School Health Curriculum Project. From a handful of small-scale studies conducted before 1980 with limited controls (usually pretest-posttest designs) and with little behavioral impact measured (usually knowledge and attitude changes only),[17] the opportunity arose in 1981 to carry out a multisite randomized evaluation of this and several other health curricula with support from the U.S. Office of Disease Prevention and Health Promotion and the Centers for Disease Control.

The School Health Education Evaluation was a pioneering 3-year prospective study, involving 30,000 students in grades 4–7 from 20 states. It revealed that students who were exposed to comprehensive school health education not only showed significant positive changes in their health-related knowledge and attitudes, compared with students in matched schools without such exposure, they also were considerably less likely to take up smoking. Especially relevant were those findings clearly demonstrating that administrative support and teacher training were directly linked to the positive student outcomes detected, as were the cumulative hours of classroom time devoted to comprehensive school health education.[18]

THE NATIONAL INSTITUTES OF HEALTH

Following the lead of other agencies in the Public Health Service, the National Institutes of Health began to lend their considerable scientific prestige to the study of school health promotion. In 1988, an expert advisory group convened by the National Cancer Institute reviewed 20 years of research on school-based efforts to prevent tobacco use. The panel found nine areas with sufficient data or experience to reach preliminary conclusions and recommendations: program, impact, focus, context, length, ideal age for intervention, teacher training, program implementation, and need for peer and parental involvement.[19]

During the mid-1980s, the National Heart Lung and Blood Institute supported a variety of school-based research efforts, 10 of which are summarized in Table 10-1.[20] As the table indicates, these studies reflect diversity in the demographic characteristics of the populations studied, in the risk-factor focus, and in methods and channels of intervention. The importance of **family and community involvement** in the coordinated school health program is reinforced by the fact that 7 of the 10 studies used the strategy of linking home and school to create a mutually reinforcing setting for the behavior of children.[21] Several of the studies applied the Precede model and emphasized the importance of a planning model to complement and organize specific theoretical models.[22]

The success of this research effort, combined with growing interest in the concept of coordinated school health programs, prompted the National Heart Lung and Blood Institute to support for a randomized intervention trial to assess the effectiveness of school-based efforts to promote cardiovascular health. The Child and Adolescent Trial for Cardiovascular Health (CATCH) was a 3-year, multicenter trial (1991–1994) involving 5,000 students from 96 schools in four states. CATCH used a multicomponent, coordinated approach focused on the school organization/environment, classroom curricula, and the family.[23] Results from the CATCH trials showed significant positive change with respect to school environment goals, including a reduction in fat in school lunches and an increase in moderate to vigorous activity in physical education classes. Results in other intervention categories were less pronounced but still showed significant changes in knowledge mediated through the family intervention component[24] and individual level changes in dietary intention, food choice, knowledge, and perceived social support for healthy food choices.[25]

TABLE 10-1

A summary of NHLBI school-based health promotion studies

Investigator Institution Study	Ethnicity[a] SES Grade State	Schools[b] Classes Students	Channel: Curriculum, Food Service, Home	Provider	Target Areas	Outcomes
Perry, Cheryl, Ph.D. Univ of Minn "Healthy Heart" "The Home Team"	W, A SES (M) Grade 3 MN, ND	24T/7C — 1405T 422C	Curr Home	Teachers Mail	Eating	Changes in knowledge, total fat, saturated fat, complex carbohydrate intake
Parcel, Guy, Ph.D. Univ of Texas "Go for Health"	W, H, B SES (L, M) Grades 3–4 TX	2T/2C 40 1156	Curr Food Serv	Teachers Food workers	Eating Exercise	Changes in knowledge, self-efficacy, behavioral expectations, food service, PE classes, diet
Walter, Heather, M.D. American Health Fdn "Know Your Body"	W, B, A, H SES (L, M, H) Grades 4–9 NY	22T/15C — 2075T 1313C	Curr Home	Teachers	Eating Exercise Smoking BP WT	Changes in knowledge, total fat, complex carbohydrate intake, chol, initiation of smoking
Bush, Patricia, Ph.D. Georgetown Univ "Know Your Body"	B SES (L, M, H) Grades 4–9 DC	6T/3C — 707T 334C	Home	Teachers	Eating Exercise Smoking BP WT	Change in knowledge, smoking attitudes, BP, HDL chol, fitness, thiocyanate
Nader, Philip, M.D. Univ of CA/SD "Family Health Project"	H, W SES (L, M) Grades 5–6 CA	6T/6C — 163T/160C	Home	Inst	Eating Exercise	Changes in diet, chol, BP, knowledge

(continued)

Investigator Institution Study	Ethnicity[a] SES Grade State	Schools[b] Classes Students	Channel: Curriculum, Food Service, Home	Provider	Target Areas	Outcomes
Cohen, Rita, Ph.D. Brownell, Kelly, Ph.D. Univ of Penn "CV Risk Reduction"	W SES (M) Grades 5–7 PA	— 1062T 992C	Curr Home	Teachers Peers	Eating BP Smoking	Changes in knowledge, initiation of smoking, peers were equally or more effective than teachers
Fors, Stuart, Ed.D. Univ of Georgia "3R's + HBP"	W, B SES (L, M) Grade 6 GA	14T/7C 60 853T 351C	Curr Home	Teachers Students	BP	Changes in knowledge, taking BP
Ellison, R. Curtis, M.D. Univ of Mass "Food Service Project"	W, B, A SES (M, H) Grade 9 MA, NH	2 — 1100	Food Serv	Food workers	BP Eating	Changes in BP, chol, and food service
Weinberg, Armin, Ph.D. Baylor College of Med "CV Curr/Family Tree"	W, H, B SES (L, M) Grades 9–10 TX	7 40 5787	Curr Home	Teachers	Eating Exercise BP	Changes in knowledge, attitudes, self-report behavior, parents used smoking + wt + exercise
Killen, Joel, Ph.D. Farquhar, John, M.D. Stanford Univ "CV Risk Reduction"	W, H, A SES (M) Grade 10 CA	2T/2C 8 1447	Curr	Inst	Eating Exercise BP Smoking	Changes in knowledge, exercise, smoking, resting heart rate, BMI, skinfolds

[a]Predominant ethnic or racial group: A = Asian, B = Black, H = Hispanic, W = White; SES = socioeconomic status

[b]T = treatment, C = control

SOURCE: "Synthesis of Cardiovascular Behavioral Research for Youth Health Promotion," by E. J. Stone, C. L. Perry, and R. V. Luepker (1989), Health Education Quarterly, 16(2), 155–169.

THE CHALLENGE OF PARENTAL PARTICIPATION

Whether from India,[26] Finland,[27] or the United States,[28] findings confirm what seems obvious: Children tend to be physically, emotionally, and socially healthy when they are raised in an environment where they are cared for and nurtured by parents and adults. Getting such participation, however, remains a formidable challenge. A Metropolitan Life Foundation survey,[29] sampling over 4,000 students from 199 public schools and 500 randomly selected parents of schoolchildren, revealed that while the majority of both teachers and parents believe that parental involvement in children's health education would be of considerable help in encouraging good health habits for children, most parents (71%) report never getting involved in the process. This lack of parental involvement may in part explain why parents do not know the extent of drinking, smoking, or drug taking by their children. While 36% of the parents indicated that their child has had at least one alcoholic drink, 66% of the students reported that they had alcohol at least once or twice. Similarly, only 14% of the parents reported that their child had smoked a cigarette, while 41% of the students said they had smoked, and 5% of the parents said that their child had used drugs, whereas 17% of the students reported having used drugs.

Findings from the CATCH trial revealed, not surprisingly, that level of parental participation is influenced by both gender and ethnicity. This finding led to the assumption that the effectiveness of parental program components are likely to depend on how well those components are tailored to relevant cultural and ethnic factors. [30]

TWO COMMON FACTORS

The common denominators for successful school-based programs are (1) a commitment to address specific problems or modifiable risk factors, often within the context of a comprehensive approach, and (2) the use of multiple intervention methods based on an assessment of the characteristics, needs, and interests of the target population. Figure 10-3 illustrates how PRECEDE was used to facilitate the application of these principles in the Bogalusa Heart Smart cardiovascular school health promotion program.[31]

POLICY ANALYSES AND ADVANCES

Progress in research has spurred progress in school health policy. A policy has three components: (1) the clear statement of a problem (or potential problem) that needs attention, (2) a goal to mitigate or prevent that problem, and (3) a set of strategic actions to accomplish that goal. This leaves tactics to the implementers

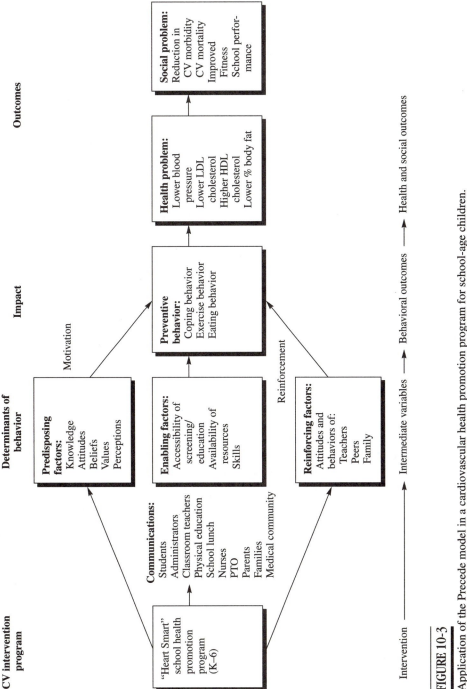

FIGURE 10-3

Application of the Precede model in a cardiovascular health promotion program for school-age children.

SOURCE: "Implementation of 'Heart Smart': A Cardiovascular School Health Promotion Program," by A. M. Downey et al., 1987, *Journal of School Health*, 57, 98–104.

of policy. Well-designed regional or national surveys provide the substance and clarity that make policy credible and influence it.

Policy Surveys. The WHO cross-national survey of health behavior in schoolchild-ren,[32] the National Children and Youth Fitness Study,[33] and the National Adolescent Student Health Survey[34] are just three examples of numerous large surveys that have begun to influence national and international policy with regard to the health of school-age youth.

School Health in America[35] provides periodic reports of state policies and program status in school health in the United States. Nationwide surveys are carried out to elicit information on seven areas akin to the expanded components of a school health program cited earlier: (1) health services, (2) health instruction, (3) a healthful school environment, (4) food services, (5) physical education, (6) guidance and counseling, and (7) school psychology from state education agencies.

In 1993, the School Health Policies and Programs Study (SHPPS) was undertaken to measure the status of policies and programs related to health education, physical education, health services, food services, and policies prohibiting the use of tobacco, alcohol, other drugs, and violence; it took measurements at the state, district, and local level. Supported and conceptualized by the U.S. Centers for Disease Control and Prevention (CDC), all 50 states and the District of Columbia were surveyed; personal interviews were used at the local school level.[36] The primary purpose of SHPPS was to fill national data gaps for measuring progress on 14 of the 111 national health objectives that address adolescents.[37]

Policy Analysis. Data from these kinds of surveys require the additional effort of investigators, policy analysts, and practitioners to translate them into action or policy. For example, Mutter describes how strategic planning and systematic analysis and dissemination of the results of two national surveys in Canada resulted in the documented emergence of policies, resources, and programs targeted at improving the health of Canadian children and youth.[38]

Table 10-2 presents data from *School Health in America* and shows the average number of hours of health education instruction per year required for each state by grade level. Note the extremely wide variation among the states in the number of hours required for health education per year (0–150). These data become especially relevant to planners and policy makers in light of evidence indicating that desirable improvements in levels of students' health knowledge, attitude, and self-reported health practices occur after 50 hours of exposure to quality health education instruction.[39] Note also that although the mean number of hours required for grades 1–6 is over 50, it steadily diminishes to 28 hours for grades 9–12, with a 26-hour mean for all grades.

Even though the state-level data mask the specific practices occurring at the local level, school health workers in those states with no or weak requirements would be well advised to consider how they can support advocacy efforts at the state level to correct what appears to be a problematic enabling factor.

TABLE 10-2

Average number of health education hours per year in states with a specific time requirement

| State | Grade Range | | | |
	1–6	7–8	9–12	1–12
Alaska	0	0	9.00[a]	3.00[a]
Arkansas	60.00	60.00	22.50	47.50
Arizona	30.00	19.00	22.50	25.67
District of Columbia	86.00	54.00	27.00	61.00
Delaware	60.00	30.00	22.50	42.50
Florida	0	0	7.50	2.50
Georgia	30.00	30.00	18.75	26.25
Hawaii	—	45.00	22.50	15.00
Idaho	0	35.00	17.50	11.67
Illinois	—	45.00	22.50	15.00
Indiana	54.00[a]	60.00[a]	150.00[a]	87.00[a]
Kentucky	60.00	30.00	22.50	42.50
Louisiana	90.00	180.00[a]	15.00	80.00[a]
Maine	0	0	17.00	5.67
Minnesota	36.00	20.00	20.00	28.00
Montana	—	72.00[a]	36.00[a]	24.00[a]
North Carolina	—	—	22.50[a]	7.50[a]
North Dakota	0	0	30.00[a]	10.00[a]
New Hampshire	0	0	9.00	3.00
New Jersey	90.00[a]	90.00[a]	90.00[a]	90.00[a]
Nevada	—	—	22.50	7.50
New York	0	30.00	15.00	10.00
Ohio	0	48.00	22.50	15.50
Oregon	0	0	45.00	15.00
Pennsylvania	—	15.00	7.50	5.00
South Carolina	45.00	37.50	0	28.75
Tennessee	—	90.00	22.50	22.50
Texas	16.00	6.00	40.00	22.33
Utah	—	45.00	22.50	15.00
Virginia	0	72.00	36.00	24.00
Wisconsin	—	15.00	15.00	7.50
West Virginia	34.00	54.00	33.75	37.25
Total	691.00	1182.00	886.00	838.08
Mean[b]	53.154	49.271	28.597	26.190
Standard deviation	24.351	35.871	27.141	24.056

NOTE: Zero indicates no hours; dash indicates health education hours required but unable to determine how many.

[a]Hours are combined with those of physical education.

[b]Mean is based on the states that reported a requirement.

SOURCE: *School Health in America*, 5th ed., by C. Y. Lovato and D. Allensworth, 1989, Kent, OH: American School Health Association. Reprinted with permission.

Other policy analyses supporting or promoting school health have emerged from national commissions[40] and international study groups for the World Health Organization.[41] The voluntary health associations have published strong advocacy statements and policy analyses in support of school health promotion.[42] Professional associations also have made their voices heard.[43]

COMPREHENSIVE SCHOOL HEALTH EDUCATION: A RESPONSE TO THE AIDS EPIDEMIC

History is full of examples where breakthroughs for public good are borne out of tragedy; behind such clouds there is sometimes a silver lining. The tragic circumstances that define the global problem of AIDS have given rise to opportunities never before afforded to school health. The severity of the epidemic and the essential role of education in the world prevention strategy, together with the public demand for action, have offered the perfect opportunity for a proactive response in the global fight against AIDS by strengthening comprehensive school health education.

"Guidelines for Effective School Health Education to Prevent the Spread of AIDS"[44] presents an excellent example of the influence strong, timely policy documents can have in focusing and implementing a nationwide health education program.[45] At the time they were presented, these guidelines legitimized the school as a credible national focal point for an important aspect of AIDS prevention. They were developed by CDC staff in close collaboration with leaders representing 16 national school or health organizations. With the support of these broad-based and influential constituencies, the guidelines were crafted such that there could be no mistake in interpreting the strategy for implementation: close collaboration between the health and education sectors, active participation and review by and with parents, and programs carried out in the context of comprehensive school health education. Specifically, "AIDS education interventions may be most effective when implemented within a more comprehensive school health education programme that establishes a foundation for understanding the relationships between personal behaviours and health."[46]

USING PRECEDE AND PROCEED FOR PLANNING IN SCHOOLS

The school setting differs from work sites most significantly in the age range of the population, although the school setting is also a work site for teachers and staff. It also differs, however, in the social functions it serves, its mission, and its ways of accounting for its successes. These latter differences pertain most to the social assessment phase of Precede-Proceed planning and evaluation.

SOCIAL ASSESSMENT

Schools have education, not health, as their mission and as their criterion of success or failure. They are accountable for improvements in the learning and preparedness of children and youth to take on a wider range of life challenges than just the preservation or enhancement of their health.

Health: An Instrumental Value for Schools. In their background justification of the School Health Policies and Programs Study, Kann and her colleagues documented the following health status profile for youth in the United States:

- Among persons aged 5–24, three quarters of all mortality is due to motor vehicle crashes (30%), other unintentional injuries (12%), homicide (19%), and suicide (11%).
- Significant physical, mental, and social problems result from the 1 million pregnancies among adolescents annually and from the 10 million cases of sexually transmitted diseases that occur each year among those aged 15–29.
- As well as being associated with the early initiation of sexual intercourse and unintended pregnancy, alcohol is a key factor in half of the deaths attributed to motor vehicle crashes, homicide and suicide.
- Six categories of behaviors make a major contribution to the leading causes of death and disability: (1) safety behaviors (use of seat belts, weapon carrying), (2) tobacco use, (3) alcohol and other drug use, (4) sexual behaviors that contribute to unintended pregnancy or STD or HIV infection, (5) unhealthy dietary behaviors, and (6) physical inactivity.[47]

Data like these, combined with the reality that school-age children constitute a huge audience, convince public health professionals that schools constitute a critical focal point for health promotion. Do educators hold that same perspective? Recall that in Chapter 2, health was described as an *instrumental* value—a resource for everyday life, not the objective of living. Thus, to the question "What is your mission?" the school administrator would respond, "To educate the students, to prepare them to be competent citizens capable of coping with the demands of daily living." A response of "to improve the health status of students and faculty" would be highly unlikely. If asked to identify the indicators that would best reflect "success" for his or her school, the administrator would likely include the following:

1. Academic progress
2. Low absenteeism (students and faculty)
3. Low rates of student dropouts
4. Competitive salary schedule
5. Minimal discipline problems

6. Parental and community support for school
7. Stable, supportive faculty and staff
8. Student pride in the school

Objective data usually available at the school level can provide insight into the kind of issues identified in items 1–5. For input on items 6–8, one could obtain valuable qualitative information through questionnaires or focus groups.[48] The latter information, often referred to as "soft data," should not be taken as lesser in value than more objective, "hard data." Experiences around the world have taught planners, sometimes quite painfully, this lesson: Failure to acknowledge and address the perceptions and feelings held by administrators, teachers, and parents, however difficult those sentiments may be to quantify, can stop the best-designed, well-intended program dead in its tracks.

For health institutions, the mission is improved health; for schools, the mission is education. While these missions are not mutually exclusive, they reflect differences in institutional priorities. Health promotion planners need to be especially sensitive to such differences. Whether it involves curriculum, counseling, food services, or community participation, efforts to promote school health programs will be problematic if they are not framed as contributing to the educational mission of the school.[49]

Reciprocally, school health personnel and advocates need to seek more aggressively the cooperation and resources of community agencies and media to support the school's mission. True, students spend one third of workweek hours in school, but they spend more than two thirds of their total hours—counting weekends, holidays, and summer vacations—outside school. Furthermore, some of the children and youth who most need health promotion have dropped out of school or have such high absenteeism that they will not be reached by school programs.

Education and Health: A Two-Way Relationship. The capsule findings presented in Table 10-3 provide a vivid reminder that health and social circumstances are inextricably tied to the school performance of school-age youth in the United States. This pattern is not unique to the U.S. For example, the 1994 Health of Young Australians report identifies child abuse, children living in poverty, and youth suicide among its top five concerns related to improving the health status of youth.[50]

In addition to documenting subjective priorities and concerns, results from a social assessment of school health promotion illuminates an important public message: that the cause-effect relationship between education and health is reciprocal.[51] The National Commission on the Role of the School and the Community in Improving Adolescent Health has declared that education and health are inextricably intertwined, that "poor health is an important reason why a large percentage of young people today are unable or not motivated to learn."[52] Furthermore, epidemiological research has consistently shown that the number of years of schooling completed by adolescents is a consistent and strong correlate to health status at any subsequent age.

Developmental Assets. Because schools cannot solve society's health and social problems alone, a meaningful commitment to the kind of community participation and collaboration highlighted in the social assessment phase of PRECEDE-PROCEED should remain a priority for planners seeking to nurture health-promoting schools. Findings emerging from research on social factors that influence children's health offer considerable promise for activating broad community support for children's health in general and school health in particular. For example, Benson and his co-workers observed that 40 quantifiable factors appeared to have a strong influence on the behavior of youth.[53] These 40 factors are called "developmental assets" because they represent the *positive* experiences, opportunities, and personal qualities of a given population.

The 40 developmental assets are grouped into two general categories: external and internal assets, as shown in Table 10-4. *External assets* refer to those factors made available through existing social circumstances in the community; they emerge as children come in contact with a community's interlocking systems of support and with the expectations of community members. Such assets appear consistent with the theory of social capital discussed in Chapter 8. *Internal assets* refer to the personal qualities of a child or adolescent—her or his personal values, commitment to learning, social competencies, and self-identity.

Using the Profiles of Student Life: Attitudes and Behaviors Survey, the Search Institute studied over 254,000 children in 460 communities and found a

---

TABLE 10-3

Selected social factors that influence school performance among students within the United States

- One third of children entering kindergarten are unprepared to learn—that is, they lack physical health, confidence, maturity, and general knowledge.[54]
- One child in four—fully 10 million—is at risk of failure in school because of social, emotional, and health handicaps.[55]
- During the 1980s, poverty among children in the United States worsened by 22%.[56]
- Between 12% and 22% of children experience mental, emotional, or behavioral disorders, yet few receive mental health services.[57]
- Twenty-two percent of ninth graders report carrying a weapon in the previous month.[58]
- Almost one fourth of high-school students report having seriously considered suicide in the previous year, and 8.6% made an attempt.[59]
- One fourth of 10–16 year olds report being assaulted or abused in the previous year.[60]
- Over 40% of children living below the poverty level have deficient intakes of iron.[61]
- On any given night, more than 100,000 children are homeless.[62]

SOURCE: Reprinted by permission of the publisher from *Health Is Academic: A Guide to Coordinated School Health Problems,* (p. 6), edited by Eva Marx and Susan Frelick Wooley, with Daphne Northrop, 1998, New York: Teachers College Press. © 1998 by Educational Development Center, Inc. All rights reserved.

TABLE 10-4

The Search Institute's 40 developmental assets

External Assets

Support

1. Family support—Family life provides high levels of love and support.
2. Positive family communication—Young person and her or his parent(s) communicate positively, and young person is willing to seek advice and counsel from parent(s).
3. Other adult relationships—Young person receives support from three or more nonparent adults.
4. Caring neighborhood—Young person experiences caring neighbors.
5. Caring school climate—School provides a caring, encouraging environment.
6. Parent involvement in schooling—Parent(s) are actively involved in helping young person succeed in school.

Empowerment

7. Community values youth—Young person perceives that adults in the community value youth.
8. Youth as resources—Young people are given useful roles in the community.
9. Service to others—Young person serves in the community one hour or more per week.
10. Safety—Young person feels safe at home, at school, and in the neighborhood.

Boundaries & Expectations

11. Family boundaries—Family has clear rules and consequences and monitors the young person's whereabouts.
12. School boundaries—School provides clear rules and consequences.
13. Neighborhood boundaries—Neighbors take responsibility for monitoring young people's behavior.
14. Adult role models—Parent(s) and other adults model positive, responsible behavior.
15. Positive peer influence—Young person's best friends model responsible behavior.
16. High expectations—Both parent(s) and teachers encourage the young person to do well.

Constructive Use of Time

17. Creative activities—Young person spends three or more hours per week in lessons or practice in music, theater, or other arts.
18. Youth programs—Young person spends three or more hours per week in sports, clubs, or organizations at school and/or in the community.
19. Religious community—Young person spends one or more hours per week in activities in a religious institution.
20. Time at home—Young person is out with friends "with nothing special to do" two or fewer nights per week.

(continued)

TABLE 10-4 *(continued)*

Internal Assets

Commitment to Learning

21. Achievement motivation—Young person is motivated to do well at school.

22. School engagement—Young person is actively engaged in learning.

23. Homework—Young person reports doing at least one hour of homework every school day.

24. Bonding to school—Young person cares about her or his school.

25. Reading for pleasure—Young person reads for pleasure three or more hours per week.

Positive Values

26. Caring—Young person places high value on helping other people.

27. Equality and social justice—Young person places high value on promoting equality and reducing hunger and poverty.

28. Integrity—Young person acts on convictions and stands up for her or his beliefs.

29. Honesty—Young person "tells the truth even when it is not easy."

30. Responsibility—Young person accepts and takes personal responsibility.

31. Restraint—Young person believes it is important not to be sexually active or to use alcohol or other drugs.

Social Competencies

32. Planning and decision making—Young person knows how to plan ahead and make choices.

33. Interpersonal competence—Young person has empathy, sensitivity, and friendship skills.

34. Cultural competence—Young person has knowledge of and comfort with people of different cultural/racial/ethnic backgrounds.

35. Resistance skills—Young person can resist negative peer pressure and dangerous situations.

36. Peaceful conflict resolution—Young person seeks to resolve conflict nonviolently.

Positive Identity

37. Person power—Young person feels he or she has control over "things that happen to me."

38. Self-esteem—Young person reports having a high self-esteem.

39. Sense of purpose—Young person reports that "my life has a purpose."

40. Positive view of personal future—Young person is optimistic about her or his personal future.

strong association between the level of developmental assets and level of health risk behaviors within a given population. Specifically, Table 10-5 shows that high levels of developmental assets are associated with fewer high-risk behaviors among youth and adolescents in Albuquerque and Minneapolis.

These data are consistent with findings from surveys administered across the United States. Based on nearly 100,000 survey questionnaires from different parts of the country, Figure 10-4 shows that youth in grades 6–12 with more assets are less likely than youth with fewer assets to engage in four different categories of risk behavior. Using data from the same sample, Figure 10-5 shows that higher levels of developmental assets are associated with higher levels of key educational goals, including both success in school and valuing diversity.

These patterns of consistency suggest that developmental assets may offer school health advocates a valuable tool for social assessment. For example, by

TABLE 10-5

40 developmental assets and high risk behavior patterns: Albuquerque and Minneapolis

	Patterns of High-Risk Behavior		Percentage of Youth Engaged in High-Risk Behavior Patterns			
Category	Definition	City	If 0–10 Assets	If 11–20 Assets	If 21–30 Assets	If 31–40 Assets
Alcohol	Has used alcohol three or more times in the past month or got drunk one or more times in the past two weeks	Albu. Minn.	53 63	35 52	16 24	4 12
Tobacco	Smokes one or more cigarettes every day or uses chewing tobacco frequently	Albu. Minn.	36 35	19 18	7 7	2 2
Sexual Intercourse	Has had sexual intercourse three or more times in lifetime	Albu. Minn.	38 44	28 32	17 17	5 4
Violence	Has engaged in three or more acts of fighting, hitting, injuring a person, carrying or using a weapon, or threatening physical harm in the past year	Albu. Minn.	65 69	41 49	21 31	7 10

NOTES: Albuquerque sample is a census of public-school students, grades six to twelve ($N = 12,440$). Minneapolis sample is a census of public-school students, grades seven, eight, ten, and eleven ($N = 5,235$).

SOURCE: *All Our Kids Are Our Kids,* (p. 57), by Peter L. Benson, 1997, San Francisco: Jossey-Bass. Copyright © 1997 Jossey-Bass Publishers Inc. Reprinted with permission from the publisher.

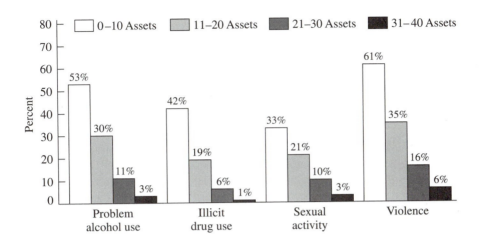

FIGURE 10-4

Developmental assets and high-risk behavior patterns: 100,000 U.S. public school students—1996–1997.

SOURCE: *Assets: The Magazine for Healthy Communities and Healthy Youth,* 1997, 2(4), 10.

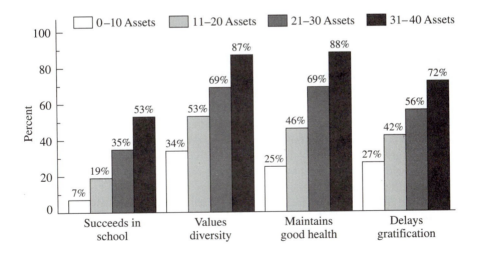

FIGURE 10-5

Developmental assets and positive attitudes/behaviors: 100,000 U.S. public school students—1996–1997.

SOURCE: *Assets: The Magazine for Healthy Communities and Healthy Youth,* 1997, 2(4), 10.

establishing a positive goal to increase their external developmental assets, community groups or coalitions, without having to focus on a specific health issue per se, would be making a commitment to influence social norms in a way that would positively affect virtually all aspects of a health-promoting school.

EPIDEMIOLOGICAL ASSESSMENT

Two Approaches. Planners can use one or a combination of two approaches to carry out the epidemiological assessment in the school setting. The first approach follows the same steps as those outlined in Chapter 3 and requires analysis of local health data to identify the current priority health problems of the children and youth served by the school(s) in question. Sources for such information might include health records from the school (school health nurse, school-based clinic), data from the local health department, social services agencies, the police department, the highway safety department, reports on pediatric health from local physicians or clinics, and special surveys covering the area or region. Information gathered through this procedure would enable planners to (1) increase the chances of detecting the incidence of extraordinary health events, (2) compare the prevalence of various health conditions within a given school population, (3) compare incidence or prevalence data of a given school population with those of the district, a neighboring region, the state, or perhaps the nation, and (4) compare the prevalence of risk factors among students with those of adults within the same community.

Because demographic characteristics, environmental conditions, and social norms together shape the unique health status of a given community, it is ideal for planners to use local data. However, local data on the health of children and youth are sometimes limited; even when available, these data are sometimes difficult to obtain or may have dubious reliability. In such cases, planners can consider a second approach—estimating the epidemiological assessment by calling attention to the leading health problems for school-age youth in the region, state, province, or nation. This approach has considerable merit, despite the obvious deficiency of not being able to detect problems unique to a given school or community.

Starfield and Budetti not only characterize the complexities inherent in gathering health information about school-age youth, they also remind us that our assessments will be accurate to the extent that we take into account perspectives from multiple sources:

> No one method is sufficient to describe the frequency of health problems in childhood. Some problems are known only to parents or families, because they are not manifested outside the home and are not brought in for medical care. Some are noticed only by teachers, who observe children under different circumstances than do their parents. Some health conditions become known only upon special questioning by qualified personnel, and some require a physician's assessment for their diagnosis.[63]

Problems are a matter of degree. For example, the rate of alcohol-related motor vehicle fatalities among teens in Community X may be 35% lower than the national average, but motor vehicle crashes remain the leading cause of death and injury for youth age 15–24 throughout the nation. A school need not await "higher than" status to address a nation's leading cause of death for youth. The same sentiment can be expressed for other problems, including teen pregnancy, sexually transmitted diseases (STDs), alcohol and drug use, smoking, obesity, and physical inactivity. There is merit in promoting a global view of the priority problems of any country. "Think globally, act locally," as the environmental movement's slogan says. "Peace starts at home," as child abuse prevention advocates say. Such a perspective emphasizes that the individual efforts of schools and communities are a part of a larger overall nationwide response to those health problems that threaten the health of all school-age youth.[64]

Health Problems and Health Behaviors. Virtually all reports listing health problems among school-age youth will mix health and health behaviors (as used within the context of the Precede-Proceed model). Such lists will include discrete health events such as motor vehicle–related deaths, suicide, asthma, sexually transmitted disease, but also include behaviors such as alcohol consumption, sexual activities, eating patterns, and levels of physical activity.

The temporal relationship between the behavior, such as not taking hypertensive medicine, and the health problem, such as stroke, is likely to be quite immediate for the 60-year-old hypertensive man. For the teenager, however, the relationship is more distal, as in the behavior smoking and the health problem lung cancer. Nevertheless, school health planners can justifiably consider smoking or chewing tobacco as health problems. Although the deleterious health effects of smoking and chewing, alcohol and drug abuse, high dietary fat intake, and lack of exercise may not be immediate, their effects on learning and school performance may be.[65] Furthermore, the more traditional application of linking a behavioral problem to a health problem remains useful because not all behavioral problems manifested by school-age youth are distant from health outcomes. For example, the time between drinking alcohol or taking drugs and an automobile fatality is tragically and dramatically short. Planned endeavors like the highly successful Project Graduation Program provide evidence that a focused, collaborative school and community effort can result in dramatic reductions in alcohol-related automobile fatalities that so often and tragically follow graduation celebrations.[66]

Emphasize Flexibility. The Precede model was never intended to be a rigid process. Rather, it was designed as an organizing framework to enable planners to sort through the complexities inherent in addressing individual and collective health behaviors. The results of that sorting should provide insights for developing or selecting effective health promotion strategies. The intermingling of health and behavioral problems for school-age youth puts both planners and PRECEDE to the test of flexibility. As the studies cited earlier in this chapter indicate, schools do not operate in a vacuum. They are part of a larger community, and their programs and activities have traditionally reflected the values, interests, and expectations of that community. Accordingly, social and epidemiological assessments will be richer if they include information about, and input from, the community as well as the school. Although amplifying the assessment in this way will demand more time and effort, the benefits are worth it.

BEHAVIORAL, ENVIRONMENTAL, AND EDUCATIONAL ASSESSMENT

What Is the Goal? Behavioral, environmental, and educational assessments in the school setting follow the same process described in Chapters 4 and 5. School health research consistently confirms the longstanding assumption that qualified teachers can greatly influence the health knowledge, attitudes, and practices of their students. Should teachers, then, be held accountable for manifest changes in students' behavior?

Because schools serve communities, school activities and teachers are clearly accountable to community members, especially parents. Parents should reasonably be able to expect their children to learn enough to matriculate each year. If fifth-grade pupils are supposed to be able to read at a certain rate and comprehend at a certain level, valid tests should be devised to ascertain those competencies. In health education, such tests would provide both a short-range evaluation of impact and evidence that progress has been made toward enabling future behavior conducive to health.

One should not expect measurable and convincing success in school health education programs that do not use epidemiological analysis to find and focus on specific problematic behaviors. Further, programs will be more successful if efforts are made to assess whether these behaviors, or suitable surrogates, increase, decrease, or remain the same over time.

Skills: A Legitimate Focus. School health educators are faced with the unique problem of linking health education activities to future behaviors, a problem confounded by the potential multitude of variables intervening over time. The Precede framework can be useful in attacking this problem, with the addition of skills as an intermediary between the behavioral construct and the educational constructs (predisposing, reinforcing, and enabling factors).

School health researchers, whose work has demonstrated positive outcomes, are unanimous in their conclusion that development of relevant cognitive skills, resistance to peer pressure, and social competence skills, in some combination, facilitates change or resistance to change.[67] Environmental changes through regulatory and policy actions further enhance the results achieved through educational processes. Figure 10-6 shows the Precede framework as it was adapted and

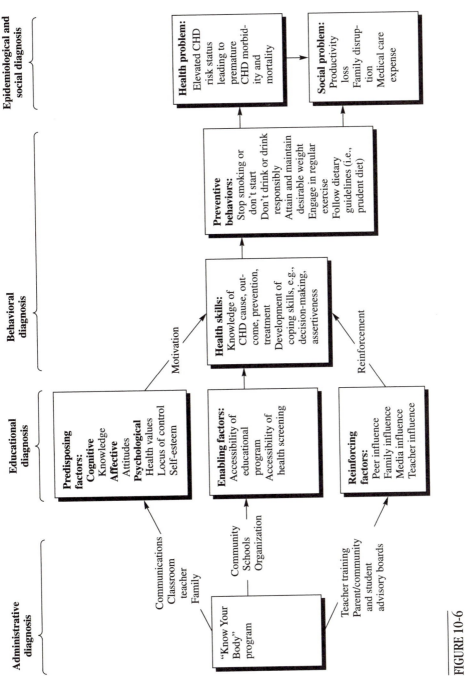

FIGURE 10-6

Application of the Precede model to the Know Your Body research project.

SOURCE: "Cardiovascular Risk Factor Prevention in Black School Children: Two-Year Results of the 'Know Your Body' Program," by P. J. Bush et al., 1989, *American Journal of Epidemiology, 129*(3), 466–482.

applied by Bush and her colleagues in a 5-year study to determine the impact of the Know Your Body Program on selected cardiovascular risk factors among students in grades 4–6 in the District of Columbia. Note that the predisposing, enabling, and reinforcing factors center on the skills linked to the target behaviors of smoking, drinking, weight management, and exercise. Note also that the program derived from the educational assessment required the participation of representative advisory boards and multiple actors, including parents.

Many investigators have applied PRECEDE in the school setting to a wide range of topics, from cardiovascular disease,[68] cancer,[69] and their attending risk factors to human sexuality,[70] infectious disease control,[71] general health promotion and wellness,[72] nutritional policy,[73] and seat-belt and helmet use,[74] and drinking.[75] Others have given particular attention to enabling and reinforcing factors contributing to a given behavior.[76]

Using Theory. Working knowledge of social, behavioral, and educational theories is essential for the expeditious identification of the predisposing, enabling, and reinforcing factors most likely to influence the skills or behaviors in question. One practical benefit from a command of theory is that it enables planners to be precise in their selection of questions to include in a survey, thus saving precious teacher time and minimizing the chance of using questionnaires that are overly burdensome. In this regard, practitioners will find Parcel's reviews of the major theories relevant to school health and school health education especially useful.[77]

In 1985, the smoking prevalence among adult male smokers (age 30–50) in China was nearly 75%.[78] Zhang and her colleagues[79] applied the steps of the Precede-Proceed model in developing a school-based approach to address the health problems associated with similar rates of smoking in Hangzhou, Zhejiang Province, People's Republic of China. The project was directed at students in primary grades 2 through 6; there were approximately 10,000 children in the intervention group and 10,000 in the reference group. Students in the former group received a special curriculum designed to enhance their knowledge about tobacco. Survey questions from stages of change theory had revealed that a substantial proportion of smokers were in the "precontemplative stage." This assessment led to the creation of a parental component for the intervention: Students brought home a personal letter to fathers expressing the child's hope that he would consider quitting to enhance the likelihood that the father would live a long life and provide wisdom and guidance as the child grew older. A community-wide campaign was also designed to heighten public awareness and public support for the program. Among the 6,843 fathers in the intervention group who were smokers, 90% reported quitting for at least 10 days; 64% were still not smoking at 20 days; 30% were not smoking by 60 days; and at 210 days, 11% were still not smoking. In the reference group, only 2% had quit after 10 days, and the quit rate was .02% after 210 days.

PRECEDE-PROCEED AND SCHOOLS: A HYPOTHETICAL CASE

The Greenfield School District provides administrative support for 10 elementary schools, 4 junior high schools, and 2 high schools. Greenfield is in a state that takes great pride in its system of public education. The state ranks in the top 15 in the nation in expenditures of state and local government resources for education expressed as percentage of personal income; the national percentage of adults 25 years of age and over who graduated from high school is 65%, the average in the state in which Greenfield lies is 71%. Within the state, however, Greenfield ranks below the mean on all of these indicators.

WHERE ARE WE?

The recently appointed superintendent of the Greenfield school district established a school health committee consisting of two students and representatives from the eight components that constitute a coordinated school health program. The committee was charged with the mission of developing a proposal to promote and maintain health in the district. The superintendent committed to support their recommendations "within reason." As a first step, the committee elected to conduct district-wide social and epidemiological assessments.[80] Their data were derived from (1) school records organized by school year and grade; (2) surveys and focus groups with school administrators, teachers, parents, students, and community gatekeepers; and (3) health statistics from school nurses, the local health department, and selected clinics and community health centers. The information obtained from the assessment was voluminous, far more than the committee imagined they would get and far more than they could handle.

WHAT MATTERS?

During the course of trying to sort the information into manageable chunks, a committee member who was a pediatrician in a health center in the Greenfield neighborhood known as the Heights asked if the information collected in her service area could be compared with data on the community in general. The Heights population is primarily low-income and about 60% Hispanic. The committee agreed that such a comparative approach made sense and would be a good way to focus their analysis. Table 10-6 compares information obtained from school records and some recent surveys. Table 10-7 provides a summary of the comparative concern expressed by school personnel and parents from both the Greenfield and Heights areas. Comparative data from the epidemiological assessment for the

TABLE 10-6

Hypothetical student social assessment information from school records and survey

Problem	Greenfield	Heights
Time missed last year (per student)		
Grades K–6 (mean days)	4.8	7.2
Grades 7–12 (mean days)	5.3	8.4
10th-graders who are 1 or more years below expected grade level (%)	17	32
Dropouts by grade (%)	5	29
Students who "don't eat breakfast"		
Grades K–6 (%)	5	15
Grades 7–12 (%)	25	34

students are displayed in Table 10-8 and student perceptions are summarized in Table 10-9.

The committee gathered additional information from various sources. For example, a health department report indicated that in the Greenfield area last year, there were 1,220 births to women under 20, 102 of which were out-of-wedlock births. This represented a 19% increase in out-of-wedlock births in the last 5 years. The rates were only slightly higher in the Heights. Also, a nutritionist on the committee presented preliminary data gathered by Greenfield's Cooperative Extension Agency, showing that the intake of total fat, saturated fat, and sodium among teenagers throughout Greenfield exceeded recommended levels. She said the Extension staff expressed their concern over poor nutritional habits, especially among younger students in the Heights area. They wondered if the general trend (both areas) of declining performance on aerobic fitness scores by students was related to low activity, poor nutrition, or both. Statistics from the state department of public safety indicated that there were 34 automobile fatalities among youth age 14–19 in the Greenfield area. Although the data did not allow for comparison between the Heights and the rest of Greenfield, 70% of the fatalities occurred among white male youth.

It may be impossible or inappropriate in some communities to compare data in this way, but the example serves to illustrate what the data-collection aspect of social and epidemiological assessment is supposed to do: get planners in a position to set priorities for programmatic action based on the best information available, including input from those for whom the program is intended.

Put yourself in the place of one of the Greenfield school health committee members. What do the data tell you? They certainly confirm what we suspect the pediatrician in the Heights already knew: the population she served bore a dispro-

TABLE 10-7

School personnel and parent response to the question "What concerns you most about your school?"

Greenfield

Availability of drugs

Low SAT scores

Lack of parental and community support

Mass media reporting only the problems

Questionable competence of some school personnel

Some of the building in disrepair

Need equipment (e.g., computers, afterschool recreational facilities)

Alcohol-related events (vandalism, auto crashes)

Heights

Violence and fighting

Increase in teen pregnancy

Absenteeism, truancy

Some students coming to school hungry

Student apathy

Low teacher morale

Poor facilities and very limited resources

portionate burden of both social and health problems. Regardless of the setting, questions of inequities and justice must be foremost in setting priorities.

The high rates of teen pregnancy are troubling because they trigger so many other problems: more low-birth-weight babies who are vulnerable to a host of immediate and future complications; mothers dropping out of school, severely compromising their future and significantly increasing their need for income maintenance and public assistance. Beyond the effects of the pregnancy, teen pregnancy implies a pattern of early unprotected sexual activity that indicates a risk of contracting STDs, including AIDS.

The tobacco, alcohol, and drug use rates are equally troubling for some of the same reasons. The short- and long-term health effects of these addictive substances are compounded by their devastating secondary effects: absenteeism; poor academic performance; loss of part-time employment; severe mood changes that can lead to depression, suicide, or violence; arrests; fines; detention; and auto crashes. Frequently, these secondary outcomes hurt others. Less spectacular in the attention they get, but problematic nonetheless, are the recurring issues of inadequate nutrition and concurrent declines in levels of physical activity.

TABLE 10-8

Epidemiological assessment: Comparative health problems in Greenfield and the Heights

Self-Reported Use	Greenfield (%)	Heights (%)
Smoking (grades 6–9)	17	22
Smoking (grades 10–12)	26	35
Alcohol (grades 6–9)	58	60
Alcohol (grades 10–12)	90	97
Drugs (grades 6–9)	29	24
Drugs (grades 10–12)	57	52
Regular seat-belt use (grades 10–12)	14	22

TABLE 10-9

Students' concerns in hypothetical case

Greenfield	Heights
Nothing to do	Nothing to do
Not enough parking spaces	Prejudice in some teachers
Cafeteria food not good	School no good
Too much drinking	Drinking and drugs
	Boring weekends

SORTING OUT THE COMPLEXITY

The committee has no shortage of problems to tackle and it is quite likely that they have more questions than they had at the outset. But, having completed this phase of PRECEDE, their questions will be qualitatively different. Questions like "What should we do as a committee to address our mission?" will be replaced by insightful questions generated by thoughtful planning, like "Here are five documented health problems affecting the children in our schools, and they need attention. Which ones are the most important, and in which ones can we make a difference?"

As the committee digs into these questions and the issues associated with them, other confounding issues will surface, such as the need for more resources, the lack of community and parent involvement and support, and attitudes that school is boring and is no good. When planners come face to face with the interplay of these very real social, behavioral, institutional, economic, and emotional factors, the complexity of it all can be overwhelming and, therefore, crippling.

Yet, it is the complexity of this challenge that calls on the ultimate strength of the Precede model: its demonstrated ability to analyze those complexities and then use the results of that analysis to develop robust programs calling for multiple strategies from multiple sectors. One might say that attention to PRECEDE is good prevention, in that it can help save the school health planner from the illusion of expecting great outcomes after making changes in only one component area.

CAN THE LITERATURE HELP US?

We can imagine planners on the Greenfield school health committee being encouraged by the findings in the literature that even the most complicated problems can be effectively addressed through a well-planned, school-based effort. Vincent and his co-workers[81] have demonstrated how a program with school, community, and church support reduced teen pregnancy in a predominantly black, low-income, South Carolina county. Over a 4-year period, teen pregnancy declined over 50% in the intervention county; the study also demonstrates a diffusion beyond the school. There were four comparison sites: one in the same county and three in separate counties. Pregnancy rates in the comparison site in the same county declined approximately 22% while the pregnancy rates increased in all three comparison counties. The researchers could not identify what element or combinations of elements accounted for the changes, including perhaps increased use of contraceptives. Nevertheless, the Greenfield planner's review of the Vincent study might call attention to a subtle but important point common in most successful programs: Credible sources *outside* the school act as a major force for change. Perhaps success is driven by the resources these outside interests bring to the problem, their credibility, or some combination of the two. As a result, the Greenfield school health committee might seek consultation from both the state education agency and faculty with school health expertise from a nearby university.

THE APPLICATION OF PROCEED

Have you ever heard the following rationale as the reason for a new idea or program floundering or not getting off the ground? "It was just too far ahead of its time!" The implication is that the idea or program in question was too innovative. Either the timing was off or resources were limited; whatever the reason, the decision makers in authority were not ready to take action. The Proceed process reviewed in Chapter 6, however, assumes that the health education or health promotion program planned in the Precede process is indeed an innovation. Furthermore, PROCEED acknowledges the reality that matters of timing, resources, or other organizational or administrative factors, including policies, must be carefully assessed as a part of the strategic planning process; failure to take these institutional and environmental forces into account could lead to implementation delays or failure. In other words, failure stems not from innovation per se but from problems of planning and implementation.

RESOURCES

All the elements of PROCEED apply to the school setting. Time constraints can be a limiting factor for all aspects of a comprehensive school health program. The school day is finite. Curricula for math, science, language, history, health, physical education, art, music, and countless other meritorious subjects or activities must compete for a part of that time. Furthermore, school or district policies or even state codes may require that certain subjects receive a specific portion of the school day.

Organizational policies can also influence program implementation. For example, while the allocation of professional and support staff obviously depends on the school budget, it is sometimes influenced by regulations or policies that govern the personnel ceiling. In some instances, such ceilings or hiring freezes may prohibit new personnel even if economic resources can be obtained.

Whether a program is new or just a logical extension of an ongoing effort, the question of budget is inescapable. Nothing is free. All aspects of a proposed program—personnel needs, space, educational materials, health services resources and equipment, teacher and staff training—are inextricably tied to budget considerations. Although health planners should not be paralyzed by budget constraints, they must be practical about costs when designing an intervention.

The planners' Proceed task then is to make a careful assessment of time, personnel, materials, and other resources needed for the proposed program, and then juxtapose those needs with two things: (1) the administrative and organizational realities of current operations in the school and (2) an assessment of the potential for making changes in those administrative and organizational elements that may bar program implementation. The identification of program needs should be a natural outgrowth of the Precede planning process. Further, while the assessment of current administrative, organizational, and policy factors can by no means be taken for granted, the steps outlined in Chapter 6 can be readily applied by members of the planning group. The question of assessing the potential for influencing change in selected administrative, organizational, or policy elements merits further consideration here.

"Within Reason." Let us return to the Greenfield scenario. Recall that the recently appointed superintendent of schools called for the formation of the school health committee, charged them with a health promotion mission, and promised support "within reason." Did "within reason" refer to resources? To public opinion? Both? The expression of support is a signal that health is high on the superintendent's agenda, and the committee would be well advised to taken prudent steps to

not only keep it there but elevate it. This is where the principles of community participation, highlighted throughout this book and incorporated in the formation of the Greenfield school health committee, are so critical.

PUBLIC OPINION

Many things influence the decisions school officials make. One of the most important is community opinion. The most obvious example is the loud and persistent opposition to sex education. Yet, in most cases, it is not the loud outcry that influences a decision on an innovative program, it is quiescence. Regardless of how good a program may be, decision makers can easily withhold support if they believe that constituents do not care one way or another about it. An uninformed, quiescent community is a barrier to change. The committee should make a concerted effort to apprise parents and local leaders and involve them in planning and implementing the proposed program.[82] This process can ensure that the community committee members understand the important problems the program is designed to mitigate. Creating a groundswell of interest and eventually support will legitimize the exploration of creative ways to obtain the resources for the program and will help implementers overcome administrative problems. One sure way to squelch an administrator's enthusiasm for school health activities is to propose programs that require large budgetary increases for personnel and materials without an accompanying plan outlining a realistic means to meet those increases.

USING POLICY

Policy issues also need special attention. A new health education curriculum, however creative and well-conceived, would by itself be no match for the problems in Greenfield. Lohrmann and Fors[83] are among many investigators whose work addresses this reality. In an analysis of recommendations for school-based education to prevent drug abuse, they conclude that many of the factors influencing adolescent drug use cannot be affected by exposure to a preventive curriculum. They call for greater attention to policy changes, teacher training, and special programs for high-risk children, as well as greater participation from social institutions outside the school.

Parcel and his colleagues[84] carried out a 3-year study directed at influencing the dietary habits and exercise behaviors of third- and fourth-grade children. The program, "Go For Health," incorporated classroom instruction, school food services, and physical education as intervention components and was consistent with the expanded concept of school health programs cited earlier in this chapter.

However, the unique aspect of this study was not the comprehensive nature of components for intervention. Rather, it was the detailed attention paid to salient issues in the Proceed process—that is, those organizational factors and dynamics that either facilitate or hinder implementation. Parcel's group made the assumption, based on prior work done by Charter and Jones,[85] that program changes in schools generally occur sequentially in four steps: first, with institutional commitment, followed by changes in policies, then alterations in the roles of staff, and finally changes in the students' learning activities. These four phases of change are illustrated in Figure 10-7. Note how looking at the change process from this organizational and policy perspective creates a natural inventory of change strategies to addresses personnel and resource needs.

SUMMARY

This chapter tests the applicability of the Precede framework to school health. A review of the current status of school health and school health education reveals a vigorous field in which the traditional innovation and diversity in the classroom has been strengthened by greater involvement with the community. Policy innovations together with remarkable research advances are beginning to give school health the national and international attention it deserves.

In developing school health programs, one must focus on the needs of the school and community when using PRECEDE and PROCEED. One must also establish a clear relationship between the quality of both community and school life. The innovative application of developmental assets is a positive means to activate community participation and support for roles the school can play in promoting community health. The analytic strength of the Precede process is maximized when applied within the context of the expanded concept of a coordinated approach to school health promotion. It is also important to address the administrative, organizational, and policy factors inherent in schools that can lead to severe problems or can facilitate program implementation.

Even though outcome evaluation research in school health is the job of the academic researchers, school health personnel and teachers should attend to the critically important task of monitoring the quality of their programs, curricula, and instructional practices. Where feasible, they should also try to measure the effects of their programs on students' knowledge, attitudes, intentions, and self-reported health practices.

EXERCISES

1. What is the ultimate goal of schools, and how does that goal influence the school health planning process?

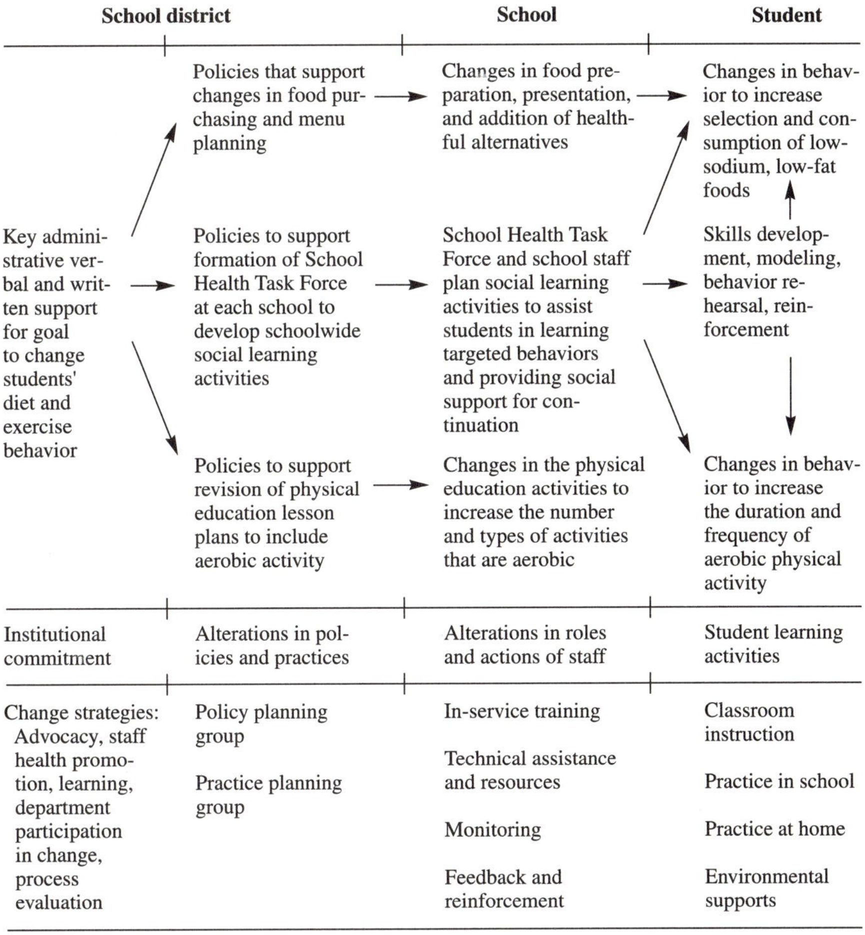

School district	School	Student
Policies that support changes in food purchasing and menu planning →	Changes in food preparation, presentation, and addition of healthful alternatives →	Changes in behavior to increase selection and consumption of low-sodium, low-fat foods ↑
Key administrative verbal and written support for goal to change students' diet and exercise behavior → Policies to support formation of School Health Task Force at each school to develop schoolwide social learning activities	School Health Task Force and school staff plan social learning activities to assist students in learning targeted behaviors and providing social support for continuation →	Skills development, modeling, behavior rehearsal, reinforcement ↓
Policies to support revision of physical education lesson plans to include aerobic activity →	Changes in the physical education activities to increase the number and types of activities that are aerobic	Changes in behavior to increase the duration and frequency of aerobic physical activity
Institutional commitment	Alterations in policies and practices	Alterations in roles and actions of staff	Student learning activities
Change strategies: Advocacy, staff health promotion, learning, department participation in change, process evaluation	Policy planning group Practice planning group	In-service training Technical assistance and resources Monitoring Feedback and reinforcement	Classroom instruction Practice in school Practice at home Environmental supports

FIGURE 10-7

Model for planned change: Go For Health.

SOURCE: Parcel, B. Simons-Morton, & Kolbe, "Health Promotion: Integrating Organizational Change and Student Outcomes and Self-Reported Behavior," 1988, *Health Education Quarterly, 15,* 435–450.

2. Traditionally, the school health program has been described as consisting of three complementary components: instruction, services, and the school environment. Recently, an expanded concept of the school health program has emerged. Even though the two share commonalities, describe the advantages of the expanded model.

3. The productivity of school health researchers in the 1980s was substantial both in quality and quantity; as a result, we can now say with confidence that well-planned school health and school health education, carried out by qualified staff, make a difference. Using the summary information in Table 10-1, interpret the nature of the intervention strategies used in the NHLBI studies in light of the components and rationale of the expanded concept of school health promotion.

4. Explain how national- and state-level school health policy can be beneficial in promoting programs at the local level.

5. Review the strategy employed by CDC in the development of the national guidelines *School Health to Prevent the Spread of AIDS.* What lessons learned from that effort can be directly applied by school health planners at the local level?

6. Using the data collected by the school health committee in Greenfield:
   a. Give an example of how a program or activity, generated by *each component* in the expanded model, could be targeted to address one or more of the problems identified.
   b. Use PROCEED to identify potential administrative, organizational, or policy barriers and give an example of how each might be addressed.
   c. List two process outcomes and two impact outcomes that could be assessed for each component program example you gave in (a).

NOTES AND CITATIONS

1. World Health Organization, 1996, frontmatter. See also World Health Organization, 1997.

2. American Council of Life Insurance, 1998.

3. The numbers and proportion of school-based people is larger if one includes colleges, universities, and the rapidly growing number of preschool and day-care centers. The principles discussed in this chapter apply similarly to college and to preschool health promotion. For applications of PRECEDE-PROCEED in college and university settings, see Bonaguro, 1981; Calabrio, Weltge, Parnell, Kouzekanani, & Ramirez, 1998; Hofford & Spelman, 1996; Hunnicutt, Perry-Hunnicutt, Newman, Davis, & Crawford, 1993; Kraft, 1988; Lee, 1992; Melby, 1986; Neef, Scutchfield, Elder, & Bender, 1991; Ostwald & Rothenberger, 1985; Shine, Silva, & Weed, 1983; B. G. Simons-Morton, Brink, Parcel, et al., 1989; B. G. Simons-Morton, Brink, Simons-Morton, et al., 1989; Sloane & Zimmer, 1992; J. R. Weiss, Wallerstein, & MacLean, 1992; Zapka & Averill, 1979; Zapka & Dorfman, 1982; Zapka & Mamon, 1982; Zapka & Mamon, 1986. Applications of PRECEDE-PROCEED in preschool settings can be found in Huang, Green, & Darling, 1997; Keintz, Fleisher, & Rimer, 1994; Lafontaine & Bedard, 1997; Mesters, Meertens, Crebolder, & Parcel, 1993; D. B. Reed, 1996; Wortel, de Geus, Kok, & van Woerkum, 1994; Wortel, de Vries, & de Geus, 1995.

4. Carnegie Council on Adolescent Development, 1989; National Commission on the Role of the School and the Community in Improving Adolescent Health, 1990. These reports also note the importance of integrating and coordinating school and community approaches. A new National Committee on Partnerships for Children's Health has been funded by the U.S. Centers for Disease Control to connect colleges, children, and communities. See Deutch, 1998.

5. American Physical Education Association, 1935.

6. Cornacchia, Olsen, & Nickerson, 1988; Creswell & Newman, 1997; Pollock, 1987; Pollock & Middleton, 1994.

7. L. Kolbe, 1986.

8. Allensworth & Kolbe, 1987.

9. Baranowski et al., 1993; Institute of Medicine, 1997; Kolbe et al., 1985; Shea et al., 1993. G. C. Frank, Vadin, & Martin, 1987, concluded, "The current challenge for child nutrition programs is to seek common threads with the other components of school health programs and to provide primary prevention to forestall chronic disease progression. The PRECEDE framework may provide the most relevant model for such a coordinated effort" (p. 451). For an application of PRECEDE in developing a national nutrition and cancer education curriculum, see Light & Contento, 1989.

10. Blair et al., 1993; Ewart, Young & Hagberg, 1998; Shea et al., 1994; Stewart, 1996. For applications of PRECEDE-PROCEED in child exercise assessments and programs, see Bush et al., 1987; B. G. Simons-Morton, Parcel, O'Hara, et al., 1988; S. Stewart, 1996.

11. Mason & McGinnis, 1985, p. 299. The continued development of interdisciplinary and intersectoral approaches to community and school planning and evaluation is seen, for example, in Barnett, Niebuhr, & Baldwin, 1998; Hoover & Schwartz, 1992; Papenfus & Bryan, 1998; Probart, McDonnell, & Anger, 1997; Rockwell & Buck, 1995. M. L. Wong et al., 1992, propose how PRECEDE-PROCEED can be applied in assuring intersectoral and interdisciplinary planning for both the behavioral and environmental aspects of health promotion at the same time that it identifies "a highly focused subset of factor as targets for intervention" (p. 341).

12. Basch, 1984; Basch, Eveland, & Portnoy, 1986; D'Onofrio, 1989; Parcel et al., 1989. For a discussion of how other sectors view the attempts of the health sector to get them to account for their policies on the basis of health impact as "health empirialism," see Ratner, Green, Frankish, Chomik, & Larsen, 1997.

13. Marx & Wooley, 1998. This book provides the scientific and theoretical rationale for the eight components of a coordinated school health program. Although the individual chapters were written by recognized scholars and practitioners, the overall framework and organization of the book was grounded on input from those representing over 50 national organizations in the United States whose constituencies have a stake in at least one of the eight components.

14. S. L. Becker et al., 1989; Hahn, Simpson, & Kidd, 1996; McKay, Levine, & Bone, 1985; Perry et al., 1988, 1989.

15. Lohrmann & Wooley, 1998.

16. Joint Committee on National Health Education Standards, 1995.

17. Green, Heit, Iverson, Kolbe, & Kreuter, 1980.

18. Connell, Turner, & Mason, 1985. In this reference, the whole issue of the journal is devoted to the School Health Education Evaluation.

19. T. J. Glynn, 1989. This article describes the 15 school-based smoking prevention studies supported by the National Cancer Institute (NCI). In the same issue, eight studies of smokeless tobacco prevention trials supported by NCI are described by G. M. Boyd & Glover, 1989. Also in this issue, the American Cancer Society's and NCI's application of the Precede model to a school nutrition and cancer education curriculum is described in Light & Contento, 1989.

20. Stone, Perry, & Luepker, 1989. All work cited in Table 10-1 appears in separate articles in this reference's issue of *Health Education Quarterly*. Another study supported by the National Heart, Lung and Blood Institute, under a separate program of grants was Heart Smart, an extension of the Bogalusa Heart Study in Louisiana, which applied the Precede model in its design. See Downey et al., 1988.

21. In the Nader study, the family is the primary locus of change rather than the school and its environment, which serve a supportive role. See Broyles, Nader, & Elder, 1996; P. R. Nader et al., 1989.

22. For commentary on these studies, see Best, 1989.

23. Stone et al., 1996.

24. P. R. Nader et al., 1996.

25. Resnicow, Robinson, & Frank, 1996.

26. Gupta, Mehortra, Arora, & Saran, 1991.

27. Vartiainen & Puska, 1987.

28. P. R. Nader et al., 1989; Perry et al., 1996.

29. Metropolitan Life Foundation, 1988.

30. See page 463 in Nader et al., 1996.

31. Downey, Frank, et al., 1987. For other details of the implementation and follow-up evaluations of this extensive application of PRECEDE-PROCEED, see Arbeit et al., 1992; Downey, Butcher, et al., 1987; Downey, Cresanta, & Berenson, 1989; C. C. Johnson, Powers, Bao, Harsha, & Berenson, 1994; Walter et al., 1987.

32. Aaro, Laberg, & Wold, 1995; Aaro, Wold, Kannas, & Rimpela, 1986; A. J. C. King & Coles, 1992; Nutbeam, Aaro, & Wold, 1991.

33. J. G. Ross & Gilbert, 1985.

34. "Results from the National Adolescent Student Health Survey," 1989. See also Children's Defense Fund, 1990; Krolnick, 1989; National Center for Children in Poverty, 1990; U.S. Department of Education, Office of Educational Research and Improvement, 1988; Zill & Rogers, 1988.

35. Lovato & Allensworth, 1989. See also Koshel, 1990; Lovick & Stern, 1988.

36. Kann, Collins, et al., 1995; Kann, Warren, & Kolbe, 1995; Lowry, Kann, & Kolbe, 1996.

37. *Healthy people 2000,* 1991.

38. Mutter, 1988.

39. Connell, Turner, & Mason, 1985.

40. State School Health Education Project, 1981. See also Carnegie Council on Adolescent Development, 1989; Deutch, 1998; National Commission on Excellence in Education, 1983; National Commission on the Role of the School and the Community, 1990.

41. World Health Organization, 1997; World Health Organization and United Nations Children's Fund, 1986.

42. Corcoran & Portnoy, 1989.

43. American College Health Association, 1986; American College of Physicians, 1989; National Professional School Health Education Organizations, 1984; Parcel, Muraskin, & Endert, 1988; P. Smith, 1989.

44. Centers for Disease Control, 1988. The President's Commission on the HIV Epidemic, in its 1988 report, also concluded that the school's contribution to AIDS education should take place in the context of comprehensive school health education: *Report of the Presidential Commission on the Human Immunodeficiency Virus Epidemic,* 1988.

45. Kolbe et al., 1988.

46. Ibid., p. 11. See also "Guidelines for School Health Programs Promote Lifelong Healthy Eating," 1996; "Guidelines on School Heath Programs to Prevent Tobacco Use and Addiction," 1994.

47. Kann et al., 1995, p. 291.

48. For indicators of these and other criteria for social, epidemiological, behavioral, environmental, organizational, and educational indicators, see Kolbe, 1989.

49. Green, 1988a; MacDonald & Green, 1994.

50. Australian Health Ministers Advisory Council, 1994.

51. Green, Simons-Morton, & Potvin, 1997; Winkleby, Fortmann, & Barrett, 1990.

52. National Commission on the Role of the School and the Community, 1990, p. 3.

53. See pages 54–76 in Benson, 1997. The Profiles of Student Life: Attitudes and Behaviors Survey yields measures of the 40 developmental assets and self-reported behavioral risk factors. The

survey instrument is proprietary and can be obtained by contacting the Search Institute, 700 South Third Street, Suite 210, Minneapolis, MN 55415; www.search.org; (612) 376–8955.

54. Boyer, 1991.

55. Dryfoos, 1994.

56. U.S. Department of Education and U.S. Department of Health and Human Services, 1993.

57. Costello, 1989; Hoagwood, 1995.

58. Kann, Warren, et al., 1995.

59. Ibid.

60. Finkelhor & Kziuba-Leatherman, 1994.

61. Pollitt, 1994.

62. U.S. Department of Education and U.S. Department of Health and Human Services, 1993.

63. Starfield & Budetti, 1985, p. 833.

64. Kolbe & Gilbert, 1984.

65. Kolbe et al., 1985.

66. Maine Department of Educational and Cultural Services, 1985.

67. Chung & Elias, 1996; R. I. Evans & Raines, 1982; Flay, 1987; Gager, Kress, & Elias, 1996; D. M. Murray, Johnson, Luepker, & Mittelmark, 1984; Schinke, 1982.

68. Arbiet et al., 1992; P. J. Bush, Zuckerman, Taggart, et al., 1989; Downey, Butcher, et al., 1987; Downey, Cressanta, & Berensen, 1989; Downey, Frank, et al., 1987; Fors et al., 1989; C. C. Johnson, Powers, Bao, Harsha, & Berenson, 1994; Meagher & Mann, 1990; Parcel, Simons-Morton, et al., 1989; Walter et al., 1987; Walter & Wynder, 1989; Zuckerman et al., 1989.

69. C. Boyd, 1993; Contento, Kell, Keiley, & Corcoran, 1992; Iverson & Scheer, 1982; Light & Contento, 1989.

70. Alteneder, 1994; Alteneder, Price, Telljohann, Didion, & Locher, 1992; de Haes, 1990; Edet, 1991; Jensen, 1997; Mathews, Everett, Binedell, & Steinberg, 1995; Nozu, Iwai, & Watanabe, 1995; Palti et al., 1997; Rubison & Baillie, 1981; Schaalma et al., 1996; Walter & Vaughan, 1993.

71. Calabro, Keltge, Parness, Kouzekanani, & Ramirez, 1998; Ekeh & Adeniyi, 1989; Lafontaine & Bedard, 1997; Zapka & Averill, 1979.

72. Bonaguro, 1981; R. R. Cottrell, Capwell, & Brannan, 1995a, 1995b; Simpson & Pruitt, 1989; Sutherland, Pittman-Sisco, Lacher, & Watkins, 1987; J. R. Weiss, Wallerstein, & MacLean, 1995.

73. G. C. Frank, Vaden, & Martin, 1987.

74. Farley, 1987; Farley, Haddad, & Brown, 1996; Jones & Macrina, 1993.

75. Fawcett et al., 1997; Higgins & McDonald, 1992; Hofford & Spelman, 1996; Hunnicutt, Perry-Hunnicutt, Newman, Davis, & Crawford, 1993; Kraft, 1988; Lipnickey, 1986; Newman, Martin, & Weppner, 1982; B. G. Simons-Morton, Brink, Simons-Morton et al., 1989; Stivers, 1994; Vertinsky & Mangham, 1991; Villas, Cardenas, & Jameson, 1994.

76. P. J. Bush, Zuckerman, Theiss, et al., 1989.

77. L. K. Bartholomew, Parcel, & Kok, 1998; Grunbaum, Gingiss, & Parcel, 1995; Parcel, 1984; Parcel et al., 1995; Parcel, Eriksen, et al., 1989; Parcel, Green, & Bettes, 1989; Parcel et al., 1991; Parcel, Simons-Morton, & Kolbe, 1988.

78. Xin-Zhi, Zhao-guang, & Dan-yang, 1987.

79. Methods and preliminary results from this study were provided during a World Bank consultation with the Chinese Ministry of Health in Hangzhou, Zhejiang Province. Information is presented here with the permission of the principle investigator, Zhang De-Xiu, M.D., Center for Health Education, Zhejiang Hygiene and Epidemic Prevention Center.

80. The strategy of conducting the social and epidemiological assessment together is often strategic and practical because it encourages those planners who typically have a strong health bias to be mindful of linking health problems to salient social problems.

81. Vincent, Clearie, & Schluchter, 1987.

82. A method for identifying community leadership to participate in planning and guiding the implementation of specific health programs has been developed in the context of a Precede application in North Carolina: Michielutte & Beal, 1990. For software to guide the process of identifying community leadership and participants in planning, see Gold, Green, & Kreuter, 1997.

83. Lohrmann & Fors, 1986.

84. Parcel, Simons-Morton, & Kolbe, 1988.

85. Charter & Jones, 1973.

Chapter 11

Applications in Health Care Settings[1]

Nowhere is the evidence stronger for the efficacy of health education and promotion than in the health care setting.[2] As in schools, work sites, and other community settings, health promotion planning in hospitals, clinics, physicians' offices, pharmacies, and other health care settings can be strengthened by the combined educational and environmental approach of PRECEDE and PROCEED, linking clinical and other community or population-based programs. This calls for several departures from the medical model that dominates health care planning in these settings, each of which will constitute a section of this chapter.

The first departure for clinical practitioners is to recognize the need, the missed opportunities, and the effectiveness they can have in improving the lives of their patients. The first section of this chapter will examine these considerations from the perspective of clinical practice, with the understanding that acute care will always take precedence in one's practice insofar as acute cases are urgent and call directly on the practitioner's skills and resources.

A second departure called for is a break from the traditional medical approach of concentrating health care diagnosis and planning on the individual patient. The Precede-Proceed model works best when applied to a population of patients or potential patients. This population-based or epidemiological approach will be outlined in the second section of the chapter.

The educational and environmental approach requires a third departure from the traditional medical model as practiced in most health care settings. It calls for a greater emphasis on self-care and patient-centered authority and responsibility for planning and controlling the health care regimen. This break from medical tradition is not a break from nursing tradition. The earliest philosophies of nursing from Florence Nightingale to the present have emphasized self-care.[3] Health care providers need to emphasize the active and informed engagement of patient decision and control from the earliest stages of seeking diagnosis to the postmedical or postsurgical self-monitoring and maintenance of lifestyle and environmental changes. The second part of this chapter offers a protocol for applying the

417

Precede-Proceed model to this style of health care. The third section examines how the same principles of behavioral and educational assessment apply to health care professionals and other personnel as apply to populations of patients.

The fourth section of this chapter addresses the health care system itself, recognizing that the culture, environment, and professional behavior of health care settings must change if they are to support health promotion and self-care objectives. In this section, we apply the Precede-Proceed model to the assessment of behavioral and environmental factors in the health care setting that can be changed through the education of health care providers and through environmental reforms of the system itself. Empowerment and patients' rights are important considerations for managed care firms seeking more satisfied and effective consumer partners and for government-sponsored care that seeks a population less dependent on the medical system. This idea does not appeal to potential consumers, however, when it is presented by the government, health insurance companies, or HMOs as a matter of patient or consumer responsibility for appropriate use of health services. The question the taxpayer or consumer reasonably asks is "Responsible to whom?" A recent study reveals that subjects' perceived control over their health, rather than their sense of responsibility, had greater impact on health-related behaviors like breast self-examination, exercise, and membership in a health promotion program.[4]

Finally, we seek to pull the strands of the last several chapters together by examining the combination of environmental factors in the community that can support the objectives of the health care system in preventing and controlling illness and promoting health.

HEALTH PROMOTION AS A PRIORITY OF CLINICAL CARE[5]

When one considers the range and pervasiveness of influences beyond the biomedical on lifestyle, behavioral, and health-related environments, one must wonder whether clinical and office-based practice is a reasonable place to invest health promotion resources. Lifestyle and behavior are influenced daily by psychological, social, cultural, occupational, recreational, economic, and political factors. Exposure of people to these influences shape the attitudes, beliefs, and values that consciously drive their personal choices of health-directed behavior, such as seeking an immunization, a physical examination, a low-fat food, or a condom. These purposeful actions are usually time limited and reasonably responsive to clinical or office-based intervention. Even so, one's history of exposure to the social and other environmental conditions also shape one's lifestyle, associated with enduring patterns of unconsciously health-related behavior such as food consumption, physical activity, ways of coping with stress, aggression, risk taking, and using alcohol and other drugs. Because such patterns of living are often deeply rooted in one's upbringing and social relationships, they resist intervention.

DEFINITIONS

We return, then, to the distinction between behavior and lifestyle developed in Chapter 1. There we defined *behavior* as a discrete act or series of acts. When a person acts consciously for health improvement or health maintenance, we may refer to such behavior as *health-directed. Lifestyle* is a pattern of behavior developed over time as a result of cultural, social, and economic conditions, usually without a specific purpose but with health consequences. Changing a lifestyle means calling on a much wider range of resources and influences than the average health care provider has at his or her disposal in relation to an individual patient. Indeed, many individuals themselves may be willing and able to make significant lifestyle changes only once or twice in a lifetime.[6]

To avoid a false dichotomy, we should view these distinctions between behavior and lifestyle as a continuum. At the extreme of simplistic behavior is the discrete, singular act that an individual performs to satisfy a specific need or drive. A patient's "**compliance**" with each step in a set of instructions for taking a urine sample, for example, illustrates how a complex behavior can be broken down into discrete actions. The specificity of instructions for the proper taking of some medications or to follow a low-sodium diet reflect the ways health care workers often disassemble complex behavior into discrete acts. The complex behavior with a specific purpose (e.g., reducing fat in the diet to lose weight) lies somewhere in the middle of the continuum. The combination of several of these complex behaviors as expressed in everyday living represents lifestyle, at the other end of the continuum. For example, daily consumption of high-fat foods from vending machines at work is part of a lifestyle related to work stress. The working circumstances may preclude time for a more nutritious lunch. This, in turn, results in fatigue at the end of the day and a preference to sit in front of the television set with a beer, a cigarette, or some potato chips rather than going out to exercise.

THE OPPORTUNITY

Health care workers can serve as powerful instigators and reinforcers of many specific behavioral changes. If sustained and integrated into an individual's pattern of living, these changes may in turn cause a change in lifestyle. The literature suggests that health care workers may reasonably expect to play a major role in strengthening the motivation and capabilities of their patients to change specific health-related behaviors; however, they should expect to play only a supporting role in the more complex, durable, and deep-seated lifestyle issues related to health. This supporting role should not be regarded as trivial or unnecessary; without support and encouragement from health care personnel, many patients will fail to start or to continue the process of change, and some of the critical community efforts to influence the broader determinants of lifestyles will falter.[7]

In Germany, physicians have a unique opportunity to enable prevention. They are expected to work in their office, at the group level within or across practices, and at the community level in cooperation with relevant agencies and associations.[8] Thus, they may expect a relatively important role as enablers and reinforcers in lifestyle behavior change.

Clinical Credibility. The opportunity for health care workers to play a part in the change process relates first to their credibility as authoritative sources of health information. Surveys asking people what was the most important source of information in their decision to change a particular health-directed behavior usually find that they single out their personal physician[9] and would respond to physician recommendations for health-related behavioral change. This tendency shows signs of increasing differentiation, however, among types of behavior and dimensions of lifestyle, as well as between sources of information and sources of help. In the most recent Canadian Health Promotion Survey, for example, respondents who reported specific improvements in their health practices or lifestyle were asked which of a list of influences helped them make the change. Increased knowledge of health risks ranked highest (67%). Only about half of those indicating increased knowledge, however, cited advice or support from a health professional as their source of influence. The percentages who cited professional advice or support ranged from a high of 69% among those who changed their cholesterol level or their blood pressure to a low of 22% for those who reduced their alcohol intake or increased their exercise.[10]

Access to Teachable Moments. Health care workers can also influence change through access to "teachable moments" or times when patients are particularly receptive to health care advice. Over 78% of the population in the United States, and a similar proportion in Canada, visits a physician at least once a year; the average North American has contact with a physician more than five times per year.[11] About 58% of visits to doctors' offices are return visits. Of course, this is far less than the time children spend in schools, adults spend in the workplace, and both spend in front of television sets, so the physician's office cannot compete with school health promotion programs, workplace wellness programs, or mass media programs for exposure time. The credibility and authority factor makes up for some of this. What matters more is that patients seek out health care workers at a time of heightened concern about their susceptibility and the potential severity of their condition. Fully 40% to 60% of patients seeing their physicians are basically well, but worried, providing enormous potential for prevention efforts by physicians.[12] According to the Health Belief Model,[13] this should make them more attentive, receptive, and responsive, to change than they might be in the school, workplace, or home. A small proportion of patients responding to recommendations from health care workers translates to a large number at the population level. For example, 8% of physicians consider themselves successful in changing the smoking habits 75% or more of the time.[14] At a practice level, this would be interpreted by most physicians as failure, but at the population level, this seemingly small effect may have a more significant impact on reducing smoking-related morbidity than most of the more purely medical interventions the physician might apply at later stages in relation to the same morbidities.

Public Interest. The recent wave of health-consciousness in the general population has enlarged the inherent interest of patients in seeking the counsel of health care workers to help them change health-directed behavior or to cope with lifestyle issues threatening their health. Today, adults who consult physicians demand more preventive medicine and health education than in the past.[15] Some studies show that patients seek and are more satisfied when they find greater physician participation in health promotion activities.[16] Further, in one half of the visits in which preventive services are provided, the patient initiates the services for periodic examination.[17] In a survey of 1,800 adults at 47 family physician practices, 72% indicated they wanted to discuss at least one wellness topic with their physician.[18] Patients perceive physician recommendations to exercise, for example, as helpful.[19] Even so, such interest appears not to have penetrated lower socioeconomic populations, where lifestyle conspires most against health.[20]

Readiness of Clinical Practitioners. The fourth opportunity for physicians to contribute to lifestyle change is the apparent readiness of the medical profession to take on this role.[21] Surveys show that physicians generally are receptive to a larger role in health promotion[22] and support its value to patients of all ages.[23] Regarding health promotion as challenging and enjoyable, they agree they should actively support legislation.[24] Many believe medical schools should devote greater attention to preventive medicine.[25] These indicators of support probably mirror broader societal trends to which physicians generally subscribe and respond.[26] The increased interest of health care workers in health promotion is consistent with patient attitudes toward health care workers as the primary source of health information and as effective agents of behavioral change.[27]

THE MISSED OPPORTUNITY

Whether health care workers seize or miss health promotion opportunities depends on several factors, including their preparation, practice environment, personal health beliefs and habits, and an understanding of effective health promotion interventions.

Health care workers are trained to diagnose and triage medical, not educational, problems. Medical and surgical specialties dominate the culture and curriculum of medical school, leaving little room for preventive medicine and health promotion.[28] As a result, physicians and other clinical or office-based practitioners under their direction may miss opportunities for intervention, underestimate patient interest or overestimate patient knowledge and skill, lack the confidence to intervene, hold unrealistic expectations about the results of interventions, or question the social and legal implications of educational interventions. For example, physicians perceive patients as unusually "noncompliant" in response to advice for health-related behavior change. One study found that almost one half of physicians estimated patient compliance with a prescribed exercise regimen to be 25% or less.[29] Whether correct or not, this perception, combined with the lack of skill to change patients' behavior, may discourage physicians from implementing prevention in practice.

Furthermore, physicians and other health care workers practice in environments unconducive to health promotion. Tight clinic schedules, limited space, weak links to supporting resources, limited tracking capabilities, and economic disincentives preclude or at best discourage effective physician involvement in health promotion.

How physicians resolve these issues depends in part on their age, location of practice, type of practice, office management practices, and willingness to accept "outsider" (nonphysician) recommendations on health promotion practice.[30] The routine use of computer-generated preventive reminders[31] and reminders from office staff for special follow-up appointments[32] are effective management practices in the clinical setting. One study found physicians practicing general internal medicine to be more aggressive in counselling than were specialists.[33] Medical school preparation may serve a major role in establishing the degree of physician involvement in preventive services.[34] Other studies identify physician attitudes, beliefs, and health promotion practices as an important determinant of physician practice patterns.[35] Physicians with good personal health habits are more likely to counsel patients on lifestyle behaviors.[36] For example, nonsmoking providers are more likely to counsel smokers than are providers who smoke,[37] and physicians with an unhealthy lifestyle are the least likely to counsel even patients suffering from alcohol-related liver disease.[38] Physicians who perceive themselves as overweight were found to practice tertiary prevention, while physicians perceiving themselves as closer to ideal weight were more likely to practice primary prevention.[39] Therefore, to prepare health care workers to offer health promotion, the first task is to change attitudes of physicians toward their own health.

Even those health care workers inclined to offer health promotion might find, however, that patients expect more than advice. One body of literature suggests that modern medicine has cultivated a society in which patients have both high expectations for the receipt of a prescription drug and a low tolerance of discomfort.[40] The act of giving and receiving a prescription holds symbolic meaning for doctors and their patients in that it represents a concrete expression of concern, inspires confidence, and legitimizes the doctor-patient relationship. Thus, physicians' readiness to change is tempered by the dominant role that pharmaceuticals convey to patients and the message it sends to the public. This accounts for much of the overprescribing of antibiotics.[41]

Health promotion research has been equivocal in providing clear direction to health care workers. As a consequence, they often use ineffective interventions at the expense of more effective behavior change strategies.[42] Until recently, scientific evidence of the potential effectiveness of patient education and counseling was not readily available in the medical literature. Recommendations to physicians about counseling too often fail to specify situations of practice and type of patient. Physicians feel uncertain of the empirical basis for implementing preventive services, especially when they perceive disagreement, for example, between recommendations from the U.S. Preventive Services Task Force, the Canadian Task Force on the Periodic Health Examination, and the American College of Physicians.[43] Information overload from professional societies, consensus conferences, and task forces has resulted in avoidance by some physicians.[44] Clearly, health promotion research can help physicians by providing a clear rationale for effective health promotion interventions.

THE RATIONALE

With biomedical science as the prevailing paradigm in clinical or office-based practice, health care workers interpret "technology," "diagnosis," and "prescription" as medical terms. Though these terms have more generic dictionary definitions, they have become synonymous with biomedical material and procedures that have acquired their credibility from clinical research. Clinical or office-based technologies are best known in the forms of drugs, instruments, and to a lesser extent medical and surgical procedures codified in the form of protocols and algorithms. As we shall show, behavioral science also offers diagnostic and prescriptive procedures, tested in clinical trials with protocols and algorithms.

Clinical or office-based technology and scientific developments in medical research have had limited effects in the primary prevention of the behavioral and environmental risk factors in chronic disease. The modest successes with smoking cessation, reductions in fat in the diet, and control of selected risk factors such as blood pressure give little consideration to the role of social and behavioral determinants in the initiation and maintenance of health-directed and health-related behaviors. The "compliance" problem in medicine has been addressed as much with pharmacological solutions such as larger doses per tablet for lapses, and surgical solutions such as implants to avoid the pill-taking problem altogether, as it has with behavioral change.

The successful implementation of patient education strategies requires more secularization of and less medicalization of health in both philosophy and practice. Health care workers are somewhat reluctant to provide preventive care services when the patient is asymptomatic. In doing so, they ignore the established 20-year latency in the development and manifestation of some chronic diseases. Reflecting the greater value placed on treatment rather than prevention, doctors are more likely to treat those smokers with a smoking-related disease rather than treat asymptomatic smokers.[45] The findings of another study suggest that over half of smokers have not received advice from doctors to stop smoking.[46] Physicians tend to reschedule a visit if the patient has a diagnosed medical problem (e.g., diabetes, hypertension), irrespective of patient motivation.[47] The same study found that physicians relegate patients who are smokers to self-care, particularly if they are poorly motivated. Primary care practitioners provide preventive services in less than a third of patient visits.[48] Physicians in practice do agree on the importance of counseling on smoking, alcohol, and other drug use. They assign less importance, however, to counseling on exercise, nutrition, and stress. These attitudes reflect an element of scientific doubt or skepticism regarding the role of these risk factors in chronic disease.[49] In one study, almost one third of physicians did not counsel about dietary fat and fiber, because they were not convinced of the value of the diet.[50]

Despite resistance, clinical disease prevention and health promotion have evolved considerably during the last decade, culminating in recommendations and guidelines from the Canadian Task Force on the Periodic Health Examination (CTF),[51] Healthy People 2000,[52] and the U.S. Task Force for Preventive Services (USTFPS).[53] These reports place education and counseling into the mainstream of clinical preventive medicine.

The USTFPS *Guide to Clinical Preventive Services* identifies patient education and counseling as one of the most important activities of clinicians, even more promising than screening for disease. Of all recommendations proposed by the USTFPS in its first edition, 54% were for patient education and counseling activities. The USTFPS report covers a wider range of preventive interventions than considered by previous groups. Its interdisciplinary committee of health experts adapted the CTF's rigorous process for evaluating the quality of research on the effectiveness of preventive services. The process identified important conditions that were clearly preventable and evaluated the strength of evidence that supported the use of various preventive interventions in clinical practice. General approaches for patient education and counseling are recommended to enhance clinicians' effectiveness in achieving patient behavioral change. These recommendations reflect consensus among the American College of Physicians (ACP), the CTF, and the USTFPS. The guidelines demonstrate movement away from the simple classification of patients by age and gender for preventive services toward a stratification that considers additional risk factors and toward the development of prevention strategies tailored to risk profiles.[54]

AN EPIDEMIOLOGICAL AND COMMUNITY APPROACH TO HEALTH CARE[55]

The changing epidemiology of diseases calls for a shift in clinical or office-based interventions within the epidemiological triad of host-agent-environment, from a primary emphasis on the agent to a greater emphasis on the **host** (patient) and the environment. Most efforts to maximize the benefits and to minimize the risks of medical interventions have concentrated on the regulation or control of the **agent**—the invading organism or pathology. Most clinical or office-based therapies employed have emphasized technological agents such as drugs and surgical procedures. With the decline in acute communicable diseases and the increasing frequency of chronic conditions in the population, single causes in the form of a controllable pathological agent have been replaced with multiple, contributing agents, many of which are embedded in normal living conditions and lifestyle. Patients must often manage their own complex, long-term regimens of drugs and lifestyle modifications. This requires a refocusing of health care attention to environments and to more autonomous patients outside hospitals and other clinical settings.

Most studies of patient "compliance"[56] begin with the medical care setting as the locus of patient identification and intervention.[57] A community approach to the problems of patient adherence to medical recommendations begins with a population in which many of the potential benefactors of medical advice have varying degrees of contact with clinical or office-based practitioners, and some have no contact. PRECEDE-PROCEED provides a rationale and a framework for an analysis of health care issues that considers the total population at risk, including those who should be but are not receiving clinical or office-based care, as well as those who are misusing their prescribed medicines or recommended preventive or self-care practices. It also allows for targeting health care personnel and others in the community whose behavior may need to change if they are to influence the factors predisposing, enabling, and reinforcing patient behavior or environmental change in the right direction (see Figure 11-1). Several reviews of the continuing medical education literature have recommended a typology of interventions based on the Precede framework to improve physicians' practices in patient counseling or prevention.[58]

The following four questions will be addressed in developing the framework:

1. What groups of people in the population have illnesses, conditions, or risk factors that would benefit from medical or nursing interventions not yet received?
2. What types of patients have illnesses or conditions that would benefit from more appropriate use of the medications or self-care procedures prescribed for them?
3. What types of patients, conditions, medical settings, drugs, and self-care regimens most likely result in error and would benefit from improved education and monitoring?
4. What means of intervention for each group of patients and type of regimen appear most effective when (a) a condition is either diagnosed or undiagnosed, (b) a regimen is either prescribed or not prescribed, (c) it is either dispensed or not dispensed, and (d) it is either followed or not followed?

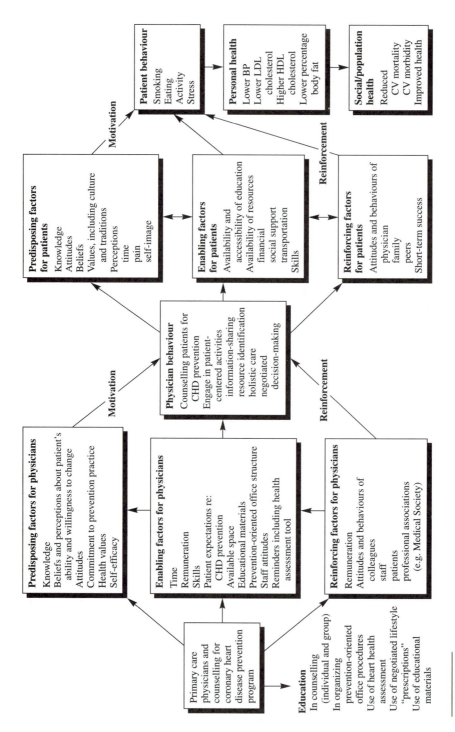

FIGURE 11-1

Primary care physicians were the initial target group in this study of physician counseling for coronary heart disease prevention, based on the Precede-Proceed model.

SOURCE: "Primary Care Physicians and Coronary Heart Disease Prevention," by L. Makrides, P. L. Veinot, J. Richard, and M. J. Allen, 1997, *Patient Education and Counseling, 32*, 207–217. Reprinted with permission.

EPIDEMIOLOGY OF HEALTH CARE ERRORS

In health care, one may make errors of commission or omission. For instance, an error of commission occurs when a patient misuses a prescribed therapeutic or preventive regimen or uses a drug prescribed for another patient. An error of omission occurs when a patient fails to receive or to apply a clinically important medication or procedure as needed. One can characterize both types of error as failures of health care professionals, failures of patients, or both. The purpose of this epidemiological approach to assessing the errors is not to affix blame but to pinpoint the most strategic points for intervention.

Figure 11-2 identifies the several points in the flow of circumstances under which patients or would-be patients might benefit from health education. At point A, an intervention to inform them about treatable signs and conditions would predispose and enable them to find care. At point B, informing them about the risks and benefits of a preventive intervention, a drug, or alternative nonpharmacological therapies or self-care procedures would predispose them to seek the benefits or avoid the risks. At point C, efforts to inform them about the proper use of a medication or procedure should enable them to follow the regimen appropriately. The figure identifies needs for patient education and broader public-health education both to prevent errors of omission (in A and B) and to prevent errors of commission (in C_1 or C_2).

HEALTH CARE ERRORS OF OMISSION

Potential patients can be classified into two groups, each of which could be the target of different health education programs to reduce health care errors of omission:

- Those who are not currently seeking or receiving medical care for their illness or condition (the undiagnosed), or a symptom or risk factor that could warrant examination and health counseling (the unscreened)
- Those who received a medical diagnosis but did not receive, fill, or use a prescription or recommendation for a procedure or medicine that could benefit them (the nonusers)

The Undiagnosed. The purpose of health education for people with undiagnosed conditions is to predispose and enable them to obtain screening, or medical diagnosis and treatment, assuming that one or more tests, medications, or procedures would help prevent or treat their condition and would be prescribed for them.[59] General communications targeted to these people would advise them that if they have certain high-risk characteristics or were experiencing specified symptoms, they should obtain periodic screening tests or consult a physician or other health care provider because medical or dental advice or treatment may be needed.

Health education of this kind has long been part of public health programs to induce high-risk populations to seek prenatal care, immunizations, contraceptives,

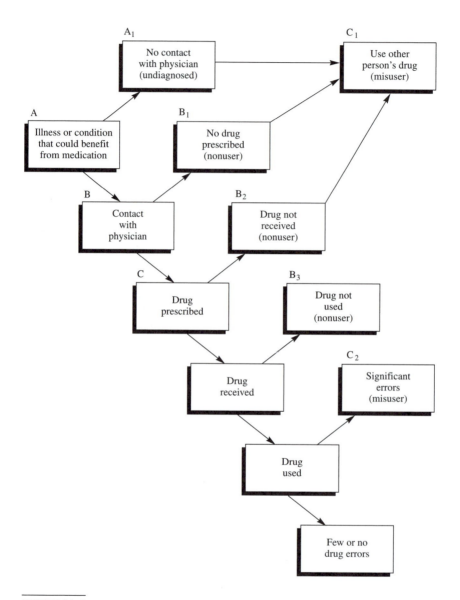

FIGURE 11-2

The flow of patients into categories of health care and health care errors can pinpoint stages in the process at which educational interventions can be strategically targeted.

SOURCE: "An Epidemiological Approach to Targeting Drug Information," by L. W. Green, P. D. Mullen, and R. B. Friedman, 1986; and Chap. 29 in Cramer & Spilker, eds., 1991, *Patient Compliance in Medical Practice and Clinical Trials,* New York: Raven. Reprinted with permission from Elsevier.

blood pressure screening, and a variety of other preventive measures.[60] The effectiveness of such efforts has been documented in primary prevention and communicable disease control,[61] accounting for the dramatic reductions in infant mortality and congenital defects, as well as the near eradication of some childhood diseases.[62] It has been the mainstay of high blood pressure control programs and campaigns,[63] accounting for dramatic reductions in the incidence of strokes and cerebrovascular death rates.[64] It has also proven pivotal to the successes of family planning,[65] cancer control,[66] mental health care,[67] and other areas of secondary prevention and early diagnosis.[68] Both those suffering overt symptoms and the "worried well"[69] will be most responsive to media messages that encourage them to seek medical care to alleviate their symptoms or worries. Those with financial constraints and those with risk factors considered normal in their family, culture, or experience[70] will require more intensive case-finding,[71] outreach,[72] and screening programs.[73]

Nonusers. The first class of nonusers (B_1 in Figure 11-2) consists of patients with preventable or treatable conditions who do not receive self-care or medical recommendations from their physicians or who receive a prescription or recommendation for the wrong therapy or self-care regimen. Such patients might benefit from information normally directed to the undiagnosed.[74] A more appropriate remedy, however, is improved quality assurance from prescribers,[75] or from pharmacists or dispensers, who could head off the incorrectly prescribed products.[76]

In another category of nonusers are those patients who do not obtain recommended self-care devices (e.g., a blood pressure cuff) or medications or who fail to fill their prescriptions (B_2). This tends to occur when patients cannot get to pharmacies, when they are exceptionally fearful of side effects, and when the price of devices or drugs is unaffordable or perceived to exceed the value of the therapy.[77]

Where the medical conditions are not life threatening, educational communications would serve to increase awareness that the patient's condition may lead to complications, spread, or recur if untreated. Education for patients with symptoms that cannot consistently be seen or felt, such as high blood pressure, would attempt to strengthen the belief that the conditions may nevertheless be serious.[78] For those who cannot afford drugs, information about less expensive medicines and sources of financial aid would be most useful. In particular, the degree of benefit from palliative regimens should be clarified so that the user can weigh potential benefits against financial and other costs, including possible side effects.[79]

HEALTH-CARE ERRORS OF COMMISSION

Two types of errors of commission are (1) those made by physicians, pharmacists, or others recommending or prescribing medications or self-care procedures and (2) those made by patients.

Professional Errors. The first type of error of commission can occur when

- A diagnosis is applied without adequate confirmation
- Drugs are sometimes prescribed in lieu of more appropriate nonpharma-cological therapies
- A new drug's potential interaction with other regimens has not been evaluated
- The proper drug is prescribed in the wrong dosage

Arguably, such errors can be reduced through professional media communication and continuing education or quality assurance for physicians and others who care for patients,[80] although general messages to high-risk subpopulations of the public may be helpful in shaping patients' expectations.[81] The benefits of effectively curtailing these errors have been documented, particularly among patients with chronic diseases.[82] We shall consider physicians' errors of commission in greater detail further in the chapter.

Patient Errors. Patients may also misunderstand instructions and make errors in their use of procedures or drugs.[83] The amount of information provided about a particular product to prevent such mistakes does not always correspond to the amount needed by the patient or, indeed, to what the patient can understand.[84] In the debate over patient packaging inserts, some proponents argue that full disclosure in a consistently available written format can at least give patients access to all the information they need.[85] In fact, however, as with any mass medium, some patients receive a great deal of unnecessary information, as with patient package inserts, while others may receive it but fail to notice, comprehend, or recall the specific information they need.[86]

Uniformly distributed communications, such as brochures or videos in waiting rooms, are to medical care what mass media are to community programs. They are, by definition, cost-effective as channels for reaching the largest numbers of people, especially those already motivated and eager to learn. However, they do not sufficiently assure the education and support of those most in need of behavioral or environmental changes. They tend to be designed with the average patient in mind, and this "average" misses the people at one end of the normal curve on any particular characteristic such as reading ability, acculturation, motivation, socioeconomic status, or age. The health care providers who use mass-produced patient educational materials also must guard against the tendency to allow them to substitute for spending personal time with the patients who have questions or concerns and for being responsive to patients' cues.[87]

A necessarily more complicated alternative to this universal informational strategy involves systematic surveying of the behavioral and educational needs of each demographic or epidemiological grouping of patients. Certainly, this should be less a complicated and burdensome procedure for practitioners than attempting to do a systematic educational diagnosis on each patient. A simplification of this approach is to estimate the probabilities of errors in each group or subpopulation of patients and the severity of consequences associated with each potential error. A specific group's relative need for drug education or counseling may be defined mathematically and estimated from a combination of national survey data[88] and local census data. Formulas for estimating drug information need in local populations have been proposed.[89] This approach has been made more practicable with computer-generated communications that take selected characteristics of individuals into account in producing tailored messages.[90]

Special Groups. Two groups present special problems of patient errors of commission—pregnant women and people who use prescription drugs obtained for another illness or by another person. For women who are or intend to become pregnant or those who are breast-feeding, an increased number of active health education campaigns need to be launched through the mass media or through fertility clinics.[91] The campaigns must urge them to report fully their use of drugs, tobacco, and alcohol to their physician or to a drug information service for evaluation, even before other needs for prenatal care arise.[92]

People who use medicines obtained for previous illnesses, or from other persons, risk making a variety of mistakes, including use of an inappropriate drug, the wrong dosage of the right drug, or the right drug at the wrong time. Only education through nonmedical channels can reach most of these consumers to warn them about these potential hazards.[93]

PATIENT CONSIDERATIONS IN TARGETING INTERVENTIONS

The preceding analysis leads to two conclusions:

- Broad-scale patient educational programs must reach beyond the clinical setting, but they can be contained and targeted to demographic groups in which the prevalence of risk factors, undiagnosed conditions, or untreated illnesses are high.
- The remaining patient education and counseling resources can be concentrated on clinical and self-help group settings.

Based on estimates of a 50% prevalence of "compliance" in patients,[94] the probability of preventing a potentially harmful error per patient per encounter could be as high as .50 if methods of patient education and counseling were 100% effective. To maximize their effectiveness, educational and counseling resources must be conserved and concentrated on those encounters with patients that represent the greatest need and opportunity to improve or protect health. The first task, then, is to determine which patients comprise these target groups and what kinds of "compliance" errors educating and counseling them effectively could prevent.

THE UNDIAGNOSED

Who are the undiagnosed? National statistics can help one identify groups or types of would-be patients who are most likely not to seek help or to receive drugs for various conditions. The prevalence of those types in a local area or population can then be estimated from census data. National statistics indicate, for instance, that women experience (or acknowledge) more symptoms than do men within most broad classifications of illness,[95] and women also more frequently seek diagnosis, medical care, and prescription therapy for the same symptoms than do men, who are more likely to "tough it out" or prefer home remedies.[96]

When they do seek care, men account for 40% of the total number of patient visits to office-based physicians and 40% of drug "mentions."[97] The same underrepresentation of men can be found in preventive care visits.[98]

Lower socioeconomic and nonwhite groups have higher incidence rates for most illnesses and lower medical and preventive care utilization rates relative to their greater need.[99] White patients tend to receive more information from physicians than do African Americans and Hispanics.[100] Low-income patients receive less than do affluent patients.[101] Of 261 women receiving primary care in an urban hospital, those patients with higher educational levels were more likely to be offered mammography screening than were those with relatively less education.[102]

Patients over 65 years of age are more often ill and require more visits and drugs than do those in younger age groups. Patients 65 years and older purchase almost 25% of all prescription and nonprescription drugs.[103] The elderly require more medication than do younger patients for the management of acute disease,[104] and they have a higher incidence of chronic disease.[105]

Although the elderly may not make more drug compliance errors than do younger patients with the same prescriptions, the deleterious consequences may be more serious,[106] less easily detected, and less easily resolved than for younger patients.[107] In addition, their complex medical regimens place the elderly at greater risk of combination drug and dietary errors.[108] For instance, dietary adherence among patients with high blood cholesterol decreases with age.[109]

The best indicators, then, for targeting broad patient education and counseling programs to reduce errors of omission in health care are male gender, lower socioeconomic status, and older age. The following are the most prevalent illnesses and conditions of older men in lower socioeconomic groups (listed from highest to lowest): high blood pressure, respiratory, mental, nervous, digestive, skin, urinary, eye and ear, arthritis, and pain in bones and joints.[110]

DIAGNOSED NONUSERS WHO RECEIVED
INAPPROPRIATE MEDICAL RECOMMENDATIONS

Those patients who received no prescription or the wrong medical advice cannot be considered uncompliant, in the strictest sense, especially if they followed the wrong advice. Nevertheless, their medical care error puts them at risk, so this class of adherence errors must be prevented or corrected. Some professionals expect the current tradition of continuing medical education of physicians and other health care providers to prevent diagnostic and prescribing errors in individual practitioners and to build a level of knowledge and skill in the medical community that might detect and correct many of the individual errors that continue. However, only weak and inconsistent evidence supports this expectation.[111] Innovative modalities of continuing education involving patients,[112] as well as more comprehensive quality assurance methods combining educational with behavioral, economic, and environmental approaches to physicians' and other professionals' practices, show greater promise but mixed results.[113]

The evidence that mass media can influence prescribing also seems conflicted. From 1973 to 1981, the national media aided a campaign by the National Institute of Mental Health targeted at physicians who were overprescribing barbiturate sedatives and minor tranquilizers. Prescriptions for these drugs declined substantially.[114] A Canadian study suggests, moreover, that some physicians have overreacted to this publicity and as a result may have underprescribed these drugs.[115] Media events such as news of Nancy Reagan's breast cancer diagnosis tend to result in exaggerated increases in the demand for selected medical or screening procedures such as mammography.[116] Thus, it appears that certain mass communications can influence clinical behavior, prescribing patterns, and public demand for certain procedures, but the appropriateness and extent of the responses are more difficult to manage or contain when using mass media.

NONUSERS WHO DID NOT OBTAIN
A RECOMMENDED DRUG OR DEVICE

For nonusers who have failed to fill prescriptions, to purchase nonprescription drugs or devices, or to adopt recommended procedures, two further strategies of targeting health education and communications can be considered. One is direct-to-public advertising of the price advantage of one product or pharmacy over another. The second is patient education directed at patients in medical-care settings including pharmacies, especially for illnesses where the cost of drugs most frequently discourages the filling or refilling of prescriptions. Such discouragement most often occurs when the illness or condition is not life threatening, the symptoms are not very painful or noticeable, the patient is averse to taking drugs generally, or the patient simply cannot afford the drug.[117] A survey of the American

Association of Retired Persons, for example, found that 20% of older patients in the United States never filled their prescriptions.[118]

POLICY CHANGES

As with all the other categories of nonusers in which financial barriers to adequate health care restrict behavior, health promotion can play a role in educating the electorate and policy makers about the need for new provisions under health insurance, medicare, medicaid, managed care, or health care reform proposals.[119] Direct political organizing with influential groups such as the Association of Retired Persons, national medical or nursing associations, and the Cancer Society or Foundation. These organizations have powerfully lobbied for legislation and regulatory changes in support of patients, providing important **advocacy** on their behalf.

Misusers. Misusers (C_2 in Figure 11-2) provide a more efficient target for "compliance"-improving strategies than do nonusers for several reasons. They can be reached more readily—through providers of medical care—than can nonpatients and nonusers (B_3). Patient education can also be tailored more closely to their information needs and learning capacities.[120] Misusers also can be assumed to be more highly motivated, on average, to respond to drug information than can nonpatients and nonusers, because they have made the effort to obtain medical care and to fill their prescription or to purchase recommended nonprescription medications or devices. The cumulative evidence from 102 published evaluations of patient education directed at drug misuse indicates that patient education reduces drug errors by an average of 40–72% and improves clinical outcomes by 23–47%.[121]

The same meta-analysis of the 72 studies of patient education directed at drug "compliance" in chronic disease treatment showed that the medium, channel, or technique of communication mattered less than did the appropriate application of learning principles such as individualization, relevance, facilitation, feedback, and reinforcement.[122] These principles can be applied more efficiently, systematically, and strategically with an algorithm that sorts or triages patients into educational groupings according to their educational needs.[123] Such an algorithm for patient education will be presented in the next section of this chapter.

ALLOCATION DECISIONS

The foregoing demonstrates some efficiencies and cost-*effectiveness* of interventions directed at patients classified as misusers or potential misusers of medical advice and prescriptions. Yet, the cost-*benefit* potential of reaching the healthy population with preventive services, the undiagnosed people with risk factors or incipient illness, and the dropouts from treatment could be much greater in the long run.[124] These nonusers represent new or lost markets for the pharmaceutical companies, who should find it beneficial to support medical and public health agencies in their efforts to reach these patients and to reduce the extent of untreated illness in the poorest populations. Pharmaceutical companies, the Food and Drug Administration (FDA), consumer groups, and advertising firms are now bringing medication information directly to the general public. Several companies have attempted to educate consumers about the signs of certain diseases—hypertension, diabetes, and depression—without mentioning products by name. Referred to as *institutional advertising,* these ads have been applauded by both consumers and the FDA. Institutional advertising could be an efficient and profitable method of reaching the undiagnosed and nonuser groups. More recent initiatives by the drug companies advertise brand names of drugs only available by prescription, encouraging potential users to consult with their physicians. Viagra is a notable recent example.

Efforts to bring more of the nonusers—the undiagnosed, the dropouts, the uninsured—into the medical care system will be frustrated if the burden on the system only makes the problems of compliance worse because of overworked staff spending too little time with patients. More widespread and more effective patient education and professional education related to the adherence problems, combined with organizational, economic, and environmental reforms of the system itself, will make the efforts to recruit the nonusers worthwhile and productive.[125]

This has been the philosophy and developing strategy of a movement within the health services professions called Community-Oriented Primary Care (COPC). It has developed methods and procedures for practicing "denominator medicine" through community analysis of the population served by the health care institution or practice. COPC seeks to apply the Precede and Proceed assessments of community perceptions and epidemiological distributions of health problems and risk factors described in this chapter. COPC has been adopted variously within the community health centers and migrant health centers funded by the Health Services and Resources Administration, the Indian Health Service, and various foundations.[126]

APPLICATION OF EDUCATIONAL ASSESSMENT TO INDIVIDUAL PATIENTS[127]

The Precede-Proceed concepts and methods have been widely applied, usually with some adaptation, to the health care or counseling setting, including patient education, nutrition counseling, smoking-cessation, and self-care or self-help programs. It suggests protocol for the stepped education and support of patients and the continuing education of health care workers.

All too often, physicians arrive at a correct medical diagnosis and nurses or dieticians devise appropriate management plans, only to be frustrated by unsatisfactory outcomes resulting from the patient's not understanding instructions or, in many instances, choosing to ignore them. What sustains an outpatient's adherence to a prescribed medical or dietary regimen between visits? The answer, apparently, is that not enough sustains their behavior. Patient adherence failure, or "noncompliance," is reflected most clearly in relapse rates ranging from 20% to 80%, not only in nonadherence to medications but even more in ignoring advice on lifestyle modifications.[128] Challenges of this nature have been documented in a variety of cultural settings and concerning a range of health conditions. Time and time again, patients make decisions affecting their health based on nonmedical aspects of their experience and other pushes and pulls in their environment, such as social influence networks, disposable income, or beliefs about their condition's origins.[129]

Reviews of patient education studies and epidemiological models suggest that more effective interaction between health care providers and patients could reduce drug errors by as much as 72% and improve clinical outcomes by as much as 40% over conventional treatment.[130] A recent Japanese study demonstrated that patient satisfaction with health care, particularly with the communication of health care providers, increased "compliance" rates.[131] Improved interaction corrects not only many patients' errors but also those attributable to the health care providers, who with better interactions become more conscious of the patient's specific needs. Allegrante and his colleagues tested several components of a program to increase walking for patients with arthritis of the knee. Based on their application of the Precede-Proceed process, they developed a comprehensive intervention strategy that addressed factors both within and beyond the control of health care providers. Examples of the former include behavioral contracting, commitment strategies, and cognitive strategies—frameworks that the provider can compose with the patient's collaboration. In the larger community context, they addressed reinforcement measures and stimulus control.[132]

THE RELAPSE CURVE

Figure 11-3 shows the typical relapse pattern in a variety of practices recommended to patients, especially those practices relating to addiction, compulsive behavior, pleasures, comforts, unpleasant side effects, inconveniences, costs, or even simple habits. For example, breast self-examination is a commonly advised practice, especially for women.[133] Assuming that 100% of the patients who leave a medical care encounter are committed to adopting the prescribed practice, studies have uncovered a characteristic drop of 40% to 80% in actual maintenance behavior during the first 6 weeks.[134]

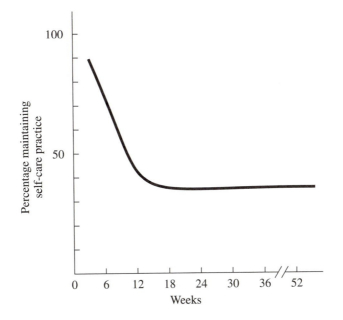

FIGURE 11-3

The typical shape of the relapse curve applies to a variety of self-care practices, especially those involving an addictive element such as smoking cessation or the addition of a complex lifestyle behavior such as physical activity.

SOURCE: "How Physicians Can Improve Patients' Participation and Maintenance in Self-Care," by L. W. Green, 1987, *Western Journal of Medicine, 147,* 346–349. Reprinted with permission.

Though the shape of the curve is highly predictable, the drop in percentage before it levels off is not. More effective intervention for selected self-care practices can alter the curve's slope and plateau levels.[135] For example, physicians can reduce a male patient's daily consumption of cigarettes by simply giving advice, as shown in a randomized clinical trial that also documented lower mortality in lung cancer compared with the control group.[136] Figure 11-4 shows how three different smoking-cessation clinics achieved identical relapse curves in terms of their shape but different levels of plateau, depending on their effectiveness in applying educational and behavioral principles.[137] Adult smokers, approximately 70% of whom visit a physician each year, reported in 1976 that their physician had counseled them to stop smoking, but nearly twice as many reported this 11 years later.[138]

PRECEDE had its earliest test as a systematic planning and evaluation model to design interventions for doctors and nurses treating patients with hypertension,

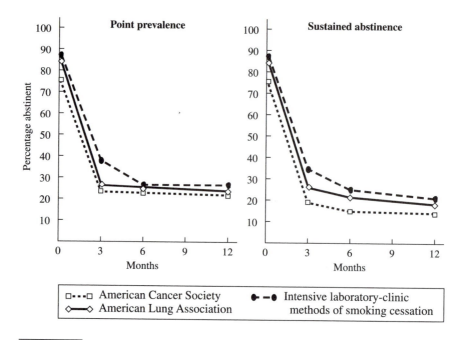

FIGURE 11-4

Three smoking-cessation clinics achieved identical patterns of quitting or relapse but slightly different levels of effectiveness depending on their populations and success in applying educational and behavioral principles.

SOURCE: "Comparative Evaluation of American Cancer Society and American Lung Association Smoking Cessation Clinics," by H. A. Lando, P. G. McGovern, F. X. Barrios, and B. D. Etringer, 1990, *American Journal of Public Health, 80,* 554–559. Reprinted with permission.

for the patients themselves, and for significant others who could support them in adjusting their medical and dietary regimens to their living circumstances.[139] In a randomized controlled trial in the Johns Hopkins outpatient clinics, significant improvements in relapse rates and blood pressure control were obtained over an 18-month period.[140] These and related improvements correlated significantly with the extent of patient, staff, and family exposure to the planned interventions to predispose, enable, and reinforce the patients in adhering to the prescribed regimens for controlling their blood pressure.[141] A long-term follow-up of the patients found lower relapse rates, greater sustained improvement in blood pressure control, and more than 50% fewer deaths in those who had received any combination of three patient education methods than in those who received the usual medical care.[142]

In another early application of PRECEDE in a family-planning clinic, women smoked less when they were exposed to a combination of a physician's counseling and waiting room media than when they were exposed only to waiting room media.[143] In a series of related smoking-cessation studies applying the Precede-Proceed model in rural public health clinics with pregnant women, significant reductions in smoking were obtained. The quit rate was more than twice as high (14% versus 6%) for the women exposed to the Precede-planned intervention than for those given a self-help manual developed by the American Lung Association. The rates were seven times greater for the Precede-planned program participants than for the control group receiving usual clinical care.[144] A simplified rendering of their application of the Precede model is shown in Figure 11-5 A and B. Since then, literally hundreds of other studies have shown the effectiveness of well-designed patient education and self-care education programs in reducing relapse of patients in adherence to medical advice, including lifestyle and home environmental modifications for primary prevention and health promotion.[145]

A more positive way of interpreting the relapse curve is to note that as much as 40% to 60% of the population does maintain its self-care practices. This fact indicates that any global intervention program designed to prevent relapse may be unnecessary and probably wasteful for a large portion of patients entering health care programs. Furthermore, the interventions designed to prevent relapse range from simplistic, inexpensive methods effective for only a few patients to complex, obtrusive, and costly methods effective for most but needed by few. Morisky and his colleagues demonstrated in the Los Angeles Tuberculosis Control Program that the rate of dropouts or relapse in adherence to antituberculosis medical regimens can be reduced from 73% to 36% in preventive therapy patients, when one applies the Precede-Proceed model in designing a targeted educational counseling and incentives program.[146] Figure 11-6 shows the relapse curves for the two groups of patients, indicating similar dropout patterns for the two groups during the first 3 months and higher rates for the usual-care group. Then, the special intervention group leveled off in its relapse rate, while the usual-care group continued to lose patients to follow-up for the next 2 years.

A HIERARCHY OF FACTORS AFFECTING SELF-CARE BEHAVIOR

Considerable study has been devoted to identifying the characteristics of patients or participants in medical care and health programs who typically drop out or fail to sustain their recommended behavioral or environmental changes. Comparative and prospective studies have identified four sets of correlates that predict adherence or relapse: (1) demographic and socioeconomic characteristics; (2) motivational characteristics; (3) physical, manual, or economic facilitators and barriers; and (4) circumstantial rewards and penalties associated with the behavior, especially in the social environment.

One can view the first of the four sets of factors as predisposing or enabling factors, but they cannot be easily changed, especially in the clinical setting. The

A.

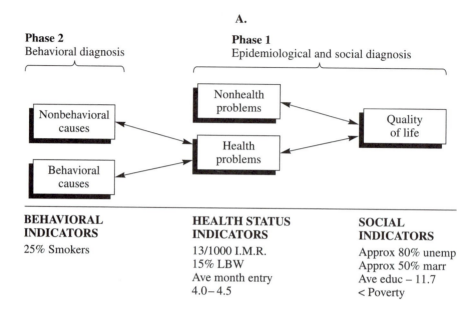

BEHAVIORAL INDICATORS	HEALTH STATUS INDICATORS	SOCIAL INDICATORS
25% Smokers	13/1000 I.M.R. 15% LBW Ave month entry 4.0–4.5	Approx 80% unemp Approx 50% marr Ave educ – 11.7 < Poverty

other three sets of factors can. These modifiable factors are the predisposing, enabling, and reinforcing factors of the Precede-Proceed model. Predisposing factors need to change before enabling factors can. A patient will not devote much effort to learning skills or pursuing resources if he or she has little motivation or commitment to the goal of the behavior. Enabling factors need to change before the reinforcing factors can. Efforts to reward a behavior that has not yet been enabled would be wasted. This hierarchy of factors influencing adherence and relapse suggests a logical order of intervention that should maximize the support to a patient while conserving the energy and time of health care staff. Logic would dictate the concentration of educational resources on patients according to which of the three changeable characteristics they possess.[147] It would further dictate that if a patient possesses more than one of the changeable characteristics predicting relapse, a combination of interventions designed to change the characteristics should be applied.[148]

The three sets of changeable characteristics predicting adherence or relapse reflect a natural hierarchy of action from wanting to do, being able to do, and being rewarded for doing. This hierarchy produces a logical flow of intervention from strengthening motivation to enabling to reinforcing the self-care behavior. A need to conserve resources, however, dictates skipping those interventions not required if a patient is already motivated, enabled, or reinforced. The skip pattern can be guided by a minimum of questions designed to detect the patient's motivational state, barriers and the potential rewards, and likely side effects. The skip pattern can also include assessments, decision nodes, and recursive loops in an

B.

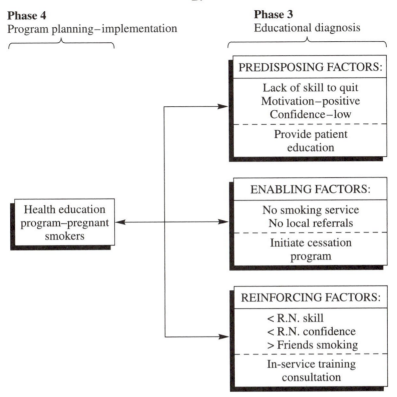

Phase 4
Program planning–implementation

Phase 3
Educational diagnosis

PREDISPOSING FACTORS:

Lack of skill to quit
Motivation–positive
Confidence–low
- - - - - - - - - - - - -
Provide patient
education

Health education
program–pregnant
smokers

ENABLING FACTORS:

No smoking service
No local referrals
- - - - - - - - - - - - -
Initiate cessation
program

REINFORCING FACTORS:

< R.N. skill
< R.N. confidence
> Friends smoking
- - - - - - - - - - - - -
In-service training
consultation

FIGURE 11-5

An early application of the Precede model in planning a program for pregnant women in rural public health clinics produced significant reductions in smoking rates. (A, p. 440) shows the indicators identified in the social and epidemiological diagnosis leading to the identification of maternal smoking as the key behavioral determinant of high infant mortality and low-birth-weight babies that the program could target. In (B), the key predisposing, enabling, and reinforcing factors influencing smoking cessation were identified.

SOURCE: "An Application of the PRECEDE Model for Planning and Evaluating Educational Methods for Pregnant Smokers," by R. A. Windsor, 1986, *Hygie, 5,* 38–43. Reprinted with permission of the International Union for Health Promotion and Education.

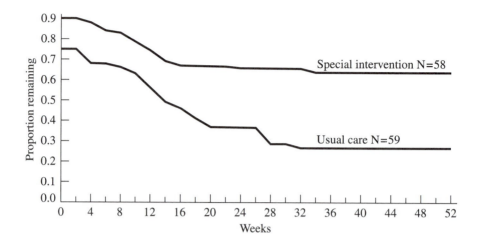

FIGURE 11-6

Here are the cumulative proportions of people receiving Precede-planned interventions or usual care who were lost to follow-up, presumably having lapsed in their antituberculosis preventive treatment.

SOURCE: "A Patient Education Program to Improve Adherence Rates with Antituberculosis Drug Regimens," by D. E. Morisky et al., 1990, *Health Education Quarterly, 17,* 253–267. Reprinted with permission of the Society for Public Health Education.

algorithm for patient education, diagnosis, and intervention as suggested in Figure 11-7.

The recommended procedure entails assessing a patient's educational needs by asking a sequence of "diagnostic" questions to ensure the relevance of the intervention to the patient's motivation, skill, and resources and to reinforce adherence to the prescribed medical regimen or lifestyle modifications. The sequence of questions and interventions minimizes the time required of staff and patients and maximizes the probability of medical benefit to the patient. Physicians, nurses, dieticians, pharmacists, counselors, and others who work with patients on a one-to-one basis can apply the protocol. It can also be adapted to work with self-help groups and counseling for behavior change in healthy individuals.

The principles of relevance (predisposing factors), facilitating (enabling factors), and feedback combined with social support (reinforcing factors) were tested prospectively in the Hopkins study.[149] The combined interventions yielded significant improvements in compliance and blood pressure control after 18 months[150] and a 50% reduction in mortality after 5 years.[151]

A more refined model of patient decisions in accepting influenza vaccination has been derived from patient questionnaires and tested prospectively with

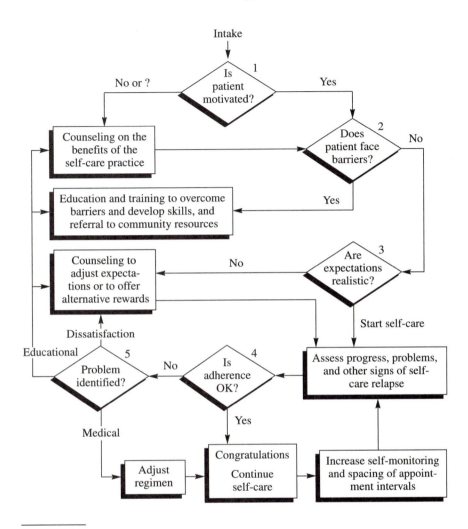

FIGURE 11-7

An algorithm for assessing predisposing, enabling, and reinforcing factors in patient education for self-care or lifestyle and environmental modification leads to a triage and stepped-care approach to patient education and counseling. This can save clinical staff time and other resources, resulting in more effective intervention.

SOURCE: "How Physicians Can Improve Patients' Participation and Maintenance in Self-Care," by L. W. Green, 1987, *Western Journal of Medicine, 147,* 346–349. Reprinted with permission.

correct prediction of vaccination behavior for 82% of high-risk patients.[152] This model questionnaire could provide the source of more specific answers to the initial questions in Figure 11-7.

TRIAGE ACCORDING TO MOTIVATION

The first question a physician, nurse, or other clinical staff needs to answer is whether a patient cares enough about the problem even to try the prescribed regimen. This can be answered on three levels, according to the Health Belief Model:[153]

1. Does the patient believe he or she is susceptible to continuing problems if the recommended behavior is not adopted?
2. Does the patient believe the problems associated with failure to comply with the recommended behavior are severe?
3. Does the patient perceive the benefits of adopting the recommended behavior to be greater than the perceived risks, costs, side effects, and barriers?

If the answer to all three questions is yes, the patient is likely to be willing to try the recommended behavior. The clinical staff need not strive to convince the patient of the importance of following the prescribed regimen. The patient has sufficient motivation.

With a willing patient, considerable time and energy otherwise spent on persuasion can be conserved for training or support. If a patient is not motivated according to these three criteria, however, then it would be premature to train the patient in skills or to counsel the patient to overcome barriers in the home environment. The time and resources of the health care worker should be spent first on educating the patient on the importance and benefits of the recommended practice. The purpose of this initial education is to strengthen the three beliefs in the patient.

In this situation, written materials are no substitute for face-to-face, two-way communication. In the meta-analysis of 102 controlled studies of patient education related to prescription drugs, the factors that predicted the magnitude of change in patient knowledge or beliefs, as well as in drug errors and clinical effects, were not the media or channels of communication. The most influential factors were individual attention, relevance, and feedback provided in the communication.[154] These findings held up in subsequent meta-analyses of clinical health promotion and counseling for lifestyle modifications.[155]

If a patient's level of prior motivation cannot be assessed after a few direct questions, the best predictor of the need for patient education and counseling at this first level is the years of school completed by the patient. Less formal education means a greater need for patient education.[156] This might seem too obvious to warrant mention, but an irony of medical practice is that physicians tend to talk more to patients who ask more questions—typically those of higher educational achievement—than to those who ask fewer questions but probably need more answers.[157] In addition, age factors can play a significant role. A Dutch study found that both young and old cancer patients often did not follow through on their intentions to seek additional information or raise difficult questions with their specialists during an office visit.[158] Cultural and language barriers similarly impede effective interaction between health care providers and patients. Regardless of the patient's level of education or the provider's level of cultural sensitivity, a health care provider can easily probe for a patient's level of understanding by asking the patient to repeat the instructions he or she is to follow.

TRIAGE ACCORDING TO ENABLING FACTORS

Once the interaction between staff and patient establishes that a patient is motivated, the next diagnostic step is to assure that the patient can carry out the prescribed behavior. Staff members need to investigate the skills, resources, and barriers in the home or work environment that the patient needs help to develop or overcome. If the patient is highly motivated and willing to try the regimen prescribed by the physician but faces inability, lack of needed resources, or barriers that cannot be overcome alone, the patient will become frustrated and ultimately discouraged. Skill deficiencies are most common in young children; arthritic patients who cannot open certain containers; illiterate, low-literate, or non-English-speaking patients who cannot read or understand directions; old patients whose eyesight or mobility makes adherence to certain regimens impossible; and other disabled or poor patients without the necessary resources to follow the recommended practices.

If patients lack any of these enabling factors, the staff recommending the unattainable regimen have some obligation to help the patient find ways to overcome the deficiency. Minimal interventions expected of the physician include some training of the patient in the necessary skills or modification of the regimen to fit the patient's circumstances. At the very least, the health care worker owes it to the patient to provide systematic referral to other agencies or resources in the community to help deal with such problems.

ASSESSING REINFORCING FACTORS
NECESSARY FOR PATIENTS' ADHERENCE

Even with the predisposing and enabling factors in place, there remains one more level of possible breakdown in a patient's "compliance" with a prescribed regimen. If the recommended behavior is met with side effects, inconvenience, derision by family or friends, criticism by employers or teachers, or other sources of discouragement, the patient will likely discontinue the practice prescribed or recommended. A 1991 study demonstrated that diabetic patients' decision making with respect to diet-related self-care could be characterized by the interactions of three distinct but overlapping categories of factors: individual, contextual, and diabetes-related.[159] The opposite of these discouraging factors are reinforcing factors. The health care staff can help build reinforcement of patient "compliance" in two ways.

First, health care personnel can provide reinforcement by assuring that the patient's expectations are realistic, so that when something happens during the course of the treatment the patient expects it rather than seeing it as a rude shock. Side effects should be anticipated. Counseling can help prevent the relapse typically associated with the first signs of side effects.[160] Difficulties in following a diet or in stopping smoking should be described in advance, coupled with encouragement for the patient to expect and cope with them rather than to give up at the first discouraging experience or event. If a patient has unrealistic expectations about the smooth course of recovery, weight loss, abstention, or adoption of a new health practice, the caregiver needs to correct these misperceptions before they become an excuse for giving up.

The second way the health care professional can help reinforce the adoption of a complex regimen requiring behavioral change at home or at work is to communicate directly or indirectly with family members or others in a patient's immediate circle of daily contacts. The critical importance of family support has been documented among patients with hypertension[161] and those with asthma.[162]

Family members can be invited to accompany the patient in discussing the prescribed regimen with the physician. Often, family members are left sitting in the waiting room when they could be participating in the discussion of home strategies to support the patient in adapting the prescribed regimen to daily routines. Cancer patients have reported that two factors influenced their decision to seek information during a physician consultation: the behavior and attitude of the physicians and the presence and disposition of a companion.[163] If the important parties cannot be influenced in the physician's office, a written message to them from the physician, carried by the patient or mailed or phoned to them with the patient's permission, could carry as much weight. The power of involving family members in reinforcing support of patients has been well established.[164]

SELF-MONITORING

Once the patient is motivated and the provider has addressed the enabling and reinforcing factors as well as the counseling, referrals, and support necessary to make the patient's self-care possible, return appointments can be spaced with increasing intervals. With each subsequent visit, some of what the provider examines as signs, symptoms, risk factors, or problems can be made the responsibility

of the patient in self-monitoring. Transferring increasing responsibility for self-care to the patient should be accompanied by an increase in the patient's self-monitoring skills.

Health care providers miss a powerful educational tool when they hoard patients' data and the methods of observation that would make patients capable of obtaining their own feedback on progress and achieving success in self-management. By transferring these skills and tools—such as self-monitoring blood pressure devices—to patients, providers enable them to obtain more immediate feedback on health adjustments. Over time, feedback from self-monitoring can become the most powerful source of reinforcement for positive behavior. A recent study on diabetes showed that self-efficacy alone could account for the diet, exercise, and home-glucose-testing behaviors of diabetics.[165] However, individual self-efficacy assessments did vary over time, implying that continuous physician adherence to the triage model described in Figure 11-7 remains critical.

If a patient continues to depend on the health care professional for this reinforcement, the patient can fail to make the conversion to self-reliance that is so essential to long-term maintenance for control of chronic or compulsive disorders. Recent assessments have emphasized that "a knowledgeable, activated patient will improve the provision of preventive services, and thus enhance community health."[166]

A recently developed model, which uses the Precede-Proceed components as a guiding framework, identifies tools that can change both physician and patient behavior.[167] Mapping the motivational and reinforcing components of physicians *and* patients in a collinear model [see Figure 11-1[168]] clarifies the interdependence of the two agents. This illustration also enumerates the pressures which make the triage model presented in Figure 11-7 necessary and effective.

In their qualitative assessment of physician practices, Makrides and associates have identified obstacles to *both* physician and patient success. Physicians' obtacles include personal, organizational, and structural factors, while those of patients involved individual and socioenvironmental components. The authors encourage physicians to acknowledge and address the socioenvironmental influences their patients face and to operationalize processes in a way similar to the process described in Figure 11-7.

CHANGING THE BEHAVIOR OF HEALTH CARE STAFF

What makes physicians, nurses, and other health care workers behave as they do with respect to prevention and health promotion? Although medical education and training have emphasized neither prevention nor promotion, physicians and allied health professionals show growing interest in enhancing their prevention practices. Physicians themselves have pointed out the influence their recommendations can have on patients' willingness to seek mammography screening[169] and the extent to which physicians' individual factors influence the use of cancer-screening procedures.[170]

Nursing education and the professional preparation of dieticians, pharmacists, and other health care workers have given greater emphasis to patient counseling, but working circumstances often conspire against enabling and reinforcing preventive practices. In addition, recent applications of the Precede-Proceed model, including its integration with health belief, behavioral, preventive, and adaptation principles, indicate that barriers to change exist for *both* patient and physician.[171]

In the concluding sections of this chapter, we present some principles of behavioral change that apply to the continuing education and support of health care workers to become more effective in counseling their patients to change lifestyles and environments.

BEHAVIORAL AND EDUCATIONAL ASSESSMENT OF PRACTITIONERS' BEHAVIOR

The following discussion could apply to any of the health care professions, but let us take the physician as the example. Other health care professionals may wish to contemplate how the Precede and Proceed concepts might be applied to behavioral changes of decision makers and policy changes in the health care system. Until recently, most people assumed that physicians routinely carried out preventive measures and patient counseling as part of their practice. They probably did until specialization and technology, along with rapidly expanding medical information and new economic circumstances, began to crowd these elements out of medical care. Now, even primary care physicians have difficulty devoting much time, attention, or effort to the education of their patients about behavioral risk factors and ways to modify them.[172] Recent studies have found large discrepancies among physician initiatives, patient expectations, and published guidelines.[173] A 1993 study of physician breast-cancer-screening behavior found no predictive link between some traits typically thought to be predictive of physician behavior and physicians' use of mammography screening.[174] The authors pointed instead to the patient's family history of breast cancer and ability to pay for a mammogram as predictive. Research has shown that even clear, concise recommendations for screening practices are not influential enough to change physician practices. Instead, many other factors influence them.[175]

In attempting to understand the practices of physicians, nurses, and other health care personnel, the three categories of behavioral influence (predisposing, enabling, and reinforcing factors) represent a convenient classification. They provide a practical grouping of the more specific influences—such as knowledge, attitudes and beliefs, skills, incentives, and rewards—under broader rubrics according to the measures that might be used to change behavior.[176]

PREDISPOSING FACTORS

The problem is partly attitudinal. Physicians and others trained in the medical tradition appear to doubt the importance of some behavioral risk factors.[177] In a survey of primary care physicians, less than half agreed that moderating or eliminating alcohol use, decreasing salt consumption, avoiding saturated fats, engaging in regular exercise, avoiding cholesterol, and minimizing sugar intake are very important for health promotion. Most of these physicians, however, agreed that reducing cigarette smoking is important. This suggests that physicians' attitudes are determined in part by the weight and general acceptance of scientific evidence.[178]

Some studies indicate large differences among medical specialties in their rates of patient counseling.[179] Physicians' preventive roles thus appear to be partly determined by their specialty; other researchers find little difference between general and family practitioners when the year of graduation from medical school is controlled for.[180]

Recent surveys indicate that health care personnel are becoming more interested in the health behavior of their patients. This probably reflects societal trends and interests, to which health professionals generally subscribe and respond. A statewide survey of primary care physicians in Texas found that most considered health promotion a challenging and enjoyable part of their practice. They considered smoking the most important risk factor.[181] A survey on nutrition counseling in private practices in Minnesota reported that physicians believe it is important to educate their patients about health risks, but they devote little time to it because they do not think patients want or would follow their advice.[182] A survey of primary care physicians found that most believe they should modify patient behavior to minimize risk factors, but only a small percentage report success in helping patients achieve behavioral change.[183]

The predisposing attitudinal factors, then, seem to be shifting toward a greater appreciation of the importance of behavioral risk factors and the importance of intervening to modify those factors. The problem now appears to center on the physician's diffidence in carrying out the intervention.[184] This, in turn, relates to a justifiable lack of self-confidence in knowing how to intervene effectively and a perception that the patients are not receptive to advice or willing to change. On the other side of the same coin, patients often perceive their physicians to be uninterested in their efforts to change, such as attempts to quit smoking.[185]

Physicians who believe the patient does not want to quit or is unable to do so are less likely to provide advice than are physicians who believe otherwise.[186] Also, physicians' beliefs about the effectiveness or importance of a particular practice technique or health behavior have repeatedly been shown to impact their use of it. This has been demonstrated regarding activities as varied as breast cancer screening[187] and the counseling of patients to continue breast-feeding.[188] Physicians consider this pessimism to be the greatest barrier to their preventive counseling.[189]

These cognitive, attitudinal, and perceptual problems can be classified as the predisposing factors influencing professional behavior. Depending on a health care provider's degree of self-confidence and his or her perception of the patient's willingness and ability to change, he or she will be more or less predisposed to take action to support the patient in making behavioral changes. Predisposing factors include the professional's values, beliefs, attitudes, and perceptions. Values include basic orientations, such as the role of the professional, patient autonomy, and issues of privacy of patient behavior or lifestyle outside the immediate medical realm. Though important, these have not been well studied. They can potentially predispose health care workers to pursue or avoid counseling and encouraging patients to pursue healthful lifestyles.

Beliefs include the more immediate and changeable viewpoints of the professional on matters such as patients' willingness to change their lifestyles or their ability to change their health practices. Related to the professional's beliefs about the patient's ability is the professional's belief in his or her own ability. This is referred to in social learning theory as a **self-efficacy** belief. Many physicians apparently feel unprepared to counsel patients about their lifestyles and consequently tend to avoid doing do.[190] Nurses' traditional adherence to the medical model has created some of the same barriers to their use of health promotion that physicians face.[191] Similar reservations about training or self-efficacy can limit nurses' attempts to educate patients.[192] In large measure, this probably reflects the training experience of physicians. Studies suggest that, compared with earlier graduates, recent graduates of family practice residencies have greater confidence in their counseling effectiveness.[193] The need for attention at the undergraduate and graduate levels of medical education to these matters should be apparent.[194]

ENABLING FACTORS

The foregoing predisposing factors account for the health care professional's motivation and confidence, but even with motivation, professionals sometimes fail to take the appropriate action, because they lack the necessary skills or resources to do so. The combination of low self-efficacy and a lack of fiscal and other resources to offer smoking-cessation services may account for most of the missed counseling opportunities reported by physicians and patients.[195] When preventive services are not reimbursed, a physician may be discouraged from both learning new skills and applying them. Predisposing factors must be quite strong to offset the disincentive of cost. In addition, while many practices might determine that preventive services could best be provided by someone other than the physician, there may not be another person available.

In a survey of 120 randomly selected primary care physicians in New York City, 87% agreed that physicians should practice more preventive medicine. However, the physicians cited lack of time, inadequate reimbursement, and unclear recommendations as the main obstacles to preventive care.[196] These obstacles represent a second class of factors influencing behavior—those that enable behaviors.

The lack of staff and space and the paucity of tested educational materials are also major barriers to preventive services.[197] A computerized health maintenance prompting system was gladly accepted by physicians in one study, and it seemed to improve their attitudes toward health promotion.[198] A twofold increase in preventive care measures was found among a group of physicians using computer-prompted reminders in another study.[199] Physicians' use of three cancer-screening techniques rose with the use of computer-generated reminders, particularly for patients over 70 years old.[200]

Actual skills in the practice of patient counseling represent another set of enabling factors. A lack of skills, usually because of education, differs from a poor "perceived self-efficacy" in that it represents a real deficit, not just a lack of confidence. Perceptions of skill predispose; competence enables.

Enabling factors, then, can be as simple as available space, materials, or reminders. They often take a more substantial form in the minds of professionals. Adequate reimbursement functions as an enabling factor by promising that the health care professionals' investment of time and effort in patient education and preventive medicine will not be wasted.

REINFORCING FACTORS

Actual reimbursement functions later as a reinforcing factor. Because it rewards behavior, it increases the probability that the behavior will recur at the next opportunity.

Reinforcing factors also include visible results, support from colleagues, and feedback from patients.[201] Colleague behavior both reinforces and eventually predisposes.

Curative treatment yields visible, usually short-term results that are satisfying to the patient and therefore rewarding to the health care professional. Because preventive measures often yield no palpable results, at least in the short term, they provide no positive feedback and reinforcement. "Treatment failures," or the absence of visible results, are more common in preventive care than in acute care. Since much illness is self-limited, the efficacy of treatment and the natural history of the illness combine to create the perception of efficacy. Preventive care has a longer time frame, and its effect—a change in prospective health status—is delayed or may never be evident to the patient.

Examinations of preventive care pressures within the managed care environment reveal opportunities to apply Precede-Proceed evaluations to the ever-expanding population of patients insured by these systems. Several critically important challenges within the sector also emerge. These must be overcome for significant change to occur.

MANAGED CARE

Individual managed care organizations or health maintenance organizations (HMOs) possess the structural tools to incorporate health promotion activities and preventive care into the practices of physicians' and other health care personnel.[202] They can effectively disseminate educational materials and practice guidelines, follow up by monitoring practice patterns through medical chart review and claims data, and generate a wide variety of data-generated tools (reminders, tracking tools, etc.) for preventive interventions. Efficiencies in this area often significantly exceed those available to government entities interested in attaining similar goals. A single HMOs tracking system, after providing physician feedback and individual patient reminders regarding immunizations for young children, based on PRECEDE-PROCEED showed an improvement in full compliance from 62% to a sustained rate of 90% within 2 years.[203]

An HMO can be particularly effective when its contractual relationship with physicians involves *capitation,* a payment mechanism that obligates a physician or medical group to provide comprehensive care in exchange for an agreed-on monthly payment. The providers of care are then motivated to prevent costly conditions rather than treat them once they emerge. Otherwise, physicians often have no financial incentive to spend the time to counsel for, perform, or interpret the results of screening procedures such as mammography.[204]

In addition, some see the impact of market forces on HMOs as advantageous to health promotion. Trends in the managed care industry indicate that competition for members will increasingly depend on demonstrated quality-of-care measures—which often include screening rates and other preventive care activities. Individual U.S. plans report data on a wide variety of preventive, administrative, and clinical activities to the National Committee for Quality Assurance (NCQA). This reporting process can occur either through the Health Plan Employer Data and Information Set (HEDIS) or accreditation procedures, both of which are becoming increasingly critical to effective competition in the marketplace and are sometimes required by state legislation.

HMO wellness programs, highlighted by some in the 1980s as a beacon of hope for health promotion advocates, incorporate need and risk assessments, which in turn often generate the delivery of educational materials.[205] Some multifactorial patient education programs, difficult or impossible to implement in a fee-for-service environment, have generated encouraging results in the managed care setting. A kit aimed at increasing medication compliance among hypertensives, for example, and including educational, nutritional, and lifestyle information can be highly effective when combined with telephone follow-up and mailed prescription reminders.[206] The primary caveat from a health promotion standpoint remains the profit motive underlying these activities. However, as competition based on quality measurement criteria continues, consumers can benefit from the continued pursuit of preventive care activities.

COMPLICATIONS AND BARRIERS

Just as individual managed care organizations can build effective structures to promote health among their own members, the larger system of managed care can make interventions more complicated for practitioners. Often, physicians and their staffs receive guidelines, tracking forms, and requests for data from a variety of managed care organizations. This can cause uncertainty and confusion regarding preferred practice patterns, which has been shown to influence negatively physician adherence to recommendations for preventive services.[207] It can also create serious impediments to implementing comprehensive tracking or reminder systems within an office setting. Generally, each managed care organization provides enough tools and logistical support only for its own members, and each may face a range of implementation or compliance problems for monitored conditions, like diabetes mellitus.[208]

Health care providers who are directly employed by an HMO, rather than operating under a contractual relationship with one or several, can avoid some of these complications. A collaborative relationship between HMOs and physicians remains crucial to the success of programs such as patient education.[209] However, most providers throughout the U.S. system continue to lack any automated data systems used in managing clinical care or coordinating screening programs.[210] This impedes the creation of enabling factors for providers and patients alike.

Challenges for these two groups also arise from two structural components of the managed care system. One of these challenges is the general pressure to provide care to more patients at lower cost.[211] Concerns have emerged regarding attention to quality of care[212] and efficacy of one-step patient education programs. A second challenge is the push to apply self-care skills to a wider array of illnesses as coverage for inpatient care continues to shrink. Research assessing the impact of this pressure on patient health remains incomplete.

In the wake of intense reevaluations in both the United States and Canada, various components of the health care system have been undergoing change, expansion, and in some cases elimination. Health promotion, disease prevention, and community-based care are now receiving more attention from Canadian officials looking to deliver more long-term health for less money.[213] Evidence that good communication and structured patient education can be cost-effective for conditions like asthma[214] and arthritis[215] will likely encourage the expansion of similar programs.

For example, recognition of Precede-Proceed interactions has shaped the re-designing of patient care at a large integrated teaching and health care system lo-cated in the southeastern United States.[216] The designers acknowledged that, traditionally, "decision making and goal setting have been the functions of the health care provider."[217] Their redesign instead uses principles of collaboration to bring patients into a position of equal stature. The principles of collaboration, ca-pacity building, and coalitions apply reciprocally to health plans, other commu-nity organizations concerned with health, and state or provincial and federal government agencies, as suggested by Figure 11-8.

PRINCIPLES OF HEALTH EDUCATION IN RELATION TO HEALTH CARE BEHAVIORS

If the determinants of health workers' preventive and health promotion practices can be distilled from the wide range of studies into the three broad categories, how can one use these categories to organize interventions to enhance preventive practices? A study of the cancer prevention practices of primary care physicians found variables that could be classified as predisposing, enabling, and reinforc-ing, but the specific mix of determinants varied with the cancer site.[218] This sug-gests that attempts to alter physician behavior should follow an assessment of the factors that require primary attention and modification.

THE PRINCIPLE OF EDUCATIONAL DIAGNOSIS

The first task in changing behavior is to determine its causes. We refer to this as the *diagnostic principle* of changing behavior. Just as the physician must diag-nose an illness before it can be properly treated, so, too, must a behavior be diag-nosed before it can be properly changed. *Properly* in this context means interventions that are essentially educational rather than coercive or manipulative. If the causes of a behavior can be understood, physicians can intervene with the most appropriate and efficient combination of education, training, resource devel-opment, and rewards to influence the factors that predispose, enable, or reinforce the behavior.

Until it is possible to diagnose each health professional, all we may know is that insufficient preventive care is being provided. If there are insufficient diag-nostic data, some analogies from medical practice may apply: (1) treating the symptom, (2) treating presumptively using broadly effective therapy, and (3) treating the specific etiological or underlying problem. In symptomatic treatment, we recognize the lack of preventive care and choose one level (e.g., predisposing, enabling, reinforcing) at which to intervene.

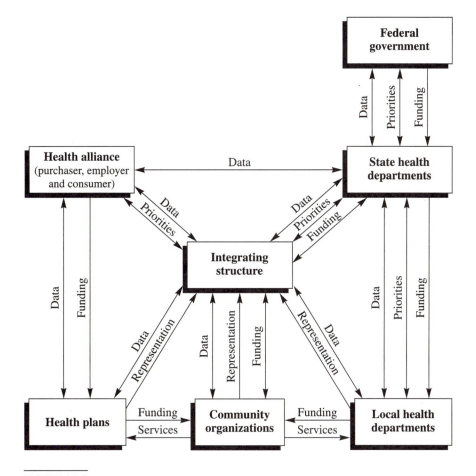

FIGURE 11-8

This model of organizational relationships for disease prevention and health promotion among public, private, and voluntary organizations suggests greater collaboration than has been characteristic of health sector organizations in medical care. An integrating structure will be needed.

SOURCE: H. H. Schauffler, M. Faer, L. Faulkner, and K. Shore, contract report to the California Wellness Foundation, University of California School of Public Health, October 1993.

Treating the problem with broad-based intervention—working at multiple levels simultaneously—is more likely to be effective than specific intervention. However, as with medication, there are potential adverse consequences. First, a broad-based approach tends to cost more. Second, it may elicit an "allergic" reaction. If health professionals consider an educational intervention inappropriate or redundant, they may perceive it as criticism and become hypersensitive. Should this occur, they will be unlikely to cooperate with efforts to change their behavior. Educational interventions that consistently elicit this response could make the professional relatively resistant to further efforts. Because of these risks, broad-based efforts to change behavior should focus on predisposing factors; if enabling or reinforcing factors are addressed, the intervention should be individualized for each health care worker.

Finally, an intervention linked to a diagnosed problem has the greatest chance of success. A program based on the Precede model to help physicians in rural western Pennsylvania assess their own learning needs was developed at Johns Hopkins University. Experimental groups of primary care physicians participated in audiovisual self-study programs tailored to their own assessments of their educational needs. Researchers measured the course's impact by using questionnaires to gauge gains in knowledge and using simulated patient visits to observe performance with patients with chronic obstructive pulmonary disease. The experimental groups retained significantly greater amounts of information 9 months after the program and used more program material in counseling patients than did the control group.[219]

THE HIERARCHICAL PRINCIPLE

The *hierarchical principle* of behavioral change states that there is a natural precedence in the sequence of factors influencing behavior; the first order of business is to ensure that predisposing factors have been addressed before enabling factors, and enabling factors before reinforcing factors. In reality, the opportunities for intervention are usually fleeting, so that all three types of factors must be addressed simultaneously in most circumstances.

In addition, a single intervention may address several factors at once. The hierarchial principle aligns the interventions (education, counseling, training, resources, feedback, rewards) so that they are expended or deployed in the most efficient and logical order.

It is inefficient and sometimes ineffective to train someone in skills to enable a behavior when he or she lacks prior motivation. We have seen evidence that many physicians lack confidence in the efficacy or importance of some preventive maneuvers; of those who accept the value of the procedures, many doubt their own competence or the ability of the patient to make changes. Unless these beliefs are in place, there is little point in training physicians in preventive or health promotion skills.

Similarly, reinforcement designed to reward a behavior for which a health care professional was not predisposed is useless. There is little point in setting up a reward system for physicians who perform sigmoidoscopies if the physicians have not been educated to understand the need for them or trained to perform them.[220]

THE PRINCIPLE OF CUMULATIVE LEARNING

Related to the hierarchical principle is the *principle of cumulative learning.* To affect the behavior of professionals or patients, a series of learning experiences must be planned in a sequence that takes into account the prior learning experiences and concurrent incidental experiences to which the learners are exposed. Learning does not occur in a vacuum. Behavior results from the cumulative learning experiences of an individual, including those that preceded and those that were incidental to the planned educational or behavioral change program. Physicians' behaviors are the products not only of medical education but of all prior education, formal and informal; of concurrent life experiences; and of the society in which physicians were raised, educated, and trained and in which they practice. In gathering data, physicians first learn a fairly rote and uniform approach. They need an equally circumscribed, basic approach to preventive medicine and patient education.

Clearly the medical curriculum of the past has not given physicians a base of learning that would predispose or enable them to take maximum advantage of new educational opportunities in preventive medicine, much less practice it effectively.[221] Preventive medicine remains one of the "orphan" areas of medical education.[222] A recent meta-analysis of continuing medical education formats indicated a continuing reliance on those methods, like conferences, which have been shown to be least effective in changing physicians' attitudes or practice patterns.[223]

However, postgraduate training appears to be changing, and new medical graduates are demanding more behavioral medicine and patient education in their residencies.[224] Federal programs in the United States that support physician training, advisory committees, certifying and accrediting organizations, and employers of physicians are all broadening their expectations of physicians' capabilities and responsibilities in this regard.

THE PRINCIPLE OF PARTICIPATION

The prospects for success in any attempt to change professional behavior will be greater if the professionals have helped identify their own need for change and have selected the method that will enable them to make the change.[225] No principle of behavioral change has greater generalizability than the *principle of participation.*[226]

This principle allows packaged behavioral change programs to adapt to the diversity of prior learning experiences and concurrent circumstances in a population of health care professionals. Physicians who adapt education materials to their own needs, for example, are more committed to using the materials than are those who do not.[227]

THE PRINCIPLE OF SITUATIONAL SPECIFICITY

The *principle of situational specificity* holds that there is nothing inherently superior or inferior about any method of intervention to achieve behavioral change. Such change always depends on the circumstances, the target audience, the timing, and the enthusiasm and commitment of the instructor or other agent of change. New methods of education or intervention often appear to have an advantage over traditional methods in randomized trials, but this advantage typically fades when the method loses its novelty. Though this novelty effect makes some methods seem superior, the history of educational research is strewn with new educational technologies that prove in the long run to be no better than the older technologies except in their strategic application to the right audience, at the right time, with enthusiasm and commitment. Thus, efforts to change behavior must rely more on the diagnostic principle and the principle of participation to match appropriate methods with the characteristics and felt needs of participants rather than on the presumed inherent superiority of any method.[228]

THE PRINCIPLE OF MULTIPLE METHODS

The *principle of multiple methods* also follows from the diagnostic principle, insofar as multiple causes will invariably be found for any given behavior. For each of the multiple predisposing, enabling, and reinforcing factors identified, a different method or component of a comprehensive behavioral change program must be provided.

Primary care physicians attempting to promote health or offer preventive services often use ineffective methods. Only one fourth of those who give advice regularly offer a systematic behavioral or educational intervention.[229] Physicians tend to use the same multiplicity of approaches in preventive medicine as they use to obtain information for therapeutic decisions.[230]

THE PRINCIPLE OF INDIVIDUALIZATION

The tailoring or *individualization* of learning essentially applies the principles of cumulative learning, participation, and situational specificity. *Tailoring* refers to the adaptation of learning experiences to each individual. This becomes impossible for large-scale programs, which is one reason why reading continues to be rated by physicians as a preferred source of information for preventive medicine decisions.[231] The physician can control the selection, pace, repetition, skipping pattern, and other aspects of the learning experience better with reading material than with any other learning method. Reading fails, however, to provide the practice and feedback necessary for successful behavior change. This leads us to the final principle.

THE FEEDBACK PRINCIPLE

The *principle of feedback* is critical. It ensures that the individual whose behavior is expected to change obtains direct and immediate feedback on the progress and effects of his or her behavior. This enables the learner to adapt to both the learning process and the behavioral responses within his or her own situation and pace. As with other principles, the feedback principle applies to both professionals and patients.

One of the reasons physicians rely on reading for their primary source of information on prevention is because there is little feedback from patients or colleagues on preventive practice. When it does exist, however, feedback can affect physicians' behaviors greatly. Peer comparison feedback on physician performance in colorectal screening was found to improve "compliance" with recommended standards of care and played an important role in quality assurance.[232]

One study demonstrated that physicians trained to give antismoking advice to their patients did it following their training but did so less frequently without feedback. A subsequent intervention in which the advice-giving rates of the physicians were monitored monthly and physicians were given immediate corrective feedback resulted in sustained antismoking advice giving by the physicians.[233]

SUMMARY

Factors predisposing, enabling, and reinforcing patients and the health care professionals who provide preventive care and education to their patients about lifestyle changes have been identified in various recent studies. The organization of these findings within a framework for planning educational and behavioral change interventions suggests a series of learning principles that can be applied with greater effect than can the standard continuing education format. Essentially the same Precede-Proceed steps and principles that apply to patients and populations apply to health care professionals.

The opportunities and needs for patient education and counseling exceed the current supply, not as much in quantity as in quality, willingness, and distribution. Much of the available energy devoted to patient education and counseling fails to reach the patients who need it most, when they need it, and in ways that would be most helpful to them. This chapter describes "compliance" problems in terms of errors of omission and errors of commission. An epidemiological assessment of needs for intervention on the various categories of such errors would segment the potential patient population into five high-risk groups:

1. Nonusers who are not under medical care but who would benefit from the use of a prescription or other medical or lifestyle regimen
2. Nonusers whose medical care provider has not recommended or prescribed a needed drug, device, or lifestyle regimen

3. Nonusers who did not purchase a recommended drug or device or adopt a recommended lifestyle modification

4. Misusers who are using someone else's drug or a medication or procedure previously recommended or prescribed for another problem

5. Misusers who are not following the schedule or dosage recommended

The environments, channels, and methods for communicating effectively with each of these groups vary systematically in ways that recommend new strategies for the support of professional, public health, and patient education.

Pharmaceutical companies and third-party payers could play a more active role in direct mass communications to the public about the risk factors, signs, and symptoms of diseases and conditions for which medical or self-care measures are available. Encouraging and enabling affected patients to seek screening or medical advice would improve the public health more in the long run than would increased efforts to eliminate "noncompliance" for those already under care. On the other hand, burdening the medical system with more patients when staff have too little time to spend understanding and interacting with patients will only make the problems worse.

The efficiency of patient education for those under care could be improved by systematic analyses of compliance error rates in various subpopulations of patients. This would lead in most settings to a greater allocation of patient education and counseling effort for older men lower on the socioeconomic scale than for younger women with high incomes. A similar epidemiological analysis of the relative rates of compliance error for specific pathologies or symptomatologies could segment the patient population for effective educational triage within demographic groups.

Medical schools and other continuing education and quality assurance resources could be targeted more sharply to those physicians who are prescribing drugs incorrectly or who remain unconvinced that underused drugs or procedures are a problem. Physicians, for example, do not have as much conviction and belief in their ability to modify dietary practices in their patients as in their ability to control blood pressure. Similarly, these educational resources could give greater emphasis to those patient education and counseling skills required by physicians in educating and strengthening the motivation of their patients to fill prescriptions and to adhere to the prescribed regimens. According to the net results of 102 published evaluations of patient education related to errors with drug regimens, such an investment would reduce drug errors by 40–72% and improve clinical outcomes such as blood pressure control and reduced emergency room visits by 23–47%.

Sufficient knowledge has now accumulated to enable health care professionals to approach the problem of patient "compliance" with greater confidence, effectiveness, and efficiency than before. Greater confidence should come from the accumulated evidence offered by studies of teaching and counseling patients on self-medication and more complex lifestyle changes. Greater effectiveness should come from the increased awareness among health professionals that basic principles of learning have been instrumental in transferring knowledge, skills, and responsibility to patients. Greater efficiency should come from the stepped-care approach to patient education and counseling. By focusing their time and effort at the level of help needed by each patient, health professionals can bypass needless motivational appeals and skill development for some patients and use the same effectively for others.

A final maneuver in consigning greater responsibility to patients for their own care and health maintenance is to transfer self-monitoring skills and tools to them. These become both enabling and reinforcing factors in patients' long-term maintenance of behaviors conducive to health. In the final analysis, they enable people to take ownership and control of their own lives—the determinants of their own health and quality of life.

EXERCISES

1. For a given clinical setting, describe the distribution of health problems presented by patients and justify the selection of a particular problem as the first priority for health education planning.
2. For the priority health problem, show the procedures you would follow in conducting a behavioral assessment and write a behavioral objective for the highest priority behavior to be addressed in this population of patients.
3. For the chosen behavior, develop an inventory of predisposing, enabling, and reinforcing factors, set priorities on one or two of each, and write educational objectives, methods of intervention, and evaluation measures for these.

NOTES AND CITATIONS

1. We thank Lacuna Williams, Fulbright Fellow at the UBC Institute of Health Promotion Research during 1998, for her helpful contributions to the updating of literature for this chapter.
2. P. D. Mullen, Green, & Persinger, 1985; P. D. Mullen, Mains, & Velez, 1992; P. D. Mullen, Ramirez, & Groff, 1994; P. D. Mullen et al., 1997. Other meta-analyses and systematic reviews of the continuing and professional education literature in medical care settings have applied PRECEDE in examining the factors influencing behavioral change in practitioners, revealing the necessity of including attention to enabling and reinforcing factors, in addition to the usual emphasis on predisposing factors: Davis, Thomson, Oxman, & Haynes, 1992, 1995; Oxman, Thomson, Davis, & Haynes, 1995; Tamblyn & Battista, 1993.
3. The Nursing Development Conference Group (1973) reviews the evolution of the self-care concept from Nightingale's "helping the helpless" and her distinction between "sick nursing and health nursing," through Shaw and Harmer's textbooks of nursing at the turn of the century, to current nursing concepts of self-care. For a broader history of the concept of self-care in contrast

to the medical model, as well as its relationship to parallel movements such as consumer partic-ipation, see Green, Werlin, Schauffler, & Avery, 1977; Levin & Idler, 1983.

4. Ziff, Conrad, & Lachman, 1995. For applications of PRECEDE in examining the issues of per-ceived control and empowerment in relating patient or community needs and capacities to those of health professionals, see Allison, 1991; Garvin, 1995; Jenny, 1993; and the control typology of Padilla & Bulcavage, 1991, including processual, contingency, cognitive, behavioral, and existential controls.

5. This section is adapted from Green, 1993; Green, Cargo, & Ottoson, 1994.

6. Okene, Lindsay, Berger, & Hymowitz, 1990–1991.

7. Green, Wilson, & Lovato, 1986.

8. Nussel et al., 1992.

9. "Adult Immunizations," 1988.

10. Health and Welfare Canada, 1992.

11. National Center for Health Statistics, 1992.

12. Institute of Medicine, 1983.

13. M. H. Becker, 1974; Harrison, Mullen, & Green, 1992. For applications of the Health Belief Model within the context of PRECEDE-PROCEED in patient education, see W. C. Bailey et al., 1987; Breckon, 1982 (esp. pp. 175–184); Deeds & Gunatilake, 1989; Green, Levine, Wolle, & Deeds, 1979; Neumark-Sztainer & Story, 1996; Padilla & Bulcavage, 1991; Street, Gold, & Manning, 1997, esp. pp. 54–65. Lorig & Laurin, 1985, critiqued the Health Belief Model and an earlier version of PRECEDE for assuming that behavior mediated the relationship between beliefs and health outcomes for patients with chronic conditions such as arthritis. She presented data showing that the beliefs can directly affect perceptions of health without changing behav-ior. The current version of PRECEDE-PROCEED attempts to take this psychosomatic connec-tion into account. See McGowan, 1995; McGowan & Green, 1995.

14. Moser, McCance, & Smith, 1991.

15. Coulter & Schofield, 1991; Risker & Christopher, 1995.

16. Kottke, Brekke, & Marquez, 1997; Wallace & Haines, 1984.

17. Battista, 1983; Battista, Palmer, Marchland, & Spitzer, 1985.

18. P. S. Williamson, Driscoll, Dvorak, Garber, & Shank, 1988.

19. Iverson, Fielding, Crow, & Christenson, 1985. See, however, Godin & Shephard, 1990.

20. Green, Simons-Morton, & Potvin, 1997.

21. Council on Scientific Affairs, 1990. Most of what we review here concerning physicians, who control or at least influence the professional practices of most other health care workers in clin-ical settings, applies also to those other professions. For applications of PRECEDE-PROCEED in assessing or influencing the health promotion practices of other clinical health workers, see Berland, Whyte, & Maxwell, 1995; DeJoy, Murphy, & Gershon, 1995; Han, Baumann, & Cim-prich, 1996; Laitakari, Miilunpalo, & Vuori, 1997; Macrina, Macrina, Horvath, Gallaspy, & Fine, 1996; Mahlock, Taylor, Taplin, & Urban, 1993; Mann et al., 1996; McKell, 1994; McKell, Chase, & Balram, 1996; Miilunpalo, Laitakari, & Vuolo, 1995; Shamian & Edgar, 1987; P. H. Smith, Danis, & Helmick, 1998; Whyte & Berland, 1993.

22. K. B. Wells, Ware, & Lewis, 1984.

23. Price, Desmond, Krol, Snyder, & O'Connell, 1987. Studies applying PRECEDE-PROCEED to assessment of physician attitudes, barriers, and practices in clinical health promotion include Battista, Williams, & MacFarlane, 1990; Burglehaus, Smith, Sheps, & Green, 1997; Costanza, 1992; Donovan, 1991; Downey, Cresanta, & Berenson, 1989; Duke, McGraw, & Avis, 1995; Green, Eriksen, & Shor, 1988; Haber, 1994; Heywood, Firman, Sanson-Fisher, & Mudge, 1996; Hiddink, Hautvast, van Woerkum, Fieren, & van't Hof, 1995, 1997a, 1997b; Langille, Mann, & Gailiunas, 1997; Love et al., 1993; Mann & Putnam, 1989, 1990; Singer, Lundsay, & Wilson, 1991; V. M. Taylor, Taplin, Urban, Mahloch, & Majer, 1994; Thamer et al., 1998; J. M. E. Walsh & McPhee, 1992; Weinberger et al., 1992.

24. McAlister et al., 1985; Price, Desmond, Krol, Snyder, & O'Connell, 1987.

25. Price, Desmond, Krol, Snyder, & O'Connell, 1987.

26. Eriksen, Green, &Fultz, 1988.

27. Trumble, 1991.

28. Gelman, 1992.

29. Reed, Jensen, & Gorenflo, 1991.

30. Radecki & Mandenhall, 1986; Wechsler, Levine, Idelson, Rothman, & Taylor, 1983.

31. C. E. Lewis, Clancy, Leake, & Schwartz, 1991.

32. Green, Eriksen, & Schor, 1988.

33. C. E. Lewis, Clancy, Leake, & Schwartz, 1991.

34. Green, Eriksen, & Schor, 1988.

35. Council on Scientific Affairs, 1990.

36. K. M. Cummings, Giovino, Sciandra, Koenigsberg, & Emont, 1987; Lewis, Clancy, Leake, & Schwartz, 1991; K. B. Wells, Lewis, Leake, & Ware, 1984; Wells, Ware, & Lewis, 1984.

37. Cummings, Giovino, Sciandra, Koenigsberg, & Emont, 1987; Lewis, Clancy, Leake, & Schwartz, 1991.

38. Wells, Lewis, Leake, & Ware, 1984.

39. Radecki & Mandenhall, 1986.

40. Schwartz, Soumerai, & Avorn, 1989.

41. Holmes, Morrow, & Pickering, 1996.

42. McArtor et al., 1992; Schwartz et al., 1991.

43. Costanza, 1992; Dodek & Ottoson, 1996; Stange et al., 1992.

44. Elford, 1992; Schriger, Baraff, & Cretin, 1997.

45. Dickinson, Wiggers, Leeder, & Sanson-Fisher, 1989.

46. Anda, Remington, Sienko, & Davis, 1987.

47. McArtor et al., 1992.

48. Radecki & Mandenhall, 1986; U.S. Preventive Services Task Force, 1996.

49. Green, Eriksen, & Schor, 1988; Love, Davoli, & Thurman, 1996.

50. Kottke, Foels, Hill, Choi, & Fendersonet, 1984.

51. Canadian Task Force on the Periodic Health Examination, 1979, 1994.

52. Tolsma, 1993; U.S. Department of Health and Human Services, 1991.

53. U.S. Preventive Services Task Force, 1989.

54. Hayward, Steinberg, Ford, Roizen, & Roach, 1991.

55. This section is based on an adaptation of Green, 1994b, and of Green, Mullen, & Friedman, 1986, updated as Chapter 29 in Cramer & Spilker, 1991. The environmental focus of this chapter is on the environment of patients, including the home, the workplace, and the health care setting itself. For consideration of the role of hospitals and health care workers in community health promotion, school health, or work-site health promotion, see the respective previous chapters. For applications of PRECEDE in hospital settings, see L. K. Bartholomew, Koenning, Dahlquist, & Barron, 1994; L. K. Bartholomew, Seilheimer, Parcel, Spinelli, & Pumariega, 1988. This project received the Award of Program Excellence from the Society for Public Health Education, 1994. Berland, Whyte, & Maxwell, 1995; Burglehaus, Smith, Sheps, & Green, 1997; Calabro, Weltge, Parnell, Kouzekanani, & Ramirez, 1998; Han, Baumann, & Cimprich, 1996; Fulmer et al., 1992; Kovar et al., 1992; Larson et al., 1991; Macrina, Macrina, Horvath, Gallaspy, & Fine, 1996; McGovern, Kochevar, Vesley, & Gershon, 1997; Macarthur, Macarthur, & Weeks, 1995; Malo & Leviton, 1987; Michalsen et al., 1997; Parcel et al., 1994; van Veenendal, Grinspun, & Adriaanse, 1996; Taggart et al., 1991.

56. We use the terms *compliance* and *patient* for convenience and convention, even though several of the types of error discussed here are not patient errors of failing to follow physicians' directions. Many are errors sometimes of physicians, nurses, or pharmacists themselves, or of patients who have not yet received appropriate directions from a physician or other health care provider. We shall introduce the phrase *health care error* to encompass the wider range of behavioral and environmental sources of medical or health care problems that PRECEDE/PROCEED attempts to address. The issue of practitioner compliance with best practices guidelines has become one of the focal points for many applications of PRECEDE-PROCEED. See for example Makrides, Veinot, Richard, & Allen, 1997; Mann & Putnam, 1989, 1990; Mann, Putnam, Lindsay, & Davis, 1996. For more on the concept and language of compliance, see P. D. Mullen, 1997.

57. Cramer & Spilker, 1991; Goldbloom & Lawrence, 1990; Green, 1990; Haynes, Taylor, & Sackett, 1979; Maes, Spielberger, Defares, & Sarason, 1988; Schmidt & Leppik, 1988; Shumaker, Parker, & Wolle, 1990. Cf. Michielutte, Dignan, Bahnson, & Wells, 1994.

58. D. A. Davis, Thomson, Oxman, & Haynes, 1992, 1995; Mann, 1994; Oxman, Thomson, Davis, & Haynes, 1995; Tamblyn & Battista, 1993.

59. Goldbloom & Battista, 1986; Goldbloom & Lawrence, 1990; Haber, 1994; Selby-Harrington et al., 1995; U.S. Preventive Services Task Force, 1996.

60. Andersen, 1968; Green & Ottoson, 1999; Green & Roberts, 1974; Mercer et al., 1997; Rimer, 1993; Zapka, Stoddard, Costanza, & Greene, 1989; Zapka et al., 1993.

61. U.S. Preventive Services Task Force, 1996.

62. Green & Ottoson, 1999, pp. 314–319; National Center for Health Statistics, 1990.

63. Lenfant & Roccella, 1984. For specific applications of the Precede model for increased use of health services for high blood pressure control, see R. L. Bertera & Cuthie, 1984; Bowler, Morisky, & Deeds, 1980; Grueninger, Duffy, & Goldstein, 1995; Haber, 1994; D. M. Levine et al., 1982; Livingston, 1985; Mamon et al., 1987; Mann, 1989; Modeste, Abbey, & Hopp, 1984–1985; Morisky, Levine, Wood et al., 1981; Salazar, 1985; Ward et al., 1982.

64. Garraway & Whisnant, 1987; Kotchen et al., 1986.

65. Cuca & Pierce, 1977; Dawson, 1986; Udry et al., 1972; Zelnik & Kim, 1982.

66. Cullen, Fox, & Isom, 1976; Green, Rimer, & Elwood, 1982. This last review uses the Precede model to assess strengths and gaps in the cancer prevention and screening efforts of the 1970s. Subsequent studies of cancer education and screening efforts that applied the Precede model include Brailey, 1986; Borgers et al., 1993; Bowen, Kinne, & Urban, 1997; Chie & Chang, 1994; Chie, Cheng, Fu, & Yen, 1993; Contento, Kell, Keiley, & Corcoran, 1992; Cretain, 1989; Dignan et al., 1991; Dignan, Beal, et al., 1990; Dignan et al., 1996; Dignan, Michielutte, et al., 1990; Dignan, Michielutte, Sharp, Young, & Daniels, 1991; Dignan, Michielutte, Wells, & Bahnson, 1995; Earp, Alpeter, Mayne, Viadro, & Omalley, 1995; Eng, 1993; Fawcett, Paine, Francisco, & Vliet, 1993; Fleisher et al., 1998; Glanz & Rimer, 1995; Haber, 1994; Han, Baumann, & Cimprich, 1996; Keintz, Rimer, Fleisher, & Engstrom, 1988; Lefebvre et al., 1995; Love et al., 1993; Mahloch, Taylor, Taplin, & Urban, 1993; Maxwell, Bastani, & Warda, 1998; McCoy, Nielsen, Chitwood, Zavertnik, & Khoury, 1991; Mercer et al., 1997; Michielutte et al., 1989; Michielutte, Dignan, Bahnson, & Wells, 1994; Morrison, 1996; Neef, Scutchfield, Elder, & Bender, 1991; Ostwald & Rothenberger, 1985; Padilla & Bulcavage, 1991; Rimer, 1993, 1995; Rimer, Keintz, & Fleisher, 1986; Rimer, Ross, Balshem, & Engstrom, 1993; Rimer, Ross, Christinzio, & Keng, 1992; Sanderson et al., 1996; Sanders-Phillips, 1996; Shamian & Edgar, 1987; Sharp et al., 1998; J. A. Smith & Scammon, 1984; Sneden, Nichols, & Gottlieb, 1997; Taplin, 1989; V. M. Taylor, Taplin, Urban, Mahloch, & Majer, 1994; R. S. Thompson, Taplin, McAfee, Mendelson, & Smith, 1995; Thomsen & Ter Maat, 1998; Ureda, 1993; M. Weinberger et al., 1992; Worden et al., 1990; Workman, 1989; Zapka, Chasen, Berth, Mas, & Costanza, 1992; Zapka et al., 1993; Zapka & Mamon, 1982; Zapka, Stoddard, Costanza, & Green, 1989.

67. Hersey, Klibanoff, Lam, & Taylor, 1984. Applications of PRECEDE-PROCEED in mental health include Kelly, 1990; R. W. Wilson, 1986; M. L. Wong, Alsagoff, & Koh, 1992.

68. Other applications of the Precede model in secondary prevention and screening or early diagnosis (besides cancer) include Bakdash, 1983; Bakdash, Lange, & McMillan, 1983; Donovan,

1991; Haber, 1994; C. C. Johnson, Powers, Bao, Harsha, & Berenson, 1994; Kraft, 1988; Lau et al., 1980; Olson, 1994; Redman, Spencer, & Sanson-Fisher, 1990; Salazar, 1985; Selby-Harrington et al., 1995.

69. Garfield, 1970.

70. Chassin, Mann, & Sher, 1988; Zapka et al., 1989.

71. Bloom, 1990; German et al., 1987.

72. E. M. Bertera & Bertera, 1981; Brimberry, 1988; Earp, Ory, & Strogatz, 1982; Fink & Shapiro, 1990; Fleisher et al., 1998; Hindi-Alexander & Cropp, 1981; Selby, Riportella-Muller; Sorenson, & Walters, 1989; Selby et al., 1990; Selby-Harrington et al., 1995.

73. Fried & Bush, 1988; Risser, Hoffman, Bellah, & Green, 1985; R. S. Thompson et al., 1988.

74. C. E. Lewis, 1988b; Silvers, Hovell, Weisman, & Mueller, 1985.

75. Eraker & Politser, 1982; Fedder, 1982; Herbert & Paluck, 1997; Paluck, 1998; Pels, Bor, & Lawrence, 1983.

76. Herbert & Paluck, 1997; Paluck, 1998; Thamer et al., 1998.

77. Cockburn et al., 1997; Halloway, 1996; O'Connor, Pennie, & Dales, 1996.

78. Bruhn, 1983; A. C. King et al., 1986; Korhonen et al., 1983; Landman, Levine, & Rappaport, 1984; Pederson & Baskerville, 1983.

79. Detullio et al., 1986; Lamb, Green, & Heron, 1994; Leickly et al., 1998.

80. For reviews of the continuing medical education literature applying PRECEDE-PROCEED, see Bertram & Brooks-Bertram, 1977; and the more recent reviews cited in endnotes 2 and 23. For other approaches based on quality control, see Canadian Council of Cardiovascular Nurses, 1993, which uses the Precede model to set clinical health promotion standards of practice and quality assurance guidelines for cardiovascular nurses; Eriksen, Green, & Fultz, 1988; Pincus, 1996; Sneden, Nichols, & Gottlieb, 1997.

81. Applications of PRECEDE in accomplishing patient education through mass media include Bakdash, 1983; Centers for Disease Control, 1987; Kroger, 1994; Meredith, O'Reilly, & Schulz, 1989.

82. Ailinger & Dear, 1993; Andersen & Genthner, 1990; Palmer, 1996; Sennett, 1998.

83. Roter, Hall, & Katz, 1988; Vickery & Fries, 1981; Vickery et al., 1983. Daltroy, 1993; Estey, Musseau, & Keehn, 1994; Holloway, 1996; Yeo, 1998 applied PRECEDE in assessing understanding and perceptions of patients with osteoarthritis who had been prescribed nonsteroidal anti-inflammatory drugs.

84. Estey, Musseau, & Keehn, 1994; Gregor, 1984; Mann & Sullivan, 1987; Tuckett, Bouleton, & Olson, 1985.

85. Green & Faden, 1977. More recent debate on informed consent emphasizes the understatement by physicians of side effects (see Katz, Daltroy, Brennan, & Liang, 1992), while recognizing that physicians could cause undue fear and even induce side effects by mentioning them: Howland, Baker, & Poe, 1990; Katz, Daltroy, Brennan, & Liang, 1992; Lamb, Green, & Heron, 1994; M. G. Myers, Cairns, & Singer, 1987.

86. Bonnet, Gagnayre, & d'Ivernois, 1998; S. Fisher, Mansbridge, & Lankford, 1982; Grenier & Grenier, 1996; Morrow, Hier, & Leirer, 1998; Pepe & Chodzko-Zajko, 1997.

87. Esdale & Harris, 1985; Maiman, Green, Gibson, & Mackenzie, 1979. The major barriers to clinical practitioners devoting more time to patient education and counseling are organizational and system (enabling and reinforcing) factors, which this chapter attempts to address. See Cooke, Mattick, & Campbell, 1998; Glanz, Brekke, Harper, Bache-Wiig, & Hunnighake, 1992; P. D. Mullen et al., 1995. On tailoring, see M. K. Campbell et al., 1994.

88. Honig & Gillespie, 1995; L. Lawrence & McLemore, 1983; W. J. Millar, 1998.

89. Green, Mullen, & Friedman, 1986.

90. Kreuter, Vehige, & McGuire, 1996; Rimer, Orleans, Fleischer et al., 1994.

91. I. T. Hill, 1988. Applications of PRECEDE in recruiting women for prenatal assessment or clinical preventive care include Donovan, 1991; V. C. Li et al., 1984; Olson, 1994; Windsor, 1984, 1986; Windsor et al., 1985.

92. Committee to Study Outreach for Prenatal Care, 1988.

93. National Research Council, 1989, pp. 78–93.

94. Sackett & Snow, 1979. Some applications of PRECEDE in assessing "compliance," "adherence," or "concordance" problems in selected care issues and settings include W. C. Bailey et al., 1987; Barnhoorn & Andriannse, 1992; Bowler & Morisky, 1983; Chwalow, Green, Levine, & Deeds, 1978; Cramer & Spilker, 1991; Eastaugh & Hatcher, 1982; Estey, 1988; Fedder, 1982; Green & Simons-Morton, 1988; Kelly, 1990; Leppik, 1990; Mann & Putnam, 1989; Morisky, 1986; Rimer et al., 1988; Roter, 1977; Tamez & Vacalis, 1989; Zapka et al., 1993.

95. Anson, Paran, Neumann, & Chernichovsky, 1993; Jeffery, 1998.

96. Povar, Mantell, & Morris, 1984. Some assessments of health care utilization patterns applying PRECEDE include W. C. Bailey, et al., 1987; Knazan, 1986; Maxwell, Bastani, & Warda, 1998; Mercer et al., 1997; Muus & Ahmed, 1991; Rimer, 1993; Zapka, Harris, Hosmer et al., 1993; Zapka, Stoddard, Costanza, & Greene, 1989.

97. Baum, Kennedy, Forbes, & Jones, 1983. By convention, the National Disease and Therapeutic Index employs the term *mentions* (including refills and renewal of prescriptions) to reflect drug usage. The term should not be interpreted as equivalent to number of patients or prescriptions.

98. Phillips, Morrison, & Aday, 1998; Stephens & Schoenborn, 1988.

99. Duncan, 1996; Feinstein, 1993; Hertzman, Frank, & Evans, 1994; Stronks, Van de Mheen, Looman, & Mackenbach, 1998. Some applications of PRECEDE in addressing the socioeconomic gradient in health care utilization include Barnhoorn & Andriaanse, 1992; C. B. McCoy, Nielsen, Chitwood, Zavertnik, & Khoury, 1991; Sun & Shun, 1995; Zuckerman et al., 1989.

100. Hall, Roter, & Katz, 1988. Applications of PRECEDE that have addressed racial or ethnic populations include Airhihenbuwa, 1995; Daniel & Green, 1995; Dignan, Michielutte, Wells, & Bahnson, 1995; Eng, 1993; Keith & Doyle, 1998; McGowan & Green, 1995; Modeste, Abbey, & Hopp, 1984–1985; Neef, Scutchfield, Elder, & Bender, 1991; O'Brien, Smith, Bush, & Peleg, 1990; Sanders-Phillips, 1996; Sutherland et al., 1989; Walter & Vaughan, 1993.

101. Morrison, 1996; Reed, 1996; Sanders-Phillips, 1996; Waitzkin, 1985.

102. Schoen, Marcus, & Braham, 1994.

103. Kayne, 1984; Yeo, 1998.

104. German, Klein, McPhee, & Smith, 1982.

105. Holloway, 1996; National Center for Health Statistics, A. J. Moss and Parsons, 1986.

106. Honig & Gillespie, 1995; Lamy & Beardsley, 1982.

107. Millar, 1998; Williamson & Chapin, 1980.

108. Green, Mullen, & Stainbrook, 1986. Applications of PRECEDE in planning and evaluating programs for the elderly include Haber, 1994; Keintz, Rimer, Fleisher, & Engstrom, 1988; Kemper, 1986; Knazan, 1986; McGowan & Green, 1995; Morisky, Levine, Green, & Smith, 1982; Opdycke, Ascione, Shimp, & Rosen, 1992; Pichora-Fuller, 1997; Rimer, Jones, Wilson, Bennett, & Engstrom, 1983; Weinberger et al., 1992; Yeo, 1998; Zapka et al., 1993.

109. Gans, Lapane, Lasater, & Carleton, 1994.

110. National Center for Health Statistics, T. Mc Lemore and J. DeLozier, "1987.

111. D. A. Davis, Thomson, Oxman, & Haynes, 1995; Haynes, Davis, McKibbon, & Tugwell, 1984.

112. Avorn & Soumerai, 1983.

113. Candeias, 1991; D. A. Davis et al., 1984; Haber, 1994; Han, Baumann, & Cimprich, 1996; Kok, 1992; Mann, 1994; Rootman, 1997; Speller, Evans, & Head, 1997.

114. Baum, Kennedy, Forbes, & Jones, 1982.

115. Rosser, 1987.

116. *Morbidity and Mortality Weekly Report,* 1989.

117. Green & Fedder, 1977; Katz, Daltroy, Brennan, & Liang, 1992.

118. Green, 1985b. See, however, Millar, 1998.

119. Schauffler, Faer, Faulkner, & Shore, 1994.

120. Inui et al., 1980.

121. P. D. Mullen & Green, 1985.

122. P. D. Mullen, Green, & Persinger, 1985.

123. Green, 1983a, 1987a.

124. National Coordinating Committee on Clinical Preventive Services, 1993.

125. Andersen, 1995; Green, 1990, 1994b; Hiatt et al., 1996.

126. Garr, 1989; F. Mullen, 1982; Nutting, 1987, 1990.

127. This section is based on an update of Green, 1987a.

128. Haynes, Taylor, & Sackett, 1979. See also references cited in endnotes 56 and 57.

129. Barnhoorn & Adriaanse, 1992.

130. Green, Mullen, & Friedman, 1986; Mullen, Green, & Persinger, 1985.

131. Imanaka, Araki & Nobutomo, 1993.

132. Allegrante, Kovar, MacKenzie, Peterson, & Gutin, 1993; Kovar et al., 1992.

133. Bottimore & Hailey, 1988–1989; Chie & Chang, 1994; Danigelis et al., 1995.

134. Marlatt & Gordon, 1985. See also Allen, Lowman, & Miller, 1996.

135. Green, Cargo, & Ottoson, 1994. See further examples and applications of relapse prevention strategies in Lowe, Windsor, & Woodby, 1997; Secker-Walker, Solomon, & Mead, 1995.

136. Rose et al., 1982.

137. Lando, McGovern, Barrios, & Etringer, 1990; Lando, Pirie, & Schmid, 1996.

138. Gilpin et al., 1992.

139. Green, Levine, & Deeds, 1975.

140. D. M. Levine, Green, Deeds, et al., 1979; D. M. Levine, Green, Russell, et al., 1979.

141. Green, Levine, & Deeds, 1977; Green, Levine, Wolle, & Deeds, 1979.

142. Morisky et al., 1983.

143. V. C. Li et al., 1984.

144. Windsor, 1984, 1986; Windsor & Cutter, 1983; Windsor et al., 1985. See also Lowe et al., 1997.

145. The literature on these hundreds of studies is summarized and critically analyzed in the series of meta-analyses cited in Note 2 of this chapter and in the Cochran Library of systematic reviews, e.g., Freemantle et al., 1977. The Freemantle review illustrates the limitations of printed material such as practice guidelines, or media only, in clinical settings.

146. Morisky et al., 1990.

147. Cantor et al., 1985; Green, 1982, 1983a.

148. Bartlett, 1985; Green, 1976a, b; Morisky, DeMuth, Field-Fass et al., 1985.

149. Green, Levine, & Deeds, 1975.

150. Green, Levine, Wolle, & Deeds, 1979; D. M. Levine, Green, Deeds, et al., 1979.

151. Morisky et al., 1983. See also Morisky et al., 1980, 1982.

152. Carter et al., 1986.

153. Janz & Becker, 1984. See Chapter 5 for detailed discussion of the Health Belief Model.

154. P. D. Mullen, Green, & Persinger, 1985. See also Green & Frankish, 1994.

155. Kok, van den Borne, & Mullen, 1997; P. D. Mullen et al., 1997.

156. Hatcher, Green, Levine, & Flagle, 1986.

157. Roter, 1977; Roter, Hall, & Katz, 1988.

158. Borgers et al., 1993.

159. Maclean, 1991.

160. Jacobs et al., 1983; O'Connor, Pennie, & Dales, 1996.

161. Morisky et al., 1980.

162. Hindi-Alexander & Cropp, 1981; Taggart et al., 1991.

163. Borgers et al., 1993.

164. Earp, Ory, & Strogatz, 1982; Morisky et al., 1985.

165. Skelly, Marshall, Haughey, Davis, & Dunford, 1995.

166. Scuttchfield, 1992.

167. Makrides, Veinot, Richard, & Allen, 1997.

168. Ibid.

169. A. K. Davis, 1994; NCI Breast Cancer Screening Consortium, 1990.

170. A. K. Davis, 1994; Dignan, Michielutte, Wells, & Bahnson, 1994.

171. Mahloch et al., 1993; Mann et al., 1996; Schapira et al., 1993; Walsh & McPhee, 1992.

172. N. H. Gottlieb, Mullen, & McAlister, 1987; Mann & Putnam, 1990; McAlister et al., 1985; Nutting, 1986; Wechsler, Levine, Idelson, Rothman, & Taylor, 1983.

173. Anda, Remington, Sienko, & Davis, 1987; McPhee, Richard, & Solkowitz, 1986; Romm, Fletcher, & Hulka, 1981; Singer, Lindsay, & Wilson, 1991; Welles, Lewis, Leake, Schleiter, & Brooks, 1986; Woo, Woo, Cook, Weisberg, & Goldman, 1985.

174. Love et al., 1993.

175. Green, Cargo, & Ottoson, 1994; Lomas et al., 1989.

176. Battista, Williams, & MacFarlane, 1990; Burglehaus et al., 1997; Green, 1987a.

177. Battista, 1983; Sobal, Valente, Muncie, Levine, & Deforge, 1986.

178. Weschler, Levine, Idelson, Rothman, & Taylor, 1983.

179. Heywood, Firman, Sanson-Fisher, & Mudge, 1996; Radecki & Mandenhall, 1986.

180. Attarian, Fleming, Barron, & Strecher, 1987.

181. McAlister et al., 1985.

182. Kottke, Foels, Hill, Choi, & Fendersonet, 1984.

183. Valente, Sobal, Muncie, Levine, & Antilitz, 1986.

184. K. M. Cummings, Giovino, Emont, Sciandra, & Koenigsberg, 1986; Love et al., 1993; Orleans, George, Houpt, & Brodie, 1985; K. B. Welles, Ware, & Lewis, 1984.

185. Anda, Remington, Sienko, & Davis, 1987.

186. K. M. Cummings, Giovino, Sciandra, Koenigsberg, & Emont, 1987.

187. Battista, Williams, & MacFarlane, 1990.

188. Burglehaus, Smith, Sheps, & Green, 1997.

189. Maheux, Pineault, & Beland, 1987; Weinberger et al., 1992.

190. Orleans, George, Houpt, & Brodie, 1985; Wechsler, Levine, Idelson, Rothman, & Taylor, 1983.

191. Han, Bauman, & Cimprich, 1996; Jenny, 1993.

192. Health and Welfare Canada, 1992c. Also in Jenny, 1993, p. 1411.

193. B. Goldstein, Fischer, Richards, Goldstein, & Shank, 1987.

194. General Professional Education of Physicians Panel, 1984.

195. Anda, Remington, Sienko, & Davis, 1987; Tamblyn & Battista, 1993.

196. Gemson & Elinson, 1986.

197. Carter, Belcher, & Inui, 1981.

198. Knight, O'Malley, & Fletcher, 1987.

199. McDonald et al., 1984. See also Schringer, Baraff, & Cretin, 1997.

200. Litzelman, Dittus, Miller, & Tierney, 1993.

201. Orlandi, 1987; Winickoff, Coltin, Morgan, Busbaum, & Barnett, 1984.

202. Schauffler & Rodriquez, 1993; R. S. Thompson, 1996.

203. R. S. Thompson, 1997. Also Thompson, Taplin, McAfee, Mandelson, & Smith, 1995.

204. A. K. Davis, 1994. See, however, Terris, 1998.

205. McQueen, 1985; Mullen & Zapka, 1981, 1982, 1989.

206. Sclar et al., 1991. See also Vickery & Fries, 1981, Vickery et al., 1983.

207. Weinberger et al., 1992.

208. Lawler & Viviani, 1997.

209. Legorreta, Hasan, Peters, Pelletier, & Leung, 1997.

210. R. S. Thompson, 1996.

211. Walsh & McPhee, 1992.

212. Reinke, 1995.

213. Makrides, Veinot, Richard, & Allen, 1997.

214. Boulet, Chapman, Green, & FitzGerald, 1994; Partridge, 1995.

215. Lorig, Mazonson, & Holman, 1993.

216. Yingling & Trocino, 1997.

217. Ibid., p. 246.

218. Battista, Williams, & MacFarlane, 1986. See also Green, 1976b.

219. Terry et al., 1981; Wang et al., 1979.

220. Perera, LoGerfo, Shulenberger, Ylvisaker, & Kirz, 1983.

221. Pokorny, Putnam, & Fryer, 1980.

222. Somers, 1987.

223. D. A. Davis, Thomson, Oxman, & Haynes, 1995. See also Dodek & Ottoson, 1996.

224. Cassatta & Kirkman-Liff, 1981; Kosch & Dallman, 1983; Lewis, 1998.

225. Westberg, 1986.

226. Green, 1986f; McGowan & Green, 1995; Milewa, 1997; Minkler & Pies, 1997.

227. Terry et al., 1981.

228. P. D. Mullen & Green, 1985; Worden, Flynn, Geller et al., 1988.

229. Orleans, George, Houpt, & Brodie, 1985.

230. Green, Lewis, & Levine, 1980; Weinberger, Mazzuca, Cohen, & McDonald, 1982.

231. Ibid. Cf. Tzung-yu, 1993.

232. Winickoff, Coltin, Morgan, Busbaum, & Barnett, 1984. See also Azevedo & Bernard, 1995.

233. Ewart, Li, & Coates, 1983.

Chapter 12

Technological Applications
of PRECEDE-PROCEED

With more than 800 published applications of PRECEDE-PROCEED in the planning, evaluation, or review of health promotion policies, programs, methods, and processes, the record shows that the model is both robust and extensible to a wide variety of issues.[1] An examination of these published applications also suggests that the model is adaptable to new trends in theory and practice that are refined and improved over time. The model allows emerging technologies for intervention design and delivery to be incorporated into the planning, implementation, and evaluation aspects of health promotion. At the same time, emerging technologies provide new ways to learn and to apply the model, along with its component assessments, more efficiently than in the past.

The complexity of designing community interventions requires attention to several more specific complexities:

- The array of social and health problems and issues, each with its own multiple and interacting determinants
- The heterogeneous nature of human populations, each with its unique culture, traditions, politics, demographic composition, and socioeconomic conditions
- The increasingly sophisticated and demanding target audiences for assessments and interventions
- The need to reconcile and integrate scientific evidence from afar with idiosyncratic data and preferences from the local situation
- The number of skills and areas of expertise necessary to plan and implement interventions effectively and to evaluate their myriad outcomes

Encompassing the entirety of the model for its most comprehensive and effective application demands participatory, collaborative, multidisciplinary efforts. Few individuals have the breadth of skills that can span the variety of assessments it calls for. In our work, as we discovered each new complexity, we escaped despair only by discovering new information technologies to help us cope with them. Technology offers new ways to process large volumes of information, to collaborate, and to receive technical assistance for complete implementation of the processes embodied in PRECEDE-PROCEED. Further, those involved in the design, development, and deployment of communications technologies such as computer-assisted instruction (CAI) can use the Precede-Proceed model as a framework. Therefore, this chapter is divided into four broad sections:

1. An overview of public health informatics
2. An examination of technology-based applications that can facilitate the conduct of assessments in each of the phases of the model
3. A description of several technology-based applications that provide comprehensive support for learning and for applying the model
4. A case report of how the model was used to develop a technology-based health education intervention

PUBLIC HEALTH INFORMATICS

HISTORY

The foreword to a book on microcomputer application in health education noted that the World Health Organization had made technological transfer and health education two of the pillars of its global strategy of "Health for All by the Year 2000." With respect specifically to technological transfer, we observed the following:

> Transfer must involve "appropriate technology," meaning technology that can be applied and managed locally to analyze and solve a people's own health problems. The caveat with respect to health education is that it must involve and enable people to take control of the determinants of their own health. These, then, are the challenges for computer applications in health today.[2]

Since then, communications technology has continued to develop as a product of three converging areas—computing, information systems, and telecommunications. As Waterworth writes:

> Systems that integrate these three powerful elements will have an impact on daily life more than equivalent to that of the introduction of telephones, television, and computer games combined into one. Application areas such as education, cooperative work, authoring, entertainment, military command and control, information access, and ideas generation will all benefit from these developments.[3]

Friede and colleagues define *public health informatics* as the "science of applying Information-Age technology to serve the specialized needs of public health."[4] Examples of serving specialized needs include access to and the application of information on populations and the determinants of their health. It also involves the effective communication, digestion, synthesis, and guided application of this growing volume of information. In *Technotrends,* Burris suggests that the appropriate application of advanced technologies can facilitate several revolutions, including the delivery systems of products and services; the way we communicate; the way we personalize and individualize education; the way we internalize, understand, and use massive amounts of information; and opportunities to provide the foundation for new products and variations of old products. Though Burris uses terms related to a variety of sectors, each of these potential revolutions clearly has a connection to public health.[5]

HOW CAN TECHNOLOGY FACILITATE PLANNING?

Most of the potential applications and contributions of new technologies remain to be exploited, but many show signs of taking root in the everyday working life of health professionals. These reflect the ways technology helps overcome the essential barriers to good planning: time, information, and communication.

1. Technology provides new opportunities for the delivery of public health programs and services by reaching out to current target audiences in new ways, both asynchronously (e.g., e-mail, CAI), synchronously (e.g., chat and discussion rooms, online focus groups, real-time delphi studies), and on demand (e.g., world wide web–based information sources).
2. Technology allows for person-to-person, person-to-group, or group-to-group communication over vast distances, reducing the long-distance telephone costs and increasing the rate at which information is transferred to a larger number of people.
3. Technology-based applications of real-time assessment, monitoring, and message tailoring enable the ultimate application of individualized attention in the delivery of public health programs.
4. With the increasing speed and memory capacity of computers, growing libraries of knowledge are becoming ever more available to the practitioner or consumer, with ever more complex and efficient search strategies.
5. Access to current and emerging technologies allows for new ways of thinking about assessments, intervention design, data gathering, and analysis.

Friede and colleagues caution, however, that the appropriate application of the potentials implied in public health informatics requires "developing a cadre of professionals with training and experience in both public health and information technology."[6] Technology can both facilitate a fuller application of PRECEDE-

PROCEED to complex problems and guide the further development of intervention technologies.

TECHNOLOGY-BASED APPLICATIONS OF PRECEDE-PROCEED

This section examines how people can use existing technological resources to conduct various assessments. Some general technologies effectively support the planning process at all phases. These include such applications as bibliographical retrieval, decision support and expert systems, and both **synchronous** and asynchronous communications.[7] Table 12-1 lists some general-purpose applications that support the planner in different phases of the Precede-Proceed model.[8]

Note that in Table 12-1 the community tool box (CTB) applies to all phases of the Precede-Proceed model. Developed by Fawcett and his co-workers, the CTB uses the latest computer technology to assist those responsible for addressing local concerns such as substance abuse, teen pregnancy, youth violence, environmental health, child abuse and neglect, and promoting independent living for older adults. It can be used to develop leadership and organizational capacities among those just beginning local efforts as well as those in the later stages of a project. The CTB contains practical information about strategic planning, promoting financial sustainability, media advocacy, and other information needed by collaborative partnerships. Users may guide their own searches for information and print information from the database within the CTB. Problem-specific information not found in the CTB can be accessed easily through gateways to other databases or networks, including the Centers for Disease Control and Prevention.

As seen in previous chapters, program planning, implementation, and evaluation for community programs is a complex endeavor. Comprehensive efforts require an understanding of the factors that influence the implementation and evaluation of those plans. The process is difficult because it is information-intensive, requires the ability to take on multidisciplinary tasks, and requires attention to interorganizational and intersectoral issues.[9] We shall now describe two examples of comprehensive applications designed to facilitate the application of the Precede-Proceed model to comprehensive planning efforts—EMPOWER and NETPOWER.

EMPOWER: ENABLING METHODS OF PLANNING AND ORGANIZING WITHIN EVERYONE'S REACH

As you have seen, *EMPOWER*[10] is a computerized software program tailored to assist local practitioners in their efforts to plan and implement community-based health promotion programs. It is built on the foundations and experiences of the

TABLE 12-1

Examples of technology used in support of Precede-Proceed planning processes are shown here for each phase of the model

Phase	Technological Support
Social assessment	Online synchronous communications capabilities for primary data collection (e.g., online chat rooms for town-hall-type meetings; online focus groups; real-time Delphi studies)
	Qualitative analysis software
	Online access to community-based social indicators data (e.g., White House Social Statistics briefing room—*http://www.whitehouse.gov/fsbr/ssbr.html* or *http://www.fedstats.gov/*)[a]
	Online asynchronous communications capability for gathering community input (e.g., e-mail communications; electronic bulletin boards; online LISTSERVs)
	Technical assistance on how to accomplish this assessment (e.g., Community Tool Box—*http://ctb.lsi.ukans.edu/*)
Epidemiological assessment	World wide web access to myriad databases for secondary data (e.g., CDCP WONDER—*http://wonder.cdc.gov/*)
	Online access to bibliographic retrieval from relevant databases (e.g., NLM's Medline—*http://www.ncbi.nlm.nih.gov/PubMed/*)
	Online access to population/demographic data (e.g., Census Bureau Map Stats—*http://www.census.gov/datamap/www/index.html*)
	Statistical software (e.g., SPSS and SAS)
	Technical assistance on how to accomplish this assessment (e.g., Community Tool Box—*http://ctb.lsi.ukans.edu/*)
Behavioral and environmental assessment	World wide web access to myriad databases for secondary data (e.g., CDCP WONDER—*http://wonder.cdc.gov/*—includes the Behavioral Risk Factor Surveillance Surveys)
	Online access to bibliographical retrieval from relevant databases (e.g., NLM's Medline—*http://www.ncbi.nlm.nih.gov/PubMed/*)
	Online access to population/demographic data (e.g., Census Bureau Map Stats—*http://www.census.gov/datamap/www/index.html*)
	Online access to collegial input and review (e.g., groupware for real-time group decision making; e-mail; synchronous and asynchronous communications)
	Statistical software
	Technical assistance on how to accomplish this assessment (e.g., Community Tool Box—*http://ctb.lsi.ukans.edu/*)

(continued)

Phase	Technological Support
Educational and ecological assessment	Online access to bibliographical retrieval from relevant databases (e.g., NLM's Medline—*http://www.ncbi.nlm.nih.gov/PubMed/*)
	Online access to attitudinal and opinion surveys (*http://www.cdc/gov/wwwnchs*)
	Online access to population/demographic data (e.g., Census Bureau Map Stats—*http://www.census.gov/datamap/www/index.html*)
	Online access to collegial input and review (e.g., groupware for real-time group decision making; e-mail; synchronous and asynchronous communications)
	Technical assistance on how to accomplish this assessment (e.g., Community Tool Box—*http://ctb.lsi.ukans.edu/*)
	Electronic simulations (e.g., University of Minnesota National Micropopulation Simulation Resource—*http://dragon.labmed.umn.edu/nmsr/NMSR.html*)
Administrative and policy assessment	Productivity tools (e.g., spreadsheets for budget projections, project management software to estimate time and resource requirements)
	Online access to collegial input and review (e.g., groupware for real-time group decision making; e-mail; synchronous and asynchronous communications)
	Technical assistance on administrative and policy assessment (e.g., Community Tool Box—*http://ctb.lsi.ukans.edu/*)
Implementation	Management tools (e.g., spreadsheets for budget monitoring, electronic Gantt charting and project management software)
	Communications tools to improve management and quality control (e.g., groupware for real-time group decision making; e-mail; online focus groups; chat rooms; electronic newsletters for project communications)
	Technical assistance administrative and evaluate programs (e.g., Community Tool Box—*http://ctb.lsi.ukans.edu/*)
Evaluation	Online access to collegial input and review (e.g., e-mail; synchronous and asynchronous communications)
	National health objectives and progress (e.g., *http://odphp.osophs.dhhs.gov/pubs/*)
	Technical assistance on how to evaluate programs (e.g., Community Tool Box—*http://ctb.lsi.ukans.edu/*)
	Online synchronous communications capability for primary data collection and interpretation (e.g., forms-based data collection over world wide web; groupware for real-time group decision making; online focus groups; real-time Delphi studies)
	Online asynchronous communications capability for gathering community input (e.g., e-mail; electronic bulletin boards, online LISTSERVs)

Precede-Proceed model for health promotion planning. The timeliness and significance of this effort stemmed from two converging developments:

1. The technology concerning artificial intelligence and expert systems provided an opportunity to extend expertise to meet unmet needs in much the same way that a group of human experts would be consulted if they were accessible.
2. A growing body of literature concerning the complexity of the determinants of health and of program planning for comprehensive health promotion interventions called for professional training and experience and access to technical assistance from multidisciplinary experts.

Expert Systems Technology. The management of myriad sources and types of information is essential in community applications of health promotion planning procedures. The program-planning process is often difficult for health professionals in the dynamic, political nature of the community. Health promotion draws from a variety of fields such as epidemiology, social and political science education, and behavioral psychology; health professionals need to apply the resources and strategies suggested by these fields. A major problem relating to the utilization of such a broad base is the difficulty inherent in attempting to apply knowledge from diverse disciplines effectively. The need to understand and apply such diverse and complex materials and processes has stimulated the use of expert systems, for example, in clinical settings and the social sciences.

Expert systems have been most helpful when human sources of information are scarce or lost or when there is a widespread, unmet need. These systems are structured to offer information and guidance to health professionals regarding decision-making strategies; they offer a process similar to the consultation of experts. Such technology combines a well-defined knowledge base with a rule-based computer program to enable a user to gain access to information and to apply complex processes to problem solving. Table 12-2 contains an overview of the types of tasks and problems to which expert systems technology has been applied.

Within the scope of the applications identified in Table 12-2, the recognized benefits of expert and decision support systems are numerous. For example, expert systems are cost effective, provide valuable training potentials, improve professional practice, are technically feasible, and provide a tool by which all professionals can have access to the expert knowledge that only a few previously had.[11] EMPOWER and NETPOWER are expert and decision support systems based on PRECEDE-PROCEED.

The Structure of EMPOWER. Figure 12-1 illustrates the principal subsystems and several external databases linked dynamically to provide guidance to program managers and directors. Five of the six subsystems are applications of the Precede-Proceed model. The sixth, situation analysis, was added as a tool for assessing the readiness and capacity of a community group to complete the plan-

---

TABLE 12-2

Tasks that expert systems help users accomplish

Task	Examples
Interpretation	Using sensors to obtain data: evaluating rock formations and chemical compounds, identifying speech and visual cues
Prediction	Determining consequences of actions: drought, oil shortages, economic changes, military buildup, and insect damage
Diagnosis	Determining causes and characteristics of states: clinical medicine, systems analysis (e.g., electrical circuits, machinery, spacecraft systems)
Design	Describing microprocessors, genes for cloning, organic molecules, industrial plans
Planning	Finding desired configuration given constraints: actions and events such as military response
Monitoring	Assuring the proper functioning of systems: comparing status to a standard (e.g., condition of patients in hospital, performance of aircraft or nuclear power plants)
Debugging	Finding problems and suggesting solutions: telecommunications systems and electrical equipment
Instruction	Diagnosis, educational prescription, and provision of appropriate instruction by building a model of student knowledge or skills

---

ning process. It does not appear as a heading on this screen but is accessible from it.

Purpose. As the current version of EMPOWER is presented as a training tool, it therefore focuses on a single application—early detection of breast cancer. As a result, all the examples found in EMPOWER are related to that example. EMPOWER provides guidance and technical assistance to its users in any component of the program planning and evaluation of community-based breast cancer prevention and control interventions. It does this by prompting the user through a series of algorithms based on the Precede-Proceed framework while at the same time providing the capacity for the user to ask about the reasoning and rule processes used during the consultation. Figure 12-2 illustrates that nature of the questioning provided in EMPOWER.

Figure 12-3 displays the support materials available to a user in the Consult on Tap menu in EMPOWER. *Consult on Tap* is a concept designed for EMPOWER that was to be consistent with the use of expert systems to provide guidance on demand to users as though human experts were available. At any point in time during the use of EMPOWER, a user may "ask" a series of questions to help provide an understanding about the nature of the processes used. Also, at any

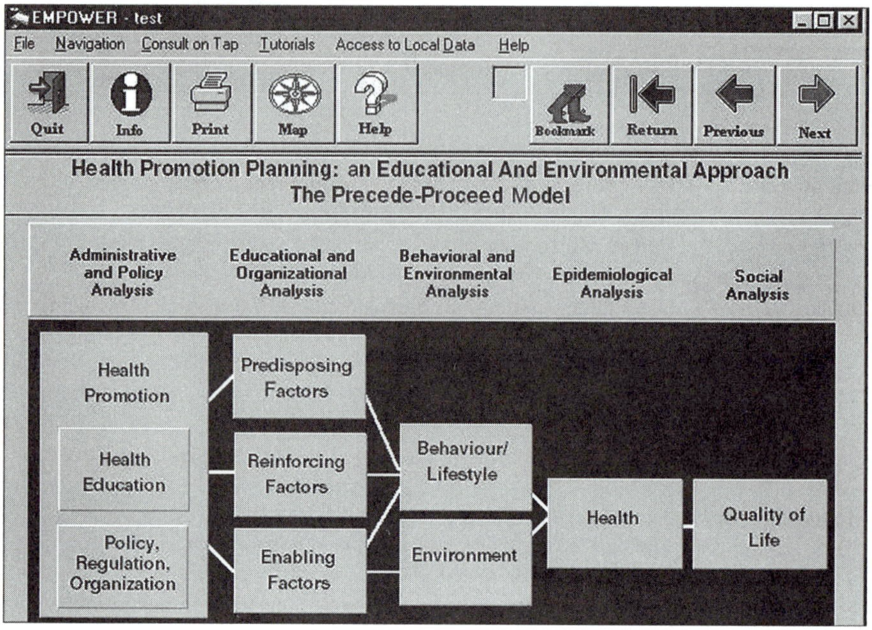

FIGURE 12-1

The opening screen of EMPOWER allows users to click on any box in the Precede-Proceed model to get to that model in the interactive software. By clicking in the dark area surrounding the boxes, users can go to the first module, situation analysis.

SOURCE: Reprinted from EMPOWER software by permission of Jones and Bartlett Publishers.

point, a user may retrieve case examples, references to additional information, or access to supporting databases (e.g., *Healthy People Objectives*).

Tasks EMPOWER Helps the User Accomplish. Examples of specific steps in the planning and community organizing process that EMPOWER addresses include the following:

1. Data-gathering procedures essential to the planning, conduct, or evaluation of community-based cancer prevention programming
2. Organizing the involvement of community residents or representatives in the planning process
3. Setting priorities and initial and long-term objectives
4. Preparing full program and evaluation plans
5. Organizing coalitions or other interagency and intersectoral collaboration arrangements

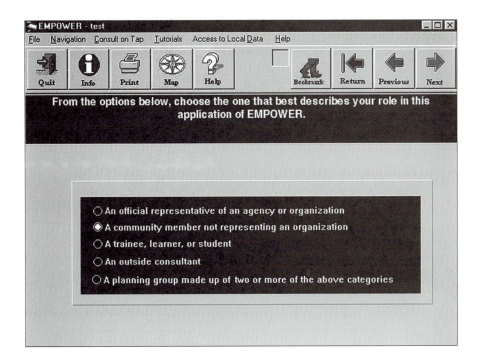

FIGURE 12-2

EMPOWER data gathering allows a user to identify his or her essential characteristics and position in the situational assessment.

SOURCE: Reprinted from EMPOWER software by permission of Jones and Bartlett Publishers.

6. Assessing the plausibility of the intended outcomes in light of the proposed activities, the level and manner of implementation of the program, and the gap between required resources and available resources
7. Assessing policies and developing proposals and strategies for policy changes
8. Identifying of elements of the plans that are at odds with each other and that reduce the plausibility of achieving the intended program outcomes
9. Assessing organizational and regulatory constraints and strategies for reorganization and making and enforcing regulations
10. Assessing whether the program has succeeded in attracting the target population in the expected numbers
11. Assessing the impact of cancer prevention programming on community awareness, interest, motivation, attitudes, beliefs, perceptions, behaviors, and environmental changes

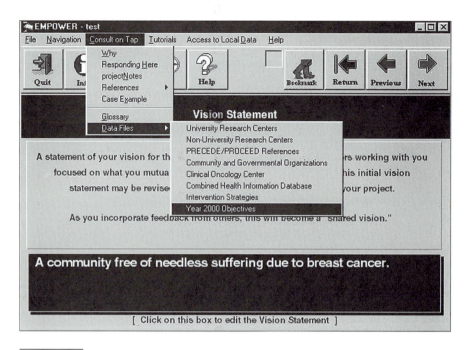

FIGURE 12-3

EMPOWER supporting materials include drop-down menus with explanations, bibliographical references, case examples, glossaries, and the various data files shown in this screen.

SOURCE: Reprinted from EMPOWER software by permission of Jones and Bartlett Publishers.

The Intended Users of EMPOWER. Although anyone involved with or learning program planning may use EMPOWER, it was originally designed for several specific intended audiences:

1. Program managers and health promotion directors and staff of provincial, state, and local health departments
2. Program managers, directors, and staff of Canadian or American Cancer Society units and divisions
3. Program managers and directors of other community-based cancer prevention programs
4. Directors of work-site health promotion programs
5. Health directors or coordinators of state education agencies, local education agencies, and school districts
6. Community organizations with little or no health science background
7. Trainees, students, and others interested in learning more about the strategies for applying the Precede-Proceed model for program planning

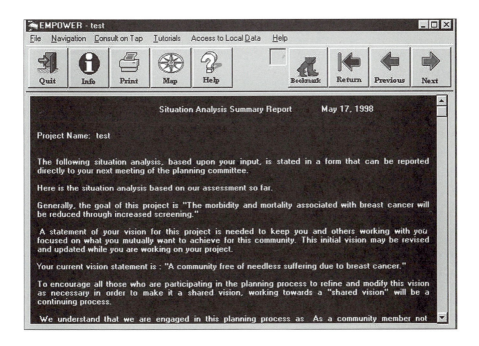

FIGURE 12-4

A "smart report" for situation analysis provides a summary of the information supplied by the user and the implications of that information for the next steps in the planning.

SOURCE: Reprinted from EMPOWER software by permission of Jones and Bartlett Publishers.

The six subsystems or modules that provide the structure for the proposed EMPOWER system are described in the sections that follow.[12] Module 1 is unique to EMPOWER. Although modules 2–6 are often seen as sequential, the benefit of the proposed system is that there is now the opportunity to conduct continuous "what if" analyses by moving dynamically back and forth among the modules.

At the end of each phase, a specific "smart report" is provided as feedback to the user. Figure 12-4 illustrates a smart report at the end of the situation analysis. A *smart report* is created in real time from a user's responses to EMPOWER. Such a report provides a restating of information provided by the user plus recommendations to the user based on those responses.

Module 1: Situation Analysis. This module allows planners to assess their initial mandate and to determine if the resources necessary for the planning process are available. Just as a human consultant would need to gather background on a project, EMPOWER needs a situational assessment to tailor output in each of the other modules.

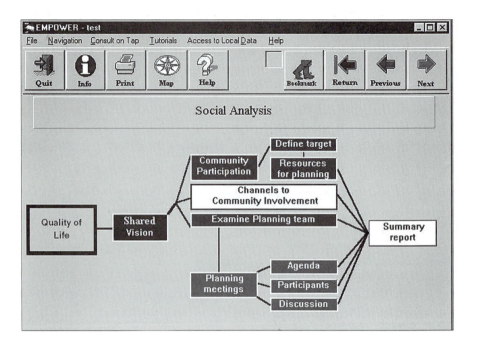

FIGURE 12-5

Flowchart for social analysis guides the user through the steps in social assessment.

SOURCE: Reprinted from EMPOWER software by permission of Jones and Bartlett Publishers.

Module 2: Guidance on Social Analysis. This module takes the user through a variety of procedures to assess the breast cancer concerns of the target population. The processes used attempt to maximize the participation and representation of the intended population in this assessment. This assessment is designed to be a fair gauge of the quality-of-life concerns of the target population as these concerns relate to breast cancer (see Figure 12-5).

Module 3: Guidance on Epidemiological Analysis. The steps taken in this module identify the specific health goals in breast cancer control or problems contributing to those issues emerging from the preceding social analysis. This phase involves several data-gathering strategies to rank the problems identified and to assign them relative priority based on limited resources and educational capabilities. In this phase, the initial crafting of objectives for breast cancer control occurs (see Figure 12-6).

Module 4: Guidance on Behavioral and Environmental Analysis. This links the breast cancer objectives of highest priority identified in Module 2 with their likely behav-

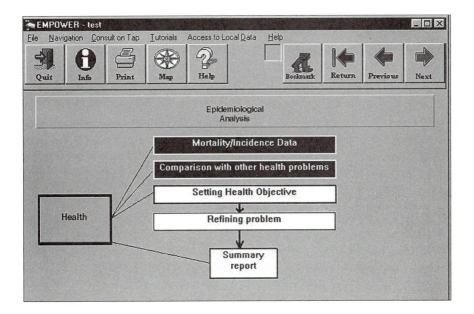

FIGURE 12-6

Flowchart for epidemiological analysis guides the user through the steps in epidemiological assessment.

SOURCE: Reprinted from EMPOWER software by permission of Jones and Bartlett Publishers.

ioral and environmental determinants. The factors identified in this step and judged to be most important and most amenable to change become the focus of proposed interventions. It is here that specific behavioral objectives and environmental targets are first formulated for the intervention (see Figure 12-7).

Module 5: Guidance on Educational and Organizational Analysis. Each of the potential factors influencing the behavioral and environmental factors identified in Module 4 are here grouped into one of three categories: predisposing factors (personal factors that influence motivation for change), enabling factors (skills, resources, barriers to making change), and reinforcing factors (rewards and feedback that positively or negatively reinforce changes made). These are then ranked according to the prevalence of the factors and their likelihood of playing a key role in bringing about change in the behavioral or environmental determinants. The results of this module are the specific educational and resource objectives that drive the activities in the proposed interventions (see Figure 12-8).

Module 6: Guidance on Administrative and Policy Analysis. Once the educational and resource objectives are formally identified, an administrative and policy analysis

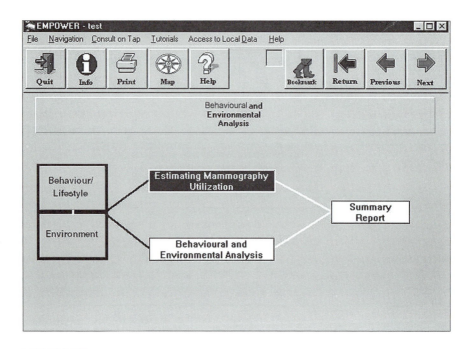

FIGURE 12-7

Flowchart for behavioral and environmental analysis guides the user through the steps in environmental assessment.

SOURCE: Reprinted from EMPOWER software by permission of Jones and Bartlett Publishers.

will carry a planner through an assessment of the likelihood that an intervention to accomplish those objectives is feasible, given available organizational resources and policy constraints. The gap between required resources and available ones identifies training strategies, policy options, and organizational or regulatory reforms required to accomplish the objectives. The results of this module provide a substantive guidebook on maximizing the implementation of a proposed intervention. Given this guidebook, the specific educational methods and strategies can be chosen for the intervention, and specific policy and regulatory enforcement options can be selected (see Figure 12-9).

Summary. Planning health programs is a complex, multidisciplinary process. It requires recognition of the role of the distinct elements of the planning process; more importantly, it demands an understanding of their interrelatedness. EMPOWER was developed to enhance an individual's ability to plan breast cancer screening programs from a global perspective by providing expert guidance

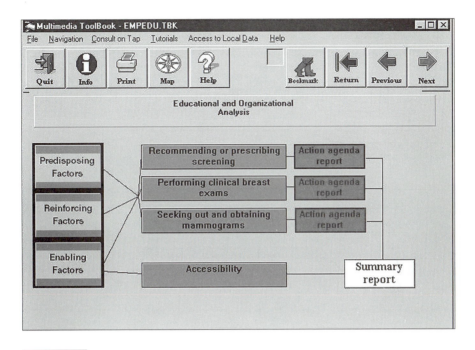

FIGURE 12-8

Flowchart of educational and organizational analysis guides the user through the steps in educational and organizational assessment.

SOURCE: Reprinted from EMPOWER software by permission of Jones and Bartlett Publishers.

during the process. With the increasing use, acceptance, and availability of computers in all fields, including the health professions, coupled with the increased development of artificial intelligence, expert systems, and decision assistance software, one can see clearly the wisdom in applying this sophisticated technology to preventable health problems such as cancer.

Expert systems technology has been found useful when human resource information is scarce or when widespread, unmet needs exists. Few practitioners today in cancer prevention have not been confronted with the difficulty of making programs sensitive, without bias, and acceptable to members of target populations. As a result, we anticipate a high interest in software that helps those in federal, state or provincial, and local public health communities, as well as those in associations, hospitals, and health settings in the private sector, to plan more effectively for population health. EMPOWER offers just one example of a system one can employ to facilitate the use of the Precede-Proceed model. NETPOWER is another.

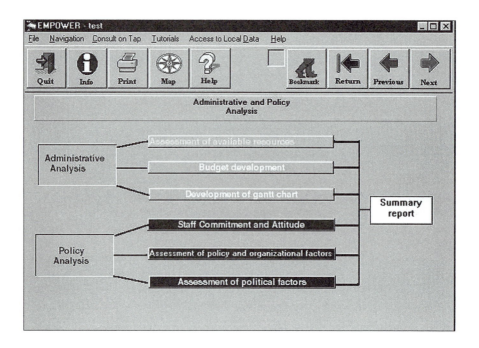

FIGURE 12-9

Flowchart for administrative and policy analysis guides the user through the steps in administrative and policy assessment.

SOURCE: Reprinted from EMPOWER software by permission of Jones and Bartlett Publishers.

NETPOWER: NETWORKED PLANNING
AND ORGANIZING WITHIN EVERYONE'S REACH

The main limitation of EMPOWER that we sought to overcome with new software based on PRECEDE-PROCEED was that EMPOWER could be applied to just one health issue, breast cancer control. Its utility was limited to planning one type of program or using that example of planning as a case for learning the Precede-Precede model.

To create a generic planning tool in software form, we had to sacrifice some of the specific guidelines that EMPOWER could offer. In place of specificity of input and output data and of guidelines, NETPOWER offers the Precede-Proceed framework as a means-ends template for the user to enter local and best-evidence data. NETPOWER is taking two forms in its development. One provides examples, but users must fill in the necessary data to link means and ends in the Precede-Proceed model for their specific case. The other anticipates the building of databases that the user can tap at a central web site or at multiple, linked web sites.

The essential data for NETPOWER's use consists of four types:

1. Data from the local situation that describe local preferences and perceived or actual problems or goals to be addressed
2. Data from best-evidence research sources that suggest causes or determinants in the means-end chain for the selected problem or goal, as well as the strength of their relationships
3. Data from the local situation that estimates the prevalence or importance of the suggested determinants in the local situation
4. Data that links interventions with the selected determinants according to the strength of evidence for their efficacy or effectiveness

USING PRECEDE AND PROCEED FOR PLANNING TECHNOLOGY-BASED INTERVENTIONS

Since the 1970s, computer applications have allowed new and compelling methods for reaching target populations.[13] At the end of the 20th century, communications technology offers a broad range of applications, from simple text-based health risk assessment appraisals to interactive multimedia and virtual reality simulations that allow users to make health decisions and experience consequences in a risk-free environment. To be truly effective, these applications must be based on a planning process that assesses the problem and its determinants and includes the affected population in various stages of development.

We shall describe the planning process as it applies to technology-based interventions, including CAI and Internet applications. Figure 12-10 shows the design process used in the development of technology-based applications. Similar to other health communications efforts, this process includes input from target audiences as well as a thorough understanding of the research literature before developing a plan (design specifications) and carrying it out (prototyping and development). A solid plan includes evaluation throughout the effort, from formative evaluation to beta testing and field testing.

This process is closely aligned with the Precede-Proceed planning model, which also begins with input from the target audience when done fully (see Figure 12-11). An understanding of the health problem, related behaviors, environmental issues, and intervention factors allows the health planner to identify intervention points and the appropriate design features that will impact the health problem.

The following sections will describe the theoretical basis as well as the application of the model to intervention development, in general and in terms of a

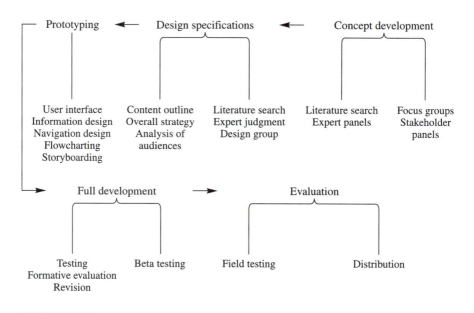

FIGURE 12-10

The design process used for technological applications.

specific health promotion program. In this example, the illustrative case is an intervention for young adults on human papillomavirus (HPV) prevention and control.[14] Figure 12-12 details the results of each stage of the Precede-Proceed planning effort.

SOCIAL ASSESSMENT: COMMUNITY PARTICIPATION

As in other applications of PRECEDE-PROCEED, community participation is a key element of technology-based intervention development. While the decision to use technology as the educational or organizational strategy may emerge from an existing community health effort, a community planner may begin with the decision to use technology to address a specific health problem. This discussion will focus on the latter course, to inform those who are interested in exploring how they can apply technology to identified problems. Community participation is important throughout concept development, formative evaluation, and outcome evaluation.

Despite beginning with the health problem, the developer must involve the community from the beginning in the planning process to ensure that the resulting

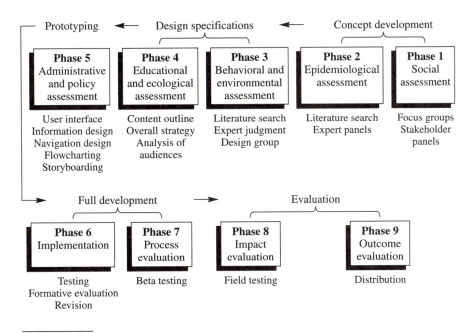

FIGURE 12-11

Technological design process compared with the Precede-Proceed planning process.

application truly reflects their viewpoints and their needs—in its content, appropriate strategies, and type of application. These efforts may begin with a feasibility study in which the community is consulted about the plans for designing a technology-based intervention to address some health disparity.[15] The community may include local residents or patients, intermediaries such as health care providers or teachers, and experts. Through focus groups and advisory panel meetings, these groups would be asked to do the following:

Identify the needs of various target audiences

Identify the characteristics of the application that the intended target audiences would perceive as useful

Review issues and problems identified in the literature review and from the experience of participants

Identify the best structural characteristics of the proposed application

Identify issues and barriers affecting the successful deployment of the technology-based application

Determining the Target Audience. Based on input from focus groups and advisory panels, the developer can refine the target audience and design a strategy.

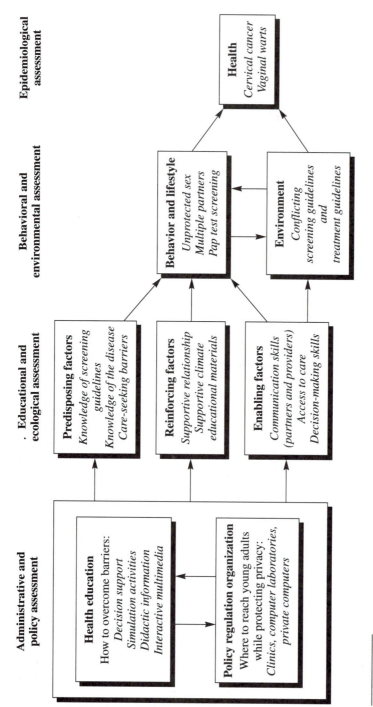

FIGURE 12-12

Application of the Precede model in a multimedia health education program on human pappillomavirus risk reduction and control for young adults.

Technology-based applications can reach a variety of audiences: members of the general public, intermediaries, and researchers. Input from these audiences will likely point to entirely different applications for each, of which one is more important or practical than the others. In some cases, this concern may change the target of the effort completely. In a feasibility study looking at the deployment of technology for reducing breast and cervical cancer among Hispanic women, the original target audience was health care providers, and the proposed application was a resource tool. The study revealed that reaching Hispanic women themselves through a multimedia educational application would be a better focus for the effort. In the case example in Figure 12-12, the feasibility study narrowed the audience of an education intervention on HPV infection from all young adults to young adults diagnosed with the disease.

Determining the Design Strategy. The type of application planned may also change as a result of community participation in the planning process. With communications technology, this is especially likely, because the advancement of more flexible, cheaper, and accessible applications means that better options may become available and feasible during the development process. In recent years, the CD-ROM has replaced other technological media, such as floppy diskettes and interactive videodiscs (IVDs), because they hold more information and are less expensive than IVD machines. More recently, the world wide web (www) provides greater access to current information. The community input will help the developer decide which application is most appropriate given which intervention attributes matter most to the target audience. For example, a CD-ROM application may be more appropriate for simulation and gaming activities because of its ability to integrate multimedia components. When the ability to update information continuously matters, the most appropriate application may involve the www.

Input from potential gatekeepers in the feasibility stage will also enable one to determine the best strategy for disseminating the application and may influence the choice of application. For example, if one plans to develop a clinic-based application but clinics are unlikely to have CD-ROM capability, the choice of medium will be narrowed accordingly.

PRECEDE-PROCEED was used to organize and incorporate health behavior theories for the development of an interactive CD-ROM for HPV risk reduction and control. Using an expansionist approach, the project started from the specified health problem of HPV infection and worked out to the larger social context in order to design a tailored intervention. Early on in the social assessment of the HPV application, the developers sought the input of young adults and their health care providers. These focus group discussions and interviews reinforced the need to develop the application on a medium that would be able to tailor information to the needs of individuals and that would be considered engaging and interesting, such as a multimedia CD-ROM.

EPIDEMIOLOGICAL ASSESSMENT: BASIS FOR TAILORING MESSAGES

Even if a health problem is already determined, an understanding of the distribution of the health problem among the target audience allows further targeting of the intervention. Knowing the epidemiology of the disease will also help in tailoring the information to different audience segments. For example, a multimedia decision support application for cystic fibrosis (CF) carrier testing had different messages for populations with higher rates of CF gene carriers than for those with lower rates.

The epidemiological assessment may also be used as a strategy within the application itself. Knowledge of a disease's incidence and prevalence may be what spurs an individual to change his or her health behavior. General rates can be presented to highlight the importance of a health problem. Specific rates can be calculated in activities such as health risk appraisals. The more specific such information is, the more users will feel that the information presented is relevant to them.

In the case example, HPV in the form of genital warts is an important health problem according to *Healthy People 2000* objective 19.5.[16] HPV is also related to cervical cancer, another priority health objective in *Healthy People 2000*. Because both genital warts and cervical displasia can recur, the prevalence of the disease is as important as new cases and points to the need to reach out to patient populations. The highest prevalence rates of genital HPV infection are found in adults 18 to 28 years of age,[17] indicating that a prime target for an intervention would be the young adult population.

BEHAVIORAL AND ENVIRONMENTAL ASSESSMENT: SETTING PRIORITIES

In the behavioral and environmental assessment, expert and community input should be augmented by other scientific evidence so that the important determinants of health problems can be identified and prioritized in the design specifications. Literature reviews, interviews with other experts, and profiles of other community efforts will uncover the important and changeable behaviors.

Once the related behaviors are identified, they must be assessed as to how amenable they are to change through specific technology-based applications. Behavioral factors are more amenable to change through technological applications that allow individuals to explore their own health behavior and learn about new behaviors, and practice them. CAI that uses interactive multimedia strategies can be developed with these issues in mind. Environmental factors may be more amenable to change through applications that facilitate discussion among stakeholders and community members, particularly methods that help reach out to underrepresented populations. Internet-based applications may help a community begin to discuss important environmental issues.

In the HPV intervention development process, several data sources—literature reviews, focus groups, expert panels, health provider interviews—pointed to the key health behaviors and environmental factors to consider in the intervention.[18] These included behaviors common to other STDs, such as unprotected intercourse and multiple sexual partners. To combat HPV-related cervical disease, the key behavior was Pap test screening. Environmentally, both screening guidelines and treatment guidelines for HPV-related disease are unclear. For example, annual Pap tests are recommended, but a woman can have them less often after she has had three or more consecutive satisfactory normal annual examinations *and* her doctor recommends fewer exams. The necessity of treating all genital warts and all HPV-related cervical disease is also unclear because these diseases can clear up on their own. This lack of clarity leads to confusion and concern among those infected with the disease.

EDUCATIONAL AND ECOLOGICAL ASSESSMENT: DESIGN SPECIFICATIONS

In this phase, planners further develop the concept and design strategy, building on the relevant health behaviors or environmental influences. Health educators must determine the predisposing, reinforcing, and enabling factors and the strategies that will be used to address them. Research has demonstrated that technological applications are effective in addressing these factors. The lessons learned from previous studies will help identify how best to intervene.

The following sections provide background on the ways CAI can be used to address health determinants. The sections on predisposing, reinforcing, and enabling factors also mention how the case example evolved in these areas. A section follows that discusses selection of factors for the intervention's focus.

Predisposing Factors. CAI can influence knowledge and attitudes, in general and related to health. General studies of CAI have shown that it has beneficial effects on learner achievement in a variety of instructional settings,[19] and it can be designed to provide reliable, consistent instruction, despite differences in environments or instructors.[20] CAI instruction is just as effective with individual students as with groups.[21] Learning retention among students who use CAI is better than among students who do not.[22] In addition, CAI learners are more interactive with the task.[23]

The effects of CAI on learner achievement has been attributed to several design features that address learning theory. Simulations that incorporate elements of challenge, control, curiosity, and fantasy enhance motivation for learning.[24] Well-designed learner control of information sequencing allows individualization of learning.[25] Organization and repetition of information maximizes memorization.[26] Realistic instruction and variety of methods increase transfer of knowledge.[27] The use of feedback allows students to recognize learning difficulties and correct his or her answers.[28] In the majority of research studies, computer games improve learning outcomes in math, language arts, and physics.[29] Intelligent CAI systems, or those that can build a knowledge base from user inputs, can learn to guide each learner toward greater success over time.[30]

CAI has also been shown to increase health-related knowledge in several studies. Many of these studies have been conducted in the area of sexually transmitted disease (STD) prevention.[31] CAI has also increased knowledge in contraception,[32] nutrition,[33] and smokeless tobacco use.[34] Compared with those who did not receive any instruction[35] and with those who received direct instruction,[36] viewed a video,[37] or used written materials,[38] learners using CIA showed significant gains in knowledge. Target audiences also perceive that they are better able to learn with CAI.[39]

Many CAI applications have been designed to address health-related attitudes and have demonstrated success in improving them.[40] Strategies used to promote positive attitudes include health risk appraisals, simulation activities, and decision-making exercises. Health risk appraisals motivate health behavior change by revealing health behaviors to users so they will perceive themselves as more susceptible to the given disease.[41] Health risk appraisals also provide reinforcement for positive behaviors, which promotes self-efficacy and positive self-esteem.[42] Simulations in which a CAI user experiences real-life situations can promote outcome and efficacy expectations in areas such as alcohol use prevention,[43] STD prevention,[44] and cessation of tobacco use.[45] Decision-making software also allows students to explore their opinions and choices, learning about their own reasons for health behavior rather than what an instructor or a peer thinks is important.[46]

Concerning our HPV case, both the focus groups[47] and the literature[48] supported that lack of HPV knowledge and barriers to seeking care for STDs were predisposing factors affecting HPV-related health behaviors. The expert panel and the interviews with health care providers revealed that knowledge of screening recommendations was another important predisposing factor among young adults at risk for HPV infection.

Reinforcing Factors. CAI can provide feedback and encouragement that reinforce health behavior. Feedback lets users know immediately whether they are on the right track. When feedback indicates that users are correct or making positive choices, it encourages them.

Simulation-based CAI can model positive and negative outcomes, thus serving as vicarious modes of reinforcement. The target audience can experience real-life situations and their consequences, which will promote outcome and efficacy expectations and reinforce the behavior.[49]

Technology can be reinforcing in itself. Use of communications technology allows health educators to take advantage of the strengths of entertainment education. Such education, or "edutainment," can be intrinsically valued by the target audience because it amuses while developing their skill or achieving their goals. Besides offering opportunities for positive role modeling, entertainment-based messages can heighten audience size, attention, and receptivity. Interactive multimedia applications initially took hold because of their entertainment value. They offer users the opportunity to customize educational experiences to their own interests and needs. Health educators are just beginning to harness this potential of interactive technologies for health behavior change.[50]

Internet applications can serve a reinforcing goal by allowing individuals in disparate areas to provide social support to each other over a bulletin board or intranet. Computer-based support groups have been used among AIDS patients,[51] Alzheimer's disease caregivers,[52] and cancer patients.[53]

In the HPV case, newsletters prepared by the American Social Health Association[54] for people infected with HPV revealed several reinforcing factors. Supportive relationships with partners was important for both positive sexual communication and risk-reduction behaviors. Positive relationships with their health care provider increases the likelihood that people will seek medical care and will adhere to screening and treatment recommendations. Few materials were available for general information on HPV; lack of educational materials may have reinforced the feeling that talking about the health problem was taboo.

Enabling Factors. Technological applications facilitate health behavior by providing resources and by improving health-related skills. Community planners can provide a broader range of materials than ever before. Telecommunications and computer technology directly facilitate access to information and people, both peers and experts.[55] Strategies such as computer bulletin boards, online databases, e-mail, and distance learning can support communication among public health workers and can channel health information to the general public. Technology can also enable intermediaries by providing them with resources and decision support previously unavailable or available only from experts too busy or too expensive to query effectively.[56] For example, a computer application called DIADS (Drug Information, Assessment and Decisions for Schools) was developed to provide a cost-effective planning resource to teachers interested in implementing drug abuse prevention programs in their schools.[57]

CAI programs provide new methods for increasing health-related skills. Many programs integrate modeling and simulations, both of which are methods that encourage self-efficacy in a target behavior.[58] Simulations provide the opportunity to explore decision making safely in dangerous or risky situations.[59] The programs offer choices, process user input, and present consequences.[60] HIV prevention applications have used modeling and simulations for both minority adolescents[61] and the military community.[62] The Marijuana Action Maze used a computerized simulation game to sensitize users to alternatives, consequences, and educational and rehabilitative resources in order to improve decision-making skills.[63]

As mentioned in the description of reinforcing factors, effective relationships with partners and health care providers are important in addressing issues related to HPV infection. Therefore, enabling factors would include improving communication skills with partners and health care providers. In this case, input from the literature review, experts, and experienced providers also confirmed that decision-making skills were important enabling factors during the treatment of HPV-related diseases.

Selecting Factors and Setting Priorities. The next step in the educational and ecological assessment is to decide which factors to address in the intervention. Whether all the factors will be addressed or only a select group of them, one must assess the importance of the various factors as indicated by the literature, experts, and the community. In addition, changeability of each factor must be assessed according to the strengths of specific technological applications.

In addition to the literature and input from experts, analysis of community input is crucial in that it further elucidates the determinants of the health problem and its related health behaviors and environmental factors, ensuring the effective tailoring of messages and teaching strategies. Keeping the community's needs and attitudes in mind during this assessment will facilitate the identification of appropriate targets, materials, and strategies.

One also needs to assess which technological application can best facilitate a given intervention strategy. For example, a decision-making exercise may require simulation so that the user can practice making decisions. A skill-building activity may require modeling so the user can observe the appropriate actions. Therefore, one must choose applications that can effect change in the desired learning objectives.[64] Table 12-3 lists various applications, their capabilities, and the intervention strategies to which they are best suited. One can find evidence for the effectiveness of all these applications except for interactive television, largely because it has not been available for very long. Community input regarding the functionality desired can also help guide one's choice of applications.[65]

In the case example, research and the community supported the facilitation of consumer health decision making and the modeling of effective patient-provider communication and communication with partners. While some of the behaviors related to STD prevention, these were seen as a lower priority than the development of communication skills. This information supported the decision to develop an interactive multimedia CD-ROM program.

ADMINISTRATIVE AND POLICY ASSESSMENT: PROTOTYPING

During this phase, by creating a prototype of the technology application, the developer assesses how the plan might work. The logic and appeal of the various

TABLE 12-3

Capabilities of technological applications and related intervention strategies

Application	Capabilities	Intervention Strategies
Distributed multimedia technologies (IVD, CD-ROM, DC-I, DVD)	High-quality video and audio	Modeling Virtual reality Simulation Gaming
Interactive television	High-quality video and audio Accessibility in the home Ease of use Ability to monitor group consensus	Modeling Virtual reality Simulation Gaming
Online communications (e-mail, chat rooms, bulletin boards, www materials)	Accessibility in public settings Education from a distance Real-time assessments Simultaneous use	Partnership building Multiplayer gaming

elements of the plan must be detailed in such a way that users can truly see what has been only imagined previously.

A key consideration in this phase is the scope of the application, given time and resources. Today, much that can be imagined can be done, but not without some tradeoffs. For example, the amount of information that can fit on a CD-ROM will determine the amount of audio, video, graphics, and text that can be included. If the health educator has enough material to cover several CD-ROMs, he or she must decide what is most important to include. Even when technology presents few constraints, the budget may not allow one to include all the features one would like. Public-domain photographs, clip art, and audio files keep costs down, but finding ones that meet a program's specific demands is often difficult. Creating new multimedia elements can be more costly than a community program's budget can bear.

In organizing information, the health educator also needs to think of the "budget" in terms of the user's time. If the application is for one-time use, the messages must be so clear that they will remain with the user after one exposure. If the user will likely use the application many times, the information must be organized so that it remains compelling, perhaps with new features or different levels of interaction, so that users will want to interact with it many times.

In addition, one must pay attention to project staff during this phase. One way to ensure that staff facilitate rather than hinder development efforts is similar to the strategy used at the community level: have them participate in the process. For example, a "design team" involves many members of a group, capitalizing on their strengths for different aspect of the project. A multimedia effort's design team may include a project manager, subject matter experts, an instructional designer familiar with health behavior theory, graphic artists, programmers, and video producers. Because each member shapes the effort, all are committed to its success.

Beginning with the understanding of HPV, its determinants, and the target population, a design team worked together to formulate the content and structure of the HPV intervention. The document that details such elements as well as where and how users will interact with a program is called the *design document*. In this case, the design document detailed the use of the application in the clinic setting by women having routine Pap test screening or STD diagnostic services. Based on community input, the clinic-based application was to be designed with appropriate privacy and confidentiality controls.

IMPLEMENTATION AND EVALUATION

As the design specifications emerge and as the intervention is developed, community participation continues to play a key role in the development process, largely as a check that the effort truly reflects the needs of the target population. Experts and advisory groups help guide the choice of educational strategies and content. The advisory panel also monitors the development to ensure that no issues will affect the dissemination of the application. For example, in the development of multimedia materials for drug abuse prevention in health care settings, reviewers can ensure that the interactive scenarios are realistic and compelling for health professionals. Inappropriate language or situations might cause a negative reaction and lead users to discount all the information being conveyed.

Similarly, the target population itself is asked to review the application at various stages of development. The initial prototype can be presented to community members and stakeholders in interviews or focus-group discussions to see if the application and its messages and strategies are appropriate. If any questions remain about design specifications (or if new ones have arisen from the development process), the community can help address them.

In the case example, the HPV application was being developed at the time this book went to press. When fully developed, it will undergo various testing methods. Alpha testing is generally an in-house test of the program's functionality to ensure that it operates correctly and smoothly. The next phase, beta testing, usually has potential users of the application determine the acceptability of the application. Expert review of the program can be conducted during this step or preceding it. Usability testing is also conducted with potential users, but the focus of this testing phase is the ability of users to understand how to use the application properly.

Once the final revisions are made, the developer will conduct a field test to determine the impact of the intervention on the learning objectives. An advantage of field testing a technology-based intervention rather than other interventions is that it can be designed to collect evaluation data as part of the intervention through electronic monitoring of user choices and through pre- and postassessment activities. This ability reduces both the expense of collecting and recording data and the chance of losing data. It also provides a way to collect very specific data about behavioral decision making, data that would otherwise not be available.[66]

SUMMARY

PRECEDE-PROCEED serves as a model for complex program planning, implementation, and evaluation. With emerging technologies, many systems are available to support the work of those applying the model. There are at least two such applications that provide guidance through the entirety of the model. One is a training tool (EMPOWER) and one is a supportive environment for guidance (Netpower). Most importantly, however, PRECEDE-PROCEED can be used to design, test, implement, evaluate, and refine complex technologies themselves.

NOTES AND CITATIONS

1. For the continuously updated, searchable bibliography of these published examples and other aspects of this and other chapters of this book, go to http://www.ihpr.ubc.ca/preapps.html

2. Green, 1983a, p. xvi. We are indebted to Mike Chiasson for further insights on this.

3. Waterworth, 1992, p. 3.

4. Friede, McDonald, & Blum, 1995, p. 239.

5. Burris, 1992.

6. Friede, McDonald, & Blum, 1995, p. 241.

7. *Synchronous communications* are those that occur in real time, with all parties able to participate concurrently. Chat rooms and instant messaging capabilities are examples of synchronous communications. *Asynchronous communications* are those in which only one party is transmitting or receiving a message at a given point in time. E-mail and message boards are examples of asynchronous communications.

8. We use the phrase *general-purpose applications* because the speed of change of technology is dramatic. By the time a textbook such as this is published, the specific names and capabilities of applications will have changed from those in use at the time the chapters were written. As a result, we talk about e-mail or chat rooms rather than specific types of e-mail or chat room programs.

9. Chiasson, 1996; Green, Gold, Tan, & Kreuter, 1994.

10. Gold, Green, & Kreuter, 1997. For its field testing, see Chiasson, 1996.

11. Jewell, Abraham, & Fitzpatrick, 1987.

12. Though named differently, these modules correspond to the stages of PRECEDE.

13. Gold, 1991; Hawkins et al., 1987; Kann 1987; Knight et al., 1987.

14. Meyer, 1995. HPV is a sexually transmitted disease related to anogenital cancers including cervical cancer.

15. Gold & Hernandez, 1992.

16. U.S. Department of Health and Human Services, 1991.

17. Koutsky, 1997.

18. Kann, 1987.

19. AMC Cancer Research Center, 1994; Azevedo & Bernard, 1995; Deardorff, 1986; Dennison, Galante, & Golaszewski, 1996; Paperny & Starn, 1989; Petri & Hyner, 1996; Reis & Tymchyshyn, 1992.

20. Boberg, Gustafson, Hawkins, & Chan, 1995; Bosworth, Gustafson, & Hawkins, 1994; Bosworth & Yoast, 1991. U.S. Congress, Office of Technology Assessment, 1995.

21. Tolman & Allred, 1991.

22. McNeil & Nelson, 1991; Petri & Hyner, 1996; Randel, Morris, Wetzel, & Whitehill, 1992.

23. Rowley & Layne, 1990.

24. Tolman & Allred, 1991.

25. Allessi & Trollip, 1985; Hannaway, Shuler, Bolte, & Miller, 1992; Tzung-yu, 1993; M. D. Williams, 1993.

26. AMC Cancer Research Center, 1994; Azvedo & Bernard, 1995; Hannaway, Shuler, Bolte, & Miller, 1992; MacKenzie, 1990.

27. AMC Cancer Research Center, 1994; Deardorff, 1986.

28. Azevedo & Bernard, 1995; Tzung-yu, 1993.

29. Randel, Morris, Wetzel, & Whitehall, 1992.

30. Azvedo & Bernard, 1995.

31. Kritch, Bostow, & Dedrick, 1995; Noell, Ary, & Duncan, 1997.

32. Reis & Tymchyshyn, 1992; Van Cura et al., 1975.

33. D. Dennison & Dennison, 1989; K. F. Dennison, Galante, & Golaszewski, 1996.

34. Levenson & Morrow, 1987.

35. Kinzie, Schorling, & Siegel, 1993; McNeil & Nelson, 1991; Meier & Sampson, 1989; Schinke, Orlandi, Schilling, & Parms, 1992.

36. C. W. Johnson, 1993; Randel, Morris, Wetzel, & Whitehill, 1992; Tolman & Allred, 1991; M. D. Williams, 1993.

37. McLean, 1996.

38. Meier & Sampson, 1989; Tzung-yu, 1993.

39. Reis & Tymchyshyn, 1992; Robinson, 1989.

40. Gold, 1991.

41. Ellis & Raines, 1983.

42. Ibid; McAuley, Michalko, & Bane, 1997.

43. Kinzie, Schorling, & Siegel, 1993.

44. Noell, Ary, & Duncan, 1997; R. Thomas, Cahill, & Santilli, 1997; Vail-Smith & White, 1992.

45. Bosworth et al., 1983, 1994.

46. Keener & Bright, 1983.

47. Meyer, 1995.

48. Gold & Hernandez, 1992.

49. Singhal, 1994.

50. Jenny, 1993; Kreuter, Vehige, & McGuire, 1998; Maibach & Holtgrave, 1995.

51. Gustafson et al., 1992.

52. P. F. Brennan, Moore, & Smyth, 1992.

53. N. Weinberg, Schmale, Uken, & Wessel, 1996.

54. American Social Health Association, 1992, 1993, 1994.

55. Laporte, 1994.

56. Randel, Morris, Wetzel, & Whitehill, 1992.

57. Bosworth & Yoast, 1991.

58. Bandura, 1977a; Parcel & Baranowski, 1981; Thomas, Cahill, & Santilli, 1997.

59. AMC Cancer Research Center, 1994.

60. Maibach & Holtgrave, 1995.

61. Meier & Sampson, 1989.

62. McGrane, Toth, & Allely, 1990.

63. Henningson, Gold, & Duncan, 1986.

64. Skinner & Kreuter, 1997.

65. Street, Gold, & Manning, 1997.

66. Chiasson, 1996.

Glossary

action Conduct of individuals, families, groups, community decision makers and administrators, government or industrial policy makers, health professionals, and others who might influence the health of themselves or others.

administrative assessment An analysis of the *policies,* resources, and circumstances prevailing in an organization to facilitate or hinder the development of the health promotion program.

advocacy Working for political, *regulatory,* or organizational change on behalf of a particular interest group or population.

age-adjusted rate The total rate for a population, adjusted to ignore the age distribution of the specific population by multiplying each of its *age-specific rates* by the proportion of a standard population (usually national) in that age group, and then adding up the products.

agent An *epidemiological* term referring to the organism or object that transmits a disease from the environment to the host.

age-specific rate The incidence (number of events during a specified period) for an age group, divided by the total number of people in that age group.

allocation A distribution of resources to specific categories of expenditure or to specific organizations or subpopulations.

assessment Estimation of the relative magnitude, importance, or value of objects observed.

attitude A relatively constant feeling, predisposition, or set of beliefs directed toward an object, person, or situation.

authorization A step in the legislative process in which the maximum amount of money to be allocated and the assignment of authority to spend it are decided.

behavior An action that has a specific frequency, duration, and purpose, whether conscious or unconscious.

behavioral assessment Delineation of the specific health-related actions that will most likely cause a health outcome.

behavioral intention A mental state in which an individual expects to take a specified action in the future.

behavioral objective A statement of desired outcome that indicates who is to demonstrate how much of what action by when.

belief   A statement or proposition, declared or implied, that is emotionally and/or intellectually accepted as true by a person or group.

benefits   Valued health outcomes or improvements in quality of life or social conditions having some known relationship to health promotion or health-care interventions.

central location intercept   A survey procedure that seeks interviews with an unsystematic sample of people on the street or in a shopping center in order to represent the opinions of those likely to be the target of a program.

coalition   A group of organizations or representatives of groups within a community, joined to pursue a common objective.

coercive strategies   Preventive methods that bypass the motivation and decisions of people by dictating or precluding choices.

community   A collective of people identified by common values and mutual concern for the development and well-being of their group or geographical area.

community organization   The set of procedures and processes by which a population and its institutions mobilize and coordinate resources to solve a mutual problem or to pursue mutual goals.

compliance   Adherence to a prescribed therapeutic or preventive regimen.

comprehensive school health education   Classroom instruction that addresses the physical, mental, emotional, and social dimensions of health; develops health knowledge, attitudes, and skills; is tailored to each age level; and is designed to predispose and enable students to maintain and improve their health, prevent disease, and reduce health-related risk behaviors.

conditions of living   The combination of behavioral and environmental circumstances that make up one's lifestyle and health-related social situation.

construct   The representation of concepts within a causal explanation or theoretical framework. For example, predisposing, enabling, and reinforcing factors are constructs for the representation of more specific concepts or variables such as health beliefs, attitudes, skills, and rewards.

cost-benefit   A measure of the cost of an intervention relative to the benefits it yields, usually expressed as a ratio of dollars saved or gained for every dollar spent on the program.

cost-effectiveness   A measure of the cost of an intervention relative to its impact, usually expressed in dollars per unit of effect.

Delphi Method   A method of sampling the opinions or preferences of a small number of experts, opinion leaders, or informants, whereby successive questionnaires are sent by mail and the results (rankings or value estimates) are summarized for further refinement on subsequent mailings.

determinants of health   The forces predisposing, enabling, and reinforcing lifestyles, or shaping environmental conditions of living, in ways that affect the health of populations.

diagnosis   Health or behavioral information that designates the "problem" or need; its status, distribution, or frequency in the person or population; and the probable causes or risk factors associated with the problem or need.

disability   The inability to perform specific functions resulting from disease, injury, or birth defects.

dose-response relationship   A term borrowed from clinical trials of drugs; when applied in epidemiology, it refers to a gradient of risk ratios corresponding to degrees of exposure; in health promotion, it refers to the increases in outcome measures associated with proportionate increases in the program resources expended or in intervention exposure.

early adopters   Those in the population who accept a new idea or practice soon after the innovators (but before the *middle majority*) who tend to be opinion leaders for the middle majority.

ecological assessment   See *environmental assessment* and *educational assessment.*

ecology   Study of the web of relationships among the behaviors of individuals and populations and their environments, social and physical.

economy of scale   The point in the growth of a program or service at which each additional element of service costs less to produce than the previous element of service.

education of the electorate   A process of political change in which those affected by policies are educated so that they will be more likely to vote for candidates or referenda that are in their best interests.

educational assessment   The delineation of factors that predispose, enable, and reinforce a specific behavior or that through behavior affect environmental changes.

educational tool   Any material or method designed to aid learning and teaching through sight and sound.

effectiveness   The extent to which the intended effect or benefits that could be achieved under optimal conditions are achieved in practice.

efficacy   The extent to which an intervention can be shown to be beneficial under optimal conditions.

efficiency   The proportion of total costs (e.g., money, resources, time) that can be related to the number of people served or benefits achieved in practice.

Employee Assistance Programs (EAPs)   A confidential, voluntary set of procedures and arrangements to provide information, referral, counseling, and support to workers and sometimes their family members to help them deal with personal problems that might interfere with their work.

empowerment education   A process of encouraging a community to take control of its own education, assess its own needs, set its own priorities, develop its own self-help programs, and, if necessary, challenge the power structure to provide resources.

enabling factor   Any characteristic of the environment that facilitates action and any skill or resource required to attain a specific behavior. Absence of the resource blocks the behavior; barriers to the behavior are included in lists of enabling factors to be developed. Skills are sometimes listed separately as predisposing factors or intermediate outcomes of education.

environment   The totality of the social, biological, and physical circumstances surrounding a defined quality of life, health, or behavioral goal or problem.

environmental assessment   A systematic assessment of factors in the social and physical environment that interact with behavior to produce health effects or quality-of-life outcomes. Also referred to as *ecological assessment.*

environmental factor   One of the specific elements or components of the social, biological, or physical environment determined during the environmental assessment to be causally linked to health or quality-of-life goals or problems identified in the social or epidemiological assessment.

epidemiology   The study of the distribution and causes of health problems in populations.

epidemiological assessment   The delineation of the extent, distribution, and causes of a health problem in a defined population.

etiology   The origins or causes of a disease or condition under study; the first steps in the natural history of a disease.

evaluation   The comparison of an object of interest with a standard of acceptability.

excise tax   A tax on the manufacture, sale, or use of certain products such as alcohol or tobacco to generate revenue for a government, to control consumption, or both.

external validity   Assurance that the results of an evaluation can be generalized to other populations or settings.

family and community involvement in schools   Partnerships among schools, families, community groups, and individuals designed to share and maximize resources and expertise in addressing the healthy development of children, youth, and their families.

fear   A mental state that motivates problem-solving behavior if an action (fight or flight) is immediately available; if not, it motivates other defense mechanisms such as denial or suppression.

focus-group method   Used in testing the perception and receptivity of a target population to an idea or method by recording the reactions of a sample of 8 to 10 people discussing it with each other.

formative evaluation   Any combination of measurements obtained and judgments made before or during the implementation of materials, methods, activities, or programs to control, assure, or improve the quality of performance or delivery. (Measurements during implementation are sometimes called *process evaluation.*)

Gannt chart   A timetable showing each activity in a program plan as a horizontal line that extends from the start to the finish date so that at any given time a program manager can see what activities should be underway, about to begin, or due to be completed.

habituation   The incorporation of a pattern of behavior into one's lifestyle to the degree that it is performed virtually without thought but does not necessarily entail physical or psychological dependence.

Health Belief Model   A paradigm used to predict and explain health behavior; based on value-expectancy theory.

health-directed behavior   The conscious pursuit of actions for the protection or improvement of health. Cf. *health-related behavior.*

health education   Any planned combination of learning experiences designed to predispose, enable, and reinforce voluntary behavior conducive to health in individuals, groups, or communities.

health enhancement   A dimension of health promotion pertaining to its goal of reaching higher levels of wellness beyond the mere absence of disease or infirmity.

health field concept   The idea that the factors influencing health can be subsumed under four categories: environment, human biology, behavior, and health-care organization.

health outcome   Any medically or epidemiologically defined characteristic of a patient or population that results from health promotion or care provided or required, as measured at one point in time.

health promotion   Any planned combination of educational, political, regulatory, and organizational supports for actions and conditions of living conducive to the health of individuals, groups, or communities.

health protection   A strategy parallel to health promotion in some national policies, that focuses on the environmental rather than behavioral determinants of health, with methods more like those of engineers and regulatory agencies than those of educational and social or health service agencies.

health-related behavior   Actions undertaken for reasons other than the protection or improvement of health but which have health effects.

healthful school environment   The physical, emotional, and social climate of a school. Designed to provide a safe physical plant as well as a healthful and supportive environment that fosters learning.

host   A concept from epidemiology referring to an individual who harbors or is at risk of harboring a disease or condition.

immediacy   A criterion for judging the importance of a factor, based on how urgent or imminent the factor is in its influence on the outcome desired.

impact evaluation   The assessment of program effects on intermediate objectives including changes in predisposing, enabling, and reinforcing factors, as well as behavioral and environmental changes.

implementation   The act of converting program objectives into actions through policy changes, regulation, and organization.

incidence   A measure of the frequency of occurrence of a disease or health problem in a population based on the number of new cases over a given period of time (usually one year). An incidence rate is obtained by dividing this number by the midyear population and multiplying the quotient by 1,000 or 100,000.

informed consent   A medical-legal doctrine that holds providers responsible for ensuring that consumers, patients, or workers understand the risks and benefits of a procedure or medicine before it is administered.

innovators   Those in a population who are first to adopt a new idea or practice, usually based on information from sources outside the community.

internal validity   Assurance that the results of an evaluation can be attributed to the object (method or program) evaluated.

intervention   The part of a strategy, incorporating method and technique, that actually reaches a person or population.

late majority   The segment of the population most difficult to reach through mass communication channels or to convince of the need to adopt a new idea or practice, either because they cannot afford it or cannot get to the source or because of cultural and linguistic differences or other difficulties.

leveraging   The use of initial investments in a program to draw larger investments.

lifestyle   The culturally, socially, economically, and environmentally conditioned complex of actions characteristic of an individual, group, or community as a pattern of habituated behavior over time that is health related but not necessarily health directed.

market testing   The placement of a message or product in a commercial context to determine how it influences consumer behavior.

middle majority   The segment of the population who adopt a new idea or practice after the *innovators* and *early adopters* but before the late adopters, usually influenced by a combination of mass media, interpersonal communications, and endorsements by famous personalities or organizations of which they are members.

morbidity   The existence or rate of disease or infirmity.

mortality   The event or rate of death.

necessity   A criterion for judging the importance of a factor, based on whether the outcome can occur without this factor.

need   (1) Whatever is required for health or comfort; (2) an estimation of the interventions required based on a diagnosis of the problem and, in populations, the number of people eligible to benefit from the intervention(s).

nominal group process   An interactive group method for assessing community needs by having opinions listed without critique from the group and then rated by secret ballot, thereby minimizing the influence of interpersonal dynamics and status on the ratings.

normative effect   The influence of perceived social patterns of and expectations for behavior on the actions taken by individuals and groups.

objective   A defined result of specific activity to be achieved in a finite period by a specified person or number of people. Objectives state *who* will experience *what* change or benefit by *how much* and by *when*.

organization   The act of marshaling and coordinating the resources necessary to implement a program.

outcome evaluation   Assessment of the effects of a program on its ultimate objectives, including changes in health and social benefits or quality of life.

planning   The process of defining needs, establishing priorities, diagnosing causes of problems, assessing resources and barriers, and allocating resources to achieve objectives.

policy   The set of objectives and rules guiding the activities of an organization or an administration, and providing authority for the allocation of resources.

positional leader   A person whose influence is based, or perceived to be based, on his or her official standing or office, such as an elected or appointed official, executive of a firm, or head of a voluntary organization.

PRECEDE   Acronym for the diagnostic planning and evaluation model outlined in this book, emphasizing *p*redisposing, *r*einforcing, and *e*nabling *c*onstructs in *e*ducational (and *e*nvironmental) *d*iagnosis and *e*valuation.

predisposing factor   Any characteristic of a person or population that motivates behavior prior to the occurrence of the behavior.

prevalence   A measure of the extent of a disease or health problem in a population based on the number of cases (old and new) existing in the population at a given time. See also *incidence.*

priority   Alternatives ranked according to feasibility or value (importance) or both.

PROCEED   Acronym for *p*olicy, *r*egulatory, and *o*rganizational *c*onstructs in *e*ducational and *e*nvironmental *d*evelopment, the phases of resource mobilization, implementation, and evaluation following the diagnostic planning phases of PRECEDE.

process evaluation   The assessment of policies, materials, personnel, performance, quality of practice or services, and other inputs and implementation experiences.

program   A set of planned activities over time designed to achieve specified objectives.

proximal risk   Those risk factors or conditions in the immediate range of influence, in time or place, over which individuals or communities could exercise control.

quality assessment   Measurement of professional or technical practice or service for comparison with accepted standards to determine the degree of excellence.

quality assurance   Formal process of implementing quality assessment and quality improvement in programs to assure stakeholders that professional activities have been performed appropriately.

quality of life   The perception of individuals or groups that their needs are being satisfied and that they are not being denied opportunities to achieve happiness and fulfillment.

reach   The number of people attending or exposed to an intervention or program.

reductionist   The approach to assessment that seeks to explain the cause of a problem or event within the person having the problem or within the immediate environment of the event.

relative risk   The ratio of mortality or incidence of a disease or condition in those exposed to a given risk factor (e.g., smokers) to the mortality or incidence in those not exposed (e.g., nonsmokers). A relative risk (RR) ratio of 1.0 indicates no greater risk in those exposed than in those not exposed.

regulation   The act of enforcing *policies,* rules, or laws.

reinforcing factor   Any reward or punishment following or anticipated as a consequence of a behavior, serving to strengthen the motivation for or against the behavior.

reputational leader   One whose leadership power is based on perceived performance as an influential person, but not necessarily on his or her position.

risk conditions   Those determinants of health that are more distal in time, place, or scope from the control of individuals than are the more proximal and malleable *risk factors* such as current behavior.

risk factors   Characteristics of individuals (genetic, behavioral, and environmental exposures and sociocultural living conditions) that increase the probability that they will experience a disease or specific cause of death as measured by population *relative risk ratios.*

risk ratio   The mortality or incidence of a disease or condition in those exposed to a given risk factor divided by the mortality or incidence in those not exposed. See also *relative risk.*

school counseling, psychological, and social services   Activities that focus on cognitive, emotional, behavioral, and social needs of individuals, groups, and families; designed to prevent and address problems, facilitate positive learning and healthful behavior, and enhance healthy development.

school food services   Integration of nutritious, affordable, and appealing meals; nutrition education; and an environment that promotes healthy eating behaviors for all children; designed to maximize each child's education and health potential for a lifetime.

school health education   Any combination of learning experiences organized in the school setting to predispose, enable, and reinforce behavior conducive to health or to prepare school-age children to be able to cope with the challenges to their health in the year ahead.

school health services   Preventive services, education, emergency care, referral, and management of acute and chronic health conditions; designed to promote the health of students, identify and prevent health problems and injuries, and ensure care for students.

school physical education   Any combination of learning experiences organized in the school setting to improve physical activity and to develop lifelong skills and a predisposition to maintain physical activity at healthful levels.

school-site health promotion for staff   Assessment, education, and fitness activities for school faculty and staff; designed to maintain and improve the health and well-being of school staff, who serve as role models for students.

self-efficacy   A construct from social learning theory referring to the belief an individual holds that he or she is capable of performing a specific behavior.

sensitivity   The ability of a test to identify all people who have a particular characteristic or condition—that is, the ability to avoid missing cases in a population screening. See also *specificity.*

settings   Organizations or institutions where health promotion is carried out. More generally, setting is a milieu in which people gather for schooling, work, cohabitation, or other mutually supportive activities, governed by rules and norms specific to the place.

social assessment   The assessment in both objective and subjective terms of high-priority problems or aspirations for the common good, defined for a population by economic and social indicators and by individuals in terms of their quality of life.

social capital   The processes and conditions among people and organizations that lead to accomplishing a goal of mutual social benefit, usually characterized by four interrelated constructs: trust, cooperation, civic engagement, and reciprocity.

social indicator   A numerical value that reflects quality of life for a population; a change in social indicators means a change in quality of life.

socialization   A process of developing behavioral patterns or *lifestyle* through modeling or imitating socially important people, including parents, peers, and media personalities.

social problem   A situation that a significant number of people believe to be a source of difficulty or unhappiness. A social problem consists of objective circumstances as well as a social interpretation of its unacceptability.

social reconnaissance   Diagnostic procedures applied to a large geographic area with the active participation of people having various levels of authority and resources, including government officials and professionals in health and other sectors, and potential recipients of new programs or services.

specificity   The ability of a test to rule out cases not possessing a particular characteristic or condition—that is, to avoid false-positive results in a population screening. See also *sensitivity.*

specific rates   Morbidity, mortality, fertility, or other rates calculated for specific age, gender, race, or other demographic groupings.

stakeholders   People who have an investment or a stake in the outcome of a program and therefore have reasons to be interested in the evaluation of the program.

stepped approach   A method of intervention, following triage, in which minimal resources or effort are expended on the first group or level, more intensive effort on the second level, and most intensive on the third.

strategy   A plan of action that anticipates barriers and resources in relation to achieving a specific objective.

surveillance   Continuous or periodic measurement and analysis to detect outbreaks or unusual patterns that might be developing in a population.

surveys   Methods of polling a group or population to estimate the norms and distribution of characteristics from a sample, using direct observations, questionnaires or interviews.

synchronous communications   Those exchanges of information in which two or more parties participate concurrently.

tactic   A method or approach employed as a part of a strategy.

triage   A method of sorting people into (usually three) groups for purposes of setting priorities on allocation of resources.

value   A preference shared and transmitted within a community.

wellness   A dimension of health beyond the absence of disease or infirmity, including social, emotional, and spiritual aspects of health.

References

Aaro, L. E., Laberg, J. C., & Wold, B. (1995). Health behaviours among adolescents: Towards a hypothesis of two dimensions. *Health Education Research, 10,* 83–94.

Aaro, L. E., Wold, D., Kannas, L., & Rimpela, M. (1986). Health behavior in school children: A WHO cross-national survey. *Health Promotion, 1,* 17–33.

Abelin, T., Brzezinski, Z. J., & Carstairs, V. D. (Eds.). (1987). *Measurement in health promotion and protection.* Copenhagen: World Health Organization Regional Publications, European Series No. 22.

Abelson, R. P., Aronson, E., McGuire, W. J., et al. (1968). *Theories of cognitive consistency: A sourcebook.* Chicago, IL: Rand McNally College.

Abma, J. C., Chandra, A., Mosher, W. D., Peterson, L. S., & Piccinino, L. J. (1997). Fertility, family planning, and women's health: New data from the 1995 National Survey of Family Growth. *Vital and Health Statistics, 30,* 4–10.

Ackerman, A., & Kalmer, H. (1977, November 1). Health education and a baccalaureate nursing curriculum: Myth or reality. Paper presented at the 105th annual meeting of the American Public Health Association, Washington, DC.

Adams, D. (1991). Planning models and paradigms. In R. V. Carlson & G. Awkerman (Eds.), *Educational planning: Concepts, strategies and practices.* New York: Longman.

Aday, L. A., Andersen, R., & Fleming, G. V. (1980). *Health care in the U.S.: Equitable for whom?* Beverly Hills, CA: Sage.

Aday, L. A., & Eichhorn, R. (1973). *The utilization of health services: Indices and correlates.* Washington, DC: National Center for Health Services Research, DHEW Pub. No. HSM 73-3003.

Aday, L.A., Pounds, M. B., Marconi, K. & Bowen, G. S. (1994). A framework for evaluating the Ryan White Care Act: Toward a CIRCLE of caring for persons with HIV/AIDS. *AIDS and Public Policy Journal, 9,* 138–145.

Adeyanju, O. M. (1987–1988). A community-based health education analysis of an infectious disease control program in Nigeria. *International Quarterly of Community Health Education, 8*(3), 263–279.

Note: Citations list all authors each time if there are up to five authors. For references that include three authors plus et al., the citation lists the first author's name plus et al., with more names included only if needed to avoid confusion. Thus, Simons-Morton, Parcel, & O'Hara, 1988, is not the same as Simons-Morton et al., 1988.

Adler, M. J. (1983). *The Paideia problems and possibilities.* New York: Macmillan.

Adler, N. E., Boyce, T., Chesney, M. A., et al. (1994). Socioeconomic status and health: The challenge of the gradient. *American Psychologist, 49,* 15–24.

Adult immunizations: Knowledge, attitudes and practices. (1988). *Morbidity and Mortality Weekly Reports, 73,* 657–661.

Ailinger, R. L., & Dear, M. R. (1993). Self-care agency in persons with rheumatoid arthritis. *Arthritis Care and Research, 6,* 134–140.

Airhihenbuwa, C. (1995). *Health and culture: Beyond the Western paradigm.* Thousand Oaks, CA: Sage.

Airhihenbuwa, C., Kamanyika, S., & Lowe, A. (1995). Perceptions and beliefs about exercise, rest, and health among African-Americans. *American Journal of Health Promotion, 9,* 426–429.

Ajzen, I., & Fishbein, M. (1980). *Understanding attitudes and predicting social behavior.* Englewood Cliffs, NJ: Prentice-Hall, 1980.

Ajzen, I., & Madden, J. T. (1986). Prediction of goal-directed behavior: Attitudes, intentions, and perceived behavioral control. *Journal of Experimental Social Psychology, 22,* 453–474.

Alcalay, R., Sabogal, F., Marin, G., et al. (1987–1988). Patterns of mass media use among Hispanic smokers: Implications for community interventions. *International Quarterly of Community Health Education, 8,* 341–350.

Alderman, M., Green, L. W., & Flynn, B. S. (1980). Hypertension control programs in occupational settings. *Public Health Reports, 90,* 158–163. Also in R. S. Parkinson, L. W. Green, M. Eriksen, & A. McGill (Eds.) (1982). *Managing Health Promotion in the Workplace: Guidelines for Implementation and Evaluation* (pp. 162–172). Palo Alto, CA: Mayfield.

Alinsky, S. D. (1972). *Rules for radicals: A pragmatic primer for realistic radicals.* New York: Vintage Books.

Allanson, J. F. (1978). School nursing services: Some current justifications and cost-benefit implications. *Journal of School Health, 48,* 603–607.

Allegrante, J. P. (1986). Potential uses and misuses of education in health promotion and disease prevention. *Teachers College Record, 86,* 359–373. Also in (1986) *Eta Sigma Gamman, 18,* 2–8.

Allegrante, J. P., & Green, L. W. (1981). When health policy becomes victim blaming. *New England Journal of Medicine, 305,* 1528–1529.

Allegrante, J. P., Kovar, P. A., MacKenzie, C. R., Peterson, M. G. E., & Gutin, B. (1993). A walking education program for patients with osteoarthritis of the knee: Theory and intervention strategies. *Health Education Quarterly, 20,* 63–81.

Allegrante, J. P., & Sloan, R. P. (1986). Ethical dilemmas in workplace health promotion. *Preventive Medicine, 15,* 313–320.

Allen, J., Lowman, C., & Miller, W. R. (1996). Introduction: Perspectives on precipitants of relapse. *Addiction, 91*(Suppl.), S3–S5.

Allen, J., & Allen, R. F. (1986). Achieving health promotion objectives through cultural change systems. *American Journal of Health Promotion, 1,* 42–49.

Allen, J., & Allen, R. F. (1990). A sense of community, a shared vision and a positive culture: Core enabling factors in successful culture-based change. In R. D. Patton & W. B. Cissel (eds.), *Community Organization: Traditional Principles and Modern Applications* (pp. 5–18). Johnson City, TN: Latchpins Press.

Allen, R. F. (1980). *Beat the system.* New York: McGraw-Hill.

Allensworth, D. (1987, October–November). Building community support for quality school health programs. *Health Education, 18,* 32–38.

Allensworth, D., & Kolbe, L. J. (Eds.) (1987). The comprehensive school health program: Exploring an expanded concept. [Special issue]. *Journal of School Health, 57*(10).

Allensworth, D., Wolford, C. A. (1988). *Achieving the 1990 objectives for the nation's schools.* Kent, OH: American School Health Association.

Allessi, S. M., & Trollip, S. R. (1985). *Computer-based instructions: Methods and development.* Englewood Cliffs, NJ: Prentice-Hall.

Allison, K. R. (1991). Theoretical issues concerning the relationship between perceived control and preventive health behaviour. *Health Education Research, 6,* 141–151.

Alteneder R. R. (1994). Use of an educational program on HIV/AIDS with junior high students. *International Conference on AIDS, 10*(2), 355 (Abstract no. PD0601).

Alteneder, R. R., Price, J. H., Telljohann, S. K., Didion, J., & Locher, A. (1992). Using the PRECEDE model to determine junior high school students' knowledge, attitudes, and beliefs about AIDS. *Journal of School Health, 62,* 464–470.

Altman, D. G. (1995). Sustaining interventions in community systems: On the relationship between researchers and communities. *Health Psychology, 14,* 526–536.

Altman, D., Flora, J., Fortmann, S., & Farquhar, J. (1987). The cost-effectiveness of three smoking cessation programs. *American Journal of Public Health, 77,* 162–165.

Altman, D. G., Endres, J., Linzer, J., et al. (1991). Obstacles to and future goals of ten comprehensive community health promotion projects. *Journal of Community Health, 16*(6), 299–314.

Altman, D. G., & Green, L. W. (1988). Area Review: Education and Training in Behavioral Medicine. *Annals of Behavioral Medicine, 10,* 4–7.

AMC Cancer Research Center. (1994). *Beyond the brochure: Alternative approaches to effective health communication.* Washington, DC: U.S. Government Printing Office.

American Association for Health, Physical Education and Recreation. (1969). Recommended standards and guidelines for teacher preparation in health education. *Journal of Health Education, 40*(2), 31–38.

American Association for Health, Physical Education and Recreation. (1974). *Professional preparation in safety education and school health education.* Washington, DC: National Conference on Undergraduate Professional Preparation.

American Cancer Society, Joint Committee on National Health Education Standards. (1995). *Achieving health literacy: An investment in the future.* Atlanta, GA: American Cancer Society.

American College Health Association. (1986). *AIDS on the college campus.* Rockville, MD: American College Health Association.

American College of Physicians. (1989). Health care needs of the adolescent. *Annals of Internal Medicine, 110,* 930–935.

American College of Preventive Medicine and Fogarty Center. (1976). *Preventive medicine USA.* New York: Prodist.

American Council of Life Insurance. (1985). *Wellness at the school worksite: Manual.* Washington, DC: Health Insurance Association of America.

American Council of Life Insurance. (1998). *Wellness at the school worksite: A manual.* Washington, DC: Health Insurance Association of America.

American Medical Association Auxiliary. (1987). *Community action: How to work in coalitions.* Chicago: American Medical Association Auxiliary.

American Physical Education Association. (1935). Health education section: Committee report, American Physical Education Association. *Journal of Health and Physical Education, 6,* 204–209.

American Public Health Association, Committee on Professional Education. (1969). Criteria and guidelines for accrediting graduate programs in community health education. *American Journal of Public Health, 59*(3), 534–542.

American School Health Association. (1976). *Professional preparation of the health educator.* Kent, OH: Author.

American Social Health Association. (1992). Coping with HPV. *HPV News, 1*(1), 1, 4.

American Social Health Association. (1993). Physician-patient relationships. *HPV News, 1*(1) 1, 5–8.

American Social Health Association. (1994). Living with HPV. *HPV News, 4*(2), 6.

Anda, R. F., Remington, P. L., Sienko, D. G., & Davis, R. M. (1987). Are physicians advising smokers to quit?: The patient's perspective. *Journal of the American Medical Association, 257,* 1916–1919.

Andersen, R. (1968). *A behavioral model of families' use of health services.* Chicago: University of Chicago, Center for Health Administration Studies, Research Series No. 25, University of Chicago Press.

Andersen, R., & Mullner, R. (1990). Assessing the health objectives of the nation. *Health Affairs, 9,* 152–162.

Andersen, R. M. (1995). Revising the behavioral model and access to medical care: Does it matter? *Journal of Health and Social Behavior, 36,* 1–10.

Andersen, R. M., & Genthner, R. W. (1990). A guide for assessing a patient's level of personal responsibility for diabetes management. *Patient Education and Counseling, 16,* 269–279.

Anderson, O. W. (1957). Infant mortality and social and cultural factors: Historical trends and current patterns. In E.G. Jaco (Ed.), *Patients, physicians and illness* (pp. 10–24). Glencoe, IL: Free Press.

Andresen, E. M., Rothenberg, B. M., & McDermott, M. P. (1998). Selecting a generic measure of health-related quality of life for use among older adults: A comparison of candidate instruments. *Evaluation and the Health Professions, 21,* 244–264.

Andrews, F. M., & Withey, S. B. (1976). *Social indicators of well-being: Americans' perceptions of life quality.* New York: Plenum.

Andrzejeswski, N., & Lagua, R. T. (1997). Use of a customer satisfaction survey by health care regulators: A tool for total quality management. *Public Health Reports, 112,* 206–210.

Anson, O., Paran, E., Neumann, L., & Chernichovsky, D. (1993). Gender differences in health perceptions and their predictors. *Social Science and Medicine, 36,* 419–427.

Arbeit, M. L., Johnson, C. C., Mott, D. S., et al., (1992). The heart smart cardiovascular school health promotion: Behavior correlates of risk factor change. *Preventive Medicine, 21,* 18–21.

Arday, D. R., Tomar, S. L., & Mowery, P. (1997). State smoking prevalence estimates: A comparison of the Behavioral Risk Factor Surveillance System and current population surveys. *American Journal of Public Health, 87,* 1665–1669.

Arkin, E. B. (1989). *Making health communication programs work: A planner's guide.* Bethesda, MD: Office of Cancer Communications, National Cancer Institute, NIH-89-1493.

Arkin, E. B. (1990). Opportunities for improving the nation's health through collaboration with the mass media. *Public Health Reports, 105,* 219–223.

Arnstein, S. R. (1969). A ladder of citizen participation. *Journal of the American Institute of Planners, 35,* 216–224.

Arsham, G. M. (1980). Behavioral diagnosis for patient education. In P. L. Vigne (Ed.), *Patient Education in the Primary Care Setting: 1979 Proceedings.* Minneapolis: University of Minnesota.

Ashford, R. A. (1998). An investigation of male attitudes toward marketing communications from dental service providers. *British Dental Journal, 184*(5), 235–238.

Ashley, M. J., Eakin, J., Bull, S. P., & Pederson, L. (1997). Smoking control in the workplace: Is workplace size related to restrictions and programs? *Journal of Occupational and Environmental Medicine, 39,* 866–873.

Ashley, N. (1993). *King County Regional Domestic Violence Public Education Campaign.* Seattle, WA: Human Services Roundtable.

Attarian, L., Fleming, M., Barron, P., & Strecher, V. (1987). A comparison of health promotion practices of general practitioners and residency-trained family physicians. *Journal of Community Health, 8,* 31–39.

Atwater, J. B. (1974). Adapting the venereal disease clinic to today's problem. *American Journal of Public Health, 64,* 433–437.

Australia, Department of Transport and Communication. (1987). *Road Crash Statistics Australia.* Canberra: Department of Transport and Communication.

Australian Bureau of Statistics. (1986). *Deaths Australia.* Canberra: Australian Bureau of Statistics Cat. No. 3302.0.

Australian Health Ministers Advisory Council. (1994). *The health of young Australians*. Canberra: Australian Government Printing Service.

Avorn, J., & Soumerai, S. B. (1983). Improving drug-therapy decisions through educational outreach: A randomized controlled trial of academically based detailing. *New England Journal of Medicine, 308*, 1457–1463.

Azevedo, R., & Bernard, R. M. (1995). A meta-analysis of the effects of feedback in computer-based instruction. *Journal of Educational Computing Research, 13*, 111–127.

Baer, D. M. (1974). A note on the absence of a Santa Claus in any known ecosystem: A rejoinder to Willems. *Journal of Applied Behavior Analysis, 7*, 167–170.

Bailey, J., & Zambrano, M. C. (1974). Contraceptive pamphlets in Colombian drugstores. *Studies in Family Planning, 5*, 178–182.

Bailey, P. H., Rukholm, E. E., Vanderlee, R., & Hyland, J. (1994). A heart health survey at the work-site: The first step to effective programming. *AAOHN Journal, 42*, 9–14.

Bailey, S. L., & Hubbard, R. L. (1990). Developmental variation in the context of marijuana initiation among adolescents. *Journal of Health and Social Behavior, 31*, 58–70.

Bailey, W. C., Richards, J. M., Manzella, B. A., et al. (1987). Promoting self-management in adults with asthma: An overview of the UAB program. *Health Education Quarterly, 14*, 345–355.

Bakdash, M. B. (1983). The use of mass media in community periodontal education. *Journal of Public Health Dentistry, 43*, 128–131.

Bakdash, M. B., Lange, A. L., & McMillan, D. G. (1983). The effect of a televised periodontal campaign on public periodontal awareness. *Journal of Periodontology, 54*, 666–670.

Baker, E. L., Melius, J. M., & Millar, J. D. (1988). Surveillance of occupational illness and injury in the United States: Current perspectives and future directions. *Journal of Public Health Policy, 9*, 198–221.

Bakker, A. B., Buunk, B. P., & van Den Eijnden, R. J. J. M. (1997). Application of a modified health belief model to HIV preventive behavioral intentions among gay and bisexual men. *Psychology and Health, 12*, 481–493.

Bandura, A. (1977a). Self-efficacy: Toward a unifying theory of behavior change. *Psychological Review, 84*, 191–215.

Bandura, A. (1977b). *Social learning theory*. Englewood Cliffs, NJ: Prentice-Hall.

Bandura, A. (1982). Self-efficacy mechanisms in human agency. *American Psychologist, 37*, 122–147.

Bandura, A. (1986). *Social foundations of thought and action: A social cognitive theory*. Englewood Cliffs, NJ: Prentice-Hall.

Bandura, A. (1997). Editorial: The anatomy of stages of change. *American Journal of Health Promotion, 12*, 8–10.

Banta, H. D., & Luce, B. R. (1983). Assessing the cost-effectiveness of prevention. *Journal of Community Health, 9*, 145–165.

Baranowski, T., Perry, C. L., & Parcel, G. S. (1997). How individuals, environments, and health behavior interact: Social cognitive theory. In K. Glanz, F. M. Lewis, & B. K. Rimer (Eds.), *Health behavior and health education: Theory, research, and practice* (pp. 153–178). San Francisco: Jossey-Bass.

Baranowski, T., Stone, E., Klesges, R., et al. (1993). Studies of child activity and nutrition (SCAN) longitudinal research on CVD risk factors and CVH behaviors in young children. *Cardiovascular Risk Factors, 2*, 4–16.

Bardach, E. (1977). *The implementation game: What happens after a bill becomes a law*. Cambridge, MA: MIT Press.

Barker, R. G. (1965). Explorations in ecological psychology. *American Psychologist, 20*, 1–14.

Barlow, J. H., Williams, B., & Wright, C. (1996). The Generalized Self-Efficacy Scale in people with arthritis. *Arthritis Care and Research, 9*, 189–196.

Barnett, S., Niebuhr, V., & Baldwin, C. (1998). Principles for developing interdisciplinary school-based primary care centers. *Journal of School Health, 68,* 99–105.

Barnhoorn, F., & Adriaanse, H. (1992). In search of factors responsible for noncompliance among tuberculosis patients in Wardha District, India. *Social Science and Medicine, 34,* 291–306.

Barratt, A., Reznik, R., Irwig, L., et al. (1994). Work-site cholesterol screening and dietary intervention: The Staff Healthy Heart Project. *American Journal of Public Health, 84,* 779–782.

Barth, P. S. (1995). Compensating workers for occupational diseases: An international perspective. *International Journal of Occupational and Environmental Health, 1,* 147–158.

Bartholomew, L. K., Czyzewski, D. I., & Seilheimer, D. K. (1997). Self-management of cystic fibrosis: Short-term outcomes of the cystic fibrosis family education program. *Health Education and Behavior, 24,* 652–666.

Bartholomew, L. K., Koenning, G., Dahlquist, L., & Barron, K. (1994). An educational needs assessment of children with juvenile rheumatoid arthritis. *Arthritis Care and Research, 7*(3), 136–143.

Bartholomew, L. K., Parcel, G. S., & Kok, G. (1998). Intervention mapping: A process for developing theory, and evidence-based health education programs. *Health Education and Behavior, 25,* 545–563.

Bartholomew, L. K., Parcel, G. S., Seilheimer, D. K., et al. (1991). Development of a health education program to promote the self-management of cystic fibrosis. *Health Education Quarterly, 18*(4), 429–443.

Bartholomew, L. K., Seilheimer, D. K., Parcel, G. S., Spinelli, S. H., & Pumariega, A. J. (1988). Planning patient education for cystic fibrosis: Application of a diagnostic framework. *Patient Education and Counseling, 13,* 57–68.

Bartlett, E. E. (1982). Behavioral diagnosis: A practical approach to patient education. *Patient Counseling and Health Education, 4,* 29–35.

Bartlett, E. E. (1985). Eight principles from patient education research. *Preventive Medicine, 14,* 667–669.

Bartlett, E. E., & Green, L. W. (1980). Selection of educational methods. Chap. 6 in L. W. Green, M. W. Kreuter, S. G. Deeds, & K. B. Partridge (Eds.), *Health education planning: A diagnostic approach* (pp. 86–115). Palo Alto, CA: Mayfield.

Basch, C. E. (1984). Research on disseminating and implementing health education programs in schools. *Journal of School Health, 54,* 57–66.

Basch, C. E. (1987). Focus group interview: An underutilized research technique for improving theory and practice in health education. *Health Education Quarterly, 14,* 411–448.

Basch, C. E. (1989). Preventing AIDS through education: Concepts, strategies, and research priorities. *Journal of School Health, 59,* 296–300.

Basch, C. E., Eveland, J. D., & Portnoy, B. (1986). Diffusion systems for education and learning about health. *Family and Community Health, 9*(2), 1–26.

Basch, C. E., Sliepcevich, E. M., Gold, R. S., et al. (1985). Avoiding Type III errors in health education program evaluations: A case study. *Health Education Quarterly, 12,* 315–331.

Basen-Enquist, K. (1992). Psychosocial predictors of "safer sex" behaviors in young adults. *AIDS Education and Prevention, 4,* 120–134.

Bates, I. J., & Winder, A. E. (1984). *Introduction to health education.* Palo Alto, CA: Mayfield.

Batey, M. V., & Lewis, F. M. (1982). Clarifying autonomy and accountability in nursing service: Part 2. *Journal of Nursing Administration, 12,* 10–15.

Battista, R. N. (1983). Adult cancer prevention in primary care: Patterns of practice in Quebec. *American Journal of Public Health, 73,* 1036–1039.

Battista, R. N., Palmer, C. S., Marchland, B. M., & Spitzer, W. O. (1985). Patterns of preventive practice in New Brunswick. *Canadian Medical Association Journal, 132,* 1012–1015.

Battista, R. N., Williams, J. L., & MacFarlane, L. A. (1986). Determinants of primary medical practice in adult cancer prevention. *Medical Care, 24,* 216–224.

Battista, R. N., Williams, J. I., & McFarlane, L. A. (1990). Determinants of private practices in fee-for-service primary care. *American Journal of Preventive Medicine, 6,* 6–11.

Baum, C., Kennedy, D. L., Forbes, M. B., & Jones, J. K. (1982). *Drug utilization in the U.S.—1981: Third annual report.* Rockville, MD: U.S. Food and Drug Administration.

Baum, C., Kennedy, D. L., Forbes, M. B., & Jones, J. K. (1983). *Drug utilization in the U.S.* Rockville, MD: U.S. Food and Drug Administration.

Bauman, K. E., & Chenoweth, R. L. (1984). The relationship between the consequences adolescents expect from smoking and their behavior: A factor analysis with panel data. *Journal of Social Psychology, 14,* 28–41.

Bausell, R. B. (Ed.). (1983). Quality assurance: Methods [Special issue]. *Evaluation and the Health Professions, 6*(3).

Beauchamp, D. (1980). Public health as social justice. In L. Hogue (Ed.), *Public Health and the Law.* Rockville: Aspen Systems.

Becker, H., Hendrickson, S. L., & Shaver, L. (1998). Nonurban parental beliefs about childhood injury and bicycle safety. *American Journal of Health Behavior, 22,* 218–227.

Becker, M. H. (Ed.). (1974). The Health Belief Model and personal health behavior [Special issue]. *Health Education Monographs, 2,* 324–473. Reprinted as a book: *The health belief model and personal health behavior,* 1974, Thorofare, NJ: Charles B. Slack.

Becker, M. H. (1986). The tyranny of health promotion. *Public Health Reviews, 14,* 15–25.

Becker, M. H., & Joseph, J. (1988). AIDS and behavioral change to reduce risk: A review. *American Journal of Public Health, 78,* 394–410.

Becker, S. L., Burke, J. A., Arbogast, R. A., et al. (1989). Community programs to enhance in-school anti-tobacco efforts. *Preventive Medicine, 18,* 221–228.

Bellingham, R. (1994). *Critical issues in worksite health promotion.* New York: Macmillan.

Belloc, N. B. (1973). Relationship of health practices and mortality. *Preventive Medicine, 3,* 125–135.

Belloc, N. B., & Breslow, L. (1972). Relationship of physical health status and health practices. *Preventive Medicine, 1,* 409–421.

Bennett, B. I. (1977). A model for teaching health education skills to primary care practitioners. *International Journal of Health Education, 20,* 232–239.

Bennett, P., & Hodgson, R. (1992). Psychology and health promotion. In R. Bunton & G. Macdonald (Eds.), *Health promotion: Disciplines and diversity* (pp. 23–41). New York: Routledge.

Bensley, L. B., & Pope, A. J. (1992). A self-study instrument for program review of graduate programs in health education. *Journal of Health Education, 23*(6), 344–346.

Benson, P. L. (1997). *All kids are our kids.* San Francisco: Jossey-Bass.

Berger, I. E. (1997). The demographics of recycling and the structure of environmental behavior. *Environment and Behavior, 29,* 515–531.

Berger, P. L., & Neuhaus, R. J. (1977). *To empower people: The role of mediating structures in public policy.* Washington, DC: American Enterprise Institute for Public Policy Research.

Bergner, M. (1985). Measurement of Health Status. *Medical Care, 23,* 696–704.

Bergner, M., & Rothman, M. L. (1987). Health status measures: An overview and guide for selection. *Annual Review of Public Health, 8,* 191–210.

Berkman L. F. (1986). Social networks, support and health: Taking the next step forward. *American Journal of Epidemiology, 123,* 559–563.

Berkman, L. F., & Breslow, L. (1983). *Health and ways of living: The Alameda County study.* New York: Oxford University Press.

Berkman L., & Syme, S. L. (1979). Social networks, host resistence, and mortality: A nine-year follow-up study of Alameda County residents. *American Journal of Epidemiology, 109,* 186–204.

Berland, A., Whyte, N. B. & Maxwell, L. (1995). Hospital nurses and health promotion. *Canadian Journal of Nursing Research, 27,* 13–31.

Berman, P., & McLaughlin, M. (1976). Implementation of educational innovation. *The Educational Forum, 40,* 347–370.

Berman, S. H., & Wandersman, A. (1990). Fear of cancer and knowledge of cancer: A review and proposed relevance to hazardous waste sites. *Social Science and Medicine, 31,* 81–90.

Bernier, M. J. (1996). Establishing the psychometric properties of a scale for evaluating quality in printed education materials. *Patient Education and Counseling, 29,* 283–300.

Bernier, M., & Avard, J. (1986). Self-efficacy, outcome, and attrition in a weight-reduction program. *Cognitive Therapy and Research, 10,* 319–338.

Bertera, E. M., & Bertera, R. L. (1981). The cost-effectiveness of telephone versus clinic counseling for hypertensive patients: A pilot study. *American Journal of Public Health, 71,* 626–629.

Bertera, R. L. (1981). *The effects of blood pressure self-monitoring in the workplace using automated blood pressure measurement.* Unpublished doctoral dissertation. Baltimore: Johns Hopkins University, School of Hygiene and Public Health.

Bertera, R. L. (1990a). The effects of workplace health promotion on absenteeism and employment costs in a large industrial population. *American Journal of Public Health, 80,* 1101–1105.

Bertera, R. L. (1990b). Planning and implementing health promotion in the workplace: A case study of the Du Pont Company experience. *Health Education Quarterly, 17,* 307–327.

Bertera, R. L. (1991). The effects of behavioral risks on absenteeism and health-care costs in the workplace. *Journal of Occupational Medicine, 33,* 1119–1124.

Bertera, R. L. (1993). Behavioral risk factor and illness day changes with workplace health promotion: Two-year results. *American Journal of Health Promotion, 7,* 365–373.

Bertera, R. L. (1999). Worksite health promotion. In B. Poland, L. W. Green, & I. Rootman (Eds.), *Settings approaches to health promotion.* Thousand Oaks, CA: Sage.

Bertera, R. L., & Cuthie, J. C. (1984). Blood pressure self-monitoring in the workplace. *Journal of Occupational Medicine, 26,* 183–188.

Bertera, R. L., & Green, L. W. (1979). Cost-effectiveness of a home visiting triage program for family planning in turkey. *American Journal of Public Health, 69,* 950–953.

Bertera, R., Levine, D. M., & Green, L. W. (1982). Behavioral effects of blood pressure self-monitoring in the workplace using automated measurements. *Preventive Medicine, 11*(3), 158-163.

Bertera, R. L., Oehl, L. K., & Telepchak, J. M. (1990). Self-help versus group approaches to smoking cessation in the workplace: Eighteen-month follow-up and cost analysis. *American Journal of Health Promotion, 4,* 187–192.

Bertram, D. A., & Brooks-Bertram, P. A. (1977). The evaluation of continuing medical education: A literature review. *Health Education Monographs, 5,* 330–362.

Berwick, D. M., Murphy, J. M., Goldman, P. A., et al. (1991). Performance of a five-item mental health screening test. *Medical Care, 29,* 169–176.

Best, J. A. (1989). Intervention perspectives on school health promotion research. *Health Education Quarterly, 16,* 299–306.

Best, J. A., Thomson, S. J., Santi, S. M., et al. (1988). Preventing cigarette smoking among school children. *Annual Review of Public Health, 9,* 161–201.

Better Health Commission. (1986). *Looking forward to better health,* vols. 1–3. Canberra: Australian Government Printing Service.

Bettes, W. A. (1976). A Method of allocating resources for health education services by the Indian health service. *Public Health Reports, 91,* 256–260.

Bezzaoucha, A., & Dekkar, N. (1990). Handicaps in Algiers according to a household survey. *International Journal of Epidemiology, 19,* 466–471.

Bibeau, D. L., Howell, K. A., Rife, J. C., & Taylor, M. L. (1996). The role of a community coalition in the development of health services for the poor and uninsured. *International Journal of Health Services, 26*(1), 93–110.

Bibeau, D. L., Mullen, K. D., McLeroy, K. R., Green, L. W., & Foshee, V. (1988). Evaluations of workplace smoking cessation programs: A critique. *American Journal of Preventive Medicine, 4,* 87–95.

Biener, L., & Siegel, M. (1997). Behavior intentions of the public after bans on smoking in restaurants and bars. *American Journal of Public Health, 87,* 2042–2044.

Bird, J. A., Otero-Sabogal, R., Ha, N.-T., & McPhee, S. J. (1996). Tailoring lay health worker interventions for diverse cultures: Lessons learned from Vietnamese and Latina communities. *Health Education and Behavior, 23*(Suppl.), S105–S122.

Bivens, E. C. (1979). Community organization: An old but reliable health education technique. In P. M. Lazes (Ed.), *The Handbook of Health Education.* Germantown, MD: Aspen.

Bjaras, G., Haglund, B., & Rifkin, S. (1991). A new approach to community participation assessment. *Health Promotion International, 6,* 199–206.

Bjurstrom, L. A., & Alexiou, N. G. (1978). A program of heart disease intervention for public employees. *Journal of Occupational Medicine, 20,* 521–531.

Black, D. R., & Cameron, R. (1997). Self-administered interventions: A health education strategy for improving population health. *Health Education Research, 12, 531–545.*

Black, D. R., Tobler, N. S., & Sciacca, J. P. (1998). Peer helping/involvement: An efficacious way to meet the challenge of reducing alcohol, tobacco, and other drug use among youth. *Journal of School Health, 68,* 87–94.

Black, R. (1980). Support for genetic services: A survey. *Health and Social Work, 5,* 27–34.

Black, T. (1983). Coalition building: Some suggestions. *Child Welfare, 42,* 264.

Blackburn, H. (1987). Research and demonstration projects in community cardiovascular disease prevention. *Journal of Public Health Policy, 4,* 398–421.

Blaine, T. M., Forster, J. L., & Pham, H. (1997). Creating tobacco control policy at the local level: Implementation of a direct action organizing approach. *Health Education and Behavior, 24,* 640-651.

Blair, S. N., Powell, K. E., Bazzare, T., et al. (1993). Physical activity: Behavior change and compliance, keys to improving cardiovascular health. *Circulation, 88,* 1402–1407.

Blake, S. M., Jeffrey, R. W., Finnegan, J. R., et al. (1987). Process evaluation of a community-based physical activity campaign: The Minnesota Heart Health experience. *Health Education Research, 2,* 115–121.

Blane, D. (1995). Social determinants of health: Socioeconomic status, social class, and ethnicity. *American Journal of Public Health, 85,* 903–905.

Block, G., Rosenberger, W., & Patterson, B. (1988). Calories, fat and cholesterol: Intake patterns in the U.S. population by race, sex and age. *American Journal of Public Health, 78,* 1150–1155.

Bloom, B. (1990). Health insurance and medical care: Health of our nation's children, United States, 1988. *Advance Data from Vital and Health Statistics* (No. 188). Hyattsville, MD: National Center for Health Statistics.

Blum, H. L. (1974). *Planning for health.* New York: Human Sciences Press.

Blum, H. L. (1981). *Planning for health* (2nd ed.). New York: Behavioral Publications.

Blum, H. L. (1983). *Expanding health care horizons: From a general systems concept of health to a national health policy* (2nd ed.). Oakland, CA: Third Party.

Blum, R., & Samuels, S. E. (Eds.). (1990). Television and teens: Health implications [Special issue]. *Journal of Adolescent Health Care, 11*(1).

Blum, H. L., et al. (1968). *Notes on comprehensive planning for health.* Berkeley: American Public Health Association and School of Public Health, University of California.

Bly, J. L., Jones, R. C., & Richardson, J. E. (1986). Impact of worksite health promotion on health care costs and utilization. *Journal of the American Medical Association, 256,* 3235–3240.

Boberg, E., Gustafson, D. H., Hawkins, R. P., & Chan, C. (1995). Development, acceptance, and use patterns of a computer-based educations and social support system for people living with AIDS/HIV infection. *Computers and Human Behavior, 11,* 289–311.

Bolan, Robert K. (1986). *Health education planning for AIDS risk reduction in the gay/bisexual male community: Use of the PRECEDE framework* (p. 162). American Public Health Association, 114th Annual Meeting Abstracts, Las Vegas.

Bolman, L. G., & Deal, T. E. (1991). *Reframing organizations: Artistry, choice, and leadership.* San Francisco: Jossey-Bass.

Bonaguro, J. A. (1981). PRECEDE for wellness. *Journal of School Health, 51,* 501–506.

Bonaguro, J. A., & Miaoulis, G. (1983, January–February). Marketing: A tool for health education planning. *Health Education, 14,* 6–11.

Bonnet, C., Gagnayre, R., d'Ivernois, J.-F. (1998). Learning difficulties of diabetic patients: A survey of educators. *Patient Education and Counseling, 35,* 139–147.

Borgers, R., Mullen, P. D., Meertens, R., et al. (1993). The information-seeking behavior of cancer outpatients: A description of the situation. *Patient Education Counseling, 22,* 35–40.

Borland, R., Chapman, S., Owen, N., & Hill, D. (1990). Effects of workplace smoking bans on cigarette consumption. *American Journal of Public Health, 80,* 178–180.

Borland, R., Owen, N., Hill, D., & Schofield, P. (1991). Predicting attempts and sustained cessation of smoking after the introduction of workplace smoking bans. *Health Psychology, 10,* 336–342.

Bosin, M. R. (1992). Priority setting in government: Beyond the magic bullet. *Evaluation and Program Planning, 15,* 33–42.

Boston, P., Jordan, S., MacNamara, E., et al. (1997). Using participatory action research to understand the meanings aboriginal Canadians attribute to the rising incidence of diabetes. *Chronic Diseases in Canada, 18,* 5–12.

Bosworth, K., Gustafson, D. H., & Hawkins, R. P. (1994). The BARN system: Use and impact of adolescent health promotion via computer. *Computers and Human Behavior, 10,* 467–482.

Bosworth, K., Gustafson, D. H., & Hawkins, R. P., et al. (1983). "Adolescents, Health Education, and Computers: The Body Awareness Resource Network (BARN)," *Health Education 14*(6): 58–9.

Bosworth, K., & Yoast, R. (1991). DIADS: Computer-based system for development of school drug prevention programs. *Journal of Drug Education, 21*(3), 231–245.

Botelho, R. J., & Richmond, R. (1996). Secondary prevention of excessive alcohol use: Assessing the prospects of implementation. *Family Practice, 13,* 182–193.

Bottimore, A. H., & Hailey, B. J. (1988–1989). Promotion of breast self-exam behavior: An attempt to modify health beliefs. *International Quarterly of Community Health Education, 9,* 273–282.

Botvin, G. J., Baker, E., Renick, N., et al. (1984). A cognitive-behavioral approach to substance abuse prevention. *Addictive Behaviors, 9,* 137–147.

Botvin, G., & Eng, A. (1980). A comprehensive school-based smoking prevention program. *Journal of School Health, 50,* 209–213.

Botvin, G.. & Eng, A. (1982). The efficacy of a multicomponent approach to the prevention of cigarette smoking. *Preventive Medicine, 11,* 199–211.

Botvin, G. J., & McAlister, A. (1982). Cigarette smoking among children and adolescents: causes and prevention. In C. B. Arnold (Ed.), *Annual Review of Disease Prevention.* New York: Springer.

Botvin, G. J., Schinke, S., & Orlandi, M. A. (1995). School-based health promotion: Substance abuse and sexual behavior. *Applied and Preventive Psychology, 4,* 167–184.

Boulet, L., Belanger, M., & Lajoie, P. (1996). Characteristics of subjects with a high frequency of emergency visits for asthma. *American Journal of Emergency Medicine, 14,* 623–628.

Boulet, L. P., Chapman, K. R., Green, L. W., & FitzGerald, J. M. (1994). Asthma education. *Chest, 106* (Suppl. 4), 184–196

Bourne, P. G. (1974). Approaches to drug abuse prevention and treatment in rural areas. *Journal of Psychedelic Drugs, 6,* 285–289.

Bowen, D. J., Kinne, S., & Urban, N. (1997). Analyzing communities for readiness to change. *American Journal of Health Behavior, 21,* 289–298.

Bowler, M. H., & Morisky, D. E. (1983). Small group strategy for improving compliance behavior and blood pressure control. *Health Education Quarterly, 10,* 57–69.

Bowler, M. H., Morisky, D. E., & Deeds, S. G. (1980). Needs assessment strategies in working with compliance issues and blood pressure control. *Patient Counselling and Health Education, 2,* 22–27.

Bowne, D. W., Russell, M. L., Morgan, J. L., et al. (1984). Reduced disability and health care costs in an industrial fitness program. *Journal of Occupational Medicine, 26,* 809–816.

Boyd, C. (1993). *Up in Smoke: Teens n' Tobacco. Tobacco-Free Canada: First National Conference on Tobacco or Health,* Toronto, Oct. Ottawa: Health Promotion Directorate, Health Canada.

Boyd, G. M., & Glover, E. D. (1989). Smokeless tobacco use by youth in the U.S. *Journal of School Health, 59,* 189–194.

Boyer, E. L. (1991). *Ready to learn: A mandate for the nation.* Princeton, NJ: Carnegie Foundation for the Advancement of Teaching.

Boyte, H. C. (1984). *Community is possible: Repairing America's roots.* New York: Harper & Row.

Bozzini, L. (1988). Local community services centers (LCSC) in Quebec: Description, evaluation, perspectives. *Journal of Public Health Policy, 9,* 346–375.

Bracht, N. (Ed.). (1990). *Health promotion at the community level.* New York: Sage.

Brailey, L. J. (1986). Effects of health teaching in the workplace on women's knowledge, beliefs, and practices regarding breast self-examination. *Research in Nursing and Health, 9,* 223–231.

Braithwaite, R. L., & Lythcott, N. (1989). Community empowerment as a strategy for health promotion for black and other minorities. *Journal of the American Medical Association, 261,* 282–283.

Brandt-Rauf, P. W., & Brandt-Rauf, S. I. (1989). The high-risk occupational disease notification and prevention act: From primary to secondary prevention, from paternalism to autonomy. *Annals of the New York Academy of Sciences, 572,* 151–154.

Breckon, D. J. (1982). *Hospital health education: A guide to program development.* Rockville, MD: Aspen.

Breckon, D. J. (1997). *Managing health promotion programs: Leadership skills for the 21st century.* Gaithersburg, MD: Aspen.

Breckon, D. J., Harvey, J. R., & Lancaster, R. B. (1998). *Community health education: Settings, roles, and skills for the 21st century* (4th ed.). Rockville, MD: Aspen.

Brennan, A. J. (1982). Health promotion: What's in it for business and industry? *Health Education Quarterly, 8*(1), 9–19.

Brennan, A. J. (1985). Health and fitness boom moves into corporate America. *Occupational Health and Safety, 54,* 38–48.

Brennan, P. F., Moore, S. M, & Smyth, K. A. (1992). Alzheimer's disease caregivers' uses of a computer network. *Western Journal of Nursing Research, 14*(5), 662–673.

Breslow, L. (1990). The future of public health: Prospects in the United States for the 1990s. *Annual Review of Public Health, 11,* 1–28.

Breslow, L., & Egstrom, J. D. (1980). Persistence of health habits and their relationship to mortality. *Preventive Medicine, 9,* 469–483.

Brieger, W. R., Onyido, A. E., & Ekanem, O. J. (1996). Monitoring community response to malaria control using insecticide-impregnated bed nets, curtains and residual spray at Nsukka, Nigeria. *Health Education Research, 11,* 133–146.

Brieger, W. R., Ramakrishna, J., & Adeniyi, J. D. (1986–87). Community involvement in social marketing: Guineaworm control. *International Quarterly of Community Health Education, 7,* 19–31.

Brigham, J., Gross, J., Stitzer, M. L., & Felch, L. J. (1994). Effects of a restricted work-site smoking policy on employees who smoke. *American Journal of Public Health, 84,* 773–778.

Brimberry, R. (1988). Vaccination of high-risk patients for influenza: A comparison of telephone and mail reminder methods. *Journal of Family Practice, 26,* 397–400.

Brindis, C., Hughes, D. C., & Newacheck, P. W. (1998). The use of formative evaluation to assess integrated services for children: The Robert Wood Johnson Foundation Child Health Initiative. *Evaluation and the Health Professions, 21,* 66–91.

Brink, S. G., Lovato, C. Y., Kolbe, L. J., & Buoy, M. E. (1989). Development and evaluation of a school-based intervention to increase the use of safety belts by adolescents. Final report to U.S. Department of Transportation.

Brink, S. G., Simons-Morton, B., & Zane, D. (1989). A hospital-based infant safety seat program for low-income families: Assessment of population needs and provider practices. *Health Education Quarterly, 16,* 45–56.

Brink, S. G., Simons-Morton, D., Parcel, G., & Tiernan, K. (1988). Community intervention handbooks for comprehensive health promotion programming. *Family and Community Health, 11,* 28–35.

British Columbia Ministry of Health, Community Health Division. (1994). *School-based prevention model handbook.* Victoria: British Columbia Ministry of Health.

Brock, G. C., & Beazley, R. P. (1995). Using the Health Belief Model to explain parents' participation in adolescents' at-home sexuality education activities. *Journal of School Health, 65,* 124–128.

Brodsky, A. E. (1996). Resilient single mothers in risky neighborhoods: Negative psychological sense of community. *Journal of Community Psychology, 24,* 347–364.

Brody, B. E. (1988). Employee assistance programs: An historical and literature review. *American Journal of Health Promotion, 2,* 13–19.

Brown, C. (1984). *The art of coalition building: A guide for community leaders.* New York: The American Jewish Committee.

Brown, E. R. (1984). Community organization influence on local public health care policy: A general research model and comparative case study. *Health Education Quarterly, 10,* 205–234.

Brown, E. R., & Margo, G. E. (1978). Health education: Can the reformers be reformed? *International Journal of Health Services, 8,* 3–25.

Brown, H. R., Carozza, N. B., Lloyd, R., & Thater, C. E. (1989). Worksite blood pressure control: The evolution of a program. *Journal of Occupational Medicine, 31,* 354–357.

Brown, W. B., Williamson, N. B., & Carlaw, R. A. (1988). A diagnostic approach to educating Minnesota dairy farmers in the prevention and control of bovine mastitis. *Preventive Veterinary Medicine, 5,* 197–211.

Brown, W. J., & Redman, S. (1995). Setting targets: A three-staged model for determining priorities in health promotion. *Australian Journal of Public Health, 19,* 263–269.

Brownell, K. D., Cohen, R., Stunkard, A., et al. (1984). Weight loss competitions at the work site: Impact on weight, morale, and cost-effectiveness. *American Journal of Public Health, 74,* 1283–1285.

Brownell, K. D., & Felix, M. R. J. (1987). Competitions to facilitate health promotion: Review and conceptual analysis. *American Journal of Health Promotion, 2*(1), 28–36.

Brownson, C. A., Dean, C., Dabney, S., & Brownson, R. (1998). Cardiovascular risk reduction in rural minority communities: The Bootheel Heart Health Project. *Journal of Health Education, 29,* 158–165.

Brownson, R. C., Smith, C.A., Pratt, M., et al. (1996). Preventing cardiovascular disease through community-based risk reduction: Five-year result of the Bootheel Heart Health Project, *American Journal of Public Health, 86,* 206–213.

Broyles, S. L., Nader, P. R., & Elder, J. P. (1996). Cardiovascular disease risk factors in Anglo and Mexican American children and their mothers. *Family and Community Health, 19,* 57–72.

Brug, J., Glanz, K., & Kok, G. (1997). The relationship between self-efficacy, attitudes, intake compared to others, consumption, and stages of change related to fruit and vegetables. *American Journal of Health Promotion, 12,* 25–29.

Bruhn, J. B. (1983, November). The application of theory in childhood asthma self-help programs. *Journal of Allergy and Clinical Immunology, 72,*(Suppl., Pt. 2), 561–577.

Brunk S. E., & Goeppinger, J. (1990). Process evaluation: Assessing re-invention of community-based interventions. *Evaluation and the Health Professions, 13,* 186–203.

Bryant, N. H., Stender, W., Frist, V., & Somers, A. R. (1976). VD hotline: An evaluation. *Public Health Reports, 91,* 231–235.

Buck, C. (1986). Beyond Lalonde: Creating health. *Journal of Public Health Policy, 20,* 444–457.

Budd R., North, D., & Spencer, C. (1984). Understanding seat-belt use: A test of Bentler and Speckart's extension of the "theory of reasoned action." *European Journal of Social Psychology, 14,* 69–78.

Budd, R., Bleiner, S., & Spencer, C. (1983). Exploring the use and non-use of marijuana as reasoned actions: An application of Fishbein and Ajzen's methodology. *Drug and Alcohol Dependence, 11,* 217–224.

Buller, D., Modiano, M. R., Zapien, J. G. de, et al. (1998). Predictors of cervical cancer screening in Mexican American women of reproductive age. *Journal of Health Care for the Poor and Under-served, 9,* 76–95.

Bunce, D. (1997). What factors are associated with the outcome of individual-focused worksite stress management interventions? *Journal of Occupational and Organizational Psychology, 70,* 1–17.

Bunker, J. P., Gomby, D. S., & Kehrer, B. H. (1989). *Pathways to health: The role of social factors.* Menlo Park, CA: Kaiser Family Foundation.

Burden, D. S., & Googins, B. K. (1987). *Balancing work life and homelife.* Boston: Boston University School of Social Work.

Burglehaus, M. J., Smith, L. A., Sheps, S. B., & Green, L. W. (1997). Physicians and breastfeeding: Beliefs, knowledge, self-efficacy and counseling practices. *Canadian Journal of Public Health, 88,* 383–387.

Burnham, J. C. (1984, Summer). Change in the popularization of health in the United States. *Bulletin of the History of Medicine, 58,* 183–197.

Burris, D. (1992). *Technotrends.* New York: HarperCollins.

Burris, S. (1997). Driving the epidemic underground? A new look at law and the social risk of HIV testing. *AIDS and Public Policy Journal, 12,* 66–78.

Burt, R. D., & Peterson, A. V., Jr. (1998). Smoking cessation among high school seniors. *Preventive Medicine, 27,* 319–327.

Bush, J. W. (1984). Relative preferences versus relative frequencies in health-related quality of life evaluations. In N. K. Wenger, M. E. Mattson, C. D. Furber, & J. Elinson (Eds.), *Assessment of Quality of Life in Clinical Trials of Cardiovascular Therapies* (pp. 118–139). New York: LaJacq.

Bush, P. J., Zuckerman, A. E., Taggart, V. S., et al. (1989). Cardiovascular risk factor prevention in black school children: The "Know Your Body" Evaluation Project. *Health Education Quarterly, 16,* 215–227.

Bush, P. J., Zuckerman, A. E., Theiss, P. K., et al. (1989). Cardiovascular risk factor prevention in black school children: Two-year results of the Know Your Body Program. *American Journal of Epidemiology, 129,* 466–482.

Butler, M. O., Abed, J., Goodman, K., Gottlieb, N., Hare, M., & Mullen, P. (1996). *A case-study evaluation of the Henry J. Kaiser Family Foundation's Community Health Promotion Grants Program in the southern states: Phase 2 final report.* Arlington, VA, Menlo Park, CA, and Atlanta, GA: Battelle Centers for Public Health Research and Evaluation, Henry J. Kaiser Family Foundation, and Centers for Disease Control.

Butterfoss, F., Goodman, R., & Wandersman, A. (1993). Community coalitions for prevention and health promotion. *Health Education Research, 8,* 315–330.

Buunk, B. P., Bakker, A. B., & Yzer, M. C. (1998). Predictors of AIDS-preventive behavioral intentions among adult heterosexuals at risk for HIV-infection: Extending current models and measures. *AIDS Education and Prevention, 10,* 149–172.

Byles, J. E., Redman, S., & Boyle, C. A. (1995). Effectiveness of two direct-mail strategies to encourage women to have cervical (Pap) smears. *Health Promotion International, 10,* 5–16.

Calabro, K., Weltge, A., Parnell, S., Kouzekanani, K., & Ramirez, E. (1998). Intervention for medical students: Effective infection control. *American Journal of Infection Control, 26,* 431–436.

California Department of Health Services. (1995, September 28). State launches counterattack against rise in youth smoking (Press release). Sacramento: California Department of Health Services.

Calnan, M., & Moss, S. (1984). The Health Belief Model and compliance with education given at a class in breast self-examination. *Journal of Health and Social Behavior, 25,* 198–210.

Campbell, D. T. (1969). Reforms as experiments. *American Psychologist, 24,* 409–429.

Campbell, M. K, Devellis, B. M., Strecher, V. J., et al. (1994). Improving dietary behavior: The effectiveness of tailored messages in primary care settings. *American Journal of Public Health, 84,* 783–787.

Canadian Council of Cardiovascular Nurses. (1993). *Standards for cardiovascular health education.* Ottawa: Heart and Stroke Foundation of Canada.

Canadian Task Force on the Periodic Health Examination. (1979). The periodic health examination. *Canadian Medical Association Journal, 121,* 1193–1254.

Canadian Task Force on the Periodic Health Examination. (1994). *Canadian guide to clinical preventive health care* (2nd ed.). Ottawa: Canada Communication Group.

Candeias, N. M. F. (1991). Evaluating the quality of health education programmes: Some comments on methods and implementation. *Hygie: International Journal of Health Education, 10*(2), 40–44.

Cantor, J. C., Morisky, D. E., Green, L. W., et al. (1985). Cost-effectiveness of educational interventions to improve patient outcomes in blood pressure control. *Preventive Medicine, 14,* 782–800.

Cardinal, B. J., & Sachs, M. L. (1995). Prospective analysis of stage-of-exercise movement following mail-delivered, self-instructional exercise packets. *American Journal of Health Promotion, 9,* 430–432.

Carlaw, R. W. (Ed.). (1982). *Perspectives on community health education: A series of case studies* (2 vols.). Oakland, CA: Third Party.

Carlaw, R. W., Mittlemark, M., Bracht, N., & Luepker, R. (1984). Organization for a community cardiovascular health program: Experiences from the Minnesota Heart Health Program. *Health Education Quarterly, 11,* 243–252.

Carlton, B., & Carlton, M. (1978, March–April). Defining a role for the health educator in the primary care setting. *Health Education, 9,* 22–23.

Carnegie Council on Adolescent Development, Task Force on Education of Young Adolescents. (1989). *Turning points: Preparing American youth for the 21st century.* Washington, DC: Carnegie Council on Adolescent Development, Carnegie Corporation of New York.

Carr, A. J., Thompson, P. W., & Kirwan, J. R. (1996). Quality of life measures. *British Journal of Rheumatology, 35,* 275–281.

Carr-Gregg, M. (1993). Interaction of public policy and research in the passage of New Zealand's Smoke-Free Environments Act 1990. *Addiction* (Suppl.), 35–41.

Carter, W. B., Beach, L. R., & Inui, T. S., et al. (1986). Developing and testing a decision model for predicting influenza vaccination compliance. *Health Service Research, 20,* 897–932.

Carter, W. B., Belcher, D. W., & Inui, T. S. (1981). Implementing preventive care in clinical practice: 2. Problems for manager, clinicians and patients. *Medical Care Review, 38,* 19–24.

Cartwright, D. (1949). Some principles of mass persuasion: Selected findings from research on the sale of United States war bonds. *Human Relations, 2,* 53–69.

Cassatta, D. M., & Kirkman-Liff, B. L. (1981). Mental health activities of family physicians. *Journal of Family Practice, 12,* 683–692.

Cassou, B., & Pissarro, B. (1988). Workers' participation and occupational health: The French experience. *International Journal of Health Services Research, 18,* 139–152.

Casswell, S., Stewart, L., & Duignan, P. (1989). The struggle against the broadcast of anti-health messages: Regulation of alcohol advertising in New Zealand 1980–87. *Health Promotion, 4,* 287–296.

Castro, K. G., Valdiserri, R. O., & Curran, J. W. (1992). Perspectives on HIV/AIDS epidemiology and prevention from the eighth international conference on AIDS. *American Journal of Public Health, 82,* 1465–1470.

Cataldo, M. F., & Coates, T. J. (Eds.). (1986). *Health and industry: A behavioral medicine perspective.* New York: Wiley.

Cataldo, M. F., Green, L. W., Herd, J. A., et al. (1986). Preventive medicine and the corporate environment: Challenge to behavioral medicine. In M. F. Cataldo & T. J. Coates (Eds.), *Health and industry: A behavioral medicine perspective* (pp. 399–419). New York: Wiley.

Catford, J. C. (1983). Positive health indicators: Toward a new information base for health promotion. *Community Medicine, 5,* 125–132.

Caulkins, J. P., & Reuter, P. (1997). Setting goals for drug policy: Harm reduction or use reduction? *Addiction, 92,* 1143–1151.

CBS Television Network. (1984). *A study of attitudes, concerns and information needs for prescription drugs and related illnesses.* New York: CBS Television Network.

Celentano, D. D., & Holtzman, D. (1983). Breast self-examination competency: An analysis of self-reported practice and associated characteristics. *American Journal of Public Health, 73,* 1321–1323.

Centers for Disease Control. (1978). *The ten leading causes of death.* Atlanta, GA: Centers for Disease Control.

Centers for Disease Control. (1986). Premature mortality in the United States: Public health issues in the use of years of potential life lost. *Morbidity and Mortality Weekly Report, 35*(Suppl.), 2S.

Centers for Disease Control. (1987). *Information/education plan to prevent and control AIDS in the United States.* Washington, DC: U.S. Public Health Service, Department of Health and Human Service.

Centers for Disease Control. (1988). Guidelines for effective school health education to prevent the spread of AIDS. *Morbidity and Mortality Weekly Report, 37*(Suppl. No. S-2.), 1–14. Also in *Health Education, 19*(3), 6–13.

Cernada, E. C., Lee, Y. J., & Lin, M. Y. (1974). Family planning telephone services in two Asian cities. *Studies in Family Planning, 5,* 111–114.

Cernada, G. P. (1974). The case of the unplanned child. *Human Organization, 33,* 106–109.

Cernada, G. P. (1982). *Knowledge into action.* New York: Baywood.

Chapman, S. (1990). Intersectoral action to improve nutrition: The roles of the state and the private sector. A case study from Australia. *Health Promotion International, 5,* 35–44.

Chapman, S., & Lupton, D. (1995). *The fight for public health: Principles and practice of media advocacy.* Sydney: University Press.

Charter, W., & Jones, J. (1973). On the risk of appraising non-events in program evaluation. *Educational Research, 2*(11), 5–7.

Chase, G. (1979). Implementing a human services program: How hard can it be? *Public Policy, 27,* 385–435.

Chassin, L., Corty, E., Presson, C., et al. (1981). Predicting adolescents' intentions to smoke cigarettes. *Journal of Health and Social Behavior, 22,* 445–455.

Chassin, L., Corty, E., Presson, C., et al. (1984). Cognitive and social influence factors in adolescent smoking cessation. *Addictive Behaviors, 9,* 383–390.

Chassin, L., Mann, L., & Sher, K. (1988). Self-awareness theory, family history of alcoholism, and adolescent alcohol involvement. *Journal of Abnormal Psychology, 97,* 206–217.

Chassin, L., Presson, C. C., Bensenberg, M., et al. (1984). Predicting adolescents' intentions to smoking cigarettes. *Journal of Health and Social Behavior, 22,* 445–455.

Chavis, D. M., Hogge, J. H., McMillan, D. W., & Wandersman, A. (1986). Sense of community through Brunswik's lens: A first look. *Journal of Community Psychology, 14,* 24–40.

Chavis, D. M., & Wandersman, A. (1990). Sense of community in the urban environment: A catalyst for participation and community development. *American Journal of Community Psychology, 18,* 55–81.

Cheadle, A., Beery, W., Woods, I., et al. (1997). Conference report: Community-based health promotion—state of the art and recommendations for the future. *American Journal of Preventive Medicine, 13,* 240–243.

Cheadle, A., Psaty, B., Wagner, E., et al. (1990). Evaluating community-based nutrition programs: Assessing the reliability of a survey of grocery store product displays. *American Journal of Public Health, 80,* 709–711.

Chen, M. K. (1979). The gross national health product: A proposed population health index. *Public Health Reports, 94,* 119–123.

Chen, M. S., Jr., & Bill, D. (1983). Statewide survey of risk factor prevalence: The Ohio experience. *Public Health Reports, 98,* 443–448.

Chen, T. L., & Cernada, G. P. (1985). *Recommended health education readings: An annotated bibliography.* Taipei: Maplewood.

Chenoweth, D. (1993). *Health care cost management: Strategies for employers* (2nd ed.). Dubuque, IA: Brown & Benchmark.

Chenoweth, D. (1994). Positioning health promotion to make an economic impact. Chap. 2 in J. P. Opatz (Ed.), *Economic impact of worksite health promotion* (pp. 33–49). Champaign, IL: Human Kinetics.

Chiasson, M. (1996). *The interaction between context and technology during information systems development (ISD): Action research investigations in two health settings.* Vancouver: Unpublished doctoral thesis, University of British Columbia.

Chie, W. C., & Chang, K. J. (1994). Factors related to tumor size of breast cancer at treatment in Taiwan. *Preventive Medicine, 23,* 91–97.

Chie W. C., Cheng, K. W., Fu, C. H., & Yen, L. L. (1993). A study on women's practice of breast self-examination in Taiwan. *Preventive Medicine, 22,* 316–324.

Children's Defense Fund. (1990). *Children 1990: A report card, briefing book, and action primer.* Washington, DC: Children's Defense Fund.

Cholat-Traquet, C. (1996). *Evaluating tobacco control activities: Experience and guiding principles.* Geneva: World Health Organization.

Chomik, T. (1998). *A case study of the development of health goals in British Columbia.* Vancouver: University of British Columbia.

Chu, C., & Simpson, R. (Eds.). (1994). *Ecological public health: From vision to practice.* Toronto: Centre for Health Promotion, University of Toronto.

Chung, H. H., & Elias, M. (1996). Patterns of adolescent involvement in problem behaviors: Relationship to self-efficacy, social competence, and life events. *American Journal of Community Psychology, 24,* 771–784.

Chwalow, A. J., Green, L. W., Levine, D. M., & Deeds, S. G. (1978). Effects of the multiplicity of interventions on the compliance of hypertensive patients with medical regimens in an inner-city population. *Preventive Medicine, 7,* 51.

Clark, J. M. (1939). *The social control of business.* New York: McGraw-Hill.

Clark, M. A., Kviz, F. J., & Warnecke, R. B. (1998). Psychosocial factors and smoking cessation behaviors among smokers who have and have not ever tried to quit. *Health Education Research, 13,* 145–153.

Clark, N. M. (1987). Social learning theory in current health education practice. In W. B. Ward, S. K. Simonds, P. D. Mullen, & M. H. Becker (Eds.), *Advances in Health Education and Promotion* (vol. 2, pp. 251–275). Greenwich, CT: JAI Press.

Clark, N. M. (1997). Editorial. *Health Education Quarterly, 24*(6), 677.

Clarke, D. O., Patrick, D. L., & Durham, M. L. (1995). Socioeconomic status and exercise self-efficacy in late life. *Behavioral Medicine, 18,* 355–376.

Clayman, G. L., Chamberlain, R. M., & Hong, W. K. (1995). Screening at a health fair to identify subjects for an oral leukoplakia chemoprevention trial. *Journal of Cancer Education, 10,* 88–90.

Cleary, H. P. (1995). *The credentialing of health educators: An historical account, 1970–1990.* Allentown, PA: National Commission for Health Education Credentialing.

Cleary, H. P., Kichen, J. M., & Ensor, P. G. (1985). *Advancing health through education: A case study approach.* Palo Alto, CA: Mayfield.

Cleary, M. J., & Neiger, B. L. (1998). *The certified health education specialist: A self-study guide for professional competency* (3rd ed.) Allentown, PA: National Commission for Health Education Credentialing.

Cleary, P. D., Rogers, T. F., Singer, E., et al. (1986). Health education about AIDS among seropositive blood donors. *Health Education Quarterly, 13,* 317–330.

Clutterbuck, R. C. (1980). The state of industrial ill-health in the United Kingdom. *International Journal of Health Services, 10,* 149–159.

Coates, T., Stall, R., & Hoff, C. (1988, May). *Changes in high risk behavior among gay and bisexual men since the beginning of the AIDS epidemic.* Washington, DC: Office of Technology Assessment, United States Congress.

Cockburn, J., Thompson, S. C., Marks, R., et al. (1997). Behavioural dynamics of a clinical trial of sunscreens for reducing solar keratoses in Victoria, Australia. *Journal of Epidemiology and Community Health, 51,* 716–721.

Cohen, A., & Murphy, L. (1989). Indicators and measures of health promotion behaviors in the workplace. In S. B. Kar (Ed.). *Health promotion indicators and actions.* New York: Springer.

Cohen, A., Smith, M. J., & Anger, W. K. (1982). Self-protective measures against workplace hazards. In R. S. Parkinson et al. (Eds.), *Managing health promotion in the workplace.* Palo Alto, CA: Mayfield.

Cohen, H., Harris, C., & Green, L. W. (1979). Cost-benefit analysis of asthma self-management educational programs in children. *Journal of Allergy and Clinical Immunology, 64,* 155–156.

Cohen, R. Y., Felix, M. R. J., & Brownell, K. D. (1989). The role of parents and older peers in school-based cardiovascular prevention programs: Implications for program development. *Health Education Quarterly, 16,* 245–253.

Colantonio, A. (1989). Assessing the effects of employee assistance programs: A review of employee assistance program evaluations. *Yale Journal of Biology and Medicine, 62,* 13–22.

Coleman, J. S. (1978). Social capital in the creation of human capital. *American Journal of Sociology, 94*(Suppl.), 95–120.

Collin, D. F. (1982–1983). Health educators: Change agents or techno/peasants? *International Quarterly of Community Health Education, 3,* 131–144.

Collings, G. H., Jr. (1982). Perspectives of industry regarding health promotion. In R. S. Parkinson et al. (Eds.), *Managing health promotion in the workplace: Guidelines for implementation and evaluation* (pp. 119–126). Palo Alto, CA: Mayfield.

Collins, J., Wagner, S., & Weissberger, L. (1986). One hundred and twenty-five teams lose 2,233 pounds in a work site weight loss competition. *Journal of the American Dietetic Association, 86,* 1578–1579.

Colton, D. (1997). The design of evaluation for continuous quality improvement. *Evaluation and the Health Professions, 20,* 265–285.

Comino, E., Bauman, A., & Hardy, A. (1995). Public education campaigns for asthma in Australia: Supplementing national media with local initiatives. *Health Promotion Journal of Australia, 5,* 57–59.

Commission on Risk Assessment and Risk Management. (1996). *Risk assessment and risk management in regulatory decision-making.* Washington, DC: Author.

COMMIT Research Group. (1995). Community intervention trial or smoking cessation (COMMIT) cohort results from a four-year community intervention. *American Journal of Public Health, 85,* 777–785

Committee on Diet and Health, National Research Council, Food and Nutrition Board. (1989). *Diet and health: Implications for reducing chronic disease risk.* Washington, DC: National Academy Press.

Committee on Risk Perception and Communication, National Research Council. (1989). *Improving risk communication.* Washington, DC: National Academy Press.

Committee on Trauma Research. (1989). *Injury in America: A continuing public health problem.* Washington, DC: National Academy Press.

Committee to Study Outreach for Prenatal Care, Institute of Medicine. (1988). *Prenatal care: Reaching infants.* Washington, DC: National Academy Press.

Condiotte, M. M., & Lichtenstein, E. (1981). Self-efficacy and relapse in smoking cessation programs. *Journal of Consulting and Clinical Psychology, 49,* 648–658.

Conference proceedings: XV World Conference on Health Promotion and Education, Tokyo, Japan. (1995). Paris: International Union for Health Promotion and Education.

Conference proceedings: XVI World Conference on Health Promotion and Education, San Juan, Puerto Rico. (1998). Paris: International Union for Health Promotion and Education.

Connell, D. B., Turner, R. R., & Mason, E. F. (1985). Summary of findings of the school health education evaluation: Health promotion effectiveness, implementation, and costs. *Journal of School Health, 55,* 316–321.

Connors, G. J., Maisto, S. A., & Donovan, D. M. (1996). Conceptualizations of relapse: A summary of psychological and psychobiological models. *Addiction, 9*(Suppl.), S6–S14.

Conrad, K. M., Campbell, R. T., Edington, D. W., et al. (1996). The worksite environment as a cue to smoking reduction. *Research in Nursing and Health, 19,* 21–31.

Conrad, P. (1987). Who comes to work-site wellness programs? A preliminary review. *Journal of Occupational Medicine, 29,* 317–320.

Conrad, P., & Walsh, D. C. (1992). The new corporate health ethic: Lifestyle and the social control of work. *International Journal of Health Services, 22,* 89–111.

Consumer self-care in health. (1977). Rockville, MD: National Center for Health Services Research Proceeding Series, DHEW Publication No. HRA 77-3181.

Contento, I. R., Kell, D. G., Keiley, M. K., & Corcoran, R. D. (1992). A formative evaluation of the American Cancer Society Changing the Course nutrition education curriculum. *Journal of School Health, 62,* 411–416.

Conway, T., Hu, T.-C., & Harrington, T. (1997). Setting health priorities: Community boards accurately reflect the preferences of the community's residents. *Journal of Community Health, 22,* 57–68.

Cook, R., & Harrell, A. (1987). Drug abuse among working adults: Prevalence rates and recommended strategies. *Health Education Research: Theory and Practice, 2,* 353–359.

Cooke, M., Mattick, R. P., & Campbell, E. (1998). The influence of individual and organizational factors on the reported smoking intervention practices of staff in 20 antenatal clinics. *Drug and Alcohol Review, 17,* 175–185.

Corcoran, R. D., & Portnoy, B. (1989). Risk reduction through comprehensive cancer education: The American Cancer Society plan for youth education. *Journal of School Health, 59,* 199–204.

Coreil, J., & Levin, J. S. (1985). A critique of the life style concept in public health education. *International Quarterly of Community Health Education, 5,* 103–114.

Cornacchia, H. J., Olsen, L. K., & Nickerson, C. J. (1991). *Health in elementary schools* (8th ed.). St. Louis, MO: Mosby.

Costanza, M. E. (1992). Physician compliance with mammography guidelines: Barriers and enhancers. *Journal of the American Board of Family Practice, 5*(2), 1–10.

Costello, E. J. (1989). Developments in child psychiatric epidemiology. *Journal of American Academy of Child Adolescent Psychiatry, 28,* 114–120.

Cottrell, L. S. (1976). The competent community. In B. H. Kaplan, R. N. Wilson, & A. H. Leighton (Eds.), *Further Exploration in Social Psychiatry* (pp. 195–209). New York: Basic Books.

Cottrell, R. R., Capwell, E., & Brannan, J. (1995a). Comprehensive school health conferences: The Ohio evaluation model. *Wellness Perspectives: Research, Theory, and Practice, 11*(4), 55-63.

Cottrell, R. R, Capwell, E., & Brannan, J. (1995b). A follow-up evaluation of non-returning teams to the Ohio Comprehensive School Health Conference. *Journal of Wellness Perspectives, 12*(1), 1–6.

Coulter, A., & Schofield, T. (1991). Prevention in general practice: The views of doctors in the Oxford region. *British Journal of General Practice, 41,* 140–143.

Council on Scientific Affairs. (1990). Education for health: A role for physicians and the efficacy of health education efforts. *Journal of the American Medical Association, 263,* 1816–1819.

Covello, V. T., von Winterfeldt, D., & Slovic, P. (1986, October). Risk communication: A review of the literature. *Risk Abstracts, 3,* 171–182.

Covington, D. L., Peoples-Sheps, M. D., Buescher, P. A., Bennett, T. A., & Paul, M. V. (1998). An evaluation of an adolescent prenatal education program. *American Journal of Health Behavior, 22,* 323-333.

Cox, C. (1979). A pilot study: Using the elderly as community health educators. *International Journal of Health Education, 22,* 49–52.

Cox, E. (1995). *A truly civil society.* Sydney: Australian Broadcasting Company.

Cramer, J. A., & Spilker, B. (Eds.). (1991). *Patient compliance in medical practice and clinical trials.* New York: Raven Press.

Crawford, R. (1977). You are dangerous to your health: The ideology and politics of victim blaming. *International Journal of Health Services, 7,* 663–680.

Creese, A., & Parker, D. (Eds.). (1994). *Cost analysis in primary health care: A training manual for programme managers.* Geneva: World Health Organizations.

Creswell, W. H. (1981). Professional preparation: An historical perspective. In *National Congress for Institutions Preparing Health Educators: Proceedings* (pp. 43–60). Birmingham, AL: U.S. Department of Health and Human Services, DHHS Publication No. 81-50171.

Creswell, W., Jr., & Newman, I. M. (1997). *School health practice* (10th ed.). St. Louis: Times Mirror/Mosby.

Cretain, G. K. (1989). Motivational factors in breast self-examination: Implications for nurses. *Cancer Nursing, 12,* 250–256.

Cromwell, J., Bartosch, W. J., & Baker, T. (1997). Cost-effectiveness of the Clinical Practice Recommendations in the AHCPR Guideline for Smoking Cessation. *Journal of the American Medical Association, 278,* 1759–1769.

Crow, R., Blackburn, H., Jacobs, D., et al. (1986). Population strategies to enhance physical activity: The Minnesota Heart Health Program. *Acta Medica Scandinavica, 711*(Suppl.), 93–112.

Crowley, S., Dunt, D., & Day, N. (1995). Cost-effectiveness of alternative interventions for the prevention and treatment of coronary heart disease. *Australian Journal of Public Health, 19,* 336–346.

Cuca, R., & Pierce, C. S. (1977). *Experiments in family planning: Lessons from the developing world.* Baltimore: Johns Hopkins University Press.

Cucherat, M., & Boissel, J.-P. (1998). A mathematical model for determination of the optimum value of the treatment threshold for a continuous risk factor. *European Journal of Epidemiology, 14,* 23–48.

Cullen, J., Fox, B., & Isom, R. (Eds.). (1976). *Cancer: The behavioral dimensions.* New York: Raven Press.

Cummings, K. M., Giovino, G., Emont, S. L., Sciandra, R., & Koenigsberg, M. (1986). Factors influencing success in counseling patients to stop smoking. *Patient Education and Counseling, 8,* 189–200.

Cummings, K. M., Giovino, G., Sciandra, R., Koenigsberg, M., & Emont, S. L. (1987). Physican advice to quit smoking: Who gets it and who doesn't. *American Journal of Preventive Medicine, 3,* 69–75.

Cummings, K. M., Hellmann, R., & Emont, S. L. (1988). Correlates of participation in a worksite stop-smoking contest. *Journal of Behavioral Medicine, 11,* 267–277.

Cummings, O. W., Nowakowski, J. R., Schwandt, T. A., et al. (1988). Business perspectives on internal/external evaluation. In J. A. McLaughlin, L. J. Weber, R. W. Covert, & R. B. Ingle (Eds.), *Evaluation Utilization.* San Francisco: Jossey-Bass.

Cuoto, R. A. (1990). Promoting health at the grass roots. *Health Affairs, 9, 144–151.*

Curry, S. J., Grothaus, L. C., & Pabiniak, C. (1998). Use and cost effectiveness of smoking-cessation services under four insurance plans in a health maintenance organization. *New England Journal of Medicine, 339,* 673–679.

Cwikel, J. M. B., Dielman, T. E., Kirscht, J. P., & Israel, B. A. (1988). Mechanisms of psychosocial effects on health: The role of social integration, coping style and health behavior. *Health Education Quarterly, 15,* 151–173.

Dahl, S., Gustafson, C., & McCullagh, M. (1993). Collaborating to develop a community-based health service for rural homeless persons. *Journal of Nursing Administration, 23*(4), 41–45.

Daltroy, L. H. (1993). Doctor-patient communication in rheumatological disorders. *Balliere's Clinical Rheumatology, 7,* 221–239.

Daltroy, L. H., Iversen, M. D., Larson, M. G., et al. (1993). Teaching and social support: Effects on knowledge, attitudes, and behaviors to prevent low back injuries in industry. *Health Education Quarterly, 20,* 43–62.

Danaher, B. G. (1982). Smoking cessation programs in occupational settings. In R. S. Parkinson et al. (Eds.), *Managing Health Promotion in the Workplace: Guidelines for Implementation and Evaluation* (pp. 217-232). Palo Alto, CA: Mayfield.

Dane, J. K., Sleet, D. A., Lam, D. J., & Roppel, C. E. (1987). Determinants of wellness in children: An exploratory study. *Health Values, 11,* 13–19.

Daneshvary, N., Daneshvary, R., & Schwer, R. K. (1998). Solid-waste recycling behavior and support for curbside textile recycling. *Environment and Behavior, 30,* 144–161.

Danforth, N., & Swaboda, B. (1978, March 17). *Agency for International Development health education study.* Washington, DC: Westinghouse Health Systems.

Daniel, M., & Green, L. W. (1995). Application of the Precede-Proceed model in diabetes prevention and control: A case illustration from a Canadian aboriginal community. *Diabetes Spectrum, 8,* 74–84.

Danigelis, N. L., Roberson, N. L., Worden, J. K., et al. (1995). Breast screening by African American women: Insights from a household survey and focus groups. *American Journal of Preventive Medicine, 11,* 311–317.

Davidson, L., Chapman, S., & Hull, C. (1979). *Health promotion in Australia 1978–1979.* Canberra: Commonwealth of Australia.

Davidson, W., & Cotter, P. (1993. Psychological sense of community and support for public school taxes. *American Journal of Community Psychology, 21,* 59–66.

Davis, A. K. (1994). Challenges in personal and public health promotion: The primary care physician perspective. *American Journal of Preventive Medicine, 10*(Suppl.), 36–38.

Davis, A. L., Faust, R., & Ordentlich, M. (1984). Self-help smoking cessation and maintenance programs: A comparative study with 12-month follow-up by the American Lung Association. *American Journal of Public Health, 74,* 1212–1219.

Davis, D. A., Haynes, R. B., & Chambers, L. W., et al. (1984). The impact of CME: A methodologic review of the continuing medical education literature. *Evaluation and the Health Professions, 7,* 251–283.

Davis, D. A., Thomson, M. A., Oxman, A. D., & Haynes, R. B. (1992). Evidence for the effectiveness of CME: A review of 50 randomized controlled trials. *Journal of the American Medical Association, 268,* 1111–1117.

Davis, D. A., Thomson, M. A., Oxman, A. D., & Haynes, B. (1995). Changing physician performance: A systematic review of the effect of continuing medical education strategies. *Journal of the American Medical Association, 274,* 700–705.

Davis, K. E., Jackson, K. L., Kronenfeld, J. J., & Blair, S. N. (1987). Determinants of participation in worksite health promotion activities. *Health Education Quarterly, 14,* 195–205.

Davis, M. F., & Iverson, D. C. (1984). An overview and analysis of the healthstyle campaign. *Health Education Quarterly, 11,* 253–272.

Davis, M. F., Rosenberg, K., Iverson, D. E., et al. (1984). Worksite health promotion in Colorado. *Public Health Reports, 99,* 538–543.

Dawley, L. T., Dawley, H. H., Jr., Glasgow, R. E., et al. (1993). Worksite smoking control, discouragement, and cessation. *International Journal of Addictions, 28,* 719–733.

Dawson, D. A. (1986). The effects of sex education on adolescent behavior. *Family Planning Perspectives, 18,* 162–170.

Dean, K. (1992). Health and social environments: Facing complexity in health promotion research. In *Supportive environments for health.* Copenhagen: World Health Organization Regional Office for Europe.

Dean, K., & Hancock, T. (1992). *Supportive environments for health: Major policy and research issues involved in creating health promoting environments.* Copenhagen: World Health Organization, Regional Office for Europe.

Deardorff, W. W. (1986). Computerized health education: A comparison with traditional formats. *Health Education Quarterly, 13,* 61–72.

Dearing, J. W., Larson, R. S., Randall, L. M., & Pope, R. S. (1998). Local reinvention of the CDC HIV prevention community planning initiative. *Journal of Community Health, 23,* 113–126.

Dedobbeleer, N., & German, P. (1987). Safety practices in construction industry. *Journal of Occupational Medicine, 29,* 863–868.

Deeds, S. G., & Gunatilake, S. (1989). Behavioural change strategies to enhance child survival. *Hygie, 8,*19–22.

Deeds, S. G., & Mullen, P. D. (1982). Managing health education in HMOs: Part II. *Health Education Quarterly, 9,* 3–95.

DeFrank, R. S., & Levenson, P. M. (1987). Ethical and philosophical issues in developing a health promotion consortium. *Health Education Quarterly, 14,* 71–77.

DeFriese, G. H. (1989). *Promoting health in America: Breakthroughs and harbingers.* Battle Creek, MI: W. K. Kellogg Foundation.

DeFriese, G. H., Crossland, C. L., Pearson, C. E., Sullivan, C. J. (Eds.). (1990). Comprehensive school health programs: Current status and future prospects [Special issue]. *Journal of School Health, 60*(4).

de Haes, W. (1990). Can prevention be achieved through health education? [La prévention par l'éducation sanitaire est-elle possible?] In N. Job-Spira, B. Spencer, J. P. Maalti, & E. Bouvel (Eds.), *Santé publique et maladies à transmission sexuelle* (pp. 217–233). Paris: John Libby Eurotext.

DeJong, W. (1996). MADD Massachusetts Versus Senator Burke: A media advocacy case study. *Health Education Quarterly, 23,* 318–329.

DeJong, W., & Atkin, C. K. (1995). A review of national television PSA campaigns for preventing alcohol-impaired driving, 1987–1992. *Journal of Public Health Policy, 16,* 59–80.

DeJong, W., & Winsten, J. A. (1990). The use of mass media in substance abuse prevention. *Health Affairs, 9,* 30–46.

DeJoy, D. M. (1986a). Behavioral-diagnostic analysis of compliance with hearing protectors. In *Proceedings of the 30th Meeting of the Human Factors Society, Vol. II* (pp. 1433–1437). Santa Monica, CA: Human Factors Society.

DeJoy, D. M. (1986b). Behavioral diagnostic model for self-protective behavior in the workplace. *Professional Safety, 31,* 26–30.

DeJoy, D. M. (1990). Toward a comprehensive human factors model of workplace accident causation. *Professional Safety, 35,* 11–16.

DeJoy, D. M., Murphy, L. M., & Gershon, R. M. (1995). The influence of employee job-task and organizational factors on adherence to universal precautions among nurses. *International Journal of Industrial Ergonomics, 16,* 43–55.

Delaney, F., & Adams, L. (1997). Preventing skin cancer through mass media: Process evaluation of a collaboration of health promotion agencies. *Health Education Journal, 56,* 274–286.

Delbecq, A. L. (1983). The nominal group as a technique for understanding the qualitative dimensions of client needs. In R. A. Bell et al. (Eds.), *Assessing Health and Human Service Needs* (pp. 191–209). New York: Human Sciences Press.

deLeeuw, E. J. J. (1989). *Health promotion: The sane revolution.* Maastricht, The Netherlands: Van Gorcum.

Demmer, H. (1966). *Worksite health promotion.* European Health Promotion Series No. 4. Copenhagen: World Health Organization, Regional Office for Europe.

Dennison, D., & Dennison, K. F. (1989). Nutrient analysis methodology: A review of DINE developmental literature. *Health Education, 20*(7), 32–36.

Dennison, K. F., Galante, D., & Golaszewski, T. (1996). A one year post-program assessment of a computer-assisted instruction (CAI) weight management program for industrial employees: Lessons learned. *Journal of Health Education, 27,* 38–42.

De Pietro, R. (1987). A marketing research approach to health education planning. In W. B. Ward & S. K. Simonds (Eds.), *Advances in Health Education and Promotion* (vol. 2, pp. 93–118). Greenwich, CT: JAI Press.

DePree, M. (1997). *Leading with power: Finding hope in serving community.* San Francisco: Jossey-Bass.

DePue, J. D., Wells, B. L., Lasater, T. M., & Carleton, R. A. (1990). Volunteers as providers of heart health programs in churches: A report on implementation. *American Journal of Health Promotion, 4,* 361–366.

Dershewitz, R. A., & Williamson, J. W. (1977). Prevention of childhood household injuries: A controlled clinical trial. *American Journal of Public Health, 67,* 1148–1153.

Des Jarlais, D. C., & Hubbard, R. L. (1997). Alcohol and drug abuse. In R. Detels, W. W. Holland, J. McEwen, & G. S. Omenn (Eds.), *Oxford Textbook of Public Health* (3rd ed., Vol. 3, pp. 1495–1515). New York: Oxford University Press.

DeTullio, P. L., Eraker, S. A., & Jepson, C., et al. (1986). Patient medication instruction and provider interactions: Effects on knowledge and attitudes. *Health Education Quarterly, 13,* 51–60.

Deutsch, C. (1998). The university and the health of children. *Promotion and Education, 5*(1), 5–8.

Devine, E. C., & Cook, T. D. (1983). A meta-analytic analysis of effects of psycho-educational interventions on length of postsurgical hospital stay. *Nursing Research, 32,* 267–274.

DeVries, H., Dijkstra, M., & Kok, G. (1992). A Dutch smoking prevention project: An overview. *Hygie, 11*(2), 14–18.

DeVries, H., Dijkstra, M., & Kuhlman, P. (1988). Self-efficacy: The third factor besides attitude and subjective norm as a predictor of behavioral intentions. *Health Education Research, 3,* 273–282.

DeVries, H., & Kok, G. J. (1986). From determinants of smoking behaviour to the implications for a prevention programme. *Health Education Research, 1,* 85–94.

Dewey, J. (1909). *Moral principles in education.* Boston: Houghton Mifflin.

Dewey, J. (1938). *Logic: The theory of inquiry.* New York: Holt.

Dewey, J. (1946). *The public and its problems: An essay in political inquiry.* Chicago: Gateway.

Dickinson, J. A., Wiggers, J., Leeder, S. R., & Sanson-Fisher, R. W. (1989). General practitioners' detection of patients' smoking status. *Medical Journal of Australia, 150,* 420–422, 425–426.

DiClemente, C. C., & Prochaska, J. O. (1982). Self-change and therapy change of smoking behavior: A comparison of process of change in cessation and maintenance. *Addictive Behaviors, 7,* 133–142.

DiClemente, C. C., Prochaska, J. O., & Gibertine, M. (1985). Self-efficacy and the stages of self-change of smoking. *Cognitive Therapy and Research, 9,* 181–200.

Dietz, T., Stern, P. C., & Rycroft, R. W. (1989). Definitions of conflict and the legitimation of resources: The case of environmental risk. *Sociological Forum, 4*(1), 47–70.

Dievler, A. (1997). Fighting tuberculosis in the 1990s: How effective is planning in policy making? *Journal of Public Health Policy, 18,* 167–187.

Dignan, M. B. (1995). *Measurement and evaluation of health education* (3rd ed.). Springfield, IL: Thomas.

Dignan, M., Bahnson, J., Sharp, P., et al. (1991). Implementation of mass media community health education: The Forsyth County Cervical Cancer Prevention Project. *Health Education Research, 6,* 259–266.

Dignan, M. B., Beal, P. E., Michielutte, R., et al. (1990). Development of a direct education workshop for cervical cancer prevention in high risk women: The Forsyth County Project. *Journal of Cancer Education, 5,* 217–223.

Dignan, M. B., & Carr, P. A. (1992). *Program planning for health education and health promotion* (2nd ed.). Baltimore: Williams & Wilkins.

Dignan, M., Michielutte, R., Blinson, K., et al. (1996). Effectiveness of health education to increase screening for cervical cancer among eastern-band Cherokee Indian women in North Carolina. *Journal of the National Cancer Institute, 88,* 1670-1676.

Dignan, M. B., Michielutte, R., Sharp, P. C., Young, L. D., & Daniels, L. A. (1991). Use of process evaluation to guide health education in Forsyth County project to prevent cervical cancer. *Public Health Reports, 106*(1), 73–77.

Dignan, M. B., & Carr, P. A. (1994). *Introduction to program planning: A basic text for community health education* (3rd ed.). Philadelphia: Lea & Febiger.

Dignan, M. B., Michielutte, R., Wells, H. B., & Bahnson, J. (1995). The Forsyth County Cancer Prevention Project: I. cervical cancer screening for black women, *Health Education Research, 4,* 411–420.

Division of Health Education, Center for Health Promotion and Education, Centers for Disease Control. (1988). *Reference Manuals: Planned Approach to Community Health.* Atlanta, GA: Centers for Disease Control.

Dobson, D., & Cook, T. J. (1980). Avoiding Type III error in program evaluation: Results from a field experiment. *Evaluation and Program Planning, 3,* 269–276.

Dodek, P., & Ottoson, J. M. (1996). The implementation link between clinical practice guidelines and continuing medical education. *Journal of Continuing Education in the Health Professions, 16,* 82–93.

Donovan, C. L. (1991). Factors predisposing, enabling and reinforcing routine screening of patients for preventing fetal alcohol syndrome: A survey of New Jersey physicians. *Journal of Drug Education, 21,* 35–42.

D'Onofrio, C. N. (1989). Making the case for cancer prevention in the schools. *Journal of School Health, 59,* 225–231.

Dore, R., & Mars, Z. (1981). *Community development.* London: Croom Helm and UNESCO.

Douglas, B., Wertley, B., & Chaffee, S. (1970). An information campaign that changed community attitudes. *Journalism Quarterly, 47,* 220–227.

Downey, A. M., Butcher, A. H., Frank, G. C., et al. (1987). Development and implementation of a school health promotion program for reduction of cardiovascular risk factors in children and prevention of adult coronary heart disease: "Heart Smart." In B. Hetzel & G. S. Berenson (Eds.), *Cardiovascular risk factors in childhood: Epidemiology and prevention* (pp. 103–121). Amsterdam: Elsevier Science Publishers.

Downey, A. M., Cresanta, J. L., & Berenson, G. S. (1989). Cardiovascular health promotion in children: "Heart Smart" and the changing role of physicians. *American Journal of Preventive Medicine, 5,* 279–295.

Downey, A. M., Frank, G. C., Webber, L. S., et al. (1987). Implementation of "Heart Smart:" A cardiovascular school health promotion program. *Journal of School Health, 57,* 98–104.

Downey, A. M., Virgilio, S. J., Serpas, D. C., et al. (1988). Heart Smart: A staff development model for a school-based cardiovascular health intervention. *Health Education, 19*(5), 64–71.

Doyle, E. I., Smith, C. A., & Hosokawa, M. C. (1989). A process evaluation of a community-based health promotion program for a minority target population. *Health Education, 20*(5), 61–64.

Doyle, E. I., Feldman, R. H. L. (1997). Factors affecting nutrition behavior among middle-class adolescents in urban area of northern region of Brazil. *Revista de Saude Publica, 31,* 342–350.

Doyle, K., Woods, S., & Deming, M. (1995). Assessment in higher education: Implications for health education professional preparation programs. *Journal of Health Education, 26,* 101–103.

Drazen, M., Nevid, J. S., Pace, N., & O'Brien, R. M. (1982). Worksite-based behavioral treatment of mild hypertension. *Journal of Occupational Medicine, 24,* 511–514.

Drellishak, R. (1997). The merits of peer education programs. *Journal of American College Health, 45,* 218.

Dryfoos, J. G. (1994). *Full-service schools: A revolution in health and social services for children, youth, and families.* San Francisco: Jossey-Bass.

DuCharme, K. A., & Brawley, L. R. (1995). Predicting the intentions and behavior of exercise initiates using two forms of self-efficacy. *Journal of Behavioral Medicine, 18,* 479–498.

Duhl, L. (1986). The healthy city: Its function and its future. *Health Promotion, 1,* 55–60.

Duke, S., McGraw, S., & Avis, N. (1995, November). *Application of the PRECEDE-PROCEED framework in the development of intervention strategies for DES exposure.* Abstract and summary from a presentation at the American Public Health Association (APHA) Conference, San Diego. Washington, DC: APHA.

Duncan, G. (1996). Income dynamics and health. *International Journal of Health Services, 26,* 419–444.

Dunlop, B. D., Piserchia, P. V., & Richardson, J. E., et al. (1989). *Evaluation of workplace health enhancement programs: A monograph.* Research Triangle Park, NC: Research Triangle Institute.

Dwore, R. B., & Kreuter, M. W. (1980). Update: Reinforcing the case for health promotion. *Family and Community Health, 2,* 103–119.

Dwyer, T., Pierce, J. P., Hannam, C. D., & Burke, N. (1986). Evaluation of the Sydney "Quit. For Life" anti-smoking campaign: Part II. Changes in smoking prevalence. *Medical Journal of Australia, 144,* 344–347.

Eakin, J. M. (1992). Leaving it up to the workers: Sociological perspective on the management of health and safety in small workplaces. *International Journal of Health Services, 22,* 689–704.

Earp, J. L., Alpeter, M., Mayne L., Viadro, C. I., & Omalley, M. S. (1995). The North Carolina breast cancer screening program: Foundations and design of a model for reaching older, minority, rural women. *Breast Cancer Research and Treatment, 35,* 7–22.

Earp, J., Ory, M. G., & Strogatz, D. S. (1982). The effects of family involvement and practitioners home visits on the control of hypertension. *American Journal of Public Health, 72,* 1146–1154.

Eastaugh, S. R., & Hatcher, M. E. (1982). Improving compliance among hypertensives: A triage criterion with cost-benefit implications. *Medical Care, 20,* 1001–1017.

Eddy, J. M., Fitzhugh, E. C., & Wang, M. Q. (1997). The impact of worksite-based safety belt programs: A review of the literature. *American Journal of Health Promotion, 11,* 281–289.

Edet, E. E. (1991). The role of sex education in adolescent pregnancy. *Journal of the Royal Society of Health, 111,* 17–18.

Eisenberg, L. (1972). The *human* nature of human nature. *Science, 176,* 123–128.

Ekeh, H. E., & Adeniyi, J. D. (1989). Health education strategies for tropical disease control in school children. *Journal of Tropical Medicine and Hygiene, 92*(2), 55–59.

Eklundh, B., & Pettersson, B. (1987). Health promotion policy in Sweden: Means and methods in intersectoral action. *Health Promotion, 2,* 177–194.

Elder, J. P., Schmid, T. L., Dower, P. & Hedlund, S. (1993). Community heart health programs: Components, rationale, and strategies for effective interventions. *Journal of Public Health Policy, 14,* 263–279.

Elford, W. E. (1992, May). *Strategies for implementing CVD prevention on practice: An Alberta perspective.* Paper presented at the International Heart Health Conference, Victoria, British Columbia.

Elinson, J. (1977). Have we narrowed the gap between the poor and the nonpoor? *Medical Care, 15,* 675–677.

Ellickson, P. L., & Bell, R. M. (1990a). Drug prevention in junior high: A multi-site longitudinal test. *Science, 247,* 1299–1305.

Ellickson, P. L., & Bell, R. M. (1990b). *Prospects for preventing drug use among young adolescents.* Santa Monica, CA: RAND, R-3896-CHF.

Ellis, L. B. M., & Raines, J. R. (1983). Health risk appraisal: A tool for health education. *Health Education, 14*(6), 30–34.

Ellison, L. F., Mao, Y., & Gibboms, L. (1995). Projected smoking-attributable mortality in Canada, 1991–2000. *Chronic Diseases in Canada, 16,* 84–89.

Ellison, R. C., Capper, A. L., Goldberg, R. J., et al. (1989). The environmental component: Changing school food service to promote cardiovascular health. *Health Education Quarterly, 16,* 285–297.

Elmore, R. (1976). Follow through planned variation. In W. Williams, and R. Elmore (Eds.), *Social Program Implementation.* New York: Academic Press.

Elwood, T. W., Ericson, E., & Lieberman, S. (1978). Comparative educational approaches to screening for colorectal cancer. *American Journal of Public Health, 68,* 135–138.

Emont, S. L., & Cummings, K. M. (1990). Organizational factors affecting participation in a smoking cessation program and abstinence among 68 auto dealerships. *American Journal of Health Promotion, 5,* 107–114.

Endres, J. (1990). Teambuilding for community health promotion, *How-To Guides on Community Health Promotion* (No. 14). Palo Alto, CA: Health Promotion Resource Center, Stanford Center for Research on Disease Prevention.

Enelow, A. J., & Henderson, J. B. (Eds.). (1975). *Applying behavioral science to cardiovascular risk.* New York: American Heart Association.

Eng, E. (1993). The Save Our Sisters Project: A social network strategy for reaching rural black women. *Cancer, 72*(3, Suppl.), 1071–1077.

Eng, E., Hatch, J., & Callan, A. (1985). Institutionalizing social support through the church and into the community. *Health Education Quarterly, 12,* 81–92.

Eng, E., & Parker, E. (1994). Measuring community competence in the Mississippi delta: The interface between program evaluation and empowerment. *Health Education Quarterly, 21,* 199–220.

Engels, R. C. M. E., Knibbe, R. A., & de Haan, Y. T. (1997). Homogeneity of cigarette smoking within peer groups: Influence or selection. *Health Education and Behavior, 24,* 801–812.

Epp, J. (1986). Achieving health for all: A framework for health promotion. *Health Promotion, 1,* 419–428.

Epstein, J. A., Botvin, G. J., & Diaz, T. (1998). Ethnic and gender differences in smoking prevalence among a longitudinal sample of inner-city adolescents. *Journal of Adolescent Health, 23,* 160–166.

Engelstad, L., Bedeian, K, Schorr, K., & Stewart, S. (1996). Pathways to early detection of cervical cancer for a multiethnic, indigent, emergency department population. *Health Education and Behavior, 23*(Suppl.), S89–S104.

Epstein, S. (1979). The stability of behavior: I. On predicting most of the people much of the time. *Journal of Personality and Social Psychology, 37,* 1097–1126.

Eraker, S. A., & Politser, P. (1982). How decisions are reached: Physician and patient. *Annals of Internal Medicine, 97,* 262–268.

Eriksen, M. P. (1986). Workplace smoking control: Rationale and approaches. In *Advances in Health Education and Promotion* (Vol. 1, Pt. A, pp. 65–103). Greenwich, CT: JAI Press.

Eriksen, M. P., & Gielen, A. C. (1983). The application of health education principles to automobile child restraint programs. *Health Education Quarterly, 10,* 30–55.

Eriksen, M. P., Green, L. W., & Fultz, F. G. (1988). Principles of changing health behavior. *Cancer, 62,* 1768–1775.

Ernst, N. D., Wu, M., Frommer, P., et al. (1986). Nutrition education at the point of purchase: The foods for health project evaluated. *Preventive Medicine, 15,* 60–73.

Esdale, A., & Harris, H. L. (1985). Evaluation of a closed-circuit television patient education program: Structure, process and outcome. *Patient Education and Counseling, 7,* 193–215.

Estey, A. L. (1988). *Follow-up intervention: Its effect on compliance with a diabetes regimen. Unpublished master's thesis.* Halifax, NS: Dalhousie University.

Estey, A., Musseau, A., & Keehn, L. (1994). Patient's understanding of health information: A multi-hospital comparison. *Patient Education and Counseling, 24,* 73–78.

Eta Sigma Gamma Monograph Series. 1985, November. Special issue, No. 4.

Evans, R. G., Barer, M. L., & Marmor, T. L. (Eds.). (1994). *Why are some people healthy and others not?* Hawthorne, NY: Alsine De Guyter.

Evans, R. I., & Raines, B. E. (1982). Control and prevention of smoking in adolescents: A psychological perspective. In T. J. Coates, A. D. Peterson, & C. Perry (Eds.), *Promoting Adolescent Health: A Dialog on Research and Practice.* New York: Academic Press.

Evans, R. I.,. Rozelle, R. M, Maxwell, S. E., et al. (1981). Social modeling films to deter smoking in adolescents: Results of a three-year field investigation. *Journal of Applied Psychology, 66,* 399–414.

Everly, G. S., & Feldman, R. H. (Eds.). (1985). *Occupational health promotion: Health behavior in the workplace.* New York: Wiley.

Evers, A. (1989). Promoting health: Localizing support structures for community health projects. *Health Promotion, 4,* 183–188.

Ewart, C. K., Li, V. C., & Coates, T. J. (1983). Increasing physicians' antismoking influence by applying an inexpensive feedback technique. *Journal of Medical Education, 58,* 468–473.

Ewart, C. K., Young, D. R., & Hagberg, J. M. (1998). Effects of school-based aerobic exercise on blood pressure in adolescent girls at risk for hypertension. *American Journal of Public Health, 88,* 949–951.

Ewles, L., & Simnett, I. (1985). *Promoting health: A practical guide to health education.* New York: Wiley.

Faden, R. R. (1987). Ethical issues in government sponsored public health campaigns. *Health Education Quarterly, 14,* 27–37.

Farley, C. (1997). Evaluation of a four-year bicycle helmet promotion campaign in Quebec aimed at children ages 8 to 12: Impact on attitudes, norms and behaviours. *Canadian Journal of Public Health, 88,* 62–66.

Farley, C., Haddad, S., & Brown, B. (1996). The effects of a 4-year program promoting bicycle helmet use among children in Quebec. *American Journal of Public Health, 86,* 46–51.

Farquhar, J. W. (1978). The community-based model of life style intervention trials. *American Journal of Epidemiology, 108,* 103–111.

Farquhar, J. W., Fortmann, S. P., Flora, J. A., et al. (1990). Effects of community-wide education on cardiovascular disease risk factors: The Stanford Five-City Project. *Journal of the American Medical Association, 264,* 359–365.

Farquhar, J. W., Fortmann, S., Maccoby, N., et al. (1984). The Stanford Five City Project: An overview. In J. D. Matarazzo et al. (Eds.), *Behavioral Health: A Handbook of Health Enhancement and Disease Prevention* (pp. 1154–65). New York: Wiley.

Farquhar, J. W., Fortman, S. P., Wood, P. D., & Haskell, W. L. (1983). Community studies of cardiovascular disease prevention. In N. M. Kaplan & J. Stamler (Eds.), *Prevention of Coronary Heart Disease: Practical Management of Risk Factors.* Philadelphia: Saunders.

Farquhar, J. W., Maccoby, N., & Wood, P. D. (1977). Community education for cardiovascular health. *Lancet, 1*(8023), 1192–1195.

Farrant, W., & Taft, A. (1988). Building healthy public policy in an unhealthy political climate: A case study from Paddington and North Kensington. *Health Promotion International, 3,* 287–292.

Fawcett, S. B., Lewis, R. K., Paine-Andrews, A., et al. (1997). Evaluating community coalitions for prevention of substance abuse: The case of Project Freedom. *Health Education and Behavior, 24,* 812–828.

Fawcett, S. B., Paine, A. L., Francisco, V. T., & Vliet, M. (1993). Promoting health through community development. In D. S. Glenwick & L. A. Jason (Eds.), *Promoting health and mental health in children, youth, and families* (pp. 233–255). New York: Springer.

Fedder, D. O. (1982). Managing medication and compliance: Physician-pharmacist-patient interactions. *Journal of the American Geriatric Society, 11*(Suppl.), 113–117.

Fedder, D., & Beardsley, R. (1979). Preparing pharmacy patient educators. *American Journal of Pharmacy Education, 43*(2), 127–129.

Federal, Provincial and Territorial Advisory Committee on Population Health. (1996). *Report on the health of Canadians.* Ottawa: Minister of Supply and Services Canada, H39-385.

Feighery, E., & Rogers, T. (1990). Building and maintaining effective coalitions. In *How-to guides on community health promotion.* Palo Alto, CA: Health Promotion Resource Center, Stanford Center for Research on Disease Prevention.

Feinstein, J. S. (1993). The relationship between socioeconomic status and health: A review of the literature. *Milbank Quarterly, 71,* 279–322.

Feldman, R. H. (1983). Strategies for improving compliance with health promotion programs in industry. *Health Education, 14*(4), 21–25.

Feldman, R. H. (1984). Increasing compliance in worksite health promotion: Organizational, educational, and psychological strategies. *Corporate Commentary, 1*(2), 45–50.

Feliz, M. R. J., Stukard, A. J., Cohen, R. Y., & Smith, W. E. (1988). Do only the healthy intend to participate in worksite health promotion? *Health Education Quarterly, 15,* 269–288.

Fellman, C., & Fellman, M. (1981). *Making sense of self: Medical advice literature in late 19th-century America.* Philadelphia: University of Pennsylvania Press.

Ferrans, C.E. (1996). Development of a conceptual model of quality of life. *Scholarly Inquiry for Nursing Practice, 10,* 293–304.

Fetterman, D. (1994). Empowerment evaluation. *Evaluation Practice, 15,* 1–15.

Fetterman, D. M. (1994). Steps in empowerment evaluation: From California to Cape Town. *Evaluation and Program Planning, 7,* 305–313.

Fetterman, D. M., Kaftarian, S. J., & Wandersman, A. (1996). *Empowerment evaluation: Knowledge and tools for self-assessment and accountability.* Thousand Oaks, CA: Sage.

Fielding, J. E. (1982). Effectiveness of employee health improvement programs. *Journal of Occupational Medicine, 24,* 907–916.

Fielding, J. E. (1984). Health promotion and disease prevention at the worksite. *Annual Review of Public Health, 5,* 237–265.

Fielding, J. E. (1990a). Worksite health promotion programs in the United States: Progress, lessons and challenges. *Health Promotion International, 5,* 75–84.

Fielding, J. E. (1990b). Worksite health promotion survey: Smoking control activities. *Preventive Medicine, 19,* 402–413.

Fielding, J. E. (1991). Smoking control at the workplace. *Annual Review of Public Health, 12,* 209–234.

Fielding, J. E., & Breslow, L. (1983). Health promotion programs sponsored by California employers. *American Journal of Public Health, 73,* 538–542.

Fielding, J. E., & Nelson, S. (1976). Health education for job corps enrollees. *Public Health Reports, 91,* 243–248.

Fielding, J. E., & Piserchia, P. V. (1989). Frequency of worksite health promotion activities. *American Journal of Public Health, 79,* 16–20.

Figa-Talamanca, I. (1975, Fall). Problems in the evaluation of training of health personnel. *Health Education Monographs, 3,* 232–250.

Fink, R., & Shapiro, S. (1990). Significance of increased efforts to gain participation in screening for breast cancer. *American Journal of Preventive Medicine, 6,* 34–41.

Finkelhor, D., & Kziuba-Leatherman, J. (1994). Children as victims of violence: A national survey. *Pediatrics, 94,* 413–420.

Finnegan, J. R., Jr., Murray, D. M., Kurth, C., McCarthy, P. (1989). Measuring and tracking education program implementation: The Minnesota Heart Health Program experience. *Health Education Quarterly, 16,* 77–90.

Fiori, F. B., de la Vega, M., & Vacarro, M. J. (1974). Health education in a hospital setting: Report of a public health service project in Newark, New Jersey. *Health Education Monographs, 2*(1), 11–29.

Fireman, P., Friday, G. A., Gira, C., Vierthaler, W. A., & Michaels, L. (1981). Teaching self-management skills to asthmatic children and their parents in an ambulatory care setting. *Pediatrics, 68,* 341–348.

First International Conference on Health Promotion. (1986). The Ottawa charter for health promotion. *Health Promotion, 1*(4), i–v.

Fisher, A., Green, L. W., McCrae, A., & Cochran, C. (1976). Training teachers in population education institutes in Baltimore. *Journal of School Health, 46,* 357–360.

Fisher, E. B., Jr. (1995). Editorial: The results of the COMMIT trial. *American Journal of Public Health, 85*(2), 159–160.

Fisher, E. B., Auslander, W., Sussman. L., et al. (1992, Summer). Community organization and health promotion in minority neighborhoods. In *Proceedings of the NIH Workshop on Health Behavior Research in Minority Populations.* Ethnicity and Disease, 2, 252–272.

Fisher, E. B., Strunk, R. C., Sussman, L. K., et al. (1996). Acceptability and feasiblity of a community approach to asthma management: The Neighborhood Asthma Coalition (NAC). *Journal of Asthma, 33,* 367–383.

Fisher, K. J., Glasgow, R. E., & Terborg, J. R. (1990). Work site smoking cessation: A meta-analysis of long-term quit rates from controlled studies. *Journal of Occupational Medicine, 32,* 429–439.

Fisher, S., Mansbridge, B., & Lankford, D. A. (1982). Public judgments of information in a diazepam patient package insert. *Archives of General Psychiatry, 39,* 707–711.

Flay, B. R. (1985). Psychosocial approaches to smoking prevention: A review of findings. *Health Psychology, 4,* 449–488.

Flay, B. R. (1986a). Efficacy and effectiveness trials in the development of health promotion programs. *Preventive Medicine, 15,* 451–474.

Flay, B. R. (1986b). Mass media linkages with school-based programs for drug abuse preventions. *Journal of School Health, 56,* 402–406.

Flay, B. R. (1987). Social psychological approaches to smoking prevention: Review and recommendations. In W. B. Ward & P. D. Mullen (Eds.), *Advances in Health Education and Promotion* (Vol. 2, pp. 121–80). Greenwich, CT: JAI Press.

Flay, B. R., & Cook, T. D. (1981). Evaluation of mass media prevention campaigns. In R. E. Rice & W. J. Paisley (Eds.), *Public Communication Campaigns* (pp. 239–264). London: Sage.

Fleisher, L., Kornfeld, J., Ter Maat, J., et al. (1998). Building effective partnerships: A national evaluation of the Cancer Information Service Outreach Program. *Journal of Health Communication, 3*(Suppl.), 21–35.

Fletcher, S. W., Morgan, T. M., O'Malley, M. S., et al. (1989). Is breast self-examination predicted by knowledge, attitudes, beliefs, or sociodemographic characteristics? *American Journal of Preventive Medicine, 5,* 207–216.

Flynn, B.S. (1995). Measuring community leaders' perceived ownership of health education programs: Initial tests of reliability and validity. *Health Education Research, 10,* 27–36.

Flynn, B. S., Gurdon, M. A., & Secker-Walker, R. H. (1995). Cigarette smoking control strategies of firms with small work forces in two northeastern states. *American Journal of Health Promotion, 9,* 202-219.

Flynn, B. S., Goldstein, A. O., & Dana, G. S. (1998). Predictors of state legislators' intentions to vote for cigarette tax increases. *Preventive Medicine, 27,* 157–166.

Flynn, B. S., Worden, J. K., Secker-Walker, R. H., Badger, G. J., et al. (1992). Prevention of cigarette smoking through mass media intervention and school programs. *American Journal of Public Health, 82,* 827–834.

Flynn, B. S., Worden, J. K., Secker-Walker, R. H., Pirie, P. L., et al. (1997). Long-term responses of higher and lower risk youths to prevention interventions. *Preventive Medicine, 26,* 389–394.

Focal Points. (1977, July). Atlanta, GA: Bureau of Health Education, Centers for Disease Control, U.S. Department of Health, Education, and Welfare.

Food and Nutrition Board, National Research Council. (1989). *Diet and Health.* Washington, DC: National Academy Press.

Ford, J. D., & Ford, J. G. (1986, March–April). Health promotion: Competitor or resource? *EAP Digest,* pp. 23–29.

Fors, S.W., Owen, S., Hall, W. D., et al. (1989). Evaluation of a diffusion strategy for school-based hypertension education. *Health Education Quarterly, 16,* 255–261

Fortmann, S. P., Flora, J. A., Winkleby, M. A., et al. (1995). Community intervention trials: Reflections on the Stanford Five-City Project experience. *American Journal of Epidemiology, 142,*476–486.

Fortmann, S. P., Williams, P. T., Hulley, S. B., et al. (1981). Effect of health education on dietary behavior: The Stanford Three-Community Study. *American Journal of Clinical Nutrition, 34,* 565–571.

Foster, G. M. (1962). *Traditional cultures and the impact of technological change.* New York: Harper.

Frank, G. C., Vaden, A., & Martin, J. (1987). School health promotion: Child nutrition. *Journal of School Health, 57,* 451–460.

Frank, J. W. (1995, May–June). Why "population health?" *Canadian Journal of Public Health, 86,*162–164.

Frank, J. W., & Mustard, J. F. (1994). Historical perspective on how prosperity has influenced health and well-being. *Daedalus, 123*(4),1–19.

Frankish, C. J., & Green, L. W. (1994). Organizational and community change as the social scientific basis for disease prevention and health promotion policy. In G. L. Albrecht (Ed.), *Advances in medical sociology: Vol. IV. A reconsideration of health behavior change models* (pp. 209–233). Ipswich, CT: JAI Press.

Frankish, C. J., & Green, L. W. (1998). Worksite smoking cessation. In L. W. Green, D. Williamson, C. J. Frankish, et al. (Eds.), *Smoking cessation: A systematic review.* Vancouver: Institute of Health Promotion Research, University of British Columbia.

Frankish, C. J., Johnson, J. L., Ratner, P. A., & Lovato, C. Y. (1997). Relationship of organizational characteristics of Canadian workplaces to anti-smoking initiatives. *Preventive Medicine, 26,* 248–256.

Franz, J. B. (1987, November). Promoting wellness and disease prevention in EAPS. *Almacan,* pp. 8–12.

Franz, M., Kresnick, A., Maschak-Carey, B., et al. (1986). *Goals for diabetes education.* Alexandria, VA: American Diabetes Association.

Frederiksen, L. W., Solomon, L. J., & Brehony, K. A. (Eds.). (1984). *Marketing health behavior: Principles, techniques, and applications.* New York: Plenum.

Freeman, H. P. (1989). Cancer in the economically disadvantaged. *Cancer, 64*(Suppl.), 324–334.

Freemantle, N., Harvey, E. L., Wolf, F., et al. (1977, June 3). Printed educational materials to improve the behaviour of health care professionals and patient outcomes. In L. Bero, R. Grilli, J. Grimshaw, & A. Oxman (Eds.), *Cochrane collaboration of effective professional practice module of the Cochrane database of systematic reviews.* Oxford: Update Software. Available in the Cochrane Library, database on disk and CD-ROM, Issue 3.

Freire, P. (1970). *Pedagogy of the oppressed.* New York: Seabury.

French, S. A., & Jeffery, R. W. (1995). Weight concerns and smoking: A literature review. *Annals of Behavioral Medicine, 17,* 234–244.

Freudenberg, N. (1978). Shaping the future of health education: From behavior change to social change. *Health Education Monographs, 6,* 372–377.

Freudenberg, N. (1984a). Citizen action for environmental health: Report on a survey of community organizations. *American Journal of Public Health, 74,* 444–448.

Freudenberg, N. (1984b). *Not in our backyards! Community action for health and the environment.* New York: Monthly Review Press.

Freudenberg, N. (1984–1985). Training health educators for social change. *International Quarterly of Community Health Education, 5,* 37–52.

Freudenberg, N. (1989). Preventing AIDS: A guide to effective education for the prevention of HIV infection. Washington, DC: American Public Health Association.

Freudenberg, N., & Golub, M. (1987). Health education, public policy and disease prevention: A case history of the New York City coalition to end lead poisoning. *Health Education Quarterly, 14,* 387–401.

Fried, L. P., & Bush, T. L. (1988). Morbidity as the focus of prevention in the elderly. *Epidemiological Review, 103,* 48–64.

Friede, A., Freedman, M. A., Paul, J. E., et al. (1994). DATA 2000: CDC WONDER information system linking Healthy People 2000 objectives to data sets. *American Journal of Preventive Medicine, 10,* 230–234

Friede, A., McDonald, M. C., & Blum, H. (1995). Public health informatics: How information age technology can strengthen public health. *Annual Review of Public Health, 16,* 239–252.

Friede, A., Rosin, P. H., Reid, J. A. (1994). CDC WONDER: A cooperative processing architecture for public health. *Journal of the American Medical Informatics Association, 1,* 303–312.

Friedman, L., Lichtenstein, E., & Biglan, A. (1985). Smoking onset among teens: An empirical analysis of initial situations. *Addictive Behaviors, 10,* 1–13.

Fries, J., Green, L. W., & Levine, S. (1989). Health promotion and the compression of morbidity. *Lancet, 1,* 481–483.

Frost, W. D., & St. Germain, P. S. (1986). Health culture assessment: A strategy for effective health behavior change. *Proceedings of the 22nd Annual Meeting of the Society of Prospective Medicine, Bethesda, MD.* Indianapolis, IN: Society of Prospective Medicine.

Fryback, D. G., Lawrence, W. F., Martin, P. A., Klein, R., & Klein, B. E. (1997). Predicting quality of well-being scores from the SF-36: Results from the Beaver Dam Health Outcomes study. *Medical Decision Making, 17,* 1–9.

Fuchs, J. A. (1988). Planning for community health promotion: A rural example. *Health Values, 12*(6), 3–8.

Fulmer, H. S., Cashman, S., Hattis, P., et al. (1992). Bridging the gap between medicine, public health and the community: PATCH and the Carney Hospital experience. *Journal of Health Education, 23,* 167–170.

Gager, P. J., Kress, J. S., & Elias, M. J. (1996). Prevention programs and special education: Considerations related to risk, social competence, and multiculturalism. *Journal of Primary Prevention, 16,* 395–412.

Gans, K. M., Lapane, K. L., Lasater, T. M., & Carleton, R. A. (1994). Effects of intervention on compliance to referral and lifestyle recommendations given at cholesterol screening programs. *American Journal of Preventive Medicine, 10,* 275–282.

Gardell, B. (1982). Worker participation and autonomy. A multilevel approach to democracy at the workplace. *International Journal of Health Services Research, 12,* 527–558.

Garfield, S. R. (1970). The delivery of medical care. *Scientific American, 222,* 15–18.

Garr, D. R. (1989). Community-oriented primary care. *Journal of Family Practice, 28,* 654.

Garraway, W. M., & Whisnant, J. P. (1987). The changing pattern of hypertension and the declining incidence of stroke. *Journal of the American Medical Association, 258,* 214–217.

Garvin, T. (1995). "We're strong women": Building a community-university research partnership. *Geoforum, 26*(3), 273–286.

Gates, C. T. (1991). Making a case for collaborative problem solving. *National Civic Review, 80,* 113–119.

Geiger, H. J. (1984). Community health centers: Health care as an instrument of social change. In V. Sidel and R. Sidel (Eds.), *Reforming medicine: Lessons of the last quarter century.* New York: Pantheon.

Gelman, S. B. (1992). Prevention, promotion and medical education. In G. Eikenberry (Ed.), *The seeds of wellness in the '90s: An anthology on health promotion.* Ottawa: Canadian College of Health Service Executives.

Gemson, D. H., & Elinson, J. (1986). Prevention in primary care: Variability in physician practice patterns in New York City. *American Journal of Preventive Medicine, 2,* 226–234.

General Professional Education of Physicians Panel. (1984). *Physicians for the twenty-first century: The GPEP report.* Washington, DC: Association of American Medical Colleges.

German, P. S., Shapiro, S., & Skinner, E. A., et al. (1987). Detection and management of mental-health problems of older patients by primary care providers. *Journal of the American Medical Association, 257,* 489–493.

Gerstein, D., & Green, L. W. (Eds.). (1993). *Preventing drug abuse: What do we know?* Washington, DC: National Academy Press.

Gerstein, D., & Harwood, H. J. (1990). *Treating drug problems,* Vol. 1. Washington, DC: National Academy Press.

Gevers, J. K. M. (1985). Worker control over occupational health services: The development of legal rights in the EEC. *International Journal of Health Services Research, 159,* 217–229.

Gielen, A. C., Mc Donald, E. M., & Auld, M. E. (1997). *Health education in the 21st century: A white paper.* Prepared for the Health Resources and Services Administration, Bethesda, Maryland.

Gielen, A. C., & Radius, S. (1984, August–September). Project KISS (Kids in Safety Belts): Educational approaches and evaluation measures. *Health Education, 15,* 43–47.

Gilbert, G. G., Davis, R. L., & Damberg, C. L. (1985). Current federal activities in school health education. *Public Health Reports, 100,* 499–507.

Gilbert, G. G., & Sawyer, R. (1996). *Health education pedagogy.* Boston: Jones and Bartlett.

Gilmore, G. D., & Campbell, M. D. (1996). *Needs assessment strategies for health education and health promotion.* Madison, WI: Brown & Benchmark.

Gilmore, G. D., Campbell, M. D., & Becker, B. L. (1989). *Needs assessment strategies for health education and health promotion.* Indianapolis, IN: Benchmark.

Gilpin, E., Pierce, J., Goodman, J., et al. (1992). Trends in physicians' giving advice to stop smoking, United States, 1974–87. *Tobacco Control, 1,* 31–36.

Girdano, D. A. (1986). Employee assistance programs. In D. A. Girdano (Ed.), *Occupational health promotion* (2nd ed., pp. 196–212). New York: Macmillan.

Gittenberg, J. (1974). Adapting health care to a cultural setting. *American Journal of Nursing, 74,* 2218–2221.

Glantz, S. A. (1997). Tobacco control in Australia: It's time to get back on top down under. *Health Promotion Journal of Australia, 7,* 72–73.

Glanz, K., Brekke, M., Harper, D., Bache-Wiig, M., & Hunnighake, D. B. (1992). Evaluation of implementation of a cholesterol management program in physicians' offices. *Health Education Research, 7,* 151–163.

Glanz, K., Lewis, F. M., & Rimer, B. K. (Eds.). (1997). *Health behavior and health education: Theory, research, and practice* (2nd ed.). San Francisco: Jossey-Bass.

Glanz, K., & Rimer, B. (1995, July). *Theory at a glance: A guide for health promotion practice.* Bethesda, MD: National Cancer Institute, NIH Pub. No. 95-3896, Public Health Service, U.S. Dept. of Health and Human Services.

Glasgow, R. E., Klesges, R., Mizes, J., & Pechacek, T. (1985). Quitting smoking: Strategies used and variables associated with success in a stop-smoking contest. *Journal of Consulting and Clinical Psychology, 53,* 905–912.

Glasgow, R. E., Schafer, L., & O'Neill, H. K. (1981). Self-help books and amount of therapist contact in smoking cessation programs. *Journal of Consulting and Clinical Psychology, 49,* 659–667.

Glenn, M. K. (1994). Preparing rehabilitation specialists to address the prevention of substance abuse problems. *Rehabilitation Counseling, 38,* 164–179.

Glik, D., Gordon, A., Ward, W., et al. (1987–1988). Focus group methods for formative research in child survival: An Ivoirian example. *International Quarterly of Community Health Education, 8,* 297–316.

Global Programme on AIDS. (1994). *Evaluation of a national AIDS programme: A methods package.* Geneva: World Health Organization.

Glynn, S. M., Gruder, C. L., & Jerski, J. A. (1986). Effects on treatment success and on mis-reporting abstinence. *Health Psychology, 5*(2), 125–136.

Glynn, S. M., & Ruderman, A. J. (1986). The development and validation of an eating self-efficacy scale. *Cognitive Therapy and Research, 10,* 403–420.

Glynn, T. J. (1989). Essential elements of school-based smoking prevention programs. *Journal of School Health, 59,* 181–188.

Glynn, T. J., Boyd, G. M., & Gruman, J. C. (1990). Essential elements of self-help/minimal intervention strategies for smoking cessation. *Health Education Quarterly, 17,* 329–345.

Gochman, D. S. (1997). *Handbook of health behavior research.* New York: Plenum.

Godin, G., Lambert, J., & Locker, D. (1997). Understanding the intention of gay and bisexual men to take the HIV Antibody Test. *AIDS Education and Prevention, 9,* 31–42.

Godin, G., & Shephard, R. J. (1990). An evaluation of the potential role of the physician in influencing community exercise behavior. *American Journal of Health Promotion, 4,* 255–259.

Goeppinger, J., & Baglioni, A. J. (1985). Community competence: A positive approach to needs assessment. *American Journal of Community Psychology, 13,* 507–523.

Goerdt, A., Koplan, J. P., Robine, J. M., Thuriaux, M. C., & van Ginneken, J. K. (1996). Non-fatal health outcomes: Concepts, instruments and indicators. Chap. 2 in J. L. Murray & A. D. Lopez (Eds.), *The global burden of disease.* Cambridge, MA: Harvard University.

Gold, R. S. (1991). *Microcomputer applications in health education.* Dubuque, IA: Brown.

Gold, R. S., & Hernandez, M. E. (1992). *Phase I final report for the IVD project.* Bethesda, MD: National Cancer Institute.

Gold, R., Green, L. W., & Kreuter, M. W. (1997). *EMPOWER: Enabling methods of planning and organizing within everyone's reach* [CD-ROM and manual]. Sudbury, MA: Jones and Bartlett.

Goldbloom, R. B., & Battista, R. N. (1986). The periodic health examination: 1. Introduction. *Canadian Medical Association Journal, 134,* 721–723.

Goldbloom, R. B., & Lawrence, R. S. (Eds.). (1990). *Preventing disease: Beyond the rhetoric.* New York: Springer-Verlag.

Goldman, L. K., & Glantz, S. A. (1998). Evaluation of antismoking advertising campaigns. *Journal of the American Medical Association, 279,* 772–777.

Goldstein, A. O., Cohen, J. E., & Munger, M. C. (1997). State legislators' attitudes and voting intentions toward tobacco control legislation. *American Journal of Public Health, 87,* 1197–1200.

Goldstein, B., Fischer, P. M., Richards, J. W., Goldstein, A., & Shank, J. C. (1987). Smoking counseling practices of recently trained family physicians. *Journal of Family Practice, 24,* 195–197.

Gomez-Rodriguez, P. (1989). Using the international classification of impairments, disabilities, and handicaps in survey: The case of Spain. *World Health Statistics Quarterly, 42,* 161–166.

Goodman, L. E., & Goodman, M. J. (1986). Prevention: How misuse of a concept can undercut its worth. *Hastings Center Report, 3,* 26–38.

Goodman, R. M., Speers, M. A., McLeroy, K., et al. (1998). Identifying and defining the dimensions of community capacity to provide a basis for measurement. *Health Education and Behavior, 25,* 258–278.

Goodman, R. M., & Steckler, A. B. (1987–1988). The life and death of a health promotion program: An institutionalization case study. *International Quarterly of Community Health Education, 8,* 5–21.

Goodman, R. M., & Steckler, A. (1989a). A framework for assessing program institutionalization. *Knowledge in Society, 2,* 57–71.

Goodman, R. M., & Steckler, A. B. (1989b). A model for the institutionalization of health promotion programs. *Family and Community Health, 11*(4), 63–78.

Goodman, R. M., & Steckler, A. B. (1990). Mobilizing organizations for health enhancement. In K. Glanz, F. M. Lewis, & B. K. Rimer (Eds.), *Health Behavior and Health Education* (pp. 314–41). San Francisco: Jossey-Bass.

Goodman, R. M., Steckler, A., & Alciati, M. H. (1997). A process evaluation of the National Cancer Institute's data-based Intervention Research Program: A study of organizational capacity building. *Health Education Research, 12,* 181–198.

Goodman, R. M., Steckler, A., Hoover, S., & Schwartz, R. (1993). A critique of contemporary community health promotion approaches: Based on qualitative review of six programs in Maine. *American Journal of Health Promotion, 7,* 208–220.

Goodman, R. M., Steckler, A., & Kegler, M. C. (1997). Mobilizing organizations for health enhancement: Theories of organizational change. In K. Glanz, F. M. Lewis, & B. K. Rimer (Eds.), *Health behavior and health education: Theory, research, and practice* (2nd ed., pp. 287–312). San Francisco: Jossey-Bass.

Goodman, R. M., Tenney, M., Smith, D. W., & Steckler, A. (1992). The adoption process for health curriculum innovations in schools: A case study. *Journal of Health Education, 23,* 215–220.

Goodman, R. M., Wandersman, A. (1994). Forecast: A formative approach to evaluating community coalitions and community-based initiatives [Special issue]. *Journal of Community Psychology.*

Goodman, R. M., Wandersman, A., Chinman, M., et al. (1996). An ecological assessment of community based interventions for prevention and health promotion: approaches to measuring community coalitions. *American Journal of Community Psychology, 24*(1), 33–61.

Goodman, R. M., Wheeler, F. C., & Lee, P. R. (1995). Evaluation of the Heart to Heart Project: Lessons from a community-based chronic disease prevention project. *American Journal of Health Promotion, 9,* 443–455.

Gordon, A. J. (1988). Mixed strategies in health education and community participation: An evaluation of dengue control in the Dominican Republic. *Health Education Research Theory and Practice, 3,* 399–419.

Gordon, N. (1986). Never smokers, triers and current smokers: Three distinct target groups for school-based antismoking programs. *Health Education Quarterly, 13,* 163–180.

Gordon, T., Fisher, M., Ernst, N., & Rifkind, B. M. (1982). Relation of diet to LDL cholesterol, VLDL cholesterol, and plasma total cholesterol and triglycerides in white adults: The lipid research clinics prevalence study. *Arteriosclerosis, 2,* 502–512.

Gottlieb, N. H., Eriksen, M. P., & Lovato, C. Y., et al. (1990). Impact of a restrictive work site smoking policy on smoking behavior, attitudes, and norms. *Journal of Occupational Medicine, 32,* 16–23.

Gottlieb, N. H., & Green, L. W. (1984). Life events, social network, life-style, and health: An analysis of the 1979 national survey of personal health practices and consequences. *Health Education Quarterly, 11,* 91–105.

Gottlieb, N. H., & Green, L. W. (1987). Ethnicity and lifestyle health risk: Some possible mechanisms. *American Journal of Health Promotion, 2,* 37–45.

Gottlieb, N. H., Lovato, C. Y., Weinstein, R., Green, L. W., & Eriksen, M. P. (1992). The implementation of a restrictive worksite smoking policy in a large decentralized organization. *Health Education Quarterly, 19,* 77–100.

Gottlieb, N. H., Mullen, P. D., & McAlister, A. L. (1987). Patients' substance abuse and the primary care physician: Patterns of practice. *Addictive Behavior, 12*(1), 23–32.

Gottlieb, N. H., & Nelson, A. (1990). A systematic effort to reduce smoking at the worksite. *Health Education Quarterly, 17,* 99–118.

Gottlieb, N. H., Wright, D., & Sneden, G. G. (1995). Using PRECEDE/PROCEED for linkage implementation planning: Diffusion of the Texas "Top Priority," a worksite health promotion program. Unpublished manuscript. Submitted to *Health Education Quarterly,* March 20, 1995. Not for quotation without permission.

Gottlieb, S. (1986). Ensuring access to health care: What communities can do to make a difference through private sector coalitions. *Inquiry, 23,* 322–329.

Governor of Mississippi. (1980). *Social reconnaissance: State of Mississippi.* Jackson, MS: Office of the Governor.

Graff, W., Pearson, D., LeVan, S., & Sofian, N. (1987). Process evaluation strengthens employee health promotion program at group health cooperative of Puget Sound. In J. P. Opatz (Ed.), *Health promotion evaluation: Measuring the organizational impact.* Stevens Point, WI: University of Wisconsin—Stevens Point Foundation, National Wellness Institute.

Great Britain Expenditures Committee. (1977). *First report from the expenditures committee: Session 1976–1977. Preventive medicine.* London: Her Majesty's Stationery Office.

Green, L. W. (1970a). Identifying and overcoming barriers to the diffusion of knowledge about family planning. *Advances in Fertility Control, 5,* 21–29.

Green, L. W. (1970b). Should health education abandon attitude-change strategies? Perspectives from recent research. *Health Education Monographs, 1*(30), 25–48.

Green, L. W. (1970c). *Status identity and preventive health behavior.* Berkeley, CA: Pacific Health Education Reports No. 1, University of California School of Public Health.

Green, L. W. (1974). Toward cost-benefit evaluations of health education: Some concepts, methods, and examples. *Health Education Monographs, 2*(Suppl. 1), 34–64.

Green, L. W. (1975). Diffusion and adoption of innovations related to cardiovascular risk behavior in the public. In A. Enelow & J. B. Henderson (Eds.), *Applying Behavioral Sciences to Cardiovascular Risk.* New York: American Heart Association.

Green, L. W. (1976a). Change process models in health education. *Public Health Reviews, 5,* 5–33.

Green, L. W. (1976b). Site- and symptom-related factors in secondary prevention of cancer. In J. Cullen, B. Fox, & R. Isom (Eds.), *Cancer: The behavioral dimensions* (pp. 45–61). New York: Raven.

Green, L. W. (1977). Evaluation and measurement: Some dilemmas for health education. *American Journal of Public Health, 67,* 155–161. Reprinted in *Nursing Digest 6:* 65–87, 1978.

Green, L. W. (1978a). Determining the impact and effectiveness of health education as it relates to federal policy. *Health Education Monographs, 6,* 28–66.

Green, L. W. (1978b). The oversimplification of policy issues in prevention. *American Journal of Public Health, 68,* 953–954.

Green, L. W. (1979a). Health promotion policy and the placement of responsibility for personal health care. *Family and Community Health, 2,* 51–64.

Green, L. W. (1979b). National policy in the promotion of health. *International Journal of Health Education, 22,* 161–168.

Green, L. W. (1979c). Toward national policy for health education. In H. Blane & M. E. Chafetz (Eds.), *Alcohol, Youth and Social Policy* (pp. 283–305). New York: Plenum.

Green, L. W. (1980a). Current report: Office of Health Information, Health Promotion and Physical Fitness and Sports Medicine. *Health Education, 11,* 28.

Green, L. W. (1980b). Healthy people: The Surgeon General's report and the prospects. In W. J. McNerney (Ed.), *Working for a Healthier America* (pp. 95–110). Cambridge, MA: Ballinger.

Green, L. W. (1980c). To educate or not to educate: Is that the question? *American Journal of Public Health, 70,* 625–626.

Green, L. W. (1981). Emerging federal perspectives on health promotion. In J. P. Allegrante (Ed.), *Health Promotion Monographs* (1). New York: Teachers College, Columbia University.

Green, L. W. (1982). Reconciling policy in health education and primary health care. *International Journal of Health Education, 24*(Suppl. 3), 1–11.

Green, L. (1983a) Foreword. In: R. S. Gold, *Microcomputer applications in health education* (pp. xv–xvi). Dubuque, IA: Brown. See also Gold, 1991.

Green, L. W. (1983b, April–May). New policies in education for health. *World Health,* pp. 13–17.

Green, L. W. (1983c). A triage and stepped approach to self-care education. *Medical Times, 111,* 75–80.

Green, L. W. (1984a). Health education models. In J. D. Matarazzo et al. (Eds.), *Behavioral Health: A Handbook of Health Enhancement and Disease Prevention* (pp. 181–198). New York: Wiley.

Green, L. W. (1984b). Modifying and developing health behavior. *Annual Review of Public Health, 5,* 215–236.

Green, L. W. (1984c). A participant-observer in a period of professional change. In H. P. Cleary, J. M. Kichen, & P. G. Ensor (Eds.), *Advancing health through education: A case study approach* (pp. 374–381). Palo Alto, CA: Mayfield.

Green, L. W. (1985a). Behavior is an inescapable product, whether we call it an objective or not. *Eta Sigma Gamma Monograph Series, 4,* 37–39.

Green, L. W. (1985b). Some challenges to health services research on children and the elderly. *Health Services Research, 19,* 793–815.

Green, L. W. (1986a). Evaluation model: A framework for the design of rigorous evaluation of efforts in health promotion. *American Journal of Health Promotion, 1*(1), 77–79.

Green, L. W. (1986b). Individuals versus systems: An artificial classification that divides and distorts. *Health Link* (National Center for Health Education), *2,* 29–30.

Green, L. W. (1986c). Health promotion and the elderly: Why do it and where does it lead? A national policy perspective. *Home Health Care Services, 1,* 271–276.

Green, L. W. (1986d). *New policies for health education in primary health care.* Geneva: World Health Organization.

Green, L. W. (1986e). Research agenda: Building a consensus on research questions. *American Journal of Health Promotion, 1*(2), 70–72.

Green, L. W. (1986f). The theory of participation: A qualitative analysis of its expression in national and international health policies. In W. B. Ward (Ed.), *Advances in health education and promotion* (Vol. 1, Pt. A, pp. 211–236). Greenwich, CT: JAI Press.

Green, L. W. (1987a). What physicians can do to increase participation and maintenance of patients in self-care. *Western Journal of Medicine, 147,* 346–349.

Green, L. W. (1987b). *Program planning and evaluation guide for lung associations.* New York: American Lung Association.

Green, L. W. (1987c, August–September). Three ways research influences policy and practice: The public's right to know and the scientist's responsibility to educate. *Health Education, 18,* 44–49.

Green, L. W. (1988a). Bridging the gap between community health and school health. *American Journal of Public Health, 78,* 1149.

Green, L. W. (1988b). Letter to the editor. *Health Education Quarterly, 15,*

Green, L. W. (1988c). Policies for decentralization and development of health education. *Revue Saude Publica* (Sao Paulo, Brazil), *22,* 217–220.

Green, L. W. (1988d). Promoting the one-child policy in China. *Journal of Public Health Policy, 9,* 273–283.

Green, L. W. (1988e). The trade-offs between the expediency of health promotion and the durability of health education. In S. Maes, C. D. Spielberger, P. B. Defares, & I. G. Sarason (Eds.), *Topics in Health Psychology* (pp. 301–312). New York: Wiley.

Green, L. W. (1989). Comment: Is institutionalization the proper goal of grantmaking? *American Journal of Health Promotion, 3,* 44.

Green, L. W. (1990). The revival of community and the public obligation of academic health centers. In R. E. Bulger & S. J. Reiser (Eds.), *Integrity in health care institutions: Humane environments for teaching, inquiry and healing* (pp. 148–164). Des Moines: University of Iowa Press.

Green, L. W. (1991). Preface. In *Healthy people 2000: National health promotion and disease prevention objectives* (pp. vii–xi). Boston, MA: Jones and Bartlett.

Green, L. W. (1992a). The health promotion research agenda revisited. *American Journal of Health Promotion, 6,* 411–413.

Green, L. W. (1992b). [Review of the book *Free to be Foolish: Politics and Health Promotion in the United States and Britain*]. *Policy Currents* (American Political Science Association), *2*(4),16–17.

Green, L. W. (1993). Modifying lifestyle to improve health. In W. D. Skelton & M. Osterweis (Eds.), *Promoting Community Health: The Role of the Academic Health Center* (pp. 54–69). Washington, DC: Association of Academic Health Centers.

Green, L. W. (1994a). Canadian health promotion: An outsider's view from the inside. In A. Pederson, M. O'Neill, & I. Rootman (Eds.), *Health promotion in Canada: Provincial, national and international perspectives* (pp. 314-326). Toronto: W. B. Saunders Canada.

Green, L. W. (1994b). Refocusing health care systems to address both individual care and population health. *Clinical and Investigative Medicine, 17,* 133–141.

Green, L. W. (1995). Commentary. In *Healthy people 2000 mid-decade review and revised objectives.* Boston: Jones and Bartlett.

Green, L. W. (1997a). Commentary: Community health promotion: Applying the science of evaluation to the initial sprint of a marathon. *American Journal of Preventive Medicine, 13*(4), 225–228.

Green, L. W. (1997b). Editorial: Taxes and the tobacco wars. *Canadian Medical Association Journal, 156*(2), 205–206.

Green, L. W. (1997c) *First John P. McGovern Award lecture.* Houston: University of Texas Health Science Center at Houston, Center for Health Promotion Research and Development.

Green, L. W. (1998a). Keynote address at the National Public Health Education Leadership Institute, San Antonio, TX.

Green, L. W. (1998b). Prevention and health education in clinical, school, and community settings. In R. B. Wallace (Ed.), *Maxcy-Rosenau-Last preventive medicine and public health* (14th ed., pp. 889-904). Stamford, CT: Appleton & Lange.

Green, L. W. (in press) "Health education's contributions to public health in the twentieth century: A glimpse through health promotion's rear-view mirror." *Annual Review of Public Health, 21.*

Green, L. W., Blakenbaker, R., Trevino, F., et al. (1987). Report of the subcommittee on data gaps in disease prevention and health promotion. In *Annual Report of the U.S. National Committee on Vital and Health Statistics.* Washington, DC: National Center for Health Statistics.

Green, L. W., & Brooks-Bertram, P. (1978). Peer review and quality control in health education. *Health Values, 2,* 191–197.

Green, L. W., & Cargo, M. (1994). The changing context of health promotion in the workplace. In M. P. O'Donnell & J. S. Harris (Eds.), *Health Promotion in the Workplace* (2nd ed., pp. 497–524). Albany, NY: Delmar Publishers.

Green, L. W., Cargo, M., & Ottoson, J. M. (1994). The role of physicians in supporting lifestyle changes. *Medicine, Exercise, Nutrition and Health, 3,* 119–130.

Green, L. W., Costagliola, D ., & Chwalow, A. J. (1991). Diagnostic éducatif et évaluation de stratégies éducatives (modèle PRECEDE): Méthodology pratique pour induire des changements de comportements et d'état de santé. *Journées Annuelles de Diabétologie de l'Hotel Dieu* (Paris: Flammarion Médecine-Sciences), pp. 227–240.

Green, L. W., Eriksen, M. P., & Schor, E. L. (1988). Preventive practices by physicians: Behavioral determinants and potential interventions. *American Journal of Preventive Medicine, 4*(Suppl. 4), 101–107. Reprinted in R. N. Battista & R. S. Lawrence (Eds.), *Implementing preventive services* (pp. 101–107). New York: Oxford University Press.

Green, L. W., & Faden, R. (1977). Potential impact of patient package inserts on patients and drug consumers. *Drug Information Journal, 2*(Suppl.), 64–70.

Green, L. W., & Fedder, D. (1977). Drug information: The pharmacist and the community. *American Journal of Pharmaceutical Education, 41,* 444–448.

Green, L. W., & Figa-Talamanca, I. (1974). Suggested designs for evaluation of patient education programs. *Health Education Monographs, 2,* 54–71.

Green, L. W., Fisher, A., Amin, R., & Shafiullah, A. B. M. (1975). Paths to the adoption of family planning: A time-lagged correlation analysis of the Dacca experiment in Bangladesh. *International Journal of Health Education, 18,* 85–96.

Green, L. W., & Frankish, C. J. (1994). Theories and principles of health education applied to asthma. *Chest, 106*(Suppl.), 195–205.

Green, L. W., & Frankish, C. J. (1996). Implementing nutritional science for population health: Decentralized and centralized planning for health promotion and disease prevention. In *Beyond nutritional recommendations: Implementing science for healthier populations.* Ithaca, NY: Cornell University.

Green, L. W., George, A., Daniel, M., et al. (1995). *Study of participatory research in health promotion.* Ottawa, Royal Society of Canada.

Green, L. W., Glanz, K., Hochbaum, G. M., et al. (1994). Can we build on, or must we replace, the theories and models in health education? *Health Education Research, 9,* 397–404.

Green, L. W., Gold, R. S., Tan, J. K. H., & Kreuter, M. W. (1994, November–December). The EMPOWER/Canadian Health Expert System. *Revue Canadienne d'Informatique Médicale,* pp. 20–23.

Green, L. W., Goldstein, R. A., & Parker, S. R. (Eds.). (1983). Research on self-management of childhood asthma. *Journal of Allergy and Clinical Immunology, 72,* 519–629.

Green, L. W., & Gordon, N. P. (1982, May–June). Productive research designs for health education investigations. *Health Education, 13,* 4–10.

Green, L. W., Gottlieb, N. H., & Parcel, G. S. (1991). Diffusion theory extended and applied. In W. Ward & F. M. Lewis (Eds.), *Advances in health education and promotion* (Vol. 3, pp. 91–117). London: Jessica Kingsley.

Green, L. W., Heit, P., Iverson, D. C., Kolbe, L. J., & Kreuter, M. (1980). The School Health Curriculum Project: Its theory, practice, and measurement experience. *Health Education Quarterly, 7,* 14–34.

Green, L. W., & Johnson, J. L. (1996). Dissemination and utilization of health promotion and disease prevention knowledge: Theory, research and experience. *Canadian Journal of Public Health, 87*(Suppl. 1), S17–S23.

Green, L. W., & Kansler, C. (1980). *The scientific and professional literature on patient education.* Detroit: Gale Information Service.

Green, L. W., & Kreuter, M. W. (1990). Health promotion as a public health strategy for the 1990s. *Annual Review of Public Health, 11,* 319–334.

Green, L. W., & Kreuter, M. W. (1991). *Health promotion planning: An educational and environmental approach* (2nd ed.). Mountain View, CA: Mayfield.

Green, L. W., & Kreuter, M. W. (1993). Are community organization and health promotion one process or two? *American Journal of Health Promotion, 7,* 221.

Green, L. W., Kreuter, M. W., Deeds, S. G., & Partridge, K. B. (1980). *Health education planning: A diagnostic approach.* Palo Alto, CA: Mayfield.

Green, L. W., & Krotki, K. J. (1968). Class and parity biases in family planning programs: The case of Karachi. *Social Biology, 15,* 235–251.

Green, L. W., Levine, D. M., & Deeds, S. G. (1975). Clinical trials of health education for hypertensive outpatients: Design and baseline data. *Preventive Medicine, 4,* 417–425.

Green, L. W., Levine, D. M., & Deeds, S. G. (1977, May 22). *Health education and control of hypertension.* Paper presented at the American Federation for Clinical Research, Washington, DC.

Green, L. W., Levine, D. M., Wolle, J., & Deeds, S. G. (1979). Development of randomized patient education experiments with urban poor hypertensives. *Patient Counseling and Health Education, 1,* 106–111.

Green, L. W., & Lewis, F. M. (1986). *Measurement and evaluation in health education and health promotion.* Palo Alto, CA: Mayfield.

Green, L. W., Lewis, F. M., & Levine, D. M. (1980). Balancing statistical data and clinician judgments in the diagnosis of patient educational needs. *Journal of Community Health, 6,* 79–91.

Green, L. W., & McAlister, A. L. (1984). Macro-intervention to support health behavior: Some theoretical perspectives and practical reflections. *Health Education Quarterly, 11,* 323–339.

Green, L. W., Mullen, P. D., & Friedman, R. (1986). An epidemiological approach to targeting drug information. *Patient Education and Counseling, 8,* 255–268. Reprinted as Chapter 29 in J. A. Cramer & B. Spilker (Eds.). (1991). *Patient compliance in medical practice and clinical trials* (pp. 373–386). New York: Raven.

Green, L. W., Mullen, P. D., & Maloney, S. (Eds.). (1984). Large-scale campaigns in health education. *Health Education Quarterly, 11,* 221–339.

Green, L. W., Mullen, P. D., & Stainbrook, G. L. (1986). Programs to reduce drug errors in the elderly: Direct and indirect evidence from patient education. *Journal of Geriatric Drug Therapy, 1,* 3–16.

Green, L. W., & Ottoson, J. M. (1999). *Community and population health* (8th ed.). Boston: WCB/McGraw-Hill.

Green, L. W., Potvin, L., & Richard, L. (1996). Ecological foundations of health promotion. *American Journal of Health Promotion, 10,* 270–281.

Green, L. W., & Raeburn, J. (1988). Health promotion: What is it? What will it become? *Health Promotion International, 3,* 151–159. Revised and reprinted as L. W. Green & J. Raeburn (1990). Contemporary developments in health promotion: Definitions and challenges. In N. Bracht (Ed.), *Health promotion at the community level* (pp. 29–44). Newbury Park, CA: Sage.

Green, L. W., Rimer, B., & Bertera, R. (1978). How cost-effective are smoking cessation strategies? *World Smoking and Health, 3,* 33–40.

Green, L. W., Rimer, B., & Elwood, T. W. (1981). Biobehavioral approaches to cancer prevention and detection. In S. Weiss, A. Herd, & B. Fox (Eds.), *Perspectives on Behavioral Medicine* (pp. 215–234). New York: Academic Press.

Green, L. W., Rimer, B., & Elwood, T. W. (1982). Public education. In D. Shottenfeld & J. Fraumeni, Jr. (Eds.), *Cancer Epidemiology and Prevention* (pp. 1100–1110). Philadelphia: Saunders.

Green, L. W., & Roberts, B. J. (1974). The research literature on why women delay in seeking medical care for breast symptoms. *Health Education Monographs, 2,* 129–177.

Green, L. W., & Simons-Morton, D. (1988). Denial, delay and disappointment: Discovering and overcoming the causes of drug errors and missed appointments. In D. Schmidt & I. E. Leppik (Eds.), *Compliance in epilepsy (Epilepsy Research,* Suppl. 1, pp. 7–21). Amsterdam: Elsevier Science Publishers B.V.

Green, L. W., & Simons-Morton, D., & Potvin, L. (1997). Education and lifestyle determinants of health and disease. In R. Detels, W. W. Holland, J. McEwen, & G. S. Omenn (Eds.), *Oxford textbook of public health* (2nd ed., pp. 181–195). London: Oxford University Press.

Green, L. W., Simons-Morton, D. G., & Potvin, L. (1997). Education and life-style determinants of health and disease. In R. Detels, W. W. Holland, J. McEwen, & G. S. Omenn (Eds.), *Oxford Textbook of Public Health* (3rd ed. Vol. 1, pp. 125–139). Oxford: Oxford University Press.

Green, L. W., Tan, J., Gold, R. S., & Kreuter, M. W. (1994, November–December). EMPOWER/Canadian health expert system: The application of artificial intelligence and expert system technology to community health program planning and evaluation. *Canadian Medical Informatics,* pp. 20–23.

Green, L. W., Wang, V. L., Deeds, S. G., et al. (1978). Guidelines for health education in maternal and child health programs. *International Journal of Health Education, 21*(Suppl.), 1–33.

Green, L. W., Wang, V. L., & Ephross, P. (1974). A three-year longitudinal study of the effectiveness of nutrition aides on rural poor homemakers. *American Journal of Public Health, 64,* 722–724.

Green, L. W., Werlin, S. H., Shauffler, H. H., & Avery, C. H. (1977). Research and demonstration issues in self-care: Measuring the decline of medicocentrism. *Health Education Monographs, 5,* 161–189. Also in J. G. Zapka (Ed.). (1981). *The SOPHE Heritage Collection of Health Education Monographs* (Vol. 3, pp. 40–69). Oakland, CA: Third Party Publishing.

Green, L. W., Wilson, A. L., & Lovato, C. Y. (1986). What changes can health promotion achieve and how long do these changes last? The tradeoffs between expediency and durability. *Preventive Medicine, 15,* 508–521.

Green, L. W., Wilson, R. W., & Bauer, K. G. (1983). Data required to measure progress on the objectives for the nation in disease prevention and health promotion. *American Journal of Public Health, 73,* 18–24.

Greenberg, J. S. (1987). *Health education: Learner centered instructional strategies.* Dubuque, IA: Brown.

Gregor, F. M. (1984). Factors affecting the use of self-instructional material by patients with ischemic heart disease. *Patient Education and Counseling, 6,* 155–159.

Griffiths, W., & Knutson, A. L. (1960). The role of mass media in public health. *American Journal of Public Health, 50,* 515–523.

Gritz, E. R., Nielsen, I. R., & Brooks, L. A. (1996). Smoking cessation and gender: The influence of physiological, psychological, and behavioral factors. *Journal of the American Medical Women's Association, 51,* 35–42.

Grueninger, U. J. (1995). Arterial hypertension: Lessons from patient education. *Patient Education and Counseling, 26,* 37–55.

Grueninger, U. J., Duffy, F. D., & Goldstein, M. G. (1995). Patient education in the medical encounter: How to facilitate learning, behavior change, and coping. In M. Lipkin, Jr., S. M. Putnam, & A. Lazare (Eds.), *The medical interview: Clinical care, education, and research* (pp. 122–133). Bern: Mack Lipkin, Jr., MD.

Grundy, S. M., Greenland, P., Herd, J. A., et al. (1987). Cardiovascular and risk factor evaluation of healthy american adults: A statement for physicians by an ad hoc committee appointed by the steering committee, American Heart Association. *Circulation, 97,* 1340A–1362A.

Grenier, K., & Grenier, J. (1996). Comprehension des allegations alimentaires par des etudiants du premier cycle universitaire. *Canadian Journal of Public Health, 87,* 351–353.

Grunbaum, J. A., Gingiss, P., & Parcel, G. S. (1995). A comprehensive approach to school health program needs assessments. *Journal of School Health, 65,* 54–59.

Guba, E. G., & Lincoln, Y. S. (1989). *Fourth generation evaluation.* Newbury Park, CA: Sage.

Guidance for conducting policy and programme evaluation in WHO: Why, what, how, when? (1997). Geneva: World Health Organization, PPE/97.3.

Guidelines for school health programs promote lifelong healthy eating. (1996). *Morbidity and Mortality Weekly Report, 45*(RR-9), 1–42.

Guidelines on school health programs to prevent tobacco use and addiction. (1994). *Journal of School Health, 64,* 353–360.

Guild, P. A. (1990). Goal-oriented evaluation as a program management tool. *American Journal of Health Promotion, 4,* 296–301.

Gupta, M. C., Mehrotra, M., Arora, S., Saran, M. (1991). Relation of childhood malnutrition to parental education and mother's nutrition related KAP. *Indian Journal of Pediatrics, 58*(2), 269–274.

Gustafson, D. (1979). *An approach to predicting the implementation potential of recommended actions in health planning.* Madison, WI: Institute for Health Planning.

Gustafson, D. H., Bosworth, K., Hawkins, R. P., et al. (1992). CHESS: A computer-based system for providing information, referrals, decision support and social support to people facing medical and other health-related crises. *Proceedings of the Annual Symposium of Computer Applications in Medical Care,* 161–165.

Guttmacher, S. L., Lieberman, D., Ward, N., et al. (1997). Condom availability in New York City public high schools: Relationships to condom use and sexual behavior. *American Journal of Public Health, 87,* 1427–1433.

Haber, D. (1994). Medical screenings and health assessments. In D. Hader (Ed.), *Health promotion and aging* (pp.41–76). New York: Springer.

Haefele, D. L. (1990). A survey of non-smoking policies in ninety-one large businesses, companies and agencies. *Health Education, 21*(4), 47–53.

Haglund, B. (1992). *We can do it! The Sundsvall handbook.* Stockholm: Karalinska Institute.

Hahn, E. J., Simpson, M. R., & Kidd, P. (1996). Cues to parent involvement in drug prevention and school activities. *Journal of School Health, 66,* 165–170.

Hall, J. A., Roter, D. L., & Katz, N. R. (1988). Meta-analysis of correlates of provider behavior in medical encounters. *Medical Care, 26,* 657–675.

Hamilton, N., & Bhatti, T. (1996). *Population health promotion: An integrated model of population health and health promotion.* Ottawa: Health Promotion Division, Health Canada.

Hammersley, M., & Atkinson, P. (1995). *Ethnography: Principles in practice.* London: Routlege.

Hammond, E. C., & Garfinkel, L. (1969). Coronary heart disease, stroke, and aortic aneurysm: Factors in the etiology. *Archives of Environmental Health, 19,* 167–182.

Han, Y., Baumann, L. C., & Cimprich, B. (1996). Factors influencing registered nurses teaching breast self-examination to female clients. *Cancer Nursing, 19,* 197–203.

Hancock, L., Reid, A., & Walsh, R. (1997). Community action for health promotion: A review of methods and outcomes 1990–1995. *American Journal of Preventive Medicine, 13,* 229–239.

Hancock, L., Sanson-Fisher, R. W., Redman, S., et al. (1997). Community action for health promotion: A review of methods and outcomes 1990–1995. *American Journal of Preventive Medicine, 13,* 229–239.

Hancock, T. (1985). Beyond health care: From public health policy to healthy public policy. *Canadian Journal of Public Health, 76,* 9–11.

Handbook for evaluating drug abuse and alcohol prevention programs. (1987). Rockville, MD: Office of Substance Abuse Prevention, U.S. Department of Health and Human Services, DHHS (ADM) 87-1512.

Handel, G., & Rainwater. L. (1964). Persistence and change in working-class life style. In A. B. Shostack & W. Gomberg (Eds.), *Blue-collar world* (pp. 36–41). Englewood Cliffs, NJ: Prentice-Hall.

Hankin, J. R. (1994). FAS prevention strategies: Passive and active measures. *Alcohol Health and Research World, 18,* 62–66.

Hannaway, D. B., Shuler, P. E., Bolte, J. P., & Miller, M. J. (1992). Development and evaluation of LEGUME ID: A ToolBook multimedia module. *Journal of Natural Resources in Life Science Education, 21*(1), 57–61.

Hanson, P. (1988–89). Citizen involvement in community health promotion: A rural application of CDC's PATCH model. *International Quarterly of Health Education, 9,* 177–186.

Hardin, G. (1968). The tragedy of the commons. *Science, 143,* 1243–1246.

Hargrove, E. (1975). *The missing link: The study of the implementation of social policy.* Washington, DC: The Urban Institute, paper 797-1.

Harris, M., & Wise, M. (1996). Can goals and targets set a radical agenda? *Health Promotion International, 11,* 63–64.

Harrison, J. A., Mullen, P. D., & Green, L. W. (1992). A meta-analysis of studies of the Health Belief Model. *Health Education Research, 7,* 107–116.

Harrison, M. I. (1987). *Diagnosing organizations: Methods, models, and processes.* Beverly Hills, CA: Sage.

Harvey, D. (1990). *The condition of post-modernity.* Cambridge, MA: Blackwell.

Haskell, W. L., & Blair, S. N. (1982). The physical activity component of health promotion in occupational settings. In R. S. Parkinson et al. (Eds.), *Managing Health Promotion in the Workplace: Guidelines for Implementation and Evaluation* (pp. 252–271). Palo Alto, CA: Mayfield.

Hatch, J. W., & Jackson, C. (1981). The North Carolina Baptist Church program. *Urban Health, 10*(4), 70–71.

Hatcher, M. E., Green, L. W., Levine, D. M., & Flagle, C. E. (1986). Validation of a decision model for triaging hypertensive patients to alternate health education interventions. *Social Science and Medicine, 22,* 813–819.

Haughton, B. (1987). Developing local food policies: One city's experiences. *Journal of Public Health Policy, 8,* 180–191.

Hausman, A. J., & Ruzek, S. B. (1995). Implementation of comprehensive school health education in elementary schools: Focus on teacher concerns. *Journal of School Health, 65,* 81–86.

Hawe, P. (1996). Needs assessment must become more change focused. *Australian and New Zealand Journal of Public Health, 20,* 473–478.

Hawe, P., Degeling, D., & Hall, J. (1990). *Evaluating health promotion: A health worker's guide.* Sydney: MacLennon and Petty.

Hawe, P., Noort, M., King, L., & Jordens, C. (1997). Multiplying health gains: The critical role of capacity-building within health promotion programs. *Health Policy, 39,* 29–42.

Hawe, P., & Shiell, A. (1995). Preserving innovation under increasing accountability pressures: The health promotion investment portfolio approach. *Health Promotion Journal of Australia, 5,* 4–9.

Hawkins, R. P., Gustafson, D.H., Chewning, B., et al (1987). Reaching hard-to-reach populations: Interactive computer programs as public information campaigns for adolescents. *Journal of Communication, 37,* 8–28.

Hawthorne, V. M., Pohl, G., & Amburg, G. V. (1984, November). *Smoking is killing your constituents: Deaths due to smoking by Michigan State senate districts.* Lansing: Division of Health Education, Michigan Department of Public Health.

Hayes, M. V., & Manson Willms, S. (1990). Healthy community indicators: The perils of the search and the paucity of the find. *Health Promotion International, 5,* 161–166.

Haynes, R. B., Davis, D. A., McKibbon, A., & Tugwell, A. P. (1984). A critical appraisal of the efficacy of continuing medical education. *Journal of the American Medical Association, 251,* 61–64.

Haynes, R. B., Taylor, D. W., & Sackett, D. L. (Eds.). (1979). *Compliance in health care.* Baltimore: Johns Hopkins University Press.

Hayward, R. S. A., Steinberg, E. P., Ford, D. E., Roizen, M. F., & Roach, K. W. (1991). Preventive care guidelines: 1991. *Annals of Internal Medicine, 114,* 758–783.

Health and Welfare Canada. (1992a). *Health promotion in the workplace: A sampling of company programs and initiatives.* Ottawa: Minister of Supply and Services.

Health and Welfare Canada. (1992b). *National Health Promotion Survey of 1990: Preliminary results.* Unpublished.

Health and Welfare Canada. (1992c). Research update: Hospital nurses and health promotion. *Health Promotion, 31*(1), 16. Also in Jenny, 1993, p. 1411.

Health and Welfare Canada. (1993). *Canada's Health Promotion Survey 1990: Technical Report,* T. Stephens & D. Fowler Graham (Eds.). Ottawa: Minister of Supply and Services Canada, H39-263/2.

Health Canada. (1998, March). Cervical cancer in Canada. *Cancer Updates,* Cancer Bureau, Laboratory Centre for Disease Control, Health Protection Branch. Web site: http://www.hc-sc.gc.ca/hpb/lcdc/bc

Health Education Center. (1977). *Strategies for health education in local health departments.* Baltimore: Maryland State Department of Health and Mental Hygiene.

Health Education Unit, Regional Office of Education, WHO Regional Office for Europe. (1986). Lifestyles and health. *Social Science and Medicine, 22,* 117–124.

Health promotion: A discussion document on the concept and principles. (1984, September). Copenhagen: World Health Organization Regional Office for Europe, ICP/HSR 602. Reprinted in (1986) *Health Promotion, 1,* 73–76.

Health Promotion: Ottawa Charter. (1998). Geneva: World Health Organization, Division of Health Promotion, Education and Communication. [Reprinted from the First International Conference on Health Promotion, Ottawa, November 1986.]

Healthy communities 2000: Model standards. (1991). (3rd ed.). Washington, DC: American Public Health Association.

Healthy people 2000. See U.S. Department of Health and Human Services, 1991.

Healthy Public Policy: 2nd International Conference on Health Promotion, Adelaide, Australia. (1988).

Heath, R. P. (1996). The frontiers of psychographics. *American Demographics, 18,* 38–47.

Helmer, D. C., Dunn, L. M., & Lubritz, L. (1995). Implementing corporate wellness programs: A business approach to program planning. *AAOHN Journal, 43,* 558-563.

Henderson, A. C. (1987). Developing a credentialing system for health educators. In W. B. Ward & S. K. Simonds (Eds.), *Advances in Health Education and Health Promotion* (Vol. 2, pp. 59–91). Greenwich, CT: JAI Press.

Henderson, A. C., Wolle, J. M., Cortese, P. A., & McIntosh, D. I. (1981). The future of the health education profession: Implications for preparation and practice. *Public Health Reports, 96,* 555–560.

Hendricson, W. D., Wood, P. R., & Parcel, G. (1996). Implementation of individualized patient education for Hispanic children with asthma. *Patient Education and Counseling, 26,* 155–166.

Henningson, K. A., Gold, R. S., & Duncan, D. F. (1986). A computerized marijuana decision maze: Expert opinion regarding its use in health education. *Journal of Drug Education, 16*(3), 243–261.

Henritze, J., Brammell, H. L., & McGloin, J. (1992). LIFECHECK: A successful, low touch, low tech, in-plant, cardiovascular disease risk identification and modification program. *American Journal of Health Promotion, 7,* 129–136.

Herbert, C. P., & Paluck, E. (1997). Can primary care physicians be a resource to their patients in decisions regarding alternative and complementary therapies for cancer? *Patient Education and Counseling, 31,* 179–180.

Hermann, D. S., & McWhirter, J. J. (1997). Refusal and resistance skills for children and adolescents: A selected review. *Journal of Counseling and Development, 75,* 177–187.

Hersey, J. C., Klibanoff, L. S., Lam, D. J., & Taylor, R. L. (1984). Promoting social support: The impact of California's "Friends Can Be Good Medicine" campaign. *Health Education Quarterly, 11,* 293–311.

Hertel, V. (1982). Changing times in school nursing. *Journal of School Health, 52,* 313–314.

Hertzman, C., Frank, J., & Evans, R. G. (1994). Heterogeneities in health status and the determinants of population health. In R. G. Evans, M. L. Barer, & T. R. Marmor (Eds.), *Why are some people healthy and others not?* (pp. 67–92). New York: Aldine de Gruyter.

Heywood, A., Firman, D., Sanson-Fisher, R., & Mudge, P. (1996). Correlates of physician counseling associated with obesity and smoking. *Preventive Medicine, 25,* 268–276.

Hiatt, R. A., Pasick, R. J., Perez-Stable, E. J., et al. (1996). Pathways to early cancer detection in the multiethnic population of the San Francisco Bay Area. *Health Education Quarterly 23*(Suppl.), S10–S27.

Hiddink, G. J., Hautvast, J. G. A. J., van Woerkum, C. M. J., Fieren, C. J., & van't Hof, M. A. (1995). Nutrition guidance by primary-care physicians: Perceived barriers and low involvement. *European Journal of Clinical Nutrition, 49,* 842–851.

Hiddink, G. J., Hautvast, J. G. A. J., van Woerkum, C. E. J., Fieren, C. J., & van't Hof, M. A. (1997a). Nutrition guidance by primary-care physicians: LISREL analysis improves understanding. *Preventive Medicine, 26,* 29–36.

Hiddink, G. J., Hautvast, J. G. A. J., van Woerkum, C. E. J., Fieren, C. J., & van't Hof, M. A. (1997b). Driving forces for and barriers to nutrition guidance practices of Dutch primary care physicians. *Journal of Nutrition Education, 29,* 36–41.

Higgins, J. W., & MacDonald, M. (1992*). The School-Based Prevention Model: A training handbook. Prepared for the Alcohol and Drug Programs,* British Columbia Ministry of Health, by M. A. MacDonald and Associates, Victoria, BC.

Hill, A. J. (1996). Predictors of regular physical activity in participants of a Canadian health promotion program. *Canadian Journal of Nursing Research, 28,* 119–141.

Hill, I. T. (1988). *Reaching women who need prenatal care.* Washington, DC: National Governors' Association.

Hindi-Alexander, M., & Cropp, G. J. (1981). Community and family programs for children with asthma. *Annals of Allergy, 46,* 143–148.

Hingson, R., McGovern, T., Howland, J., et al. (1996). Reducing alcohol-impaired driving in Massachusetts: The Saving Lives Program. *American Journal of Public Health, 86,* 791–797.

Hinthorne, R. A., & Jones, R. (1978). Coordinating patient education in the hospital. *Hospitals, 52,* 85–88.

Hoagwood, K. (1995). Issues in designing and implementing studies of non-mental health care sectors. *Journal of Clinical Child Psychology, 23,* 114–120.

Hochbaum, G. M. (1956). Why people seek diagnostic X-rays. *Public Health Reports, 71,* 377–380.

Hochbaum, G. M. (1959). *Public participation in medical screening programs: A social-psychological study.* Washington, DC: Public Health Service, PHS-572.

Hochbaum, G. M., Conley, V., Green, L. W., et al. (1986). Health education and cancer control in the workplace. In *American Public Health Association 114th Annual Meeting abstracts,* Las Vegas, p. 161.

Hoffman, L. M. (1989). *The politics of knowledge: Activist movements in medicine and planning.* Albany: State University of New York Press.

Hoffman, S. B. (1983). Peer counselor training with the elderly. *Gerontologist, 23,* 358–360.

Hofford, C. W., & Spelman, K. A. (1996). The community action plan: Incorporating health promotion and wellness into alcohol, tobacco and other drug abuse prevention efforts on the college campus. *Journal of Wellness Perspectives, 12(2),* 70–79.

Hollander, R. B., & Hale, J. G. (1987). Worksite health promotion programs: Ethical issues. *American Journal of Health Promotion, 2*(2), 37–43.

Holloway, A. (1996). Patient knowledge and information concerning medication on discharge from hospital. *Journal of Advanced Nursing, 24,* 1169–1174.

Holmes, S., Morrow, A., & Pickering, L. (1996). Child-care practices: Effects of social change on the epidemiology of infectious diseases and antibiotic resistance. *Epidemiologic Reviews, 18,* 10–28.

Holtzman, N. (1979). Prevention: Rhetoric or reality. *International Journal of Health Services, 9,* 25–39.

Honig, D. B., & Gillespie, B. K. (1995). Drug interactions between prescribed and over-the-counter medication. *Drug Safety, 13,* 296–303.

Hoover, S., & Schwartz, R. (1992). Diffusing PATCH through interagency collaboration. *Journal of Health Education, 23,* 160–163.

House, J. S. (1981). *Work stress and social support.* Reading, MA: Addison-Wesley.

Hovland, C., Janis, I. L., & Kelley, H. H. (1953). *Communication and persuasion.* New Haven, CT: Yale University Press.

Howland, J. S., Baker, M. G., & Poe, T. (1990). Does patient education cause side effects? A controlled trial. *Journal of Family Practice, 31,* 62–64.

Howse, J. D. (1991). *Lessons learned from the Babies and You Program.* White Plains, NY: March of Dimes Birth Defects Foundation.

Hu, J. C. (1990). Hobbies of retired people in the People's Republic of China: A preliminary study. *International Journal of Aging and Human Development, 31,* 31–44.

Huang, Y. W., Green, L. W., & Darling, L. F. (1997, July). Moral education and health education for elementary school and preschool children in Canada. *Journal of the National School Health Association* [Taiwan], *30,* 23–35.

Hubball, H. (1996). *Development and evaluation of a worksite health promotion program: Application of critical self-directed learning for exercise behaviour change.* Unpublished doctoral dissertation. University of British Columbia, Vancouver.

Hubbard, L., & Ottoson, J. M. (1997). When a bottom-up innovation meets itself as a top-down policy: The AVID untracking program. *Science Communication, 19,* 41–55.

Huberman, A. M., & Miles, M. B. (1984). *Innovation up close: How school improvement works.* New York: Plenum.

Hunnicutt, D. M., Perry-Hunnicutt, C., Newman, I. M., Davis, J. L., & Crawford, J. (1993). Use of the Delphi Technique to support a comprehensive campus alcohol abuse initiative. *Journal of Health Education, 24,* 88–96.

Hunt, M. K., Lefebvre, C., Hixson, M. L., et al. (1990). Pawtucket Heart Health Program point-of-purchase nutrition education program in supermarkets. *American Journal of Public Health, 80,* 730–731.

Imanaka, Y., Araki, S., & Nobutomo, K. (1993). Effects of patient health beliefs and satisfaction on compliance with medication regimens in ambulatory care at general hospitals. *Japanese Journal of Hygiene, 48,* 601–611.

Ingledew, D. (1989). Target setting for the health of populations: Some observations. *Health Promotion, 4,* 357–369.

Institute of Medicine. (1983). *Medical education and societal needs: A planning report for the health professions.* Washington, DC: National Academy Press.

Institute of Medicine. (1997). *Schools and health: Our nation's investment.* Washington, DC: National Academy Press.

Integration of risk factor interventions. (1986). Washington, DC: ODPHP Monograph Series, U.S. Department of Health and Human Services.

Inui, T. S., Carter, W. B., Pecoraro, R. E., et al. (1980). Variations in patient compliance with common long-term drugs. *Medical Care, 17,* 986–993.

IOX Assessment Associates. (1988). *Program evaluation handbook: Diabetes education, drug abuse education, nutrition education, alcohol abuse education, physical fitness programs, stress management.* Los Angeles, CA: IOX Assessment Associates.

Israel, B. A. (1985). Social networks and social support: Implications for natural helper and community level interventions. *Health Education Quarterly, 12,* 65–80.

Israel, B. A., Schulz, A. J., Parker, E. A., & Becker, A. B. (1998). Review of community-based research: Assessing partnership approaches to improve public health. *Annual Review of Public Health, 19,* 173–202.

Iverson, D. C., Fielding, J. E., Crow, R. S., & Christenson, G. M. (1985). The promotion of physical activity in the United States population: The status of programs in medical, worksite, community, and school settings. *Public Health Reports, 100,* 212–224.

Iverson, D. C., & Green, L. W. (1981). Drug abuse prevention from a public health perspective: A proposal for the 1980s. In W. Bukowski (Ed.), *NIDA Drug Abuse Prevention Monograph.* Washington, DC: National Institute of Drug Abuse.

Iverson, D. C., & Kolbe, L. J. (1983). Evaluation of the national disease prevention and health promotion strategy: Establishing a role for the schools. *Journal of School Health, 53,* 294–302.

Iverson, D. C., & Scheer, J. K. (1982). School-based cancer education programs: An opportunity to affect the national cancer problem. *Health Values: Achieving High Level Wellness, 6(3),* 27–35.

Jaccard, J. (1975). A theoretical analysis of selected factors important to health education strategies. *Health Education Monographs, 3,* 152–167.

Jacobs, C., Ross, R., Walker, I. M., et al. (1983). Behavior of cancer patients: A randomized study of the effects of education and peer support groups. *American Journal of Clinical Oncology, 6,* 347–350.

Jaffe, J. M. (1997). Media interactivity and self-efficacy: An examination of hypermedia first aid instruction. *Journal of Health Communication, 2,* 235–252.

The Jakarta declaration on leading health promotion into the 21st century. (1997). Geneva: World Health Organization, WHO/HPR/HEP/41CHP/BR/97.4, 1997).

Janz, N. K., & Becker, M. H. (1984). The Health Belief Model: A decade later. *Health Education Quarterly, 11,* 1–47.

Jasnoski, M. L., & Schwartz, G. E. (1985). A synchronous systems model for health. *American Behavioral Scientist, 28,* 468–485.

Jason, L. A., Jayaraj, S., Blitz, C. C., et al. (1990). Incentives and competition in a worksite smoking cessation intervention. *American Journal of Public Health, 80,* 205–206.

Jeffery, B. (1998). *Gender and socioeconomic interactions with perceptions of health.* Unpublished doctoral dissertation. Vancouver, BC: University of British Columbia.

Jenkins, C. D. (1979). An approach to the diagnosis and treatment of problems of health-related behavior. *International Journal of Health Education, 22*(Suppl.), 1–24.

Jenny, J. (1993). A future perspective on patient/health education in Canada. *Journal of Advanced Nursing, 18,* 1408–1414.

Jensen, K. L. (1997). *Lesbian and bisexual epiphanies: Identity deconstruction and reconstruction.* Unpublished doctoral dissertation. Cincinnati, OH: Union Institute Graduate School. (Also in press: Haworth).

Jette, A. M. (1993). Using health related quality of life measures in physical therapy outcomes research. *Physical Therapy, 73,* 528–537.

Jewell, J. A., Abraham, I. L., & Fitzpatrick, J. J. (1987). Selecting an appropriate problem for nursing expert system development. William W. Stead (Ed.), *Proceedings of the Eleventh Annual Symposium on Computer Applications in Medical Care* (pp. 85–87). Washington, DC: Computer Society Press.

Johnson, C. C., Powers, C. R., Bao, W., Harsha, D. W., & Berenson, G. S. (1994). Cardiovascular risk factors of elementary school teachers in a low socio-economic area of a metropolitan city: The Heart Smart Program. *Health Education Research, 9,* 183–191.

Johnson, C. W. (1993). *Effectiveness of a computer-based AIDS education game: BlockAIDS.* ERIC Document Reproduction Service No. 363 277.

Johnson, J. A. (1996). Self-efficacy theory as a framework for community pharmacy-based diabetes education programs. *Diabetes Educator, 22,* 237–244.

Johnson, J. V., & Johansson, G. (Eds.). (1991). *Psychosocial work environment: Work organization, democratization and health.* Amityville, NY: Baywood.

Johnston, D. R. (1991). Health promotion: The challenge to industry. In S. M. Weiss, J. E. Fielding & A. Baum (Eds.), *Perspectives in behavioral medicine: Health at work.* Hillsdale, NJ: Erlbaum.

Joint Committee on National Health Education Standards. (1995). *Achieving health literacy: An investment in the future.* Atlanta, GA: American Cancer Society.

Jones, C. S., & Macrina, D. (1993). Using the PRECEDE model to design and implement a bicycle helmet campaign. *Wellness Perspectives: Research, Theory and Practice, 9*(2), 68–95.

Kagan, N. J., Kagan, H., & Watcon, M. G. (1995). Stress reduction in the workplace: The effectiveness of psychoeducational programs. *Journal of Counseling Psychology, 42,* 71–78.

Kaiser Family Foundation. (1987). *The Community Health Promotion Grant Program. Menlo Park, CA: Henry J. Kaiser Family Foundation.*

Kaiser Family Foundation. (1989). *Strategic plan for the health promotion program, 1989–1991.* Menlo Park, CA: Henry J. Kaiser Family Foundation.

Kaiser Family Foundation. (1990). *The health promotion program of the Henry J. Kaiser Family Foundation.* Menlo Park, CA: Henry J. Kaiser Family Foundation.

Kaluzny, A. D., Schenck, A., & Ricketts, T. (1986). Cancer prevention in the workplace: An organizational innovation. *Health Promotion, 1,* 293–299.

Kanfer, F. H., & Saslow, G. (1969). Behavioral diagnosis. In C. M. Franks (Ed.), *Behavior Therapy: Appraisal and Status.* New York: McGraw-Hill.

Kann, L. K. (1987). Effects of computer-assisted instruction on selected interaction skills related to responsible sexuality. *Journal of School Health, 57,* 282–287.

Kann, L. K., Collins, J. L., Pateman, B. C., et al. (1995). The School Health Policies and Programs Study (SHPPS): Rationale for a nationwide status report on school health programs. *Journal of School Health, 65,* 291–294.

Kann, L. K., Warren, C. W., Harris, W. A., et al. (1995). Youth risk behavior surveillance—United States, 1993. *Morbidity and Mortality Weekly Report, 44,* 1–56.

Kann, L., Warren, C. W., & Kolbe, L. J. (1995). Youth risk behavior surveillance: United States, 1993. *Journal of School Health, 65,* 163–171.

Kannas, L. (1982). The dimensions of health behavior among young men in Finland. *International Journal of Health Education, 24,* 146–155.

Kannel, W. B., Doyle, J. T., Ostfeld, A. M., et al. (1984). Optimal resources for primary prevention of atherosclerotic diseases. *Circulation, 70,* 155A–205A.

Kantor, R. (1983). *The change masters.* New York: Simon & Schuster.

Kaplan, G. A., & Lynch, J. W. (1997). Editorial: Whither studies on the socioeconomic foundations of population health. *American Journal of Public Health, 87,* 1409–1410.

Kaplan, R. M. (1988). Health-related quality of life in cardiovascular disease. *Journal of Consulting and Clinical Psychology, 56,* 382–392.

Kar, S. B. (1986). Communication for health promotion: A model for research and action. In W. B. Ward & S. B. Kar (Eds.), *Advances in Health Education and Promotion* (Vol. 1, Pt. A, pp. 267–302). Greenwich, CT: JAI Press.

Kar, S. B. (Ed.). (1989). *Health promotion indicators and actions.* New York: Springer.

Karasek, R., & Theorell, T. (1990). *Healthy work: Stress, productivity, and the reconstruction of working life.* New York: Basic Books.

Kass, D., & Freudenberg, N. (1997). Coalition building to prevent childhood lead poisoning: A case study from New York City. In M. Minkler (Ed.), *Community Organizing and Community Building for Health.* New Brunswick, NJ: Rutgers University Press.

Katz, J. N., Daltroy, L. H., Brennan, T. A., & Liang, M. H. (1992). Informed consent and the prescription of nonsteroidal anti-inflammatory drugs. *Arthritis and Rheumatism, 35,* 1257–1263.

Kawachi, I., Kennedy, B. P., Lochner, K., & Prothro-Stith, D. (1997). Social capital, income inequality, and mortality. *American Journal of Public Health, 87,* 1491–1498.

Kay, J. J., & Schneider, E. (1994). Embracing complexity: The challenge of the ecosystem approach. *Alternatives, 20*(3), 32–39.

Kayne, R. (Ed.). (1984). *Drugs and the elderly.* Los Angeles: University of Southern California Press.

Keener, J. R., & Bright, L. K. (1983). Micros and interactive videodiscs for improving access to health education. *Health Education, 14*(6), 47–50.

Keesling, B., & Friedman, H. S. (1995). Interventions to prevent skin cancer: Experimental evaluation of information and fear appeals. *Psychology and Health, 10,* 447–490.

Kegler, M. C., Steckler, A., & McLeroy, K. (1998). A multiple case study of implementation in 10 local Project ASSIST coalitions in North Carolina. *Health Education Research, 13,* 225–239.

Keil, J. E. (1984). Incidence of coronary heart disease in blacks in Charleston, South Carolina. *American Heart Journal, 108,* 779.

Keintz, M. K., Fleisher, L., & Rimer, B. K. (1994). Reaching mothers of preschool-aged children with a targeted quit smoking intervention. *Journal of Community Health, 19, 25–40.*

Keintz, M. K., Rimer, B. K., Fleisher, L., & Engstrom, P. (1988). Educating older adults about their increased cancer risk. *Gerontologist, 28,* 487–490.

Keintz, M. K., Rimer, B. K., Fleisher, L., Fox, L., & Engstron, P. F. (1988). Use of multiple data sources in planning a smoking cessation program for a defined population. In P. F. Engstron, P. N. Anderson, & L. E. Mortsenson (Eds.), *Advances in cancer control: Cancer control research and the emergence of the oncology product line* (pp. 31-42). New York: Alan R. Liss.

Keith, S. E., & Doyle, E. I. (1998). Using PRECEDE/PROCEED to address diabetes within the Choctaw Nation of Oklahoma. *American Journal of Health Behavior, 22,* 358–367.

Kelinman, G. D. (1984). Occupational health and safety: The Swedish model. *Journal of Occupational Medicine, 26,* 901–905.

Kellogg Foundation. (1989). *Promoting health in America: Breakthroughs and harbingers.* Battle Creek, MI: W. H. Kellogg Foundation.

Kellogg Foundation. (1997). *Community-based public health: A 1997 progress report on the national initiative.* Battle Creek, MI: W.W. Kellogg Foundation.

Kelly, G. R. (1990). Medication compliance and health education among outpatients with chronic mental disorders. *Medical Care, 28,* 1181–1197.

Kemper, D. (1986). The Healthwise Program: Growing younger. In K. Dychtwald (Ed.), *Wellness and health promotion for the elderly* (pp. 263–273). Rockville, MD: Aspen.

Kerlinger. F. N. (1979). *Behavioral research: A conceptual approach.* New York: Holt, Rinehart & Winston.

Kernaghan S. G., & Giloth, R. E. (1988). *Tracking the impact of health promotion on organizations: A key to program survival.* Chicago, IL: American Hospital Association.

Key, M., & Kilian, D. (1983). Counseling and cancer prevention programs in industry. In G. R. Newell (Ed.), *Cancer Prevention in Clinical Medicine.* New York: Raven.

Kickbusch, I. (1986a). Health promotion: A global perspective. *Canadian Journal of Public Health, 77,* 321–326.

Kickbusch, I. (1986b). Lifestyle and health. *Social Science and Medicine, 22,* 117–124.

Kickbusch, I. (1989). Approaches to an ecological base for public health. *Health Promotion, 4,* 265–268.

Kickbusch, I. (1997a). New players for a new era: Responding to the global public health challenges. *Journal of Public Health Medicine, 19,* 171–178.

Kickbusch, I. (1997b). Think health: What makes the difference? *Health Promotion International, 12,* 265–272.

Kielhofner, G., & Nelson, C. (1983). A study of patient motivation and cooperation/participation in occupational therapy. *Occupational Therapy Journal of Research, 3,* 35–46.

King, A. J. C., Martin, J. E., Morrell, E. M., et al. (1986). Highlighting specific patient education needs in an aging cardiac population. *Health Education Quarterly, 13,* 29–38.

King, A. J. C., & Coles, B. J. (1992). *The health of Canada's youth: Views and behaviors of 11-, 13- and 15-year-olds from 11 countries.* Ottawa: Health and Welfare Canada.

King, A. W. (1993). Considerations of scale and hierarchy. In S. Woodley, J. J. Kay, & G. Francis (Eds.), *Ecological integrity and the management of ecosystems* (pp. 19–46). Delray, FL: St. Lucie Press.

King, J. (1984). Psychology in nursing: II. The Health Belief Model. *Nursing Times, 80,* 53–55.

Kingery, P. M. (1995). Cholesterol screening: A practical guide to implementation. *Journal of Health Education, 26,* 227–231.

Kingsley, R. G., & Shapiro, J. (1977). A comparison of three behavioral programs for the control of obesity in children. *Behavioral Theory, 8,* 30–33.

Kinzie, M. B., Schorling, J. B., & Siegel, M. (1993). Prenatal alcohol education for low-income women with interactive multimedia. *Patient Education and Counseling, 21*(1–2), 51–60.

Kirscht, J. P. (1974). The Health Belief Model and illness behavior. *Health Education Monographs, 2,* 387–408.

Kizer, K. W., Pelletier, K. R., & Fielding, J. E. (1995). Work-site health promotion programs and health care reform. *Western Journal of Medicine, 162,* 467–468.

Klerman, L. V. (1993). *Promoting the health of adolescents: New dimensions for the twenty-first century.* Oxford: Oxford University Press.

Klesges, R., Vasey, M., & Glasgow, R. (1986). A worksite smoking modification competition: Potential for public health impact. *American Journal of Public Health, 76,* 198–200.

Klitzner, M. (1989). Youth impaired driving: Causes and countermeasures. In *Surgeon General's workshop on drunk driving: Background papers.* Rockville, MD: Office of the Surgeon General, U.S. Department of Health and Human Services.

Knazan, Y. L. (1986). Application of PRECEDE to dental health promotion for a Canadian well-elderly population. *Gerodontics, 2,* 180–185.

Knight, B. P., O'Malley, M. S., & Fletcher, S. W. (1987). Physician acceptance of a computerized health maintenance prompting program. *American Journal of Preventive Medicine, 3,* 19–24.

Knox, S. R., Mandel, B., & Lazarowicz, R. (1981). Profile of callers to the VD national hotline. *Sexually Transmitted Diseases, 8,* 245–254.

Kok, G. J. (1992). Quality of planning as a decisive determinant of health education effectiveness. *Hygie, 11,* 5–9.

Kok, G. J., & Siero, S. (1985). Tin-recycling: Awareness, comprehension, attitude, intention and behavior. *Journal of Economic Psychology, 6,* 157–173.

Kok, G., van den Borne, B., & Mullen, P. D. (1997). Effectiveness of health education and health promotion: Meta-analyses of effect studies and determinants of effectiveness. *Patient Education and Counseling, 30,* 19–27.

Kolbe, L. J. (1982). What can we expect from school health education? *Journal of School Health, 52,* 145–150.

Kolbe, L. J. (1984). Improving the health of children and youth: Frameworks for behavioral research and development. In G. Campbell (Ed.), *Health Education and Youth: A Review of Research and Development* (pp. 7–32). Philadelphia: Falmer.

Kolbe, L. J. (1986). Increasing the impact of school health promotion programs: Emerging research perspectives. *Health Education, 17*(5), 47–52.

Kolbe, L. J. (1989). Indicators for planning and monitoring school health programs. In S. B. Kar (Ed.), *Health Promotion Indicators and Actions* (pp. 221–248). New York: Springer.

Kolbe, L. J. (1997). The application of health behavior research: Health education and health promotion. In D. S. Gochman (Ed.), *Handbook of health behavior research.* New York: Plenum.

Kolbe, L. J., & Gilbert, G. G. (1984). Involving the school in the national strategy to improve the health of Americans. In *Proceedings, Prospects for a Healthier America.* Washington, DC: U.S. Department of Health and Human Services, Office of Disease Prevention and Health Promotion.

Kolbe, L. J., Green, L. W., Foreyt, J., et al. (1985). Appropriate function of health education in schools. In N. Krasnagor, J. Arasteh, & M. Cataldo (Eds.), *Child Health Behavior* (pp. 171–209). New York: Wiley.

Kolbe, L., Iverson, D. C., Kreuter, M. W., et al. (1981, May–June). Propositions for an alternate and complementary health education paradigm. *Health Education, 12,* 24–30.

Kolbe, L. J., Jones, J., Nelson, G., et al. (1988). School health education to prevent the spread of AIDS: Overview of a national programme. *Hygie, 7,* 10–13.

Korhonen, T., Huttunen, J. K., Aro, A., et al. (1983). A controlled trial on the effects of patient education in treatment of insulin-dependent diabetes. *Diabetes Care, 6,* 256–261.

Kosch, S. G., & Dallman, J. J. (1983). Essential areas for behavioral science training: A needs assessment approach. *Journal of Medical Education, 58,* 619–626.

Koshel, J. J. (1990). *An overview of state policies affecting adolescent pregnancy and parenting.* Washington, DC: National Governors' Association.

Kotchen, J. M., McKean, H. E., Jackson-Thayer, S., et al. (1986). Impact of a rural high blood pressure control program on hypertension control and cardiovascular mortality. *Journal of the American Medical Association, 255,* 2177–2182.

Kotler, P. (1989). *Marketing for non-profit organizations* (3rd ed.). Englewood Cliffs, NJ: Prentice-Hall.

Kotler P., & Roberto, E. L. (1989). *Social marketing: Strategies for changing public behavior.* New York: Free Press.

Kottke, T. E., Brekke, M. L., & Marquez, M. (1997). Will patient satisfaction set the preventive services implementation agenda? *American Journal of Preventive Medicine, 13,* 309–316.

Kottke, T. E., Foels, J., Hill, C., Choi, T., & Fendersonet, D. (1984). Nutrition counseling in private practice: attitudes and activities of family physicians. *Preventive Medicine, 13,* 219–225.

Kottke, T. E., Puska, P., Solonen, J. T., et.al. (1985). Projected effects of high-risk versus population-based prevention strategies in coronary heart disease. *American Journal of Epidemiology, 121,* 697–704.

Koutsky, L. (1997). Epidemiology of genital human papillomavirus infection. *American Journal of Medicine, 102*(5A), 3–8.

Kovar, P. A., Allegrante, J. P., MacKenzie, R., et al. (1992). Supervised fitness walking in patients with osteoarthritis of the knee: A randomized, controlled trial. *Annals of Internal Medicine, 116,* 529–534.

Kraft, D. P. (1988). The prevention and treatment of alcohol problems on a college campus. *Journal of Alcohol and Drug Education, 34,* 37–51.

Kretzmann, J. P., & McKnight, J. L. (1993). *Building communities from the inside out: A path toward finding and mobilizing a community's assets.* Chicago: ACTA Publications.

Kreuter, M. W. (1984). Health promotion: The public health role in the community of free exchange. J. M. Dodds (Ed.), *Health Promotion Monographs* (4). New York: Teachers College, Columbia University.

Kreuter, M. W. (Ed.). (1985a). Results of the School Health Education Evaluation [Special issue]. *Journal of School Health 55*(8).

Kreuter, M. W. (1985b, February 5). Statement to the Michigan Senate Health Committee on Senate Bills 4 and 5. Unpublished. Atlanta, GA: Centers for Disease Control.

Kreuter, M. W. (1989). Activity, health, and the public. Chapter 15 in *Academy Papers.* Reston, VA: Academy of Physical Education, Alliance for Health, Physical Education, Recreation, and Dance.

Kreuter, M. W. (1993). Human behavior and cancer: Forget the magic bullet! *Cancer, 72*(Suppl.), 996–1001.

Kreuter, M. W., Christenson, G. M., & Davis, R. (1984). School health education research: Future uses and challenges. *Journal of School Health, 54,* 27–32.

Kreuter, M. W., Christenson, G. M., & DiVincenzo, A. (1982). The multiplier effect of the Health Education-Risk Reduction Grants Program in 28 states and 1 territory. *Public Health Reports, 97,* 510–515.

Kreuter, M. W., Christianson, G. M., Freston, M., & Nelson, G. (1981). In search of a baseline: The need for risk prevalence surveys. *Proceedings of the Annual National Risk Reduction Conference.* Atlanta, GA: Centers for Disease Control.

Kreuter, M. W., & Green, L. W. (1978, April). Evaluation of school health education: Identifying purpose, keeping perspective. *Journal of School Health, 48,* 228–235.

Kreuter, M. W., & Lezin, N. (1998). *Are consortia/collaboratives effective in changing health status and health systems?* Contract Report. Rockville, MD: Office of Planning, Evaluation and Legislation, Health Resources and Services Administration.

Kreuter, M. W., & Lezin, N. (1997, June). *Are consortia/collaboratives effective in changing health status and health systems? A critical review of the literature.* Prepared for the Office of Planning, Evaluation and Legislation (OPEL), Health Resources and Services Administration, Rockville, MD.

Kreuter, M. W., Lezin, N., Kreuter, M. W., & Green, L. W. (1998). *Community health promotion ideas that work: A field-book for practitioners.* Sudbury, MA: Jones and Bartlett.

Kreuter, M. W., Vehige, E., & McGuire, A. G. (1996). Using computer-tailored calendars to promote childhood immunization. *Public Health Reports, 111,* 176–178.

Krieger, N. (1994). Epidemiology and the web of causation: Has anyone seen the spider? *Social Science and Medicine, 39,* 887–903.

Krieger, N., & Lashof, J. C. (1988). AIDS, policy analysis, and the electorate: The role of schools of public health. *American Journal of Public Health, 78,* 411–415.

Krieger, N., Rowley, D. L., Herman, L. L., et al. (1993). Racism, sexism, and social class: Implications for studies of health, disease, and well-being. In D. Rowley & H. Tosteson (Eds.), *Racial differences in preterm delivery: Developing a new research paradigm. American Journal of Preventive Medicine, 9*(Suppl.).

Kristal, A. R., Goldenhar, L., & Morton, R. F. (1997). Evaluation of a supermarket intervention to increase consumption of fruits and vegetables. *American Journal of Health Promotion, 11,* 422–425.

Kristal, A. R., Patterson, R. E., Glanz, K., et al. (1995). Psychosocial correlates of healthful diets: Baseline results from the working well study. *Preventive Medicine, 24,* 221–228.

Kritch, K. M., Bostow, D. E., & Dedrick, R. F. (1995). Level of interactivity of videodisc instruction on college students' recall of AIDS information. *Journal of Applied Behavior Analysis, 28,* 85–86.

Kroger, F. (1991). Preventing HIV infection: Educating the general public. *Journal of Primary Prevention 12,* 7–17.

Kroger, F. (1994). Toward a healthy public. *American Behavioral Scientist, 38,* 215–223.

Krolnick, R. (1989). *Adolescent health insurance status: Analyses of trends in coverage and preliminary estimates of the effects of an employer mandate and Medicaid expansion on the uninsured.* Washington, DC: U.S. Congress, Office of Technology Assessment, Government Printing Office.

Kronenfeld, J. J. (1986). Self-help and self-care as social movements. In W. B. Ward & Z. Salisbury (Eds.), *Advances in Health Education and Promotion* (Vol. 1, Pt. A, pp. 105–127). Greenwich, CT: JAI Press.

Krueger, R. A. (1988). *Focus groups: A practical guide for applied research.* Newbury Park, CA: Sage.

Kumpfer, K., Turner, C., Hopkins, R., & Librett, J. (1993). Leadership and team effectiveness in community coalitions for the prevention of alcohol and other drug abuse. *Health Education Research, 20*(4), 359–374.

Kurtz, N. R., Googins, B., & Howard, W. C. (1984). Measuring the success of occupational alcoholism programs. *Journal of Studies on Alcohol, 45,* 33–45.

Labonte, R. (1994). Death of program, birth of metaphor: The development of health promotion in Canada. In A. Pederson, M. O'Neill, & I. Rootman (Eds.), *Health promotion in Canada.* Toronto: Saunders.

Lafontaine G., & Bedard, L. (1997). La prevention des infections dans les services de garde a l'enfance: Les facteurs potentiels d'influence. *Canadian Journal of Public Health, 88,* 250–254.

Laframboise, H. L. (1973). Health policy: Breaking the problem down into more manageable segments. *Canadian Medical Association Journal, 108,* 388–393.

Laitakari, J. (1998). On the practical applicability of stage models to health promotion and health education. *American Journal of Health Behavior, 22,* 28–38.

Laitakari, J., Miilunpalo, S., & Vuori, I. (1997). The process and methods of health counseling by primary health care personnel in Finland: A national survey. *Patient Education and Counseling, 30,* 61–70.

Lalonde, M. A. (1974). *A new perspective on the health of Canadians.* Ottawa: Ministry of National Health and Welfare.

Lamb, G. C., Green, S. S., & Heron, J. (1994). Can physicians warn patients of potential side effects without fear of causing those side effects? *Archives of Internal Medicine, 154,* 2753–2756.

Lamy, P., & Beardsley, R. S. (1982). The older adult and the pharmacist educator. *American Pharmacist, 22*(5), 40.

Landgreen, M., & Baum, W. (1984). Adhering to fitness in the corporate setting. *Corporate Commentary, 1,* 30–35.

Landman, G. B., Levine, M. D., & Rappaport, L. (1984). A study of treatment resistance among children referred for encopresis. *Clinical Pediatrics, 8,* 449–452.

Lando, H. A., Loken, B., Howard-Pitney, B., & Pechacek, T. (1990). Community impact of a localized smoking cessation contest. *American Journal of Public Health, 80,* 601–603.

Lando, H. A., McGovern, P. G., Barrios, F. X., & Etringer, B. D. (1990). Comparative evaluation of American Cancer Society and American Lung Association smoking cessation clinics. *American Journal of Public Health, 80,* 554–559.

Lando, H. A., Jeffery, R., McGovern, P., Forster, J., & Baxter, J. (1993). Factors influencing participation in worksite smoking cessation and weight loss programs: The Healthy Worker Project. *American Journal of Health Promotion, 8*(1), 22–24.

Lando, H. A., Pirie, P. L., & Schmid, L. A. (1996). Promoting abstinence among relapsed chronic smokers: The effect of telephone support. *American Journal of Public Health, 96,* 1786–1790.

Landrigan, P. J. (1989). Occupational health in the 1990's: Developing a platform for disease prevention. *Annals of the New York Academy of Medicine, 572,* 1–3.

Landry, F. (Ed.). (1983). *Health risk estimation, risk reduction and health promotion.* Ottawa: Canadian Public Health Association.

Langille, D. B., Mann, K. V., & Gailiunas, P. N. (1997). Primary care physicians' perceptions of adolescent pregnancy and STD prevention practices in a Nova Scotia county. *American Journal of Preventive Medicine, 13,* 324–330.

Langlie, J. (1977). Social networks, health beliefs, and preventive health behavior. *Journal of Health and Social Behavior, 18,* 244–260.

LaPorte, R. E., Adams, L. L., Savage, D. D., et al. (1984). The spectrum of physical activity and cardiovascular health: An epidemiologic perspective. *American Journal of Epidemiology, 120,* 507–517.

LaPorte, R. E., Montoye, H. J., & Caspersen, C. J. (1985). Assessment of physical activity in epidemiologic research: Problems and prospects. *Public Health Reports, 100,* 131–146.

LaPorte, R. E. (1994). Global public health and the information superhighway: Global health network university proposed. *British Medical Journal, 308*(6945), 1651–1652.

Laraque, D., Barlow, B., Durkin, M., & Heagarty, M. (1995). Injury prevention in an urban setting: Challenges and successes. *Bulletin of the New York Academy of Medicine, 72,* 16–30

Larson, E., McGee, A., Quraishi, Z. A., et al. (1991). Effect of an automated sink on handwashing practices and attitudes in high-risk units. *Infection Control and Hospital Epidemiology, 12,* 422–427.

Lasater, T., Abrams, D., Artz, L., et al. (1984). Lay volunteer delivery of a community-based cardiovascular risk factor change program: The Pawtucket experiment. In J. D. Matarazzo et al. (Eds.), *Behavioral health: A handbook of health enhancement and disease prevention.* New York: Wiley.

Last, J. M. (1995). *A dictionary of epidemiology* (3rd ed.). Oxford, England: Oxford University Press, 1995.

Lau, R., Kane, R., Berry, S., et al. (1980). Channeling health: A review of the evaluation of televised health campaigns. *Health Education Quarterly, 7,* 56–89.

Law, M., & Tang, J. L. (1995). An analysis of the effectiveness of interventions intended to help people stop smoking. *Archives of Internal Medicine, 155,* 1933–1941.

Lawler, F. H., & Viviani, N. (1997). Patient and physician perspectives regarding treatment of diabetes: Compliance with practice guidelines. *Journal of Family Practice, 44,* 396–373.

Lawrence, L., & McLemore, T. (1983). National ambulatory medical care survey. *Vital and Health Statistics Series, 88.* Washington, DC: National Center for Health Statistics.

Lawrence, R. S. (1988). Summary of workshop sessions of the International Symposium on Preventive Services in Primary Care: Issues and strategies. *American Journal of Preventive Medicine, 4*(Suppl. 4), 188–189.

Lechner, L., Brug, J., & Mudde, A. (1998). Stages of change for fruit, vegetable and fat intake: Consequence of misconception. *Health Education Research, 13,* 1–12.

Lee, M. S. (1992). *Curriculum development for health education on college level* [in Korean]. Seoul, Korea: Seoul National University School of Public Health.

Lee, M., Lee, F., & Stewart, S. (1996). Pathways to early breast and cervical detection for Chinese American women. *Health Education and Behavior, 23*(Suppl)., S76–S88.

Lefebvre, R. C., Doner, L., Johnston, C., et al. (1995). Use of database marketing and consumer-based health communication in message design: An example from the Office of Cancer Communications' "5 a Day for Better Health" program. Chapter 12 in E. Maibach & R. L. Parrott (Eds.), *Designing health messages: Approaches from communication theory and public health practice* (pp. 217–246). Thousand Oaks, CA: Sage.

Lefebvre, R. C., & Flora, J. A. (1988). Social marketing and public health intervention. *Health Education Quarterly, 15,* 299–315.

Lefebvre, R. C., Peterson, G. S., McGraw, S. A., et al. (1986). Community intervention to lower blood cholesterol: The "Know Your Cholesterol" campaign in Pawtucket, Rhode Island. *Health Education Quarterly, 13,* 117–129.

Lefebvre, R. C., & Rochlin, L. (1997). Social marketing. In K. Glanz, F. M. Lewis, & B. K. Rimer (Eds.), *Health behavior and health education: Theory, research and practice* (pp. 384–402). San Francisco: Jossey-Bass.

Legorreta, A. P., Hasan, M. M., Peters, A. L., Pelletier, K. R., & Leung, K. M. (1997). An intervention for enhancing compliance with screening recommendations for diabetic retinopathy. *Diabetes Care, 20,* 520–523.

Leichter, H. M. (1991). *Free to be foolish: Politics and health promotion in the United States and Britain.* Princeton, NJ: Princeton University Press.

Leickly, F. E., Wade, S. L., Crain, E., et al. (1998). Self-reported adherence, management behavior, and barriers to care after an emergency department visit by inner city children with asthma. *Pediatrics, 101*(5), E81–E88.

Lenfant, C., & Roccella, E. J. (1984). Trends in hypertension control in the United States. *Chest, 86,* 459–462.

Leo, R. (1996). Research note: Managing workplace stress: A Canadian study among resource managers. *Work and Stress, 10,* 183–191.

Leppik, I. E. (1990). How to get patients with epilepsy to take their medication: The problem of noncompliance. *Postgraduate Medicine, 88,* 253–256.

Leppo, K., & Melkas, T. (1988). Toward healthy public policy: Experiences in Finland 1972–1987. *Health Promotion, 3,* 195–203.

"Let's take it outside." (1988, May). In *Focus 97.* Wichita: Kansas Health Foundation.

Leupker, R. V., Pallonen, V. E., Murray, D. M., & Pirie, P. L. (1989). Validity of telephone surveys in assessing cigarette smoking in young adults. *American Journal of Public Health, 79,* 202–204.

Lev, E. L., & Owen, S. V. (1996). A measure of self-care self-efficacy. *Research in Nursing and Health, 19,* 421–430.

Levenson, P. M., & Morrow, J. R. (1987). Learner characteristics associated with responses to film and interactive video lessons on smokeless tobacco. *Preventive Medicine, 16*(1), 52–62.

Levin, D., & Coronel, G. (1997). The role of quality assessment in planning, implementation and evaluation of national health promotion strategies for youth. *Promotion and Education, 4*(2), 16–18.

Levin, L. S. (1982). Forces and issues in the revival of interest in self-care: Impetus for redirection in health. In B. P. Mathews (Ed.), *The SOPHE Heritage Collection of Health Education Monographs: Vol. 2. The Practice of Health Education* (pp. 268–273). Oakland, CA: Third Party Associates.

Levin, L. S. (1983). Lay health care: The hidden resource in health promotion. In K. A. Gordon (Ed.), *Health Promotion Monographs* (3). New York: Teachers College, Columbia University.

Levin, L. S., & Idler, E. L. (1983). Self-care in health. *Annual Review of Public Health, 4,* 181–201.

Levin, L. S., Katz, A., & Holst, E. (1978). *Self-care: Lay initiatives in health.* New York: Prodist.

Levine, D. M., & Green, L. W. (1981). Cardiovascular risk reduction: An interdisciplinary approach to research training. *International Journal of Health Education, 24,* 20–25.

Levine, D. M., & Green, L. W. (1983). Behavioral change through health education. In N. M. Kaplan & J. Stamler (Eds.), *Prevention of coronary heart disease: Practical management of the risk factors* (pp. 161–169). Philadelphia: Saunders.

Levine, D. M., & Green, L. W. (1985). Patient education: State of the art in research and evaluation. *Bulletin of the New York Academy of Medicine, 61,* 135–143.

Levine, D. M., Green, L. W., Deeds, S. G., et al. (1979). Health education for hypertensive patients. *Journal of the American Medical Association, 241,* 1700–1703.

Levine, D. M., Green, L. W., Russell, R. P., et al. (1979). Compliance in hypertension management: What the physician can do. *Practical Cardiology, 5,* 151–160.

Levine, D. M., Morisky, D. E., Bone, L. R., et al. (1982). Data-based planning for educational interventions through hypertension control programs for urban and rural populations in Maryland. *Public Health Reports, 97,* 107–112.

Levine, S., White, P., & Scotch, N. (1963). Community interorganizational problems in providing medical care and social services. *American Journal of Public Health, 53,* 1183–1195.

Levit, K. R., & Cowan, C. A. (1991). Business, households, and governments: Health care costs, 1990. *Health Care Financing Review, 13,* 83–93.

Levit, K. R., Freeland, M. S., & Waldo, D. R. (1989). Health spending and ability to pay: Business, individuals, and government. *Health Care Financing Review, 10*(2), 1–11.

Leviton, L., Mrazek, P., & Stoto, M. (1996). Social marketing to adolescents and minority populations. *Social Marketing Quarterly, 3,* 6–23.

Leviton, L., Needleman, C. E., & Shapiro, M. A. (1997). *Confronting public health risks: A decision maker's guide.* Thousand Oaks, CA: Sage.

Leviton, L. C., & Valdiserri, R. O. (1990). Evaluating AIDS prevention: Outcome, implementation, and mediating variables. *Evaluation and Program Planning, 13,* 55–66.

Lewin, K. (1943). Forces behind food habits and methods of change. *Bulletin of the National Research Council, 108,* 35–65.

Lewis, B., Mann, J. I., & Mancini, M. (1986). Reducing the risks of coronary heart disease in individuals and in the population. *Lancet, 14,* 956–959.

Lewis, C. E. (1988b). Disease prevention and health promotion practices of primary care physicians in the United States. *American Journal of Preventive Medicine, 4*(4, Suppl.) 9–16.

Lewis, C. E. (1998). Continuing medical education: Past, present, future. *Western Journal of Medicine, 168,* 334–340.

Lewis, C. E., Clancy, C., Leake, B., & Schwartz, J. S. (1991). The counseling practices of internists. *Annals of Internal Medicine, 114,* 54–58.

Lewis, F. M. (1987). The concept of control: A typology and health-related variables. In W. Ward & M. H. Becker (Eds.), *Advances in Health Education and Promotion* (Vol. 2, pp. 277–309). Greenwich, CT: JAI Press.

Lewis F. M., & Batey, M. V. (1982, October). Clarifying autonomy and accountability in nursing service: Part 2. *Journal of Nursing Administration, 12,* 10–15.

Lewis, R. K., Paine-Andrews, A., Fawcett, S. B., et al. (1996). Evaluating the effects of a community coalition's efforts to reduce illegal sales of alcohol and tobacco products to minors. *Journal of Community Health, 21*(6), 429–436.

Lewit, E. M., Hyland, A., Kerrebrock, N., & Cummings, K. M. (1997). Price, public policy, and smoking in young people. *Tobacco Control, 6*(Suppl.), S17–S24.

Li, V. C., Coates, T. J., & Spielberg, L. A., et al. (1984). Smoking cessation with young women in public family planning clinics: The impact of physician messages and waiting room media. *Preventive Medicine, 13,* 477–489.

Li, F. P., Schlief, N. Y., Chang, C. J., & Gaw, A. C. (1972). Health care for the Chinese community in Boston. *American Journal of Public Health, 62,* 536–539.

Liberatos, P., Link, B. C., & Kelsey, J. L. (1988). The measurement of social class in epidemiology. *Epidemiologic Reviews, 10,* 87–121.

Liburd, L. C., & Bowie, J. V. (1989). Intentional teenage pregnancy: A community diagnosis and action plan. *Health Education, 20*(5), 33–38.

Liefooghr, R., Michiels, N., & De Muynck, A. (1995). Perception and social consequences of tuberculosis: A focus group study. *Social Science and Medicine, 41,* 1685–1692.

Light, L., & Contento, I. R. (1989). Changing the course: A school nutrition and cancer education program by the American Cancer Society and the National Cancer Institute. *Journal of School Health, 59,* 205–209.

Lightner, M. D. (1976, November–December). The health education coordinating council. *Health Education, 7,* 25–26.

Lillquist, P. P., Haenlein, M., & Mettlin, C. (1996). Cancer control planning and establishment of priorities for intervention by a state health department. *Public Health Reports, 109,* 791–803.

Lindsey, B. J. (1997). Peer education: A viewpoint and critique. *Journal of American College Health, 45,* 187–190.

Linstone, H. A., & Turoff, M. (1975). *The delphi method: Techniques and applications.* Reading, MA: Addison-Wesley.

Lipnickey, S. C. (1986). *Application of the PRECEDE model to a school-based program of drug, alcohol and tobacco education* [microform: ED281126 Gov't Publications/Microforms Div., 12pp.). Paper presented at the 114th Annual Meeting of the American Public Health Association, Las Vegas, NV.

Lippitt, G. L., Langseth, P., & Mossop, J. (1985). *Implementing organizational change.* San Francisco: Jossey-Bass.

Litzelman, D. K., Dittus, R. S., Miller, M. E., & Tierney, W. M. (1993). Requiring physicians to respond to computerized reminders improves their compliance with preventive care protocols. *Journal of General Internal Medicine, 8,* 311–317.

Livingood, W. C., Woodhouse, L. D., & Waring, B. (1995). Integrating individual and program credentialing: The East Stroudsburg University experience. *Journal of Health Education, 26,* 104–106.

Livingston, I. L. (1985, April). Hypertension and health education intervention in the Caribbean: A public health appraisal. *Journal of the National Medical Association, 77*(4), 273–280.

Lohr, K., Squyres, W., et al. (1985). *Patient education and health promotion in medical care.* Palo Alto, CA: Mayfield.

Lohrmann, D. K., & Fors, S. W. (1986). Can school-based programs really be expected to solve the adolescent drug problem? *Journal of Drug Education, 16*(4), 327–339.

Lohrmann, D. K., & Wooley, S. F. (1998). Comprehensive school health education. In E. Marx & S. Wooley (Eds.), *Health is academic: A guide to coordinated school health programs.* New York: College Press.

Lollis, C. M., Johnson, E. H., & Antoni, M. H. (1997). The efficacy of the Health Belief Model for predicting condom usage and risky sexual practices in university students. *AIDS Education and Prevention, 9,* 551–563.

Lomas, J. (1993). Diffusion, dissemination, and implementation: Who should do what? In K. S. Warren & F. Mosteller (Eds.), *Doing more good than harm: The evaluation of health care interventions* (Vol. 703, pp. 226–237). New York: Annals of the New York Academy of Sciences.

Lomas, J., Anderson, G. M., Domnick-Pierre, K., et al. (1989). Do practice guidelines guide practice? The effect of a consensus statement on the practice of physicians. *New England Journal of Medicine, 313,* 1306–1310.

Lomas, J., & Haynes, R. B. (1988). A taxonomy and critical review of tested strategies for the application of clinical practice recommendations: From "official" to "individual" clinical policy. *American Journal of Preventive Medicine, 4,* (4, Suppl.), 77–94.

London, F. B. (1982). Attitudinal and social normative factors as predictors of intended alcohol abuse among fifth- and seventh-grade students. *Journal of School Health, 52,* 244–249.

Longabaugh, R., Rubin, A., & Lowman, C. (1996). The reliability of Marlatt's taxonomy for classifying relapses. *Addiction, 91*(Suppl.), S73–S87.

Longe, M. (1985). *Innovative hospital-based health promotion.* Chicago: American Hospital Association.

Lorig, K. (1996). Use of PRECEDE model and self-efficacy in arthritis education programs. In K. Lorig et al. (Eds.), *Patient education: A practical approach* (2nd ed., pp. 216–223). Thousand Oaks, CA: Sage.

Lorig, K., & Laurin, J. (1985). Some notions about assumptions underlying health education. *Health Education Quarterly, 12,* 231–243.

Lorig, K. R., Mazonson, P. D., & Holman, H. R. (1993). Evidence suggesting that health education for self-management in patients with chronic arthritis has sustained health benefits while reducing health care costs. *Arthritis and Rheumatism, 36,* 439–446.

Lorig, K., Stewart, A., Ritter, P., et al. (1996). *Outcome measures for health education and other health care interventions.* Thousand Oaks, CA: Sage.

Lorion, R. P., & Newbrough, J. R. (1996). Psychological sense of community: The pursuit of a field's spirit. *Journal of Community Psychology, 24,* 311–314.

Louis Harris and Associates. (1996). *The getting involved survey.* Commissioned by the California Center for Health Improvement, Karen Bodenhorn, Executive Director, under a grant from the California Wellness Foundation.

Louis Harris and Associates. (1997). *"Public health": Two words few people understand even though almost everyone thinks public health functions are very important.* New York: Louis Harris and Associates, for the California Wellness Foundation.

Lovato, C. Y., & Allensworth, D. (1989). *School health in America: An assessment of state policies to protect and improve the health of students* (5th ed.). Kent, OH: American School Health Association.

Lovato, C. Y., & Green, L. W. (1984). Consultation report for the workers institute for safety and health, Washington, D.C. Houston: University of Texas Center for Health Promotion Research and Development.

Lovato, C. Y., & Green, L. W. (1986). *Consultation report for National Cancer Institute's grant to five unions to develop cancer control programs.* Paper presented at the annual meeting of the American Public Health Association, New Orleans, LA. Houston, University of Texas Center for Health Promotion Research and Development.

Lovato, C. Y., & Green, L. W. (1990). Maintaining employee participation in workplace health promotion programs. *Health Education Quarterly, 17,* 73–88.

Lovato, C. Y., Green, L. W., & Conley, V. (1986). *Development and evaluation of occupational health education programs to reduce exposure to cancer hazards.* Paper presented at the annual meeting of the American Society for Preventive Oncology, Bethesda, MD.

Lovato, C. Y., Green, L. W., & Stainbrook, G. (1993). The benefits perceived by industry in supporting health promotion programs in the worksite. In J. P. Opatz (Ed.), *Economic impact of worksite health promotion* (pp. 3–31). Champaign, IL: Human Kinetics.

Love, M. B., Davoli, G. W., & Thurman, Q. C. (1996). Normative beliefs of health behavior professionals regarding the psychosocial and environmental factors that influence health behavior change related to smoking cessation, regular exercise, and weight loss. *American Journal of Health Promotion, 10,* 371–379.

Love, R. R., Brown, R. L., Davis, J. E., et al. (1993). Frequency and determinants of screening for breast cancer in primary care group practice. *Archives of Internal Medicine, 153,* 2113–2117.

Lovick, S. R, & Stern, R. F. (1988). *School-based clinics: 1988 update.* Houston, TX: Support Center for School-Based Clinics.

Lowe, J. (Ed.). (1992). Editorial: The Fourth Annual Health Promotion Conference. *Health Promotion Journal of Australia, 2,* 3.

Lowe, J. B., Windsor, R., & Woodby, L. (1997). Smoking relapse prevention methods for pregnant women: A formative evaluation. *American Journal of Health Promotion, 11,* 244–246.

Lowry, R., Kann, L., & Kolbe, L. J. (1996). The effect of socioeconomic status on chronic disease risk behaviors among US adolescents. *Journal of the American Medical Association, 276,* 792–797.

Luepker, R. V., Murray, D. M., Jacobs, D. R., et al. (1994). Community education for cardiovascular disease prevention: Risk factor changes in the Minnesota Heart Health Program. *American Journal of Public Health, 84*(9), 1383–1393.

Lux, K. M., & Petosa, R. (1994). Preventing HIV infection among juvenile delinquents: Educational diagnosis using the Health Belief Model. *International Quarterly of Community Health Education, 15,* 145–164.

Macarthur, A., Macarthur, C., & Weeks, S. (1995). Epidural anaesthesia and low back pain after delivery: A prospective cohort study. *British Medical Journal, 311,* 1336–1339.

Macaulay, A. C., Paradis, G., Potvin, L., et al. (1997). The Kahnawake schools diabetes prevention project: Intervention, evaluation, and baseline results of a diabetes primary prevention program with a native community in Canada. *Preventive Medicine, 26,* 779–790.

Maccoby, N., Farquhar, J. W., & Wood, P. D. (1977). Reducing the risk of cardiovascular disease: Effects of a community-based campaign on knowledge and behavior. *Journal of Community Health, 23,* 100–114.

Macdonald, A. J., Roberecki, S. A., & Cosway, N. L. (1996). Influenza immunization surveillance in rural Manitoba. *Canadian Journal of Public Health, 87,* 163–165.

Macdonald, G. (1997a). The development and measurement of quality in health promotion. *Promotion and Education, 4*(2), 3–4.

Macdonald, G. (1997b). Quality indicators and health promotion effectiveness. *Promotion and Education, 4*(2), 5–9.

Macdonald, G., & Bunton, R. (1992). Health promotion, discipline or disciplines? In R. Bunton & G. Macdonald (Eds.), *Health promotion: Disciplines and diversity* (pp. 6–19). London: Routledge.

MacDonald, M., & Green, L. W. (1994). Health education. In A. Lewy (Ed.), *International encyclopedia of education.* London: Pergamon Press.

Mackenback, J. P. (1991). Health care expenditures and mortality from amenable conditions in the European community. *Health Policy, 19,* 245–255.

MacKenzie, I. S. (1990). Courseware evaluation: Where's the intelligence? *Journal of Computer Assisted Learning, 6,* 273–285.

Maclean, H. M. (1991). Patterns of diet-related self-care in diabetes. *Social Science and Medicine, 32,* 689–696.

Maclean, H. M., & Eakin, J. M. (1992). Health promotion research methods: Expanding the repertoire—conference overview and selected papers. *Canadian Journal of Public Health, 83*(Supp. 1), S1–S72.

Macrina, D., Macrina, N., Horvath, C., Gallaspy, J., & Fine, P. R. (1996). An educational intervention to increase use of the Glasgow Coma Scale by emergency department personnel. *International Journal of Trauma Nursing, 2,* 7–12.

Macrina, D. M., & O'Rourke, T. W. (1986–1987). Citizen participation in health planning in the U.S. and the U.K.: Implications for health education strategies. *International Quarterly of Community Health Education, 7,* 225–239.

Maes, S., Spielberger, C. D., Defares, P. B., & Sarason, I. G. (Eds.). (1988). *Topics in health psychology.* New York: Wiley.

Mahaffey M., & Hanks, J. W. (Eds.). (1982). *Practical politics: Social work and political responsibility.* Silver Springs, MD: National Association of Social Workers.

Maheux, B., Pineault, R., & Beland, F. (1987). Factors influencing physicians' orientation toward prevention. *American Journal of Preventive Medicine, 3,* 12–18.

Mahlock, J., Taylor, V., Taplin, S., & Urban, N. (1993). A breast cancer screening educational intervention targeting medical office staff. *Health Education Research, 8,* 567–579.

Maibach, E., & Holtgrave, D. R. (1995). Advances in public health communication. *Annual Reviews in Public Health, 16,* 219–238.

Maibach, E., & Murphy, D. A. (1995). Self-efficacy in health promotion research and practice: Conceptualization and measurement. *Health Education Research, 10,* 37–50.

Maiman, L. A., Becker, M. H., Kirscht, J. P., et al. (1977). Scales for measuring Health Belief Model dimensions: A test of predictive value, internal consistency and relationships among beliefs. *Health Education Monographs, 5,* 215–230.

Maiman, L. A., Green, L. W., Gibson, G., & MacKenzie, E. J. (1979). Education for self-treatment by adult asthmatics. *Journal of the American Medical Association, 241,* 1919–1922.

Maine Department of Educational and Cultural Services. (1985). Project graduation. *Morbidity and Mortality Weekly Report, 34,* 233–235.

Makrides, L., Veinot, P. L., Richard, J., & Allen, M. J. (1997). Primary care physicians and coronary heart disease prevention: A practice model. *Patient Education and Counseling, 32,* 207–217.

Males, M. (1995). The influence of parental smoking on youth smoking: Is the recent downplaying justified? *Journal of School Health, 65,* 228–231.

Malilay, J., Real, M. G., & Sinks, T. (1996). Public health surveillance after a volcanic eruption: Lessons from Cerro Negro, Nicaragua, 1992. *Bulletin of the Pan American Health Organization, 30,* 218–226.

Malo, E., & Leviton, L. C. (1987). Decision points for hospital-based health promotion. *Hospital and Health Services Administration, 32,* 49–61.

Mamon, J., Green, L. W., Gibson, G., Gurley, H. T., & Levine, D. M. (1987). Using the emergency department as a screening site for high blood pressure control: Development of a methodology to improve hypertension detection and appropriate referral. *Medical Care, 25,* 770–780.

Mamon, J. A., & Zapka, J. G. (1986). Breast self-examination by young women: I. Characteristics associated with frequency. *American Journal of Preventive Medicine, 2,* 61–69.

Manfredi, C., Lacey, L., & Balch, G. (1997). Method effects in survey and focus group findings: Understanding smoking cessation in low-SES African American women. *Health Education and Behavior, 24,* 786–800.

Mann, K. V. (1989). Promoting adherence in hypertension: A framework for patient education. *Canadian Journal of Cardiovascular Nursing 1*(1), 8–14.

Mann, K. V. (1994). Educating medical students: Lessons from research in continuing education. *Academic Medicine, 69,* 41–47.

Mann, K. V., & Putnam, R. W. (1989). Physicians' perceptions of their role in cardiovascular risk reduction. *Preventive Medicine, 18,* 45–58.

Mann, K. V., & Putnam, R. W. (1990). Barriers to prevention: Physician perceptions of ideal versus actual practices in reducing cardiovascular risk. *Canadian Family Physician, 36,* 665–667.

Mann, K. V., Putnam, R. W., Linsday, E. A., & Davis, D. A. (1990). Cholesterol: Decreasing the risk. An educational program for physicians. *Journal of Continuing Education in the Health Professions, 10,* 211–222.

Mann, K. V., Putnam, R. W., Linsday, E. A., & Davis, D. A. (1996). Increasing physician involvement in cholesterol-lowering practices. *Journal of Continuing Education in the Health Professions, 16,* 225–240.

Mann, K. V., & Sullivan, P. L. (1987). Effect of task-centered instructional programs on hypertensives' ability to achieve and maintain reduced dietary sodium intake. *Patient Education and Counseling, 10,* 53–72.

Mann, K. V., Viscount, P. W., Cogdon, A., et al. (1996). Multidisciplinary learning in continuing professional education: The Heart Health Nova Scotia experience. *Journal of Continuing Education in the Health Professions, 16,* 50–60.

Manoff, R. K. (1985). *Social marketing: New imperative for public health.* New York: Praeger.

Mantell, J. E., DiVittis, A. T., & Auerbach, M. I. (1997). *Evaluating HIV prevention interventions.* New York: Plenum.

Marcus, A. C., Reeder, L. G., Jordan, L. A., & Seeman, T. E. (1980). Monitoring health status, access to health care, and compliance behavior in a large urban community. *Medical Care, 18,* 253–265.

Mark, M. M., Henry, G. T., & Julnes, G. (1998). A realist theory of evaluation practice. *New Directions for Evaluation, 78,* 3–32.

Mark, M. M., & Pines, E. (1995). Implications of continuous quality improvement for program evaluation and evaluators. *Evaluation Practice, 16,* 131–140.

Marketing core functions: Summary of focus group findings and implications for message concepts. (1994, August). Atlanta, GA: Macro International and Westat.

Markland, R. E., & Vincent, M. L. (1990). Improving resource allocation in a teenage sexual risk reduction program. *Socio-Economic Planning Science, 24,* 35–48.

Marlatt, G. A., & Gordon, J. R. (Eds.). (1985). *Relapse prevention: Maintenance strategies in the treatment of addictive behaviors.* New York: Guilford.

Marlenga, B. (1995). The health beliefs and skin cancer prevention practices of Wisconsin dairy farmers. *Oncology Nursing Forum, 22,* 681–686.

Marmot, M. G., Kogevinas, M. A., & Elston, M. (1987). Social/economic status and disease. *Annual Review of Public Health, 8,* 111–135.

Marmot, M. G., Rose, G., Shipley, M., & Hamilton, P. J. (1978). Employment grade and coronary heart disease in british civil servants. *Journal of Epidemiology and Community Health, 3,* 244–249.

Marmot, M., Ryff, C. D., Bumpass, L. L., et al. (1997). Social inequalities in health: Next questions and converging evidence. *Social Science and Medicine, 44,* 901–910.

Marsick, V. J. (1987). Designing health education programs. Chapter 1 in P. M. Lazes, L. H. Kaplan, & K. A. Gordon (Eds.), *Handbook of health education* (2nd ed.). Rockville, MD: Aspen.

Marx E., & Wooley, S. (Eds.). (1998). *Health is academic: A guide to coordinated school health programs.* New York: Teachers College Press.

Masi, D. (1984). *Designing employee assistance programs.* New York: American Management Association.

Mason, J. O. (1984). Health promotion and disease prevention: The federal and state roles. *Focal Points, 1,* 1–2.

Mason, J. O. (1989). Dr. Mason outlines goals for improving the nation's health. *Journal of School Health, 59,* 289–290.

Mason, J. O. (1990). A prevention policy framework for the nation. *Health Affairs, 9,* 22–29.

Mason J. O., & McGinnis, J. M. (1985). The role of school health. *Journal of School Health, 55,* 299.

Mathews, C., Everett, K., Binedell, J., & Steinberg, M. (1995). Learning to listen: Formative research in the development of AIDS education for secondary school students. *Social Science and Medicine, 41,* 1715–1724.

Matson, D. M., Lee, J. W., & Hopp, J. W. (1993). The impact of incentives and competitions on participation and quit rates in worksite smoking cessation programs. *American Journal of Health Promotion, 7,* 270–280, 295.

Mattarazzo, J. D. (1984). Behavioral health: A 1990 challenge for the health sciences professions. In J. D. Mattarazzo et al. (Eds.), *Behavioral health: A handbook of health enhancement and disease prevention.* New York: Wiley.

Mattarazzo, J. D., Weiss, S. M., Herd, J. A., et al. (Eds.). (1984). Behavioral health: A handbook of health enhancement and disease prevention. New York: Wiley.

Maxwell, A. E., Bastani, R., & Warda, U. S. (1998). Mammography utilization and related attitudes among Korean-American women. *Women and Health, 27,* 89–107.

Mayer, J. A., Dubbert, P. M., & Elder, J. P. (1989). Promoting nutrition at the point of choice: A review. *Health Education Quarterly, 16,* 31–43.

Mazmanian, D., & Sabatier, P. (1983). *Implementation and public policy.* Glenview, IL: Scott, Foresman.

Mazzuca, S. A. (1982). Does patient education in chronic disease have therapeutic value? *Journal of Chronic Disease, 35,* 521–529.

McAlister, A., Mullen, P. D., & Nixon, S. A., et al. (1985). Health promotion among primary care physicians in Texas. *Texas Medicine, 81,* 55–58.

McAlister, A. L., Perry, C., Killen, J., et al. (1980). Pilot study of smoking, alcohol, and drug abuse prevention. *American Journal of Public Health, 70,* 719–721.

McAlister, A., Puska, P., Salonen, J. T., et al. (1982). Theory and action for health promotion: Illustrations from the North Karelia Project. *American Journal of Public Health, 72,* 43–50.

McArtor, R. E., Iverson, D. C., Benken, D. E., et al. (1992). Physician assessment of patient motivation: Influence on disposition for follow-up care. *American Journal of Preventive Medicine, 8,* 147–149.

McAuley, E., Mihalko, S. L., & Bane, S. M. (1997). Exercise and self-esteem in middle-aged adults: Multidimensional relationships and physical fitness and self-efficacy influences. *Journal of Behavioral Medicine, 20,* 67–84.

McCarty, D., Morrison, S., & Mills, K. C. (1983). Attitudes, beliefs and alcohol use: An analysis of relationships. *Journal of Studies on Alcohol, 2,* 328–341.

McCaul, K. D., & Glasgow, R. E. (1985). Preventing adolescent smoking: What have we learned about treatment construct validity? *Health Psychology, 4,* 361–387.

McCaul, K. D., Glasgow, R., O'Neill, H., et al. (1982). Predicting adolescent smoking. *Journal of School Health, 52,* 342–346.

McCormick, L. K., Steckler, A. B., & McLeroy, K. R. (1995). Diffusion of innovations in schools: A study of adoption and implementation of school-based tobacco prevention curricula. *American Journal of Health Promotion, 9,* 210–219.

McCoy, C. B., Nielsen, B. B., Chitwood, D. D., Zavertnik, J. J., & Khoury, E. L. (1991). Increasing the cancer screening of the medically underserved in South Florida. *Cancer, 67,* 1808–1813.

McCoy, H. V., Dodds, S. E., & Nolan, C. (1990). AIDS intervention design for program evaluation: The Miami Community Outreach Project. *Journal of Drug Issues, 20,* 223–243.

McCoy, W. J. (1991). Building coalitions for the future in Charlotte-Mecklenburg. *National Civic Review, 80,* 120–134.

McCuan, R., & Green, L. W. (1991). Multivariate statistical methods for evaluation of health education and health promotion programs. In W. Ward & F. M. Lewis (Eds.), *Advances in health education and promotion* (Vol. 3, pp. 153–197). London: Jessica Kingsley.

McDonald, C. J., Hui, S. L., & Smith, D. M., et al. (1984). Reminders to physicians from an introspective computer medical record: A two-year randomized trial. *Annals of Internal Medicine, 100,* 130–138.

McDonnell, S., & Vossberg, K. (1998). Using YPLL in health planning. *Public Health Reports, 113,* 55–61.

McDowell, I., & Newell, C. (1996). *Measuring health: A guide to rating scales and questionnaires* (2nd ed). New York: Oxford University Press.

McGinnis, J. M. (1982). Targeting progress in health. *Public Health Reports, 97,* 295–307.

McGinnis, J. M. (1990). Setting objectives for public health in the 1990s: Experience and prospects. *Annual Review of Public Health, 11,* 231–249.

McGinnis, J. M., & Foege, W. H. (1993). Actual causes of death in the United States. *Journal of the American Medical Association, 270,* 2207–2212.

McGinnis, J. M., Harrell, J., Artz, L., Files, A., & Maiese, D. (1997). Objectives-based strategies for disease prevention. In R. Detels, W. Holland, J. McEwen, & G. S. Omenn (Eds.), *Oxford textbook of public health* (3rd ed., Vol. 3, pp. 1621–1631). Oxford, England: Oxford University Press.

McGovern, P. M., Kochevar, L. K., Vesley, D., & Gershon, R. R. M. (1997). Laboratory professionals' compliance with universal precautions. *Laboratory Medicine, 28,* 725–730.

McGowan, P. (1995). *The relationships of self-efficacy, pain and health status in the Arthritis Self-Management Program.* Unpublished doctoral dissertation. Vancouver: University of British Columbia.

McGowan, P., & Green, L. W. (1995). Arthritis self-management in native populations of British Columbia: An application of health promotion and participatory research principles in chronic disease control. *Canadian Journal of Aging, 14,* 201–212.

McGrane, W. L., Toth, F. J., & Allely, E. B. (1990). The use of interactive media for HIV/AIDS prevention in the military community. *Military Medicine, 155*(6), 235–240.

McGuire, F. A., O'Leary, J. T., Alexander, P. B., & Dottavio, F. D. (1987). A comparison of outdoor recreation preferences and constraints of black and white elderly. *Activities, Adaptation, and Aging, 9,* 95–104.

McKay, R. B., Levine, D. M., & Bone, L. R. (1985). Community organization in a school health education program to reduce sodium consumption. *Journal of School Health, 55,* 364–366.

McKell, C. J. (1994). *A profile of the New Brunswick Association of Dietitians: Results of the Educational Needs Assessment Survey, 1993* (42 pp. with questionnaire). Fredericton: New Brunswick Health and Community Services and Health Canada.

McKell, C. J., Chase, C., & Balram, C. (1996). Establishing partnerships to enhance the preventive practices of dietitians. *Journal of the Canadian Dietetic Association, 57,* 12–17.

McKeown, T. (1979). *The role of medicine: Dream, mirage or nemesis* (2nd ed.). Princeton, NJ: Princeton University Press.

McKinlay, J. B. (1975). A case for refocusing upstream: The political economy of illness. In A. J. Enelow & J. B. Henderson (Eds.), *Applying behavioral science to cardiovascular risk* (pp. 7–17). New York: American Heart Association.

McKinney, M. M. (1993). Consortium approaches to the delivery of HIV services under the Ryan White CARE Act. *AIDS and Public Policy Journal, 8,* 115–125.

McKnight, J. L., & Kretzmann, J. P. (1977). Mapping community capacity. Chap. 10 in M. Minkler (Ed.), *Community organizing and community building for health.* New Brunswick, NJ: Rutgers University Press.

McLean, D. D. (1996). *Use of computer-based technology in health, physical education, recreation, and dance* [Contract No. RR93002015]. Washington, DC: Office of Educational Research and Improvement, U.S. Department of Education, ERIC Document Reproduction Service No. 390 874.

McLemore, T., & DeLozier, J. (1987). 1985 summary: National ambulatory medical care survey. In *Advance data from vital and health statistics* (No. 128). National Center for Health Statistics, Washington, DC: DHHS-PHS 87-1250, Government Printing Office.

McLeroy, K. R., Bibeau, D., Steckler, A., & Glanz, K. (1988). An ecological perspective on health promotion programs. *Health Education Quarterly, 15,* 351–377.

McLeroy, K. R., Gottlieb, N. H., & Burdine, J. N. (1987). The business of health promotion: Ethical issues and professional responsibilities. *Health Education Quarterly, 14,* 91–109.

McLeroy, K., Green, L. W., Mullen, K., & Foshee, V. (1984). Assessing the effects of health promotion in worksites: A review of the stress program evaluations. *Health Education Quarterly, 11,* 379–401.

McLeroy, K. R., Steckler, A., & Bibeau, D. (Eds.). (1988). The social ecology of health promotion interventions. *Health Education Quarterly, 15,* 351–486.

McLeroy, K. R., Steckler, A. B. Simons-Morton, B. G., & Goodman, R. M. (1993). Social science theory in health education: Time for a new model? *Health Education Research: Theory and Practice, 8,* 305–312.

McMillan, D. W. (1996). Sense of community. *Journal of Community Psychology, 24,* 315–326.

McMillan, D. W., & Chavis, D. M. (1986). Sense of community: A definition and theory. *Journal of Community Psychology, 14,* 6–23.

McNeil, B. J., & Nelson, K. R. (1991). Meta-analysis of interactive video instruction: A 10 year review of achievement effects. *Journal of Computer-Based Instruction, 18*(1), 1–6.

McPhee, S. J., Bird, J. A., Ha, N.-T., et al. (1996). Pathways to early cancer detection for Vietnamese women: Suc Khoe La Vang! (Health is Gold!). *Health Education Quarterly 23*(Suppl.), S76–S88.

McPhee, S. J., Richard, R. J., & Solkowitz, S. N. (1986). Performance of cancer screening in a university general internal medicine practice. *Journal of General Internal Medicine, 1,* 275–281.

McQueen, D. (1994). Health promotion research in Canada. In A. Pederson, M. O'Neill, & I. Rootman (Eds.). *Health Promotion in Canada.* Toronto: Saunders.

McQueen, R. J. C. (1985). Attitudes toward health show a gratifying change. *Health Care, 27,* 66.

Meagher, D., & Mann, K. V. (1990). The effect of an educational program on knowledge and attitudes about blood pressure by junior high school students: A pilot project. *Canadian Journal of Cardiovascular Nursing, 1(5),* 15–22.

Mechanic, D. (1979). The stability of health and illness behavior: Results from a 16-year follow-up. *American Journal of Public Health, 69,* 1142–1145.

Meek, J. (1996). An analysis of comprehensive health promotion programs' consistency with the systems model of health. *American Journal of Health Promotion, 7,* 443–451.

Meier, S. T., & Sampson, J. P. (1989). Use of computer-assisted instruction in the prevention of alcohol abuse. *Journal of Drug Education, 19,* 245–256.

Melby, C. L. (1986). The personal laboratory for health behavior change. *Health Education, 16(6),* 29–31.

Mendelsohn, H. (1973). Some reasons why information campaigns can succeed. *Public Opinion Quarterly, 39,* 50–61.

Mercer, S. L., Goel, V., Levy, I. G., et al. (1997). Prostate cancer screening in the midst of controversy: Canadian men's knowledge, beliefs, utilization, and future intentions. *Canadian Journal of Public Health, 88,* 327–332.

Meredith, K., O'Reilly, K., & Schulz, S. L. (1989, November 28–30). *Education for HIV risk reduction in the hemophilia community: Report of the meeting, convening a panel of expert consultants.* Atlanta, GA: Centers for Disease Control and Prevention.

Mergenhagen, P. (1997). People behaving badly. *American Demographics, 19,* 37–44.

Mesters, I., Meertens, R., Crebolder, H., & Parcel, G. (1993). Development of a health education program for parents of preschool children with asthma. *Health Education Research, 8,* 53–68.

Metropolitan Life Foundation. (1988). *An evaluation of comprehensive health education in American public schools.* New York: Louis Harris and Associates, for the Metropolitan Life Foundation.

Meyer, N. A. (1995). *Human papillomavirus risk reduction and control for college students: Phase I final report.* Bethesda, MD: National Cancer Institute.

Miaoulis, G., & Bonaguro, J. (1980–1981). Marketing strategies in health education. *Journal of Health Care Marketing, 1,* 35–44.

Michaels, J. M. (1982). The second revolution in health: Health promotion and its environmental base. *American Psychologist, 37,* 936–941.

Michalsen A., Delclos G. L., Felknor S. A., et al. (1997). Compliance with universal precautions among physicians. *Journal of Occupational and Environmental Medicine, 39(2),* 130–137.

Michielutte, R., & Beal, P. (1990). Identification of community leadership in the development of public health education programs. *Journal of Community Health, 15,* 59–68.

Michielutte, R., Dignan, M., Bahnson, J., & Wells, H. B. (1994). The Forsyth County cancer prevention project: II. Compliance with screening follow-up of abnormal cervical smears. *Health Education Research, 4,* 421–432.

Michielutte, R., Dignan, M. B., Wells, H. B., et al. (1989). Development of a community cancer education program: The Forsyth County, NC, Cervical Cancer Prevention Project. *Public Health Reports, 104(6),* 542–551.

Michigan Department of Health. (1987). *Health promotion can produce economic savings.* Lansing: Center for Health Promotion, Michigan Department of Health.

Mico, P. R. (1965). Community self-study: Is there a method to the madness? *Adult Leadership, 13,* 288–292.

Mico, P. R. (Ed.). (1982). *The heritage collection of health education monographs* (4 vols.). Oakland, CA: Third Party Associates.

Miilunpalo, S., Laitakari, J., & Vuori, I. (1995). Strengths and weaknesses in health counseling in Finnish primary health care. *Patient Education and Counseling 25,* 317–328.

Milewa, T. (1997). Community participation and health care priorities: Reflections on policy, theatre and reality in Britain. *Health Promotion International, 12,* 161–169.

Milio, N. (1976). A framework for prevention: Changing health-damaging to health-generating life patterns. *American Journal of Public Health, 66,* 435–439.

Milio, N. (1983). *Promoting health through public policy.* Philadelphia: Davis. Reprinted (1987) by the Canadian Public Health Association.

Millar, J. D. (1989). The right to know in the workplace. *Annals of the New York Academy of Sciences, 572,* 113–121.

Millar, W. J. (1998). Multiple medication use among seniors. *Health Reports, 9,* 11–17.

Millar, W. J., & Naegele, B. E. (1987). Time to Quit Program. *Canadian Journal of Public Health, 78,* 109–114.

Miller, I. (1987). Interpreneurship: A community coalition approach to health care reform. *Inquiry, 24,* 266–275.

Miller, J. R. (1984). Liaisons: Using health education resources effectively. In H. P. Cleary, J. M. Kichen, & P. G. Ensor (Eds.), *Advancing health through education: A case study approach* (pp. 112–114). Palo Alto, CA: Mayfield.

Miller, L. V., & Goldstein, J. (1972). More efficient care of diabetic patients in a county-hospital setting. *New England Journal of Medicine, 286,* 1383–1391.

Miller, N. E. (1984). Learning: Some facts and needed research relevant to maintaining health. In J. D. Matarazzo et al. (Eds.), *Behavioral health: A handbook of health enhancement and disease prevention* (pp. 199–208). New York: Wiley.

Miller, R. L., Klotz, D., & Eckholdt, H. M. (1998). HIV prevention with male prostitutes and patrons of hustler bars: Replication of an HIV preventive intervention. *American Journal of Community Psychology, 26,* 97–132.

Miller, S. (1983). Coalition etiquette: Ground rules for building unity. *Social Policy, 14*(2), 49.

Miller, W. L., Crabtree, B. F., & Stange, K. C. (1998). Understanding change in primary care practice using complexity theory. *Journal of Family Practice, 46,* 369–376.

Minaire, P. (1992). Disease, illness and health: Theoretical models of the disablement process. *Bulletin of the World Health Organization, 70,* 373–379.

Minkler, M. (1980–1981). Citizen participation in health in the Republic of Cuba. *International Quarterly of Community Health Education, 1,* 65–78.

Minkler, M. (1985). Building supportive ties and sense of community among the inner-city elderly: The Tenderloin Senior Outreach Project. *Health Education Quarterly, 12,* 303–314.

Minkler, M. (1986). The social component of health. *American Journal of Health Promotion, 1,* 33–38.

Minkler, M. (1989). Health education, health promotion and the open society: An historical perspective. *Health Education Quarterly, 16,* 17–30.

Minkler, M. (1990). Improving health through community organization. In K. Glanz, F. M. Lewis, & B. K. Rimer (Eds.), *Health Behavior and Health Education* (p. 257). San Francisco: Jossey-Bass.

Minkler, M. (1994). Challenges for health promotion in the 1990s: Social inequalities, empowerment, negative consequences, and the common good. *American Journal of Health Promotion, 8,* 403–413.

Minkler, M. (Ed.). (1997). *Community organization and community building for health.* New Brunswick, NJ: Rutgers University Press.

Minkler, M., & Checkoway, B. (1988). Ten principles for geriatric health promotion. *Health Promotion International, 3,* 277–286.

Minkler, M., Frantz, S., & Wechsler, R. (1982–1983). Social support and social action organizing in a "grey ghetto": The tenderloin experience. *International Quarterly of Community Health Education, 3,* 3–15.

Minkler, M., & Pies, C. (1997). Ethical issues in community organization and community participation. In M. Minkler (Ed.), *Community Organizing and Community Building for Health.* Piscataway, NJ: Rutgers University Press.

Minnesota Department of Health. (1982). Workplace health promotion survey. Minneapolis: Minnesota Department of Health.

Mirotznik, J., Ginzler, E., & Baptiste, A. (1998). Using the Health Belief Model to explain clinic appointment-keeping for the management of a chronic disease condition. *Journal of Community Health, 23,* 195–209.

Mittelmark, M. B., Hunt, M. K., Health, G., & Schmid, T. L. (1993). Realistic outcomes: Lessons from community-based research and demonstration programs for the prevention of cardiovascular diseases. *Journal of Public Health Policy, 14,* 437–462.

Model standards: A guide for community preventive health services. (1985). (2nd ed.). Washington DC: American Public Health Association.

Modeste, N. N. (1996). *Dictionary of public health promotion and education: Terms and concepts.* Thousand Oaks, CA: Sage.

Modeste, N. N., Abbey, D. E., & Hopp, J. W. (1984–1985). Hypertension in a Caribbean population. *International Quarterly of Community Health Education, 5,* 203–211.

Morbidity and Mortality Weekly Report. (1989a). 38, 137.

Morbidity and Mortality Weekly Report. (1989b). 38, 147–150.

Moreno, C., Alvarado, M., & Forrest, M. (1997). Heart disease education and prevention program targeting immigrant Latinos: Using focus group responses to develop effective interventions. *Journal of Community Health, 22,* 435–450.

Morgan, L. S., & Horning, B. G. (1940). The community health education program. *American Journal of Public Health, 30,* 1323–1330.

Morisky, D. E. (1986). Nonadherence to medical recommendations for hypertensive patients: Problems and potential solutions. *Journal of Compliance in Health Care, 1,* 5–20.

Morisky, D. E., DeMuth, N. M., Field-Fass, M., et al. (1985). Evaluation of family health education to build social support for long-term control of high blood pressure. *Health Education Quarterly, 12,* 35–50.

Morisky, D. E., Levine, D. M., Green, L. W., et al. (1980). The relative impact of health education for low- and high-risk patients with hypertension. *Preventive Medicine, 9,* 550–558.

Morisky, D. E., Levine, D. M., Green, L. W., et al. (1983). Five-year blood-pressure control and mortality following health education for hypertensive patients. *American Journal of Public Health, 73,* 153–162.

Morisky, D. E., Levine, D. M., Green, L. W., & Smith, C. (1982). Health education program effects on the management of hypertension in the elderly. *Archives of Internal Medicine, 142,* 1835–1838.

Morisky, D. E., Levine, D. M., Wood, J. C., et al. (1981). Systems approach for the planning, diagnosis, implementation and evaluation of community health education approaches in the control of high blood pressure. *Journal of Operations Research, 50,* 625–634.

Morisky, D. E., Malotte, C. K., Choi, P., et al. (1990), A patient education program to improve adherence rates with antituberculosis drug regimens. *Health Education Quarterly, 17,* 253–267.

Morone, J. A. (1990). *The democratic wish: Popular participation and the limits of American government.* New York: Harper Collins.

Morrison, C. (1996). Using PRECEDE to predict breast self-examination in older, lower-income women. *American Journal of Health Behavior, 20*(2), 3–14.

Morrow, D. G., Hier, C. M., & Leirer, V. O. (1998). Icons improve older and younger adults' comprehension of medication information. *Journals of Gerontology, Series B, Psychology, 53,* 240–254.

Moser, R., McCance, K. L., & Smith, K. R. (1991). Results of a national survey of physicians' knowledge and application of prevention capabilities. *American Journal of Preventive Medicine, 7,* 384–390.

Mosher, J. F. (1990). *Community responsible beverage service programs: An implementation handbook.* Palo Alto, CA: Health Promotion Resource Center, Stanford Center for Research in Disease Prevention.

Mosher, J. F., & Jernigan, D. H. (1989). New directions in alcohol policy. *Annual Review of Public Health, 10,* 245–279.

Mowatt, C., Isaly, J., & Thayer, M. (1985). Project Graduation: Maine. *Morbidity and Mortality Weekly Report, 34,* 233–235.

Moynihan, D. P. (1969). *Maximum feasible misunderstanding: Community action in the war on poverty.* New York: Free Press.

Mucchielli, R. (1970). *Introduction to structural psychology.* New York: Funk & Wagnalls.

Mulford, C. L., & Klonglan, G. E. (1982). *Creating coordination among organizations: An orientation and planning guide.* Ames, IA: Cooperative Extention Service, Iowa State University, North Central Regional Extension Pub. No. 80.

Mullen, F. (1982). Community-oriented primary care: An agenda for the '80s. *New England Journal of Medicine, 307,* 1076–1078.

Mullen, P. D. (1997). Compliance becomes concordance. *British Medical Journal, 314,* 691–692.

Mullen, P. D., & Culjat, D. (1980). Improving attendance in weight-control programs. *Health Education Quarterly, 7,* 4–13.

Mullen, P. D., Evans, D., Forster, J., et al. (1995). Settings as an important dimension in health education/promotion policy, programs, and research. *Health Education Quarterly, 22,* 329–345.

Mullen, P. D., & Green, L. W. (1985). Meta-analysis points way toward more effective medication teaching. *Promoting Health, 6*(6), 6–8.

Mullen, P. D., Green, L. W., & Persinger, G. (1985). Clinical trials of patient education for chronic conditions: A comparative meta-analysis of intervention types. *Preventive Medicine, 14,* 753–781.

Mullen, P. D., Hersey, J., & Iverson, D. C. (1987). Health behavior models compared. *Social Science and Medicine, 24,* 973–981.

Mullen, P. D., & Iverson, D. C. (1982). Qualitative methods for evaluative research in health education programs. *Health Education, 13*(3), 11–18.

Mullen, P. D., Kukowski, K., & Mazelis, S. (1979). Health education in health maintenance organizations. In P. M. Lazes (Ed.), *Handbook of Health Education* (pp. 53–76). Germantown, MD: Aspen Systems.

Mullen, P. D., Mains, D. A., & Velez, R. (1992). A meta-analysis of controlled trials of cardiac patient education. *Patient Education and Counseling, 19,* 143–162.

Mullen, P. D., Ramirez, G., & Groff, J. Y. (1994). A meta-analysis of randomized trials of prenatal smoking cessation interventions. *American Journal of Obstetrics and Gynecology, 171,* 1328–1334.

Mullen, P. D., Simons-Morton, D. G., Ramirez, et al. (1997). A meta-analysis of trials evaluating patient education and counseling for three groups of preventive health behaviors. *Patient Education and Counseling, 32,* 157–173.

Mullen, P. D., & Zapka, J. G. (1981). Health education and promotion in HMOs: The recent evidence. *Health Education Quarterly, 8,* 292–315.

Mullen, P. D., & Zapka, J. G. (1982). *Guidelines for health promotion and education services in HMOs.* Washington, DC: U.S. Government Printing Office.

Mullen, P. D., & Zapka, J. G. (1989). Assessing the quality of health promotion programs. *HMO Practice, 3,* 98–103.

Mullis, R. M., Hunt, M. K., Foster, M., et al. (1987). The Shop Smart for Your Heart grocery program. *Journal of Nutrition Education, 19,* 225–228.

Mumford, E., Schlesinger, H. J., & Glass, G. V. (1982). The effects of psychological intervention on recovery from surgery and heart attacks: An analysis of the literature. *American Journal of Public Health, 72,* 141–151.

Murray, D. M. (1986). Dissemination of community health promotion programs: The Fargo-Moorhead heart health program. *Journal of School Health, 56,* 375–381.

Murray, D. M., Kurth, C. L., Finnegan, J. R., Jr., et al. (1988). Direct mail as a prompt for follow-up care among persons at risk for hypertension. *American Journal of Preventive Medicine, 4,* 331–335.

Murray, D. M., Johnson, C. A., Luepker, R. V., & Mittelmark, M. B. (1984). The prevention of cigarette smoking in children: A comparison of four strategies. *Journal of Applied Social Psychology, 14,* 274–288.

Murray, D. M., & Perry, C. L. (1987). The measurement of substance use among adolescents: When is the "bogus pipeline" method needed? *Addictive Behaviors, 12,* 225–233.

Murray, J. L., & Lopez, A. D. (Eds.). (1996). *The global burden of disease: Vol. 1. The global burden of disease.* Cambridge, MA: Harvard University Press.

Mustard, H. S. (1945). *Government in public health.* New York: Commonwealth Fund.

Muus, K. J., Mutter, G. (1988). Using research results as a health promotion strategy: A five-year case study. *Health Promotion, 3,* 393–399.

Muus, K. J., & Ahmed K. A., (1991, Fall). Physician utilization behavior among rural residents. *Focus on Rural Health,* pp. 10–12.

Mwanga, J. R., Mugashe, C. L., & Aagaard-Hansen, J. (1998). Experiences from video-recorded focus group discussion on schistosomiases in Magu, Tanzania. *Qualitative Health Research, 8,* 707–717.

Myers, D. (1985). *Establishing and building employee assistance programs.* Westport, CT: Quorum.

Myers, M. G., Cairns, J. A., & Singer, J. (1987). The consent form as a cause of possible side effects. *Journal of Clinical and Pharmacological Therapy, 42,* 250–253.

Nader, D. E., Sellers, C. C., Johnson, C. L., et al. (1996). Effect of adult participation in a school-based family intervention to improve children's diet and physical activity: The child and adolescent trial for cardiovascular health. *Preventive Medicine, 25,* 455–464.

Nader, P. R., Sallis, J. G., Patterson, T. L., et al. (1989). A family approach to cardiovascular risk reduction: Results from the San Diego Family Health Project. *Health Education Quarterly, 16,* 229–244.

Naisbitt, J. (1982). *Megatrends: Ten new directions transforming our lives.* New York: Warner Books.

Naisbitt, J., & Aburdene, P. (1990). *Megatrends 2000: Ten new directions for the 1990's.* New York: Morrow.

Nangawe, E., Shomet, F., Rowberg, E., et al. (1986–1987). Community participation: The Maasai Health Services Project, Tanzania. *International Quarterly of Community Health Education, 7,* 343–351.

National adolescent student health survey. (1988). *Health Education, 19*(4), 4–8.

National Association of County and City Health Officials and the Centers for Disease Control and Prevention. (1995). *1992–1993 national profile of local health departments.* Atlanta, GA: Centers for Disease Control.

National Center for Children in Poverty. (1990). *Five million children: A statistical profile of our poorest young citizens.* New York: School of Public Health, Columbia University, 1990.

National Center for Health Statistics. (1990). *Health United States, 1989.* Hyattsville, MD: Public Health Service, DHHS Publication No. (PHS) 90-1232.

National Center for Health Statistics. (1992). *Health United States, 1991.* Washington, DC: U.S. Department of Health and Human Services, Publication No. (PHS) 90-1232.

National Center for Health Statistics. (1996a). *Health, United States, 1995.* Hyattsville, MD: Public Health Service, DHHS-PHS-89-1232.

National Center for Health Statistics. (1996b). *Healthy people 2000 review, 1995–96.* Hyattsville, MD: Public Health Service, DHHS-PHS-96-1256.

National Center for Health Statistics. (1998). *Health, United States, 1998 and socioeconomic status and health.* Washington, DC: Public Health Service, Publication No. PHS 98-1232.

National Center for Health Statistics, T. McLemore & J. DeLozier. (1987). *1985 summary: National Ambulatory Medical Care Survey.* Advance data from Vital and Health Statistics Series 10, No. 128. Washington, DC: U.S. Government Printing Office, DHHS-PHS 87-1250.

National Center for Health Statistics, A. J. Moss & V. L. Parsons. (1986). *Current estimates from the National Health Interview Survey, United States, 1985.* Vital and Health Statistics Series 10, No. 160. Washington, DC: U.S. Government Printing Office, DHHS-PHS 86-1588.

National Commission on Excellence in Education. (1983). *A nation at risk: The imperative for educational reform.* Washington, DC: National Commission on Excellence in Education.

National Commission on the Role of the School and the Community in Improving Adolescent Health. (1990). *Code blue: Uniting for healthier youth.* Washington, DC: National Association of State Boards of Education and the American Medical Association.

National Committee for Injury Prevention and Control. (1989). *Injury prevention: Meeting the challenge.* New York: Oxford University Press. Printed as a supplement to the *American Journal of Preventive Medicine, 5*(3).

National Conference for Institutions Preparing Health Educators: Proceedings. (1981). Washington, DC: U.S. Office of Health Information and Health Promotion, PHS 92-1232.

National Coordinating Committee on Clinical Preventive Services. (1993). *Preventive services in the clinical setting: What works and what costs.* Washington, DC: Office of Disease Prevention and Health Promotion, Public Health Service.

National Professional School Health Education Organizations. (1984). Comprehensive School Health Education. *Journal of School Health, 54,* 312–315.

National Research Council. (1989). *Improving Risk Communication.* Washington, DC: National Academy Press.

National Resource Center on Worksite Health Promotion. (1992, Spring). *Benefits of worksite health promotion.* In *Promoting Health at Work* [newsletter; Washington, DC].

National Restaurant Association. (1989). *Foodservice industry forecast.* Washington, DC: Malcolm M. Knapp Research.

National Safety Council. (1995). *Accident facts.* Chicago: National Safety Council.

National survey of worksite health promotion activities: A summary. (1987). Washington, DC: U.S. Department of Health and Human Services, Public Health Service, Office of Disease Prevention and Health Promotion.

National Task Force on the Preparation and Practice of Health Educators. (1985). *A framework for the development of competency-based curricula for entry-level health educators.* New York: National Commission for Health Education Credentialing.

NCI Breast Cancer Screening Consortium. (1990). Screening mammography: A missed clinical opportunity. *Journal of the American Medical Association, 264,* 54–58.

Neef, N., Scutchfield, F. D., Elder, J., & Bender, S. J. (1991). Testicular self examination by young men: An analysis of characteristics associated with practice. *Journal of American College Health, 39,* 187–190.

Nelson, C. F., Kreuter, M. W., & Watkins, N. B. (1986). A partnership between the community, state, and federal government: Rhetoric or reality. *Hygie, 5*(3), 27–31.

Nelson, C. F., Kreuter, M. W., Watkins, N. B., & Stoddard, R. R. (1987). Planned approach to community health: The PATCH Program. Chapter 47 in P. A. Nutting (Ed.), *Community-oriented primary care: From principle to practice.* (Washington, DC: U.S. Government Printing Office, U.S. Department of Health and Human Services, HRS-A-PE 86-1.

Nelson, D. J., Sennett, L., Lefebvre, R. C., et al. (1987). A campaign strategy for weight loss at worksites. *Health Education Research, 2,* 27–31.

Neufeld, V. R., & Norman, G. R. (Eds.). (1985). *Assessing clinical competence.* New York: Springer.

Neugebauer, R. (1996). Review: World mental health: Problems and priorities in low-income countries. *American Journal of Public Health, 86,* 1654–1655.

Neuhauser, L. Schwab, M., Syme, S. L., Bieber, M., & King Obarski, S. (1998). Community participation in health promotion: Evaluation of the California wellness guide. *Health Promotion International, 13,* 211–222.

Neumark-Sztainer, D., & Story, M. (1996). The use of health behavior theory in nutrition counseling. *Topics in Clinical Nutrition, 11,* 60–73.

New approaches to health education in primary health care: Report of a WHO expert committee. (1983). Geneva: World Health Organization, Technical Report Series 690.

Newman, I. M., & Martin, G. L. (1982). Attitudinal and normative factors associated with adolescent cigarette smoking in Australia and the USA: A methodology to assist health education planning. *Community Health Studies, 6,* 47–56.

Newman, I. M., Martin, G. L., & Farrell, K. A. (1978). Changing health values through public television. *Health Values, 2*(2), 92–95.

Newman, I. M., Martin, G. L., & Weppner, R. (1982). A conceptual model for developing prevention programs. *The International Journal of the Addictions, 17,* 493–504.

Nguyen, M. N., Grignon, R., Tremblay, M., & Delisle, L. (1995). Behavioral diagnosis of 30 to 60 year-old men in the Fabreville Heart Health Program. *Journal of Community Health, 20,* 257–269.

Nguyen, M. N., Potvin, L., O'Loughlin, J., et al. (1995). L'épicerie aide-t-elle le consommateur a choisir les aliments qui favorisent la santé du coeur? Une étude exploratoire. *Canadian Journal of Public Health, 86,* 185–187.

Nickens, H. W. (1990). Health promotion and disease prevention among minorities. *Health Affairs, 9,* 133–143.

Nix, H. L. (1969). Concepts of community and community leadership. *Sociology and Social Research, 53,* 500–510.

Nix, H. L. (1970). *Identification of leaders and their involvement in the planning process.* Washington, DC: U.S. Public Health Service, Pub. No. 1998.

Nix, H. L. (1977). *The community and its involvement in the study action planning process.* Atlanta, GA: U.S. Department of Health, Education and Welfare, Centers for Disease Control, HEW-CDC-78-8355.

Nix, H. L., & Seerly, N. R. (1971, Fall). Community reconnaissance method: A synthesis of functions. *Journal of Community Development Society, 11,* 62–69.

Nix, H. L., & Seerly, N. R. (1973). Comparative views and actions of community leaders and nonleaders. *Rural Sociology, 38,* 427–428.

Noell, J., Ary, D., & Duncan, T. (1997). Development and evaluation of a sexual decision-making and social skills program: "The choice is yours—Preventing HIV/STDs." *Health Education and Behavior, 24*(1), 87–101.

Norman, S. A., Greenberg, R., Marconi, K., et al. (1990). A process evaluation of a two-year community cardiovascular risk reduction program: What was done and who knew about it? *Health Education Research, 5,* 87–97.

Novelli, W. D. (1990). Applying social marketing to health promotion and disease prevention. In K. Glanz, F. M. Lewis, & B. K. Rimer (Eds.), *Health behavior and health education: Theory, research, and practice.* San Francisco: Jossey-Bass.

Nozu, Y., Iwai, K., & Watanabe, M. (1995, August). *AIDS-related knowledge, attitudes, beliefs and skills among high school students in Akita: Results from Akita AIDS Education for Adolescent Survey. Abstract No. 234. Proceedings.* XV World Conference of the International Union for Health Promotion and Education, Makuhari, Japan.

Nursing Development Conference Group. (1973). *Concept formalization in nursing: Process and product.* Boston: Little, Brown.

Nussel, E., Wiesemann, W., Scheuermann, R., et al. (1992, May). *Health status as a tool to translate research results into policy.* Paper presented at the International Heart Health Conference in Victoria, British Columbia.

Nutbeam, D. (1985, July). *Health promotion glossary.* Copenhagen: World Health Regional Office for Europe.

Nutbeam, D. (1996). Improving the fit between research and practice in health promotion: Overcoming structural barriers. *Canadian Journal of Public Health, 87*(Suppl. 2), S18–S23.

Nutbeam, D. (1998). *Health promotion glossary.* Geneva: World Heath Organization, WHO/HPR/HEP/98.1.

Nutbeam, D., Aaro, L., & Wold, B. (1991). The lifestyle concept and health education with young people: Results from a WHO international survey. *World Health Statistics Quarterly, 44,* 55–61.

Nutbeam, D., & Catford, J. (1987). The Welsh Heart Programme evaluation strategy: Progress, plans and possibilities. *Health Promotion, 2,* 5–18.

Nutbeam, D., & Harris, E. (1995). Creating supportive environments for health: A case study from Australia in developing national goals and targets for healthy environments. *Health Promotion International, 10,* 51–59.

Nutbeam, D., Smith, C., & Catford, J. (1990). Evaluation in health education: A review of possibilities and problems. *Journal of Epidemiology and Community Health, 44,* 83–89.

Nutbeam, D., Smith, C., Murphy, S., & Catford, J. (1993). Maintaining evaluation designs in long term community based health promotion programmes: Heartbeat Wales case study. *Journal of Epidemiology and Community Health, 47*(2), 127–133.

Nutbeam, D., & Wise, M. (1996). Planning for Health for All: International experience in setting health goals and targets. *Health Promotion International, 11,* 219–226.

Nutbeam, D., Wise, M., Bauman, A., Harris, E., & Leeder, S. (1993). *Goals and targets for Australia's health in the year 2000 and beyond.* Portland, OR: International Specialized Books Services. Also published 1993, Canberra: Australian Government Publishing Service.

Nutting, P. A. (1986). Health promotion in primary medical care: Problems and potential. *Preventive Medicine, 15,* 537–548.

Nutting, P. A. (Ed.). (1987). *Community-oriented primary care: From principle to practice.* Washington, DC: U.S. Department of Health and Human Services, Health Resources and Services Administration, HRS-A-PE 86-1.

Nutting, P. A. (1990). Community-oriented primary care: A critical area of research for primary care. In *Primary care research: An agenda for the 90s.* Washington, DC: U.S. Department of Health and Human Services, Agency for Health Care Policy and Research.

Nyswander, D. (1942). *Solving school health problems.* New York: Oxford University Press.

Nyswander, D. (1967). The open society: Its implications for health educators. *Health Education Monographs, 1*(1), 3–13.

O'Brien, R. W., Smith, S. A., Bush, P. J., & Peleg, E. (1990). Obesity, self-esteem, and health locus of control in black youths during transition to adolescence. *American Journal of Health Promotion, 5,* 133–139.

O'Connor, A. M., Pennie, R. A., & Dales, R. E. (1996). Framing effects on expectations, decisions, and side effects experienced: The case of influenza immunization. *Journal of Clinical Epidemiology, 49,* 1271–1276.

O'Donnell, M. P. (1985). Research on drinking locations of alcohol-impaired drivers: Implication for prevention policies. *Journal of Public Health Policy, 6,* 510–525.

O'Donnell, M. P. (1986). Definition of health promotion. *American Journal of Health Promotion, 1,* 4–5.

O'Donnell, M. P. (1989). Definition of health promotion: Part III. Expanding the definition. *American Journal of Health Promotion, 3,* 5.

O'Donnell, M. P., & Harris, J. S. (Eds.). (1994). *Health promotion in the workplace* (2nd ed.). New York: Delmar.

Office of Disease Prevention and Health Promotion. (1981). *Toward a healthy community: Organizing events for community health promotion.* Washington, DC: U.S. Department of Health and Human Services, Pub. No. PHS 80-50113.

Office of Disease Prevention and Health Promotion. (1993). *Health promotion goes to work: Programs with an impact.* Washington, DC: U.S. Department of Health and Human Services.

Office on Smoking and Health. (1987). *Health consequence of smoking: Cardiovascular disease.* Washington, DC: U.S. Government Printing Office.

Okafor, F. C. (1985). Basic needs in Nigeria. *Social Indicators Research, 17,* 115–125.

Okene, J. K., Lindsay, E., Berger, L., & Hymowitz, N. (1990–1991). Health care providers as key change agents in the community intervention trial for smoking cessation (COMMIT). *International Quarterly of Community Health Education, 11,* 223–237.

Oldridge, N. B. (1984). Adherence to adult exercise fitness programs. In J. D. Matarazzo et al. (Eds.), *Behavioral Health* (pp. 467–487). New York: Wiley.

Oldridge, N. (1982). Compliance and exercise in primary and secondary prevention of coronary heart disease: A review. *Preventive Medicine, 11,* 56–70.

O'Loughlin, J., Paradis, G., & Gray-Donald, K. (1998). Prevalence and correlates of overweight among elementary schoolchildren in multiethnic, low income, inner-city neighbourhoods in Montreal, Canada. *Annals of Epidemiology, 8,* 422–432.

O'Loughlin, Paradis, G., Kishchuk, N., et al. (1995). Coeur en Santé St-Henri—a heart health promotion programme in Montreal, Canada: Design and methods for evaluation. *Journal of Epidemiology and Community Health, 49,* 495–502.

Olson, C. M. (1994). Promoting positive nutritional practices during pregnancy and lactation. *American Journal of Clinical Nutrition 59*(Suppl.), 525S–531S.

O'Neill, C., Normand, C., & McKnight, A. (1996). Cost effectiveness of personal health education in primary care for people with angina in the Greater Belfast area of Northern Ireland. *Journal of Epidemiology and Community Health, 50,* 538–540.

O'Neill, M., Rootman, I., & Pederson, A. (1994), Beyond Lalonde: Two decades of Canadian health promotion. In A. Pederson, M. O'Neill, & I. Rootman (Eds.), *Health Promotion in Canada.* Toronto: Saunders.

Opdycke, R. A. C., Ascione, F. J., Shimp, L. A., & Rosen, R. I. (1992). A systematic approach to educating elderly patients about their medications. *Patient Education and Counseling, 19,* 43–60.

Ordin, D. L. (1992). Surveillance, monitoring, and screening in occupational health. In J. M. Last & R. B. Wallace (Eds.), *Public health and preventive medicine* (13th ed., pp. 551–558). Norwalk, CT: Appleton & Lange.

Orlandi, M. A. (1986). Community-based substance abuse prevention: A multicultural perspective. *Journal of School Health, 56,* 394–401.

Orlandi, M. A. (1987). Promoting health and preventing disease in health care settings: An analysis of barriers. *Preventive Medicine, 16,* 119–130.

Orleans, C. T., George, L. K., Houpt, J. L., & Brodie, K. H. (1985). Health promotion in primary care: A survey of U.S. family practitioners. *Preventive Medicine, 14,* 636–647.

Orleans, C. T., & Shipley, R. (1982). Worksite smoking cessation initiatives: Review and recommendations. *Addictive Behaviors, 7,* 1–16.

O'Rourke, T. W., & Macrina, D. M. (1989). Beyond victim blaming: Examining the micro-macro issue in health promotion. *Wellness perspectives: Research, theory and practice, 6,* 7–17.

Orth-Gomer K., Rosingren, A., & Wilhelmsen, L. (1993). Lack of social support and incidence of coronary health disease in middle-aged Swedish men. *Psychosomatic Medicine, 55,* 37–43.

Orthoefer, J., Bain, D., Empereur, R., & Nesbit, T. (1988). Consortium building among local health departments in northwest Illinois. *Public Health Reports, 103,* 500–507.

Osgood, G. E., Cuci, G. J., & Tannenbaum, P. H. (1961). *The measurement of meaning.* Urbana: University of Illinois Press.

Ostrow, D. G. (1989). AIDS prevention through effective education. *Daedalus: Journal of the American Academy of Arts and Sciences, 118,* 229–254.

Ostwald, S. K., & Rothenberger, J. (1985). Development of a testicular self-examination program for college men. *Journal of the American College Health, 33*(6), 234–239.

Ottoson, J. M., & Green, L. W. (1987). Reconciling concept and context: Theory of implementation. In W. B. Ward & M. H. Becker (Eds.), *Advances in health education and promotion* (Vol. 2, pp. 353–382). Greenwich, CT: JAI Press.

Oxman, A. D., Thomson, M. A., Davis, D. A., & Haynes, R. B. (1995). No magic bullets: A systematic review of 102 trials of interventions to improve professional practice. *Canadian Medical Association Journal, 153,* 1423–1431.

Oxman, A. D., Thompson, R. S., Taplin, S. H., Carter, A. P., et al. (1988). A risk based breast cancer screening program. *HMO Practice, 2,* 177–191.

Padilla, G. V., & Bulcavage, L. M. (1991). Theories used in patient/health education. *Seminars in Oncology Nursing, 7*(2), 87–96.

Paehlke, R. C. (1989). *Environmentalism and the future of progressive politics.* New Haven, CT: Yale University Press.

Page, R. M., & Gold, R. S. (1983). Assessing gender differences in college cigarette smoking: Intenders and non-intenders. *Journal of School Health, 53,* 531–535.

Pahkala, K., Kivela, S. L., & Laippala, P. (1991). Relationships between social and health factors and major depression in old age in a multivariate analysis. *Nordisk Psykiatrisk Tidsskrift, 45,* 299–307.

Paine-Andrews, A., Fancisco, V. T., & Coen, S. (1996). Health marketing in the supermarket: Using prompting, product sampling, and price reduction to increase customer purchases of lower-fat items. *Health Marketing Quarterly, 14,* 85–95.

Palmer, R. H. (1996). Quality health care: Measuring physician performance. *Journal of the American Medical Association, 275,* 1851–1852.

Palti, H., Knishkowy, B. Epstein, Y., et al. (1997). Reported health concerns of Israeli high school students: Differences by age and sex. *Israel Journal of Medical Sciences, 33,* 123–128.

Paluck, E. C. M. (1998). *Pharmacist-client communication: A study of quality and client satisfaction. Unpublished dissertation. Vancouver:* University of British Columbia.

Papenfus, H., & Bryan, A. (1998). Nurses' involvement in interdisciplinary team evaluations: Incorporating the family perspective into child assessment. *Journal of School Health, 68,* 184–189.

Paperny, D. M. N., & Starn, J. R. (1989). Adolescent pregnancy prevention by health education computer games: Computer-assisted instruction of knowledge and attitudes. *Pediatrics, 83,* 742–752.

Paradis, G., O'Loughlin, J., Elliott, M., et al. (1995). Coeur en Santé St-Henri—a heart health promotion programme in a low income, low education neighbourhood in Montreal, Canada: Theoretical model and early field experience. *Journal of Epidemiology and Community Health, 49,* 503–512.

Parcel, G. S. (1976). Skills approach to health education: A framework for integrating cognitive and affective learning. *Journal of School Health, 66,* 403–406.

Parcel, G. S. (1984). Theoretical models for application in school health education research. *Journal of School Health, 54,* 39–49.

Parcel, G. S., & Baranowski, T. (1981). Social learning theory and health education. *Health Education, 12*(3), 14–18.

Parcel, G. S., Edmundson, E., Perry, C. L., et al. (1995). Measurement of self-efficacy for diet-related behaviors among elementary school children. *Journal of School Health, 65,* 23–27.

Parcel, G. S., Eriksen, M. P., Lovato, C. Y., et al. (1989). The diffusion of school-based tobacco-use prevention programs: Project description and baseline data. *Health Education Research, 4,* 111–124.

Parcel, G. S., Green, L. W., & Bettes, B. (1989). School-based programs to prevent or reduce obesity. In N. A. Krasnagor, G. D. Grave, & N. Kretchmer (Eds.), *Childhood obesity: A biobehavioral perspective* (pp. 143–157). Caldwell, NJ: Telford Press.

Parcel, G. S., Muraskin, L. D., & Endert, C. M. (1988). Community education: Study group report [of Society for Adolescent Medicine]. *Journal of Adolescent Health Care, 9,* 41S–45S.

Parcel, G. S., Ross, J. G., Lavin, A. T., et al. (1991). Enhancing implementation of the teenage health teaching modules. *Journal of School Health, 61,* 35–38.

Parcel, G. S., O'Hara-Tompkins, N. M., Harrist, R. B., et al. (1995). Diffusion of an effective tobacco prevention program: Part II. Evaluation of the adoption phase. *Health Education Research, 10,* 297–307.

Parcel, G. S., Simons-Morton, B. G., & Kolbe, L. J. (1988). Health promotion: Integrating organizational change and student learning strategies. *Health Education Quarterly, 15,* 435–450.

Parcel, G. S., Simons-Morton, B. G., O'Hara, N. M., et al. (1989). School promotion of healthful diet and physical activity: Impact on learning outcomes and self-reported behavior. *Health Education Quarterly, 16,* 181–199.

Parcel G. S., Swank P. R., Mariotto M. J., et al. (1994). Self-management of cystic-fibrosis: A structural model for educational and behavioral variables. *Social Science and Medicine, 38,* 1307–1315.

Parham, D. L., Goodman, R. M., Steckler, A., Schmid, J., & Koch, G. (1993). Adoption of health education: Tobacco use prevention curricula in North Carolina school districts. *Family and Community Health, 16*(3), 56–67.

Park, R. E., Burgess, E. W., & McKenzie, R. D. (Eds.). (1925). *The city.* Chicago: University of Chicago Press.

Park, P., Brydon-Miller, M., Hall, B., & Jackson, T. (Eds.). (1993). *Voices of change: Participatory research in Canada and the United States.* Toronto: Ontario Institute for Studies in Education.

Parkinson, R. S., Green, L. W., Eriksen, M., & McGill, A. (Eds.). (1982). *Managing health promotion in the workplace: Guidelines for implementation and evaluation.* Palo Alto, CA: Mayfield.

Parle, M., Maguire, P., & Heaven, C. (1997). The development of a training model to improve health professionals' skills, self-efficacy and outcome expectancies when communicating with cancer patients. *Social Science and Medicine, 44,* 231–241.

Parlette, N., Glogow, E., & D'Onofrio, C. N. (1981). Public health administration and health education training need more integration. *Health Education Quarterly, 8,*123–146.

Parsons, T. (1964). The superego and the theory of social systems. In R. L. Coser (Ed.), *The family: Its structure and functions* (pp. 433–449). New York: St. Martin's Press.

Partridge, M. R. (1995). Delivering optimal care to the person with asthma: What are the key components and what do we mean by patient education? *European Respiratory Journal, 8,* 298–305.

Parvanta, C. F., Cottert, P., Anthony, R., & Parlato, M. (1997). Nutrition promotion in Mali: Highlights of a rural integrated nutrition communication program (1989–1995). *Journal of Nutrition Education, 29,* 274–280.

Pasick, R. (1997). Socioeconomic and cultural factors in the development and use of theory. In K. Glanz, F. M. Lewis, & B. K. Rimer (Eds.), *Health behavior and health education: Theory, research, and practice* (2nd ed., pp. 425–440). San Francisco: Jossey-Bass.

Pasick, R. J., D'Onofrio, C. N., & Otero-Sabogal, R. (1996). Similarities and differences across cultures: Questions to inform a third generation for health promotion research. *Health Education Quarterly 23*(Suppl.), S142–S161.

PATCH: Planned approach to community health. (1985). Atlanta, GA: Centers for Disease Control.

Pate, R. R. (1983). A new definition of fitness. *Physician and Sports Medicine, 11,* 77–82.

Patient information and prescription drugs: Parallel surveys of physicians and pharmacists. (1983). New York: Harris and Associates.

Patton, C. (1985). *Sex and germs: The politics of AIDS.* Boston: South End Press.

Patton, M. Q. (1990). *Qualitative evaluation and research methods* (2nd ed.). Newbury Park, CA: Sage.

Patton, M. Q. (1997). *Utilization-focused evaluation: The new century text* (3rd ed.). Thousand Oaks, CA, Sage.

Patton, R. D., & Cissell, W. B. (Eds.). (1989). *Community organization: Traditional principles and modern application.* Johnson City, TN: Latchpins Press.

Paul, B. D. (Ed.). (1955). *Health, culture and community.* New York: Russell Sage Foundation.

Pearce, N. (1996). Traditional epidemiology, modern epidemiology, and public health. *American Journal of Public Health, 86,* 678–683.

Pearse, W., & Refshauge, C. (1987). Workers' health and safety in Australia: An overview. *International Journal of Health Services, 17,* 635–650.

Pechacek, T. F., Fox, B. H., Murray, D. M., & Luepker, R. V. (1984). Review of techniques for measurement of smoking behaviors. In J. Matarazzo et al. (Eds.), *Behavioral health: A handbook of health enhancement and disease prevention.* New York: Wiley.

Pederson, L. L., & Baskerville, J. C. (1983). Multivariate prediction of smoking cessation following physician advice to quit smoking: A validation study. *Preventive Medicine, 12,* 430–436.

Pelletier, K. R. (1993). A review and analysis of the health and cost-effective outcome studies of comprehensive health promotion and disease prevention programs at the worksite: 1991–1993 update. *American Journal of Health Promotion, 8,* 50–62.

Pelletier, K. R. (1996). A review and analysis of the health and cost-effective outcome studies of comprehensive health promotion and disease prevention programs at the worksite: 1993–1995 update. *American Journal of Health Promotion, 10,* 380–388.

Pelletier, K. R., Klehr, N. L., & McPhee, S. J. (1988, February). Town and gown: A lesson in collaboration. *Business and Health,* pp. 34–39.

Pelletier, K. R., & Lutz, R. (1988). Healthy people—healthy business: A critical review of stress management programs in the workplace. *American Journal of Health Promotion, 2*(3), 5–12.

Pels, R. J., Bor, D. H., & Lawrence, R. S. (1989). Decision making for introducing clinical preventive services. *Annual Review of Public Health, 10,* 363–383.

Pennington, J. T., Wisniowski, L. A., & Logan, G. B. (1988). In-store nutrition information programs. *Journal of Nutrition Education, 20,* 5–10.

Pentz, M. A. (1986). Community organization and school liaisons: How to get programs started. *Journal of School Health, 56,* 382–388.

Pentz, M. A., Dwyer, J. H., MacKinnon, D. P., et al. (1989). A multicommunity trial for primary prevention of drug abuse. *Journal of the American Medical Association, 261,* 3259–3266.

Pentz, M. A., MacKinnon, D. P., Dwyer, J. H., et al. (1989). Longitudinal effects of the Midwestern Prevention Project on regular and experimental smoking in adolescents. *Preventive Medicine, 18,* 304–321.

Pentz, M. A., & Trebow, E. (1991). Implementation issues in drug abuse prevention research. In *Drug abuse prevention intervention research: Methodological issues* [NIDA Research Monograph 107]. Rockville, MD: National Institute of Drug Abuse, DHHS Publ No. 91-1761.

Pepe, M. V., & Chodzko-Zajko, W. J. (1997). Impact of older adults' reading ability on the comprehension and recall of cholesterol information. *Journal of Health Education, 28,* 21–27.

Perera, D. R., LoGerfo, J. P., Shulenberger, E., Ylvisaker, J. T., & Kirz, H. L. (1983). Teaching sigmoidoscopy to primary care physicians: A controlled study of continuing medical education. *Journal of Family Practice, 16,* 785–799.

Permut, S. (1986). Corporate liability for occupational medicine programs. In S. Wolf & A. Finestone (Eds.), *Occupational stress: Health and performance at work* (pp. 136–152). Littleton, MA: PSG Publishing.

Perry, C. L., Luepker, R. V., Murray, D. M., et al. (1988). Parent involvement with children's health promotion: The Minnesota home team. *American Journal of Public Health, 78,* 1156–1160.

Perry, C. L., Luepker, R. V, Murray, D. M., et al. (1989). Parent involvement with children's health promotion: A one year follow-up of the Minnesota Home Team. *Health Education Quarterly, 16,* 171–180.

Perry, C. L., Sellers, D. E., & Cook, K. (1997). The Child and Adolescent Trial for Cardiovascular Health (CATCH): Intervention, implementation, and feasibility for elementary schools in the United States. *Health Education and Behavior, 24,* 716–735.

Perry, C. L., Williams, C. L,, Veblen-Mortenson, S., et al. (1996). Project Northland: Outcomes of a community-wide alcohol use prevention program during early adolescence. *American Journal of Public Health, 86*(7), 956–965.

Perspectives on Health Promotion and Disease Prevention in the United States. (1978). Washington, DC: Institute of Medicine, National Academy of Sciences.

Pertschuk, M., & Erikson, A. (1987). *Smoke fighting: A smoking control movement building guide.* New York: American Cancer Society.

Pertschuk, M., & Schaetzel, W. (1989). *The people rising: The campaign against the Bork nomination.* New York: Thunder's Mouth Press.

Peterson, C., & Stunkard, A. J. (1989). Personal control and health promotion. *Social Science and Medicine, 28,* 819–828.

Petri, C. J., & Hyner, G. C. (1996). The effects of affective versus informative computer-assisted HIV/AIDS instruction. *Journal of Wellness Perspectives, 12*(1), 29–34.

Phillips, K. A., Morrison, K. R., & Aday, L. A. (1998). Understanding the context of healthcare utilization: Assessing environmental and provider-related variables in the behavioral model of utilization. *Health Services Research, 33,* 571–596.

Pichora-Fuller, M. K. (1997). Assistive listening devices in accessibility programs for the elderly: A health promotion approach. In R. Lubinski & J. Higginbothan (Eds.), *Communication technologies for the elderly* (pp. 161–202). San Diego, CA: Singular Press.

Pierce, J. P., Macaskill, P., & Hill, D. (1990). Long-term effectiveness of mass media led antismoking campaigns in Australia. *American Journal of Public Health, 80,* 565–569.

Pigg, R. M. (1989). The contribution of school health programs to the broader goals of public health: The American experience. *Journal of School Health, 59,* 25–30.

Pilisuk, M., Parks, S., Kelly, J., & Turner, E. (1982). The helping network approach: Community promotion of mental health. *Journal of Primary Prevention, 3,* 116–132.

Pincus, T. (1996). Documenting quality management in rheumatic disease: Are patient questionnaires the best (and only) method? *Arthritis Care and Research, 9,* 339–348.

Pittman, D. J. (1993). The new temperance movement in the United States: What happened to macrostructural factors in alcohol problems? *Addiction, 88,* 167–170.

Plante, T. G., & Schwartz, G. E. (1990). Defensive and repressive coping styles: Self-presentation, leisure activities, and assessment. *Journal of Research in Personality, 24,* 173–190.

Plas, J. M., & Lewis, S. E. (1996). Environmental factors and sense of community in a planned town. *American Journal of Community Psychology, 24,* 109–144.

Plough, A., & Olafson, F. (1994). Implementing the Boston Healthy Start Initiative: A case study of community empowerment and public health. *Health Education Quarterly, 21,* 221–234.

Pokorny, A., Putnam, P., & Fryer, J. E. (1980). Drug abuse and alcoholism teaching in U.S. medical and osteopathic schools, 1975–77. In M. Galanter (Ed.), *Alcohol and drug abuse in medical education.* Washington, DC: U.S. Government Printing Office, DHEW Pub. No. (ADM)79-81.

Poland, B., Green, L., & Rootman, I. (Eds.). (in press). *Settings for health promotion.* Thousand Oaks, CA: Sage.

Polcyn, M. M., Price, J. H., Jurs, S. G., & Roberts, S. M. (1991). Utility of the PRECEDE model in differentiating users and nonusers of smokeless tobacco. *Journal of School Health, 61,* 166–171.

Polissar, L., Sim, D., & Francis, A. (1981). Survival of colorectal cancer patients in relation to duration of symptoms and other prognostic factors. *Diseases of the Colon and Rectum, 24,* 364–369.

Pollitt, E. (1994). Poverty and child development: Relevance of research in developing countries to the United States. *Child Development, 65,* 283–295.

Pollock, M. (1987). *Planning and implementing health education in schools.* Palo Alto, CA: Mayfield.

Pollock, M. B., & Middleton, K. (1994). *School health instruction* (3rd ed.). St Louis, MO: Mosby.

Popham, W. J., Potter L. D., Bal, D. G., et al. (1993). Do antismoking media campaigns help smokers quit? *Public Health Reports, 108,* 510–513.

Popham W. J., Potter, L. D., Bal, D. G., et al. (1994). Effectiveness of the 1990–1991 tobacco education media campaign. *American Journal of Preventive Medicine, 10,* 319–326.

Popkin, B., Haines, P., & Reidy, K. (1989). Food consumption trends of U.S. women: Patterns and determinants between 1977 and 1985. *American Journal of Clinical Nutrition, 49,* 1307–1319.

Porras, J., & Hoffer, S. (1986). Common behavior changes in successful organization development efforts. *Journal of Applied Behavioral Science, 22,* 477–494.

Porter, P. J. (1981). Realistic outcomes of school health service programs. *Health Education Quarterly, 8*(1), 81–87.

Posavac, E. J. (1980). Evaluations of patient education programs: A meta-analysis. *Evaluation and the Health Professions, 3,* 47–62.

Potapchuk, W. R., Crocker, J., & Schechter, W. H. (1997, February). *Systems reform and local government: Improving outcomes for children, families, and neighborhoods—a working paper.* Report to the Annie E. Casey Foundation.

Povar, G. J., Mantell, M., & Morris, L. A. (1984). Patients' therapeutic preferences in an ambulatory care setting. *American Journal of Public Health, 74,* 1395–1397.

Powell, K. E., Caspersen, C. J., Koplan, J. P., & Ford, E. S. (1989). Physical activity and chronic diseases. *American Journal of Clinical Nutrition, 49,* 999–1006.

Powell, K. E., Christenson, G. M., & Kreuter, M. W. (1984). Objectives for the Nation: Assessing the role physical education must play. *Journal of Physical Education, Recreation, and Dance, 55,* 18–20.

Powell, K. E., Thompson, P. D., Caspersen, C. J., et al. (1987). Physical activity and the incidence of coronary heart disease. *Annual Review of Public Health, 8,* 253–287.

Preparation and practice of community, patient and school health educators: Proceedings on commonalties and differences. (1978). Bethesda, MD: Bureau of Health Manpower, U.S. Department of Health, Education, and Welfare, HRA 78-71.

Pressman, J., & Wildavsky, A. (1973). *Implementation* (2nd ed.). Berkeley: University of California Press.

Preston, M. A., Baranowski, T., & Higginbotham, J. C. (1988–1989). Orchestrating the points of community intervention. *International Quarterly of Community Health Education, 9,* 11–34.

Price, J. H., Desmond, S. M., Krol, R. A., Snyder, F. F., & O'Connell, J. K. (1987). Family practice physicians' beliefs, attitudes, and practices regarding obesity. *American Journal of Preventive Medicine, 3,* 339–345.

Probart, C., McDonnell, E., & Anger, S. (1997). Evaluation of implementation of an interdisciplinary nutrition curriculum in middle schools. *Journal of Nutrition Education, 29,* 203–209.

Prochaska, J. O. (1989, August 9–10). What causes people to change from unhealthy to health enhancing behavior? Paper presented at the American Cancer Society meeting on Behavioral Research in Cancer, Bloomington, IN.

Prochaska, J. O. (1994). Strong and weak principles for progressing from precontemplation to action based on 12 problem behaviors. *Health Psychology, 13,* 47–51.

Prochaska, J. O., & DiClemente, C. (1983). Stages and processes of self-change in smoking: Towards an integrative model of change. *Journal of Consulting and Clinical Psychology, 5,* 390–395.

Prochaska, J. O., DiClemente, C. C., & Norcross, J. C. (1992). In search of how people change: Applications to the addictive behaviors. *American Psychologist, 47,* 1102–1114.

Prochaska, J. O., Norcross, J. C., & DiClemente, C. C. (1994). *Changing for good.* New York: Morrow.

Prochaska, J. O., Redding, C. A., & Evers, K. E. (1997). The transtheoretical model and stages of change. In K. Glanz, F. M. Lewis, & B. K. Rimer (Eds.), *Health behavior and health education: Theory, research, and practice* (2nd ed., pp. 60–84). San Francisco: Jossey-Bass.

Promoting health through schools: The World Health Organization's global school health initiative. (1996) Geneva: World Health Organization.

Pucci, L. G., & Haglund, B. (1994). "Naturally Smoke Free": A support program for facilitating worksite smoking control policy implementation in Sweden. *Health Promotion International, 9,* 177–187.

Pucci, L. G., Joseph, H. M., Jr., & Siegel, M. (1998). Outdoor tobacco advertising in six Boston neighborhoods: Evaluating youth exposure. *American Journal of Preventive Medicine, 15,* 155–159.

Pulley, L., McAlister, A. L., & O'Reilly, K. (1996). Prevention campaigns for hard-to-reach populations at risk for HIV infection: Theory and implementation. *Health Education Quarterly 23,* 488–496.

Puska, P., McAlister, A., Pekkola, J., & Koskela, K. (1981). Television in health promotion: Evaluation of a national programme in Finland. *International Journal of Health Education, 24,* 2–14.

Puska, P., Nissinen, A., Tuomilehto, J., et al. (1985). The community-based strategy to prevent coronary heart disease: Conclusions from the ten years of the North Karelia Project. *Annual Review of Public, 6,* 147–193.

Puska, P., Tuomilehto, J., Nissinen, A., & Vartianinen, E. (1995). The North Karelia Project: Twenty year results and experiences. Helsinki: Helsinki University Printing House.

Putnam, R. D. (1995). Bowling alone: America's declining social capital. *Journal of Democracy, 6,* 65–78.

Quick, J. C., Murphy, L. R., & Hurrell, J. H. (1992). *Stress and well-being at work: Assessments and interventions for occupational mental health.* Washington, DC: American Psychological Association.

Quirk, M., & Seymour, W. (1991). Notes on an organismic-developmental, systems perspective for health education. *Health Education Research, 6,* 203–210.

Radecki, S. E., & Mandenhall, R. C. (1986). Patient counseling by primary care physicians: Results of a nationwide survey. *Patient Education and Counseling, 8,* 165–177.

Raeburn, J. M., & Rootman, I. (1988). Towards an expanded health field concept: Conceptual and research issues in a new era of health promotion. *Health Promotion: An International Journal, 3,* 383–392.

Raeburn, J. M., & Rootman, I. (1997). *People centered health promotion.* Chichester: John Wiley & Sons.

Rafferty, Y., & Radosh, A. (1997). Attitudes about AIDS education and condom availability among parents of high school students in New York City: A focus group approach. *AIDS Education and Prevention, 9,* 14–30.

Ramirez, A. G., & McAlister, A. L. (1989). Mass media campaign: *A Su Salud. Preventive Medicine, 17,* 608–621.

Randel, J. M., Morris, B. A., Wetzel, C. D., & Whitehill, B. V. (1992). The effectiveness of games for educational purposes: A review of recent research. *Simulation and Gaming, 23*(3), 261–276.

Ransdell, L. B., & Rehling, S. L. (1996). Church-based health promotion: A review of the literature. *American Journal of Health Behavior, 20,* 195–207.

Ratcliff, J., & Wallack, L. (1986). Primary prevention in public health: An analysis of basic assumptions. *International Quarterly of Community Health Education, 6,* 215–237.

Ratner, P., Green, L. W., Frankish, C. J., Chomik, T., & Larsen, C. (1997). Setting the stage for health impact assessment. *Journal of Public Health Policy, 18*(1), 67–79.

Rayant, G., & Sheiham, A. (1980). An analysis of factors affecting compliance with tooth-cleaning recommendations. *Journal of Clinical Periodontology, 7,* 289–299.

Redman, S., Spencer, E. A., & Sanson-Fisher, R. W. (1990). The role of mass media in changing health-related behaviour: A critical appraisal of two models. *Health Promotion International, 5,* 85–102.

Reed, D. B. (1996). Focus groups identify desirable features of nutrition programs for low-income mothers of preschool children. *Journal of the American Dietetic Association, 96,* 501–503.

Reed, B. D., Jensen, J. D., & Gorenflo, D. W. (1991). Physicians and exercise promotion. *American Journal of Preventive Medicine, 7,* 410–415.

Rein, M., & Rabinovitz, F. (1977). Implementation: A theoretical perspective. Cambridge, MA: Joint Center for Urban Studies of MIT and Harvard University, Working Paper No. 43.

Reinke, W. A. (1995). Quality management in managed care. *Health Care Management, 2,* 79–88.

Reis, J., & Tymchyshyn, P. (1992). A longitudinal evaluation of computer-assisted instruction on contraception for college students. *Adolescence, 27,* 803–811.

Rejeski, W. J., Brawley, L. R., & Thompson, C. (1997). Compliance to exercise therapy in older participants with knee osteoarthritis: Implications for treating disability. *Medicine and Science in Sports and Exercise, 29,* 977–985.

Renaud, L., Chevalier, S., Dufour, R., et al. (1997). Evaluation of the implementation of a school curriculum: Intervention methods for optimizing the adoption and implementation of health education programs in elementary schools [published in French]. *Canadian Journal of Public Health, 88,* 351–353.

Report of the Presidential Commission on the Human Immunodeficiency Virus Epidemic. (1988, June 24). Washington, DC: The White House.

Report of the President's Committee on Health Education. (1973). New York: Public Affairs Institute.

Resnick, L. B. (1987). *Education and learning to think.* Washington, DC: National Academy Press.

Resnicow, K., Robinson, T., & Frank, E. (1996). Advances and future directions for school-based health promotion research: Commentary on the CATCH intervention trial. *Preventive Medicine, 25,* 378–383.

Results from the National Adolescent Student Health Survey. (1989). *Morbidity and Mortality Weekly Report, 38,* 147.

Reuter, P., & Caulkins, J. P. (1995). Redefining the goals of national drug policy: Recommendations from a working group. *American Journal of Public Health, 85,* 1059–1064.

Rezmovic, E. L. (1982). Program implementation and evaluation results: A reexamination of Type III error in a field experiment. *Evaluation and Program Planning, 5,* 111–118.

Richard, L., Potvin, L., Kischuk, N., Prlic, H., & Green, L. W. (1996). Assessment of the integration of the ecological approach in health promotion programs. *American Journal of Health Promotion, 10,* 318–328.

Richardson, M. A., Simons-Morton, B. G., & Annegers, J. F. (1993). Effect of perceived barriers on compliance with anti-hypertension medication. *Health Education Quarterly, 20,* 489–504.

Richie, N. D. (1976). Some guidelines for conducting a health fair. *Public Health Reports, 91,* 261–264.

Richmond, J. B., & Kotelchuck, M. (1991). Coordination and development of strategies and policy for public health promotion in the United States. In W. Holland, R. Detels, & G. Knox (Eds.), *Oxford textbook of public health* (2nd ed., Vol. 3, pp. 441–454). Oxford, England: Oxford University Press.

Riger, S., & Lavrakas, P. J. (1981). Community ties: Patterns of attachment and social interaction in urban neighborhoods. *American Journal of Community Psychology, 9,* 55–66.

Riggs, R., & Noland, M. (1983). Awareness, knowledge, and perceived risk for toxic shock syndrome in relation to health behavior. *Journal of School Health, 53,* 303–307.

Rimer, B. K. (1993). Improving the use of cancer screening in older women. *Cancer, 72*(Suppl.), 1084–1087.

Rimer, B. K. (1995). Audience and messages for breast and cervical cancer screenings. *Wellness Perspectives: Research, Theory and Practice, 11*(2), 13–39.

Rimer, B. K. (1997). Part two: Models of individual health behavior. In K. Glanz, F. M. Lewis, & B. K. Rimer (Eds.), *Health behavior and health education: Theory, research, and practice* (pp. 37–40). San Francisco: Jossey-Bass.

Rimer, B. K. (1997). Perspectives on intrapersonal theories of health behavior. In K. Glanz, F. M. Lewis, & B. K. Rimer (Eds.), *Health behavior and health education: Theory, research, and practice* (pp. 139–147). San Francisco: Jossey-Bass.

Rimer, B. K., Davis, S. W., Engstrom, P. F., et al. (1988). Some reasons for compliance and noncompliance in a health maintenance organization breast cancer screening program. *Journal of Compliance in Health Care, 3,* 103–114.

Rimer, B. K., Jones, W., Wilson, C., Bennett, D., & Engstrom, P. (1983). Planning a cancer control program for older citizens. *Gerontologist, 23,* 384–389.

Rimer, B. K., Keintz, M. K., & Fleisher, L. (1986). Process and impact of a health communications program. *Health Education Research, 1,* 29–36.

Rimer, B. K., Keintz, M., Glassman, B., & Kinman, J. (1986). Health education for older persons: Lessons from research and program evaluations. In Z. Salisbury, J. G. Zapka, & S. B. Kar (Eds.), *Advances in Health Education and Promotion* (Vol. 1, Pt. B, pp. 369–396). Greenwich, CT: JAI Press.

Rimer, B. K., Orleans, C. T., Fleisher, L., et al. (1994). Does tailoring matter? The impact of a tailored guide on ratings and short-term smoking-related outcomes for older smokers. *Health Education Research, 9,* 69-84).

Rimer, B. K., Ross, E., Balshem, A., & Engstrom, P. F. (1993). The effect of a comprehensive breast screening program on self-reported mammography use by primary care physicians and women in a health maintenance organization. *Cancer, 62,* 934–943.

Rimer, B. K., Ross, E., Christinzio, C. S., & Keng, E. (1992). Older women's participation in breast screening. *Journal of Gerontology, 47,* 85–91.

Ringen, K. (1989). The case for worker notification. *Annals of the New York Academy of Sciences, 572,* 133–141.

Rise, J., & Wilhelmsen, B. U. (1998). Prediction of adolescents' intention not to drink alcohol. *American Journal of Health Behavior, 22,* 206–217.

Risker, D., & Christopher, A. (1995). Segmentation analysis of consumer uses of health information. *Health Marketing Quarterly, 12,* 39–48.

Risser, L. W., Hoffman, H. M., Bellah, G. G., & Green, L. W. (1985). A cost-benefit analysis of preparticipation sports examinations of adolescent athletes. *Journal of School Health, 55,* 270–273.

Roberts, M. C. (1987). Public health and health psychology: Two cats of Kilkenny? *Professional Psychology: Research and Practice, 18,* 145–149.

Robinson, T. N. (1989). Community health behavior change through computer network health promotion: Preliminary findings from Stanford Health-Net. *Computer Methods and Programs in Biomedicine, 30*(2–3), 137–144.

Roccella, E. J., & Ward, G. W. (1984). The national high blood pressure campaign: A description of its utility as a generic program model. *Health Education Quarterly, 11,* 225–242.

Rockwell, S. K., & Buck, J. S. (1995). An interdisciplinary and interagency evaluation team: Benefits for other-discipline specialists. *Evaluation Practice, 16,* 239–246.

Rogers, E. M. (1973). *Communication strategies for family planning.* New York: Free Press.

Rogers, E. M. (1995). *Diffusion of innovations* (4th ed.). New York: Free Press.

Rogers, E. S. (1960). *Human ecology and health: An introduction for administrators.* New York: Macmillan.

Rokeach, M. (1970). *Beliefs, attitudes and values.* San Francisco: Jossey-Bass.

Roman, P. M., & Blum, T. C. (1996). Alcohol: A review of the impact of worksite interventions on health and behavioral outcomes. *American Journal of Health Promotion, 11,* 136–149.

Romer, D., & Kim, S. (1995). Health interventions for African American and Latino youth: The potential role of mass media. *Health Education Quarterly, 22,* 172–189.

Romm, R. J., Fletcher, S. W., & Hulka, B. S. (1981). The periodic health examination: Comparison of recommendations and internists' performance. *Southern Medical Journal, 74,* 265–271.

Rootman, I. (1988). Canada's health promotion survey. In I. Rootman, R. Warren, T. Stephens, & L. Peters (Eds.), *Canada's health promotion survey: Technical report.* Ottawa: Minister of Supply and Services.

Rootman, I. (1997). Continuous quality improvement in health promotion: Some preliminary thoughts from Canada. *Promotion and Education, 4*(2), 23–25.

Rose, G. (1992). *A Strategy of Preventive Medicine.* Oxford: Oxford University Press.

Rose, G., Hamilton, P. J., & Colwell, L., et al. (1982). A randomized controlled trial of anti-smoking advice: Ten year results. *Journal of Epidemiology and Community Health, 36,* 102–108.

Rosen, G. (1958). *A history of public health.* New York: MD Publications.

Rosen, J. B., & Schulkin, J. (1998). From normal fear to pathological anxiety. *Psychological Review, 105,* 325–350.

Rosenstock, I. M. (1966). Why people use health services. *Milbank Memorial Fund Quarterly, 44,* 94–127.

Rosenstock, I. M. (1974). The historical origins of the Health Belief Model. *Health Education Monographs, 2,* 354–395.

Rosenstock, I. M., Derryberry, M., & Carriger, B. (1959). Why people fail to seek poliomyelitis vaccination. *Public Health Reports, 74,* 98–103.

Rosenstock, I. M., Strecher, V. J., & Becker, M. H. (1994). The Health Belief Model and HIV risk behavior change. In J. Peterson & R. DiClemente (Eds.), *Preventing AIDS: Theory and practice of behavioral interventions.* New York: Plenum.

Ross, H. S., & Mico, P. R. (1980). *Theory and practice in health education.* Palo Alto, CA: Mayfield.

Ross, J. G., & Gilbert, G. G. (1985). The national children and youth fitness study. *Journal of Health, Physical Education, Recreation, and Dance, 56*(1), 45–50.

Ross, M. (1955). *Community organization: Theory and principles.* New York: Harper & Row.

Ross, M., & Lappin, B. W. (1967). *Community organization: Theory, principles, and practice.* New York: Harper & Row.

Ross, M. W., & Rosser, B. R. S. (1989). Education and AIDS risks: A review. *Health Education Research, 4,* 273–284.

Rosser, W. W. (1987). Benzodiapazine use in a family medicine center. *Drug Protocol, 2*(10), 9–15.

Rossi, P. H., & Freeman, H. E. (1993). *Evaluation: A systematic approach* (5th ed.). Thousand Oaks, CA: Sage.

Roter, D. L. (1977). Patient participation in the patient-provider interaction: The effects of patient question-asking on the quality of interaction, satisfaction and compliance. *Health Education Monographs, 5,* 281–315.

Roter, D. L., Hall, J. A., & Katz, N. R. (1988). Patient-physician communication: A descriptive summary of the literature. *Patient Education and Counseling, 12,* 99–119.

Rothman, J., & Brown, E. R. (1989). Indicators of societal action to promote social health. In S. B. Kar (Ed.), *Health Promotion Indicators and Actions* (pp. 202–220). New York: Springer.

Rothman, J., & Tropman, J. E. (1987). Models of community organization and macro practice: Their mixing and phasing. In F. M. Cox, J. Erlich, J. L. Rothman, & J. E. Tropman (Eds.), *Strategies of Community Organization* (4th ed., pp. 3–26). Itasca, IL: Peacock.

Rowe, M. M. (1998). Self-report measures of dental fear: Gender differences. *American Journal of Health Behavior, 22,* 243–247.

Rowley, T. H., & Layne, B. H. (1990). *Evaluation of CBI in accounting education.* International Conference of the Association for the Development of Computer-Based Instructional Systems, San Diego, CA., ERIC Document Reproduction Service No. 329 223.

Rubinson, L., & Baillie, L. (1981). Planning school based sexuality programs using the Precede model. *Journal of School Health, 51,* 282–287.

Ruchlin, H. S., & Alderman, M. H. (1980). Cost of hypertension control at the workplace. *Journal of Occupational Medicine, 22,* 795–800.

Rundall, T. G., & Phillips, K. A. (1990). Informing and educating the electorate about AIDS. *Medical Care Review, 47,* 3–13.

Rundall, T. G., & Wheeler, J. R. C. (1979a). The effect of income on use of preventive care: An evaluation of alternative explanations. *Journal of Health and Social Behavior, 20,* 397–406.

Rundall, T. G., & Wheeler, J. R. C. (1979b). Factors associated with utilization of the swine flu vaccination program among senior citizens in Tompkins County. *Medical Care, 17,* 191–200.

Runyan, D. K., Hunter, W. M., Socolar, R. S., et al. (1998). Children who prosper in unfavorable environments: The relationship to social capital. *Pediatrics, 101,* 12–18

Russell, A., Voas, R. B., & Chaloupka, M. (1995). MADD rates the states: A media advocacy event to advance the agenda against alcohol-impaired driving. *Public Health Reports, 110,* 240–245.

Rutten, A. (1995). The implementation of health promotion: A new structural perspective. *Social Science and Medicine, 41,* 1627–1639.

Ryan C. (1991). *Prime time activism: Media strategies for grassroots organizing.* Boston: South End Press.

Rychetnik, L., Nutbeam, D., & Hawe, P. (1997). Lessons from a review of publications in three health promotion journals from 1989 to 1994. *Health Education Research, 12,* 491–504.

Saan, H. (1997). Quality revisited. *Promotion and Education, 4*(2), 34–35.

Sackett, D., & Haynes, R. B. (1976). *Compliance with therapeutic regimens.* Baltimore: Johns Hopkins University Press.

Sackett, D. L., & Snow, J. C. (1979). The magnitude of compliance and noncompliance. In R. B. Haynes, D. W. Taylor, & D. L. Sackett (Eds.), *Compliance in Health Care.* Baltimore: Johns Hopkins University Press.

Salazar, M. K. (1985). Dealing with hypertension: Using theory to promote behavioral change. *AAOHN Journal, 43,* 313–318.

Sallis, J. F., Haskell, W. L., Fortmann, S. P., et al. (1986). Predictors of adoption and maintenance of physical activity in a community sample. *Preventive Medicine, 15,* 331–341.

Sallis, J. F., Hovell, M. F., & Hoffstetter, C. R., et al. (1990). Distance between homes and exercise facilities related to frequency of exercise among San Diego residents. *Public Health Reports, 105,* 179–185.

Sallis, J. F., Pinski, R. B., Grossman, R. M., et al. (1988). The development of self-efficacy scales for health-related diet and exercise behaviors. *Health Education Research, 3,* 283–292.

Salonen, J. T., Puska, P., & Mustaniemi, H. (1979). Changes in morbidity and mortality during comprenhensive community programme to control cardiovascular disease during 1972–1977 in North Karelia. *British Medical Journal, 2,* 1178–1183.

Saltz, R. (1987). The role of bars and restaurants in preventing alcohol-impaired driving: An evaluation of server intervention. *Evaluation and Health Professions, 10,* 5–27.

Salzer, M. S., Nixon, C. T., & Bickman, L. (1997). Quality as relationship between structure, process, and outcome. *Evaluation Review, 21,* 292–309.

Sampson, R. J., Raudenbush, S. W., & Earls, F. (1997). Neighborhoods and violent crime: A multilevel study of collective efficacy. *Science, 277,* 918–924.

Samuels, S. E. (1990). Project LEAN: A national campaign to reduce dietary fat consumption. *American Journal of Health Promotion, 4,* 435–440.

Sanders, I. T. (1950). *Preparing a community profile: The methodology of a social reconnaissance.* Lexington: Kentucky Community Series No. 7, Bureau of Community Services, University of Kentucky.

Sanderson, C., Haglund, B., Tillgren, P., et al. (1996). Effect and stage models in community intervention programmes; and the development of the model for management of intervention programme preparation (MMIPP). *Health Promotion International, 11,* 143–156.

Sanders-Phillips, K. (1991). *A model for health promotion in ethnic minority families.* Wellness Lecture Series. Oakland, CA: University of California President's Office.

Sanders-Phillips, K. (1996). Correlates of health promotion behaviors in low-income black women and Latinas. *American Journal of Preventive Medicine, 12,* 450–458.

Sargent, J. D., Mott, L. A., & Stevens, M. (1998). Predictors of smoking cessation in adolescents. *Archives of Pediatrics and Adolescent Medicine, 152,* 388–393.

Sarvela, P. D., & McDermott, R. J. (1993). *Health education evaluation: A practitioner's perspective.* Madison, WI: Brown & Benchmark.

Sass, R. (1989). The implications of work organization for occupational health policy: The case of Canada. *International Journal of Health Services Research, 19,* 153–173.

Sayegh, J., & Green, L. W. (1976). Family planning education: Program design, training component and cost-effectiveness of a post-partum program in Beirut. *International Journal of Health Education, 19*(Suppl.), 1–20.

Schaalma, H. P., Kok, G., Bosker, R. J., et al. (1996). Planned development and evaluation of AIDS/STD education for secondary school students in the Netherlands: Short-term effects. *Health Education Quarterly, 23,* 469–487.

Schaeffer, M. (1985). *Designing and implementing procedures for health and human services.* Beverly Hills, CA: Sage.

Schapira, D. V., Pamies, R. J., Kumar, N. B., et al. (1993). Cancer screening: Knowledge, recommendations, and practices of physicians. *Cancer, 71,* 839–843.

Schauffler, H. (1994). Health promotion and disease prevention in health care reform. *American Journal of Preventive Medicine, 10*(1), 1–31.

Schauffler, H. H., Faer, M., Faulkner, L., & Shor, K. (1994). Health promotion and disease prevention in health care reform. *American Journal of Preventive Medicine, 10*(Suppl.), 1–31.

Schauffler, H., & Rodriguez, T. (1993). Managed care for preventive services: A review of policy options. *Medical Care Review, 50,* 153–198.

Schauffler, H., & Rodriguez, T. (1996). Exercising purchasing power for preventive care. *Health Affairs, 15,* 73–85.

Schechter, J. H., Green, L. W., Olsen, L., et al. (1997). Application of Karasek's demand/control model in a Canadian occupational setting during a period of reorganization and downsizing. *American Journal of Health Promotion, 11,* 394–399.

Schellstede, W. P., & Ciszewski, R. L. (1984). Social marketing of contraceptives in Bangladesh. *Studies in Family Planning, 15*(1), 30–39.

Scheirer, M. A., Shediac, M. C., & Cassady, C. E. (1995). Measuring the implementation of health promotion programs: The case of the Breast and Cervical Cancer Program in Maryland. *Health Education Research, 10,* 11–26.

Schiller, P. L., & Levin, L. S. (1983). Is self-care a social movement? *Social Science and Medicine, 17,* 1343–1352.

Schiller, P., Steckler, A., Dawson, L., & Patton, F. (1987). *Participatory planning in community health education: A guide based on the McDowell County, West Virginia experience.* Oakland, CA: Third Party Publishing.

Schilling, R. F., Gilchrist, L. D., & Schinke, S. P. (1985). Smoking in the workplace: Review of critical issues. *Public Health Reports, 100,* 473–479.

Schinke, S. P. (1982). A school-based model for teenage pregnancy prevention. *Social Work in Education, 4,* 34–42.

Schinke, S. P., Orlandi, M. A., Schilling, R. F., & Parms, C. (1992). Feasibility of interactive videodisc technology to teach minority youth about preventing HIV infection. *Public Health Reports, 107*(3), 323–330.

Schlesinger, M. (1988). The perfectibility of public programs: Real lessons from the large-scale demonstration projects [Editorial]. *American Journal of Public Health, 78,* 899–902.

Schmidt, D., & Leppik, I. E. (Eds.). (1988). *Compliance in epilepsy.* Amsterdam: Elsevier Science Publishers.

Schnall, P. L., Landsbergis, P. A., & Baker, D. (1994). Job strain and cardiovascular disease. *Annual Review of Public Health, 15,* 381–411.

Schoen, R. E., Marcus, M., & Braham, R. L. (1994). Factors associated with the use of screening mammography in a primary care setting. *Journal of Community Health, 19,* 239–252.

"The school health education evaluation study" [Special issue]. (1985). *Journal of School Health, 55*(6).

Schooler, C., Farquhar, J. W., Fortmann, S. P., & Flora, J. A. (1997, October). Synthesis and issues from community prevention trials. *Annals of Epidemiology,* pp., S7, S54–S68.

Schorr, L. (1988). *Within our reach: Breaking the cycle of disadvantage.* New York: Doubleday/ Anchor.

Schorr, L. B., & Kubisch, A. C. (1995, September 9). *New approaches to evaluation.* Paper presented at the Annie E. Casey Foundation Annual Research/Evaluation Conference.

Schott, F. W. (1985). WELCOM: The wellness council of the midlands. In *A decade of survival: Past, present, future. Proceedings of the 20th annual meeting.* Washington, DC: Society of Prospective Medicine.

Scholer, C., Sundar, S., & Flora, J. (1996). Effects of the Stanford Five-City Project Media Advocacy Program. *Health Education Quarterly, 23,* 346–364.

Schriger, D. L., Baraff, L. J., & Cretin, S. (1997). Implementation of clinical guidelines using a computer charting system: Effect on the initial care of health care workers exposed to body fluids. *Journal of the American Medical Association, 278,* 1585–1590.

Schuckman, F. (1986). The history and practice of occupational medicine in the Federal Republic of Germany. *Journal of Occupational Medicine, 28,* 212–216.

Schultz, A. J., Parker, E. A., Israel, B. A., et al. (1998). Conducting a participatory community-based survey for a community health intervention in Detroit's East Side. *Journal of Public Health Management and Practice, 4,* 10–24.

Schumann, D. A., & Mosley, W. H. (1994). The household production of health: Introduction. *Social Science and Medicine, 38,* 201–204.

Schunk, D. H., & Carbonari, J. P. (1984). Self-efficacy models. In J. D. Matarazzo et al. (Eds.), *Behavioral health: A handbook of health enhancement and disease prevention* (pp. 230–247). New York: Wiley.

Schuurman, J., & de Haes, W. (1980). Sexually transmitted diseases: Health education by telephone. *International Journal of Health Education, 23,* 94–106.

Schwab, M., & Syme, S. L. (1997). On paradigms, community participation, and the future of public health. *American Journal of Public Health, 87,* 2049–2050.

Schwartz, J. L. (Ed.). (1978). *Progress in smoking cessation.* New York: American Cancer Society.

Schwartz, J. L. (1987). *Review and evaluation of smoking cessation methods: The United States and Canada 1978–1985.* Washington, DC: Department of Health and Human Services, National Institutes of Health, NIH 87-2940.

Schwartz, J. S., Lewis, C. E., Clancy, C., et al. (1991). Internists' practices in health promotion and disease prevention. *Annals of Internal Medicine, 114,* 46–53.

Schwartz, R. K., Soumerai, S. B., & Avorn, J. (1989). Physician motivations for non-scientific drug prescribing. *Social Science and Medicine, 28,* 577–582.

Schwarzer, R., & Scroder, K. (1997). Effects of self-efficacy and social support on postsurgical recovery of heart patients. *Irish Journal of Psychology, 18,* 88–104.

Sclar, D. A., Chin, A., Sklar, T. L., et al. (1991). Effect of health education in promoting prescription refill compliance among patients with hypertension. *Clinical Therapeutics, 13,* 489–495.

Scriven, M. (1972). Pros and cons about goal-free evaluation. *Evaluation Comment, 3*(4), 1–5.

Scriven, M. (1998). Minimalist theory: The least theory that practice requires. *American Journal of Evaluation, 19,* 57–70

Scuttchfield, F. D. (1992). Clinical preventive services: The physician and the patient. *Clinical Chemistry, 38*(8B, Part 2), 1547–1551.

Secker-Walker, R. H., Flynn, B. S., Solomon, L. J. (1996). Helping women quit smoking: Baseline observations for a community health education project. *American Journal of Preventive Medicine, 12,* 367–377.

Secker-Walker, R. H., Solomon, L. J., & Mead, P. B. (1995). Smoking relapse prevention counseling during prenatal and early postnatal care. *American Journal of Preventive Medicine, 11,* 86–93.

Secretary's Task Force on Black and Minority Health. (1985). *Report of the Secretary's Task Force on Black and Minority Health.* Washington, DC: U.S. Department of Health and Human Services.

Sederburg, W., Ortwein, R., & Durr, W. (1985). *Michigan's health initiative.* Lansing: Michigan State Legislature.

Segall, M. E., & Wynd, C. A. (1990). Health conception, health locus of control, and power as predictors of smoking behavior change. *American Journal of Health Promotion, 4,* 338–344.

Seiden, T. M., & Blonna, R. (1983, Spring). A profile of volunteers at the VD National Hotline. *Hotliner* (American Social Health Association, VD National Hotline, 260 Sherican Ave., Palo Alto, CA 94306), p. 6.

Selby, M. L., Riportella-Muller, R., Sorenson, J. R., & Walters, C. R. (1989). Improving EPSDT use: Development and application of a practice-based model for public health nursing research. *Public Health Nursing, 6,* 174–181.

Selby, M. L., Riportella-Muller, R., Sorenson, J. R., et al. (1990). Public health nursing interventions to improve the use of a health service: Using a pilot study to guide research. *Public Health Nursing, 7,* 3–12.

Selby-Harrington, M., Sorenson, J. R., Quade, D., et al. (1995). Increasing medicaid child health screenings: The effectiveness of mailed pamphlets, phone calls, and home visits. *American Journal of Public Health, 85,* 1412–1417.

Self-study course 3030-G: Principles of epidemiology (2nd ed.). (1992). Atlanta, GA: Centers for Disease Control and Prevention.

Sells, S. B. (1969). Ecology and the science of psychology. In E. P. Willems & H. L. Raush (Eds.), *Naturalistic viewpoints in psychological research* (pp. 15–30). New York: Holt, Rinehart, & Winston.

Sennett, C. (1998). Perspective: Moving ahead, measure by measure. *Health Affairs, 17,* 36–37.

Shamian, J., & Edgar, L. (1987). Nurses as agents for change in teaching breast self-examination. *Public Health Nursing, 4,* 29–34.

Shannon, B. M., Smickiklas-Wright, H., Davis, B. W., & Lewis, C. A. (1983). Peer educator approach to nutrition for the elderly. *Gerontologist, 23,* 123–126.

Shannon, J., Kirkley, B., Ammerman, A., & Simpson, R. J. (1997). Self-efficacy as a predictor of dietary change in a low-socioeconomic-status southern adult population. *Health Education and Behavior, 24,* 357–369.

Sharp, P. C., Dignan, M. B., Blinson, K., et al. (1998). Working with lay health educators in a rural cancer-prevention program. *American Journal of Health Behavior, 22,* 18–27.

Shaw, G. B. (1930). *The apple cart: A political extravaganza.* London: Constable.

Shea, S., & Basch, C. E. (1990). A review of five major community-based cardiovascular disease prevention programs: Part I. Rationale, design, and theoretical framework. *American Journal of Health Promotion, 4,* 203–213.

Shea, S., Basch, C. E., Gutin, B., et al. (1994). The rate of increase in blood pressure in children 5 years of age is related to changes in aerobic fitness and body mass index. *Pediatrics, 94,* 465–469.

Shea, S., Basch, C. E., Stein, A. D., et al. (1993). Is there a relationship between dietary fat and stature or growth in children three to five years of age? *Pediatrics, 92,* 579–586.

Shediac-Rizkallah, M. C., & Bone, L. R. (1998). Planning for the sustainability of community-based health programs: Conceptual frameworks and future directions for research, practice and policy. *Health Education Research, 13*(1), 87–108.

Shefer, A., Mezoff, J., & Herrick, P. (1998). What mothers in the Women, Infants, and Children (WIC) Program feel about WIC and immunization linkage activities: A summary of focus groups. *Archives of Pediatrics and Adolescent Medicine, 152,* 65–70.

Shephard, R. J., Corey, P., Renzland, P., et al. (1982). The influence of an employee fitness and lifestyle modification program upon medical care costs. *Canadian Journal of Public Health, 73,* 259–263.

Shiffman, S., Mason, K. M., & Henningfield, J. E. (1998). Tobacco dependence treatments: Review and prospects. *Annual Review of Public Health, 19,* 335–358.

Shimkin, D. (1986–1987). Improving rural health: The lessons of Mississippi and Tanzania. *International Quarterly of Community Health Education, 7,* 149–165.

Shine, M. S., Silva, M. C., & Weed, F. S. (1983). Integrating health education into baccalaureate nursing education. *Journal of Nursing Education, 22,* 22–27.

Shipley, R. (1987). Smoking reduction programs help business snuff out health problems. *Occupational Health and Safety, 56,* 73–77.

Shoemaker, J., & Nix, H. L. (1972). A study of reputational leaders using the concepts of exchange and coordinative positions. *Sociological Quarterly, 13,* 516–524.

Shor, I., & Freire, P. (1987). *A pedagogy for liberation.* Boston: Bergin and Garvey.

Shoveller, J. A., & Langille, D. B. (1993). Cooperation and collaboration between a public health unit and midsized private industry in health promotion programming: The Polymer Heart Health Program experience. *Canadian Journal of Public Health, 84,* 170–173.

Shumaker, S. A., Parker, S., & Wolle, J. (Eds.). (1990). *The handbook of health behavior change.* New York: Springer.

Sigelman, C. K., Goldenberg, J. L., & Dwyer, K. M. (1998). Parental drug use and the socialization of AIDS knowledge and attitudes in children. *AIDS Education and Prevention, 10,* 180–189.

Sigerist, H. E. (1946). *The university at the crossroads: Addresses and essays.* New York: Henry Schuman.

Silverfine, E., Brieger, W., & Churchill, R. (1990). *Community-based initiatives to eradicate guinea worm: A manual for Peace Corps volunteers.* Washington, DC: U.S. Peace Corps and Agency for International Development.

Silvers, I. J., Hovell, M. F., Weisman, M. H., & Mueller, M. R. (1985). Assessing physician-patient perceptions in rheumatoid arthritis: A vital component in patient education. *Arthritis and Rheumatism, 28,* 300–307.

Simmons, J. (Ed.). (1975, October). Making health education work. *American Journal of Public Health, 65*(Suppl.), 1–49.

Simons-Morton, B. G., Brink, S. G., Parcel, G. S., et al. (1989). *Preventing alcohol-related health problems among adolescents and young adults: A CDC intervention handbook.* Atlanta, GA: Centers for Disease Control.

Simons-Morton, B. G., Brink, S. G., Simons-Morton, D. G., et al. (1989). An ecological approach to the prevention of injuries due to drinking and driving. *Health Education Quarterly, 16,* 397–411.

Simons-Morton, B. G., Greene, W. H., & Gottlieb, N. H. (1995). *Introduction to health education and health promotion* (2nd ed.). Prospect Heights, IL: Waveland Press.

Simons-Morton, B. G., Parcel, G. S., & O'Hara, N. M. (1988a). Implementing organizational changes to promote healthful diet and physical activity at school. *Health Education Quarterly, 15,* 115–130.

Simons-Morton, B. G., Parcel, G. S., O'Hara, N. M., et al. (1988b). Health-related physical fitness in childhood: Status and recommendations. *Annual Review of Public Health, 9,* 403–425.

Simons-Morton, D. G., Parcel, G. S., Brink, S. G., Harvey, C. M., & Tiernan, K. M. (1991). Smoking control among women: Needs assessment and intervention strategies. In W. B. Ward & F. M. Lewis (Eds.), *Advances in health education and promotion* (Vol. 3, pp. 199–240). London: Jessica Kingsley.

Simons-Morton, D. G., Parcel, G. S., Brink, S. G. et al. (1988). *Promoting physical activity among adults: A CDC community intervention handbook.* Atlanta, GA: Centers for Disease Control.

Simons-Morton, D. G., Simons-Morton, B. G., Parcel, G. S., & Bunker, J. G. (1988). Influencing personal and environmental conditions for community health: A multilevel intervention model. *Family and Community Health, 11,* 25–35.

Simpson, G. W., & Pruitt, B. E. (1989). The development of health promotion teams as related to wellness programs in Texas schools. *Health Education, 20*(1), 26–28.

Singer, J., Lindsay, E. A., & Wilson, D. M. C. (1991). Promoting physical activity in primary care: Overcoming the barriers. *Canadian Family Physician, 37,* 2167–2173.

Singhal, A. (1994). *Social change through entertainment.* Newbury Hills, CA: Sage.

Skelly, A. H., Marshall, J. R., Haughey, B. B., Davis, P. J., & Dunford, R. G. (1995). Self-efficacy and confidence in outcomes as determinants of self-care practices in inner-city, African-American women with non-insulin-dependent diabetes. *Diabetes Educator, 21,* 38–46.

Skiff, A. W. (1974). Experiences with methods for patient teaching from a public health service hospital. *Health Education Monographs, 2*(1), 48–53.

Skinner, C. S., & Kreuter, M. W. (1997). Using theories in planning interactive computer programs. Chapter 3 in R. L. Street, Jr., W. R. Gold, & T. Manning (Eds.), *Health promotion and interactive technology: Theoretical applications and future directions* (pp. 39–65). Mahwah, NJ: Lawrence Erlbaum.

Sleet, D. A. (1987). Health education approaches to motor vehicle injury prevention. *Public Health Reports, 102,* 606–608.

Sloan, R. P. (1987). Workplace health promotion: A commentary of an evolution of a paradigm. *Health Education Quarterly, 14,* 181–194.

Sloan, R. P., & Gruman, J. C. (1988). Participation in workplace health promotion programs: The contribution of health and organizational factors. *Health Education Quarterly, 15,* 269–288.

Sloan, R. P., Gruman, J. C., & Allegrante, J. P. (1987). *Investing in employee health: A guide to effective health promotion in the workplace.* San Francisco: Jossey-Bass.

Sloane, B. C., & Zimmer, C. H. (1992). Health education and health promotion on campus. In H. M. Wallace, K. Patrick, & G. S. Parcel (Eds.), *Principles and practices of student health: Vol. 3. College health* (pp. 540–557). Oakland, CA: Third Party Press.

Slobodkin, L. B. (1988). Intellectual problems of applied ecology. *Bioscience, 38,* 337–342.

Slovic, P. (1986). Informing and educating the public about risk. *Risk Analysis, 6,* 403–415.

Smith, C. E., Kleinbeck, S. V. M., Fernengel, K., & Mayer, L. S. (1997). Efficiency of families managing home health care. *Annals of Operations Research, 73,* 157–175.

Smith, C., Roberts, J. L., & Pendleton, L. L. (1988). Booze on the box—the portrayal of alcohol on British television: A content analysis. *Health Education Research, 3,* 267–272.

Smith, G. D., Shipley, M., & Rose, G. (1990). Magnitude and causes of socioeconomic differentials in mortality: Further evidence from the Whitehall study. *Journal of Epidemiology and Community Health, 44,* 465–470.

Smith, G. S., & Kraus, J. F. (1988). Alcohol and residential, recreational, and occupational injuries: A review of the epidemiologic evidence. *Annual Review of Public Health, 9,* 99–122.

Smith, H. (1988). *The power game: How Washington works.* New York: Random House.

Smith, J. A., & Scammon, D. L. (1984). Strategies for increasing attendance at cancer screening clinics. In S. M. Smith & M. Venkatesan (Eds.), *Advances in health care research.* Provo, UT: Institute of Business Management, College of Business Administration, Brigham Young University.

Smith, J. A., & Scammon, D. L. (1987). A market segment analysis of adult physical activity: Exercise beliefs, attitudes, intentions and behaviors. *Advances in nonprofit marketing* (Vol. 2). Greenwich, CT: JAI Press.

Smith, K. W., McGraw, S. S., & McKinlay, J. B. (1996). A self-efficacy scale for HIV risk behaviors: Development and evaluation. *AIDS Education and Prevention, 8,* 97–105.

Smith, P. (1989). National School Boards Association, and Center for Chronic Disease Prevention and Health Promotion, CDC, school policies and programs on smoking and health—United States, 1988. *Morbidity and Mortality Weekly Report, 38,* 202–203. Also in (1989) *Journal of the American Medical Association, 261,* 2488.

Smith, P. H., Danis, M., & Helmick, L. (1998). Changing the health care response to battered women: A health eduction response. *Family and Community Health, 2,* 1–18.

Smith, T. (1973). Policy roles: An analysis of policy formulators and policy implementors. *Policy Sciences, 4,* 297–307.

Sneden, G. G., Nichols, D. C., & Gottlieb, N. H. (1997, November 7–9). What happens after the diagnosis? A practitioner's intervention model [Published abstract]. 48th Annual Meeting of the Society for Public Health Education, Indianapolis, IN.

Sobal, J., Valente, C. M., Muncie, H. L., Jr., Levine, D. M., & Deforge, B. R. (1986). Physicians' beliefs about the importance of 25 health promoting behaviors. *American Journal of Public Health, 75,* 1427–1428.

Sobel, D., & Hornbacher, F. (1973). *An everyday guide to your health.* New York: Grossman.

Society for Public Health Education. (1977). Guidelines for the preparation and practice of professional health educators. *Health Education Monographs, 5,* 75–89.

Soen, D. (1981). Citizen and community participation in urban renewal and rehabilitation: Comments on theory and practice. *Community Development Journal, 16,* 105–117.

Sogaard, A. J. (1988). The effect of a mass-media dental health education campaign. *Health Education Research, 3,* 243–255.

Solomon, M. Z., & DeJong, W. (1986). Recent sexually transmitted disease prevention efforts and their implications for AIDS health education. *Health Education Quarterly, 13,* 301–316.

Somers, A. (Ed.). (1976). *Health promotion and consumer health education.* Greenbelt, MD: Aspen Systems.

Somers, A. (1987). Four "orphan" areas in current medical education: What hope for adoption? *Family Medicine, 19,* 137–140.

Sommers, J. M., Andres, F., & Price, J. H. (1995). Perceptions of exercise of mall walkers utilizing the Health Belief Model. *Journal of Health Education, 26,* 158–166.

Sorensen, A. A., & Sinacore, J. S. (1979). Developing a regional health education program. *Regional Health Education, 3*(2), 79–84.

Sorensen, G., Emmons, K., Hunt, M. K., & Johnston, D. (1998). Implications of the results of community intervention trials. *Annual Review of Public Health, 19,* 379–416.

Sorensen, G., Youngstrom, R., Maclachlan, C., et al. (1997). Labor positions on worksite tobacco control policies: A review of arbitration cases. *Journal of Public Health Policy, 18,* 433–452.

Sorenson, G., Glasgow, R., Corbett, K., & Topor, M. (1992). Compliance with worksite nonsmoking policies: Baseline results from the COMMIT study of worksites. *American Journal of Health Promotion, 7,* 103–109.

Sorenson, G., Glasgow, R. E., Topor, M., & Corbett, K. (1997). Worksite characteristics and changes in worksite tobacco-control initiatives: Results from the Commit study. *Journal of Occupational and Environmental Medicine, 39,* 520–526.

Soubhi, H., & Potvin, L. (1999). Homes and families as health promotion settings. In B. Poland, L. W. Green, & I. Rootman (Eds.), *Settings for health promotion.* Thousand Oaks, CA: Sage.

Source book of health insurance data. (1989). New York: Health Insurance Association of America.

Spain, C., Eastman, E., & Kizer, K. (1989). Model standards impact on local health department performance in California. *American Journal of Public Health, 79,* 969–974.

Speller, V., Evans, D., & Head, M. J. (1997). Developing quality assurance standards for health promotion practice in the UK. *Health Promotion International, 12,* 215–224.

Spiegel, C. V., & Lindaman, F. C. (1977). Children can't fly: A program to prevent childhood morbidity and mortality from window falls. *American Journal of Public Health, 67,* 1143–1146.

Spivak, H., Prothrow-Stith, D., & Hausman, A. J. (1995). Implementation of violence prevention education in clinical settings. *Patient Education and Counseling, 25, 205–210.*

Spoon, M. P. D., Benedict, J. A., & Buonamici, A. M. (1997). Using community health fairs to target high-risk clientele. *Journal of Nutrition Education, 29,* 356A.

Spretnak, C., & Capra, F. (1984). *Green politics.* New York: Dutton.

Squyres, W. (Ed.). (1980). *Patient education: An inquiry into the state of the art.* New York: Springer.

Stachenko, S. (1996). The Canadian Heart Health Initiative: Dissemination perspectives. *Canadian Journal of Public Health, 87*(Suppl. 2), S57–S59.

Stainbrook, G., & Green, L. W. (1982, Nov–Dec). Behavior and behaviorism in health education. *Health Education, 13,* 14–19.

Standards for the preparation of graduate-level health educators. (1997). Washington, DC: Society for Public Health Education; American Association of Health Education.

Stange, K. C., Kelly, R., Chao, J., et al. (1992). Physician agreement with U.S. Preventive Services Task Force recommendations. *Journal of Family Practice, 34,* 409–416.

Starfield, B. (1982). Family income, ill health and medical care of U.S. children. *Journal of Public Health Policy, 3,* 244–259.

Starfield, B., & Budetti, P. (1985). Child health risk factors. *Health Services Research, 19*(6, Pt. II), 817–886.

State School Health Education Project. (1981). *Recommendations for school health education: A handbook for state policymakers.* Denver, CO: Education Commission of the States.

Statistics Canada and Department of the Secretary of State of Canada. (1995). *Report of the Canadian Health and Disability Survey.* Ottawa: Minister of Supply and Services Canada.

Steckler, A. (1989). The use of qualitative evaluation methods to test internal validity: An example in a work site health promotion program. *Evaluation and the Health Professions, 12,* 115–133.

Steckler, A., & Dawson, L. (1978). Determinants of consumer influence in a health systems agency. *Health Education Monographs, 6,* 377–393.

Steckler, A., & Dawson, L. (1982). The role of health education in public policy development. *Health Education Quarterly, 9,* 275–292.

Steckler, A., Dawson, L., Goodman, R. M., & Epstein, N. (1987). Policy advocacy: Three emerging roles for health education. In W. B. Ward (Ed.), *Advances in health education and promotion* (Vol. 2, pp. 5–27). Greenwich, CT: JAI Press.

Steckler, A., Dawson, L., & Williams, A. (1981). Consumer participation and influence in a health systems agency. *Journal of Community Health, 6,* 181–193.

Steckler, A., & Goodman, R. M. (1989a). How to institutionalize health promotion programs. *American Journal of Health Promotion, 3,* 34–44.

Steckler, A., & Goodman, R. M. (1989b). A model for the institutionalization of health promotion programs. *Family and Community Health, 11,* 63–78.

Steckler, A., Goodman, R. M., & Alciati, H. (1997). The impact of the National Cancer Institute's data-based intervention research program on state health agencies. *Health Education Research, 12,* 199–212.

Steckler, A., Orville, K., Eng, E., & Dawson, L. (1989). *PATCHing it together: A formative evaluation of CDC's Planned Approach to Community Health (PATCH) Program.* Chapel Hill: Department of Health Behavior and Health Education, School of Public Health, University of North Carolina.

Steckler, A., Orville, K., Eng, E., & Dawson, L. (1992). Summary of a formative evaluation of PATCH. *Journal of Health Education, 23,* 174–178.

Steinfeld, J., Griffiths, W., Ball, K., & Taylor, R. M. (Eds.). (1977). *Smoking and health: Health consequences, education, cessation activities, and government action* (Vol. 2). Washington, DC: Department of Health, Education, and Welfare, NIH 77-1413.

Stephens, T. (1987). Secular trends in adult physical activity: Exercise boom or bust. *Research Quarterly for Exercise and Sport, 58,* 95.

Stephens, T., Jacobs, D. R., Jr., & White, C. C. (1985). A descriptive epidemiology of leisure-time physical activity. *Public Health Reports, 100,* 147–158.

Stephens, T., & Schoenborn, C. A. (1988). Adult health practices in the United States and Canada. In National Center for Health Statistics, *Vital and Health Statistics* (Ser. 5, No. 3.). Washington, DC: U.S. Government Printing Office, DHHS-PHS 88-1479.

Steuart, G.W. (1965). Health, behavior and planned change: An approach to the professional preparation of the health education specialist. *Health Education Monographs, 1*(20), 3–26.

Steuart, G. W. (1969). Planning and evaluation in health education. *International Journal of Health Education, 12,* 65–76.

Stevenson, M., Jones, S., Cross, D., Howat, P., & Hall, M. (1996). The child pedestrain injury prevention project. *Health Promotion Journal of Australia, 3,* 32–36.

Stewart, A. J., & Ware, J. E. (Eds.). (1992). *Measuring functioning and well-being: The medical outcomes study approach.* Durham, NC: Duke University Press.

Stewart, S. (1996). *The effects of an 18-month weight-training and calcium supplementation program on bone mineral of adolescent girls.* Unpublished doctoral dissertation. Vancouver: University of British Columbia.

Stine, R. A., & Ellefson, P. V. (1997). Organizational effects on policy implementation in a geographically dispersed natural resources organization. *Evaluation Review, 21,* 419–438.

Stivers, C. (1994). Drug prevention in Zuni, New Mexico: Creation of a teen center as an alternative to alcohol and drug use. *Journal of Community Health, 19,* 343–359.

Stoddard, J. L., Johnson, C. A., & Boley-Cruz, T. (1998). Tailoring outdoor tobacco advertising to minorities in Los Angeles County. *Journal of Health Communication, 3,* 137–148.

Stokols, D. (1992). Establishing and maintaining healthy environments: Toward a social ecology of health promotion. *American Psychologist, 47,* 6–22.

Stone, E. J., Perry, C. L., & Luepker, R. V. (1989). Synthesis of cardiovascular behavioral research for youth health promotion. *Health Education Quarterly, 16,* 155–169.

Stonecipher, L. J., & Hyner, G. C. (1993). The effects of a comprehensive health risk appraisal, basic screening, and interpretation session on employee health practices: Differences between participants and nonparticipants. *American Journal of Health Promotion, 7,* 167–169.

Stone, E. J., Osganian, S., McKinlay, S., et al. (1996). Operational design and quality control in the CATCH multicenter trial. *Preventive Medicine, 25,* 384–399.

Strategies for promoting health in special populations. (1987). Washington, DC: Office of Disease Prevention and Health Promotion. Reprinted (1987) *Journal of Public Health Policy, 8,* 369–423.

Strecher, V. J., DeVellis, B. M., Becker, M. H., & Rosenstock, I. M. (1986). The role of self-efficacy in achieving health behavior change. *Health Education Quarterly, 13,* 73–92.

Strecher, V. J., Rimer, B. K., & Monaco, K. D. (`989). Development of a new self-help guide: Freedom From Smoking for You and Your Family. *Health Education Quarterly, 16,* 101–112.

Strecher, V. J., & Rosenstock, I. M. (1997). The health belief model. In K. Glanz, F. M. Lewis, & B. K. Rimer (Eds.), *Health behavior and health education: Theory, research, and practice* (pp. 41–59). San Francisco: Jossey-Bass.

Street, R. L., Jr., Gold, W. R., & Manning, T. (1997). *Health promotion and interactive technology: Theoretical applications and future directions.* Mahwah, NJ: Erlbaum.

Strehlow, M. S. (1983). *Education for health.* London: Harper & Row.

Stronks, K., Van de Mheen, H., Looman, C. W. N., & Mackenbach, J. P. (1998). The importance of psychosocial stressors for socio-economic inequalities in perceived health. *Social Science and Medicine, 46,* 611–623.

Sun, W. Y., & Shun, J. (1995). Smoking behavior amongst different socioeconomic groups in the workplace in the People's Republic of China. *Health Promotion International, 10,* 261–266.

Supportive environments for health: Sundsvall statement. (1998). Geneva: World Health Organization, Division of Health Promotion, Education and Communication. Reprinted from the Third International Conference on Health Promotion, Sundsvall, Sweden, June 1991.

Susser, M. (1985). Epidemiology in the United States after World War II: The evolution of technique. *Epidemiological Review, 7,* 147–177.

Susser, M. (1995). Editorial: The tribulations of trials—intervention in communities. *American Journal of Public Health, 85*(2), 156–158.

Sutherland, M. S., Barber, M., Harris, G. L., et al. (1989). Planning preventive health programming for rural blacks: Development processes of a model PATCH program. *Wellness Perspectives, 6,* 57–58.

Sutherland, M., Pittman-Sisco, C., Lacher, T., & Watkins, N. (1987). The application of a health education planning model to a school based risk reduction model. *Health Education, 18*(3), 47–51.

Sydenstricker, E. (1933). *Health and environment.* New York: McGraw-Hill.

Syme, L. W. (1986). Strategies for health promotion. *Preventive Medicine, 15,* 492–507.

Szykman, L. R., Bloom, P. N., & Levy, A. S. (1997). A proposed model of the use of package claims and nutrition labels. *Journal of Public Policy and Marketing, 16,* 228-241.

Taal, E., Rasker, J. J., & Wiegman, O. (1996). Patient education and self-management in the rheumatic diseases: A self-efficacy approach. *Arthritis Care and Research, 9,* 229–238.

Taggart, V. S., Bush, P. J., Zuckerman, A. E., & Theiss, P. K. (1990). A process evaluation of the District of Columbia "Know Your Body" Project. *Journal of School Health 60*(2), 60–66.

Taggart, V. S., Zuckerman, A. E., Sly, R. M., et al. (1991). You can control asthma: Evaluation of an asthma education program for hospitalized inner-city children. *Patient Education and Counseling, 17,* 35–47.

Tamblyn, R., & Battista, R. (1993). Changing clinical practice: Which interventions work? *Journal of Continuing Education in the Health Professions, 13,* 273–288.

Tamez, E. G., & Vacalis, T. D. (1989). Health beliefs, the significant other and compliance with therapeutic regimens among adult Mexican American diabetics. *Health Education, 20*(6), 24–31.

Taplin, S. H. (1989). Breast cancer screening: A curious problem in primary care. *Journal of Family Practice, 29,* 247–248.

Targets for health for all. (1986). Copenhagen: World Health Organization, Regional Office for Europe.

Tarlov, A. R., Kehrer, B. H., Hall, D. P., et al. (1987). Foundation work: The Health Promotion Program of the Henry J. Kaiser Family Foundation. *American Journal of Health Promotion, 2,* 74–80.

Tarrow, S. (1996). Making social science work across space and time: A critical reflection on Robert Putnam's Making Democracy Work. *American Political Science Review, 90,* 389–397.

Taylor, C. W. (1984). Promoting health and strengthening wellness through environmental variables. In J. D. Matarazzo et al. (Eds.), *Behavioral health: A handbook of health enhancement and disease prevention* (pp. 130–149). New York: Wiley.

Taylor, V. M., Taplin, S. H., Urban, N., Mahloch, J., & Majer, K. A. (1994). Medical community involvement in a breast cancer screening promotional project. *Public Health Reports, 109,* 491–499.

Tengs, T. O., Adams, M. E., Pliskin, J. S., et al. (1995). Five-hundred life-saving interventions and their cost-effectiveness. *Risk Analysis, 15,* 369–390.

Terris, M. (1975). Approaches to an epidemiology of health. *American Journal of Public Health, 65,* 1037–1045.

Terris, M. (1976). The epidemiologic revolution, national health insurance and the role of health departments. *American Journal of Public Health, 66,* 1155–1164.

Terris, M. (1978). Public health in the United States: The next 100 years. *Journal of Public Health Policy, 93,* 602–608.

Terris, M. (1986). What is health promotion? *Journal of Public Health Policy, 7,* 147–151.

Terris, M. (1987). Epidemiology and the public health movement. *Journal of Public Health Policy, 7,* 315–329.

Terris, M. (1998). Lean and mean: The quality of care in the era of managed care. *Journal of Public Health Policy, 19,* 5–14.

Terry, P. B., Wang, V. L., Flynn, B. S., et al. (1981). A continuing medical education program in chronic obstructive pulmonary diseases: Design and outcome. *American Review of Respiratory Distress, 123,* 41–46.

Thamer, M., Fox Ray, N., Henderson, S. C., et al. (1998). Influence of the NIH Consensus Conference on Helicobacter Pylori on physician prescribing among a medicaid population. *Medical Care, 36,* 646–660.

Thomas, R., Cahill, J., & Santilli, L. (1997). Using an interactive computer game to increase skill and self-efficacy regarding safer sex negotiation: Field test results. *Health Education and Behavior, 24*(1), 71–86.

Thomas, S. B. (1990). Community health advocacy for racial and ethnic minorities in the United States: Issues and challenges for health education. *Health Education Quarterly, 17,* 13–19.

Thomas, S., Quinn, S., Billingsley, A., & Caldwell, C. (1994). Community health outreach programs conducted by 635 black churches in the northern U.S. *American Journal of Public Health, 84,* 575–579.

Thompson, B., & Kinne, S. (1990). Social change theory: Applications to community health. In N. Bracht (Ed.), *Health promotion at the community level.* Newbury Park, CA: Sage.

Thompson, M. A., Davis, D. A., & Haynes, R. B. (1995). No magic bullets: A systematic review of 102 trials of interventions to improve professional practice. *Canadian Medical Association Journal, 153,* 1423–1431.

Thompson, N. J. (1993). What is surveillance? In D. Murray (Ed.), *Proceedings from the Conference on Sports Injuries in Youth: Surveillance strategies* (pp. 15–18). Washington, DC: National Institute of Arthritis and Musculoskeletal and Skin Disease.

Thompson, R. S. (1996). What have HMOs learned about clinical preventive services? An examination of the experience at Group Health Cooperative of Puget Sound. *Milbank Quarterly, 74,* 469–509.

Thompson, R. S. (1997). Systems approaches and the delivery of health services. *Journal of the American Medical Association, 277,* 670–671.

Thompson, R .S., Taplin, S. H., McAfee, T. A., Mandelson, M. T., & Smith, A. E. (1995). Primary and secondary prevention in clinical practice: Twenty years' experince in development, implementation and evaluation. *Journal of the American Medical Association, 273*(14), 1130–1135.

Thomsen, C. A., & Ter Maat, J. (1998). Evaluating the Cancer Information Service: A model for health communications. Part 1. *Journal of Health Communication, 3*(Suppl.), 1–13.

Thoresen, C. E., & Kirmil-Gray, K. (1983, November). Self-management psychology and the treatment of childhood asthma. *Journal of Allergy and Clinical Immunology, 72*(Suppl.), 596–606.

Thornton, M. A. (1979). Preventive dentistry in the veterans administration. *Dental Hygiene, 53,* 121–124.

Thorogood, N. (1992). What is the relevance of sociology for health promotion? In R. Bunton & G. MacDonald (Eds.), *Health promotion: Disciplines and diversity* (pp. 42–65). London: Routledge.

Tillgren, P., Haglund, B. J. A., & Romelsjo, A. (1996). The sociodemographic pattern of tobacco cessation in the 1980s: Results from a panel study of living condition surveys in Sweden. *Journal of Epidemiology and Community Health, 50,* 625–630.

Timmreck, T. C. (1998). *An introduction to epidemiology* (2nd ed.). Boston: Jones and Bartlett.

Timmreck, T. C. (1995). *Planning, program development, and evaluation: A handbook for health promotion, aging, and health services.* Boston: Jones and Bartlett.

Tirrell, B., & Hart, L. (1980). The relationship of health beliefs and knowledge to exercise compliance in patients after coronary bypass. *Heart and Lung, 9,* 487–493.

Tjerandsen, C. (1980). *Education for citizenship: A foundation's experience.* Santa Cruz, CA: Emil Schwarzhaupt Foundation.

Todaro, V., Denard, J., Clarke, P., et al. (1987). Survey of worksite smoking policies. *Morbidity and Mortality Weekly Report, 36,* 177–179.

Tolman, M., & Allred, R. A. (1991). *The computer and education: What research says to the teacher* (2nd ed.). West Haven. CT: NEA Professional Library, Report No. ISBN-0-8106-1090-6, ERIC Document Reproduction Service No. 335 344.

Tolsma, D. D. (1993). Patient education objectives in *Healthy People 2000:* Policy and research issues. *Patient Education and Counseling, 22,* 7–14.

Tones, B. K. (1979). Past achievement and future success. Chapter 12 in I. Sutherland (Ed.), *Health education: Perspectives and choices.* London: Allen & Unwin.

Tones K. (1994). Marketing and the mass media: Theory and myth: Reflections of social marketing. *Health Education Research, 9,* 165–169.

Tones, K., & Tilford, S. (1994). *Health education: Effectiveness, efficiency and equity* (2nd ed.). London: Chapman & Hall.

Tonin, M. O. (1980). Concepts in community participation. *International Journal of Health Education, 23*(Suppl.), 1–13.

Toward a healthy community: Organizing events for community health promotion. (1980). Washington, DC: U.S. Department of Health and Human Services, Office of Disease Prevention and Health Promotion, PHS 80-50113.

Trends: Consumer attitudes and the supermarket. (1989). Washington, DC: Food Marketing Institute.

Trepka, M. J., Davidson, A. J., & Douglas, J. M., Jr. (1996). Extent of undiagnosed HIV infection in hospitalized patients: Assessment by linking of seroprevalence and surveillance methods. *American Journal of Preventive Medicine, 12,* 195–202.

Trice, H. M., & Beyer, J. M. (1984). Work-related outcomes of the constructive-confrontation strategy in a job-based alcoholism program. *Journal of Studies on Alcohol, 45,* 393–404.

Trumble, S. (1991). The GP as a teacher. *Medical Journal of Australia, 155,* 322–324.

Trussell, J., Koenig, J., & Stewart, F. (1997). Preventing unintended pregnancy: The cost-effectiveness of three methods of emergency contraception. *American Journal of Public Health, 87,* 932–936.

Trussler, T. & Marchand, R. (1997). *Taking care of each other: Field guide to community HIV health promotion.* Vancouver, BC: AIDS Vancouver and Health Canada.

Tuckett, D. A., Boulton, M., & Olson, M. (1985). A new approach to the measurement of patients' understanding of what they are told in medical consultations. *Journal of Health and Social Behavior, 26,* 27–38.

Tudor-Smith, C., Nutbeam, D., Moore, L., & Catford, J. (1998). Effects of the Heartbeat Wales programme over five years on behavioural risks for cardiovascular disease: Quasi-experimental comparison of result from Wales and a matched reference area. *British Medical Journal, 316,* 818–822.

Tzung-yu, C. (1993). *Comparing the use of computers with traditional print in reading instruction: What the research says.* Unpublished paper. ERIC Document Reproduction Service No. 362 831.

Udry, J., Clark, L., Chase, C., et al. (1972). Can mass media advertising increase contraceptive use? *Family Planning Perspectives, 4,* 37–44.

Ureda, J. R. (1993). Community intervention: Creating opportunities and support for cancer control behaviors. *Cancer, 72*(Suppl.), 1125–1131.

U.S. Bureau of the Census. (1996). *Statistical abstract of the United States: 1997* (116th ed.). Washington, DC: U.S. Government Printing Office.

U.S. Bureau of the Census. (1998). *Statistical abstract of the United States: 1999* (118th ed.). Washington, DC: U.S. Government Printing Office.

U.S. Congress, Office of Technology Assessment. (1995). *Teachers and technology: Making the connection.* Washington, DC: U.S. Government Printing Office, OTA-EHR-616.

U.S. Department of Education and U.S. Department of Health and Human Services. (1993). *Together we can: A guide for crafting a profamily system of education and human services.* Washington, DC: U.S. Government Printing Office.

U.S. Department of Education, Office of Educational Research and Improvement. (1988). *Youth indicators 1988: Trends in the well-being of American youth.* Washington, DC: U.S. Government Printing Office.

U.S. Department of Health and Human Services. (1980, April). *Initial role delineation for health education: Final report.* Washington, DC: Health Resources Administration, DHHS Publication 80-44.

U.S. Department of Health and Human Services. (1981a). *National conference for institutions preparing health educators: Proceedings.* Washington, DC: U.S. Office of Health Information and Health Promotion, PHS 81-50171.

U.S. Department of Health and Human Services. (1981b). *Promoting health in special populations.* Washington, DC: Office of Disease Prevention and Health Promotion. Reprinted (1987). *Journal of Public Health Policy, 8,* 369–423.

U.S. Department of Health and Human Services. (1985). *Report of the secretary's task force on black and minority health.* Washington, DC: U.S. Government Printing Office.

U.S. Department of Health and Human Services. (1986). *The 1990 health objectives for the nation: A midcourse review.* Washington, DC: Office of Disease Prevention and Health Promotion.

U.S. Department of Health and Human Services. (1988a). *CDC and minority communities stopping the spread of HIV infection and AIDS.* Atlanta, GA: Office of the Deputy Director (AIDS), Centers for Disease Control, Public Health Service, National Conference on the Prevention of HIV Infection and AIDS Among Racial and Ethnic Minorities in the United States.

U.S. Department of Health and Human Services. (1988b). *Surgeon general's report on nutrition and health.* Washington, DC: Public Health Service, Publ. No. 88-50210.

U.S. Department of Health and Human Services. (1990). *The health consequences of smoking cessation: A report of the surgeon general.* Washington DC: PHS, Office on Smoking and Health.

U.S. Department of Health and Human Services. (1991). *Healthy people 2000.* Washington, DC: Office of the Assistant Secretary for Health, Public Health Service. Also published (1992). *Healthy people 2000: National health promotion and disease prevention objectives, full report, with commentary.* Boston: Jones and Bartlett.

U.S. Department of Health and Human Services. (1993). *1992 national survey of worksite health promotion activities: Summary report.* Washington, DC: U.S. Government Printing Office.

U.S. Department of Health and Human Services. (1996). *Healthy people 2000: Midcourse review and 1995 revisions.* Sudbury, MA: Jones and Bartlett.

U.S. Department of Health, Education and Welfare. (1979). *Healthy people: Surgeon general's report on health promotion and disease prevention.* Washington, DC: Public Health Service, DHEW-PHS-79-55071.

U.S. Department of Labor, Bureau of Labor Statistics. (1995). *Census of fatal occupational injuries, 1994.* Washington, DC: U.S. Department of Labor.

U.S. Department of Labor, Bureau of Labor Statistics. (1998). *Monthly labor review.* Washington, DC: U.S. Government Printing Office.

U.S. Preventive Services Task Force. (1996). *Guide to clinical preventive services* (2nd ed.). Baltimore: Williams & Wilkins.

University of Michigan. (1995, December 11). Cigarette smoking among American teens rises again in 1995 (Press Release). Ann Arbor: University of Michigan News and Information Services.

Vaillant, G. E. (1983). *The natural history of alcoholism.* Cambridge, MA: Harvard University Press.

Vail-Smith, K., & White, D. M. (1992). Risk level, knowledge, and preventive behavior for human papillomaviruses among sexually active college women. *Journal of American College Health, 40,* 227–230.

Valente, C. M., Sobal, J., Muncie, H. L., Jr., Levine, D. M., & Antilitz, A. M. (1986). Health promotion: Physicians' beliefs, attitudes, and practices. *American Journal of Preventive Medicine, 2,* 82–88.

Van Cura, L. J., Jensen, N. M., Greist, J. H., et al. (1975). Venereal disease: Interviewing and teaching by computer. *American Journal of Public Health, 65*(11), 1159–1164.

van Assema, P., Steenbakkers, M., & Kok, G. (1994). The process evaluation of a Dutch community health project. *International Quarterly of Community Health Education, 15,* 187–208.

Van den Broucke, S., & Lenders, F. (1997). Monitoring the planning quality of health promotion projects in Flanders. *Promotion and Education, 4*(2), 26–28.

van der Pligt, J. (1998). Perceived risk and vulnerability as predictors of precautionary behaviour. *British Journal of Health Psychology, 3*(1), 1–14.

Van de Ven, A. H., & Delbecq, A. L. (1972). The nominal group as a research instrument for exploratory health studies. *American Journal of Public Health, 62,* 337–342.

Van Meter, D., & Van Horn, C. (1975). The policy implementation process: A conceptual framework. *Administration and Society, 6,* 445–488.

van Veenendal, H., Grinspun, D. R., & Adriaanse, H. P. (1996). Educational needs of stroke survivors and their family members, as perceived by themselves and by health professionals. *Patient Education and Counseling, 28,* 265–276.

Vartiainen, E., & Puska, P. (1987). The North Karelia Youth Project 1978–80: Effects of two years of educational intervention on cardiovascular risk factors and health behavior in adolescence. In B. Hetzel & G. S. Berenson (Eds.), *Cardiovascular risk factors in childhood: Epidemiology and prevention* (pp. 183–202). Dublin: Elsevier.

Vartiainen, E., Puska, P., Jousilahti, P., et al. (1994). Twenty-year trends in coronary risk factors in North Karelia and in other areas of Finland. *International Journal of Epidemiology, 23,* 495–504.

Vass, M., & Walsh-Allis, G. A. (1990). Employee dependents: The future focus of worksite health promotion programs and the potential role of the allied health professional. *Journal of Allied Health, 19,* 39–48.

Vasse, R. M., Nijhuis, F. J. N., Kok, G., & Kroodsma, A. T. (1997). Process evaluation of two worksite alcohol programs. In R. Vasse (Ed.), *The development, implementation and evaluation of two worksite health programs aimed at preventing alcohol problems* (pp. 71-88). Maastricht: Maastricht University.

Ventura, S. J., Curtin, S. C., & Mathews, T. J. (1998). Teenage births in the United States: National and state trends, 1990–96. In *National vital statistics system.* Hyattsville, MD: National Center for Health Statistics.

Vertinsky, P. A., & Mangham, C. (1991). *Making it fit: Matching substance-abuse prevention strategies.* Victoria: Alcohol and Drug Programs, Ministry of Health, British Columbia.

Viadro, C. I., Earp, J. A. L., & Altpeter, M. (1997). Designing a process evaluation for a comprehensive breast cancer screening intervention: Challenges and opportunities. *Evaluation and Program Planning, 20,* 237–250.

Vickers, G. (1958). What sets the goals of public health. *New England Journal of Medicine, 258,* 12.

Vickery, D. M., & Fries, J. F. (1981). Effect of self-care book. *Journal of the American Medical Association, 245,* 341–342.

Vickery, D. M., Kalmer, H., Lowry, D., et al. (1983). Effect of a self-care education program on medical visits. *Journal of the American Medical Association, 250,* 2952–2956.

Viet, C. T., & Ware, J. E., Jr. (1982). Measuring health and health-care outcomes: Issues and recommendations. In R. L. Kane & R. A. Kane (Eds.), *Values and long-term care.* Lexington, MA: Lexington Books.

Villas, P., Cardenas, M., & Jameson, C. (1994). Instrument development using the PRECEDE model to distinguish users/triers from non-users of alcoholic beverages. *Wellness Perspectives: Research, Theory and Practice, 10*(2), 46–53.

Vincent, M. L., Clearie, A. F., Johnson, C. G., & Sharpe, P. A. (1988). *Reducing unintended adolescent pregnancy through school/community education interventions: A South Carolina case study.* Columbia: School of Public Health, University of South Carolina.

Vincent, M. L., Clearie, A. F., & Schluchter, M. D. (1987). Reducing adolescent pregnancy through school and community based education. *Journal of the American Medical Association, 257,* 3382–3386.

Viseltear, A. (1976). A short history of P.L. 94-317. In American College of Preventive Medicine and Fogerty Center (Eds.), *Preventive Medicine USA.* New York: Prodist.

Vissandjee, B., Barlow, R., & Fraser, D. W. (1997). Utilization of health services among rural women in Gujarat, India. *Public Health, 111,* 135–148.

Vojtecky, M. A. (1986). Commentary: A unified approach to health promotion and health protection. *Journal of Community Health, 11,* 219–221.

Wade, R. (1982). The evolution of occupational health and the role of government. *Western Journal of Medicine, 6,* 577–580.

Wagner, E. H., & Guild, P. A. (1989). Primer on evaluation methods: Choosing an evaluation strategy. *American Journal of Health Promotion, 4,* 134–139.

Waitzkin, H. (1985). Information giving in medical care. *Journal of Health and Social Behavior, 26,* 81–101.

Walker, R. (1992). The solution or the problem? The role of schools in drug education. *Health Promotion Journal of Australia, 2,* 43–49.

Wallace, P. G., & Haines, A. P. (1984). General practitioners and health promotion: What patients think. *British Medical Journal, 289,* 534–536.

Wallack, L. M. (1980). Assessing effects of mass media campaigns: An alternative perspective. *Alcohol, Health and Research World, 5,* 17–29.

Wallack, L. M. (1981). Mass media campaigns: The odds against finding behavior change. *Health Education Quarterly, 8,* 209–260.

Wallack, L. M. (1983). Mass media campaigns in a hostile environment: Advertising as anti-health education. *Journal of Drug Addiction, 28,* 51–63.

Wallack, L. M. (1985). Health educators and the new generation of strategies. *Hygie, 4*(2), 23–30.

Wallack, L. (1994). Media advocacy: A strategy for empowering people and communities. *Journal of Public Health Policy, 15,* 420–436.

Wallack, L., & Dorfman, L. (1996). Media advocacy: A strategy for advancing policy and promoting health. *Health Education Quarterly, 23,* 293–317.

Wallack, L., M., Dorfman, L., Jernigan, D., & Themba, M. (1993). *Media advocacy and public health: Power for prevention.* Newbury Park: Sage.

Wallerstein, N. (1990). [Review of the book *Participatory planning in community health education: A guide based on the McDowell County, West Virginia experience*]. *Health Education Quarterly, 17,* 119–121.

Wallerstein, N., & Bernstein, E. (1988). Empowerment education: Freire's ideas adapted to health education. *Health Education Quarterly, 15,* 379–394.

Wallerstein, N., & Bernstein, E. (1996) Introduction to [special issue on] community empowerment, participatory education, and health. *Health Education Quarterly, 21,* 141–148.

Wallerstein, N., & Sanchez-Merki, V. (1994). Freirian praxis in health education: Research results from an adolescent prevention program. *Health Education Research, 9,* 105–118.

Walsh, D. C. (1984). Corporate smoking policies: A review and an analysis. *Journal of Occupational Medicine, 26,* 17–22.

Walsh, D. C. (1992). Worksite drug testing. *Annual Review of Public Health, 13,* 197–221.

Walsh, D. C., & Egdahl, R. H. (1989). Corporate perspectives on work site wellness programs: A report on the Seventh Pew Fellows Conference. *Journal of Occupational Medicine, 31,* 551–556.

Walsh, D. C., & Kelleher, S. E. (1987). *Preventing alcohol and drug abuse through programs at the workplace.* Washington, DC: Washington Business Group on Health and Office of Disease Prevention and Health Promotion, Department of Health and Human Services.

Walsh, D. C., & McDougall, V. (1988). Current policies regarding smoking in the workplace. *American Journal of Industrial Medicine, 13,* 181–190.

Walsh, D. C., Rudd, R. E., Biener, L., & Mangione, T. (1993). Researching and preventing alcohol problems at work: Toward an integrative model. *American Journal of Health Promotion, 7,* 289–295.

Walsh, D. C., Rudd, R. E., Moeykens, B. A., & Maloney, T. W. (1993). Social marketing for public health. *Health Affairs, 12,* 104–119.

Walsh, J. M. E., & McPhee, S. J. (1992). A systems model of clinical preventive care: An analysis of factors influencing patient and physician. *Health Education Quarterly, 19*(2), 157–175.

Walter, H. J. (1989). Primary prevention of chronic disease among children: The school-based "Know Your Body" intervention trials. *Health Education Quarterly, 16,* 201–214.

Walter, H. J., Hofman, A., Barrett, L. T., et al. (1987). Primary prevention of cardiovascular disease among children: One-year results of a randomized intervention study. In B. Hetzel & G. S. Berenson (Eds.), *Cardiovascular risk factors in childhood: Epidemiology and prevention* (pp. 161-181). Rotterdam: Elsevier Science Publishers B.V.

Walter, H. J., & Vaughan, R. D. (1993). AIDS risk reduction among a multiethnic sample of urban high-school students. *Journal of the American Medical Association, 270,* 725–730.

Walter, H. J., & Wynder, E. L. (1989). The development, implementation, evaluation, and future directions of a chronic disease prevention program for children: The "Know Your Body" studies. *Preventive Medicine, 18,* 59–71.

Wandersman, A. (1981). A framework of participation in community organization. *Journal of Applied Behavioral Science, 17,* 27–58.

Wandersman, A., Goodman, R., & Butterfoss, F. (1997). Understanding coalitions and how they operate: An "open systems" organizational framework. In M. Minkler (Ed.), *Community organizing and community building for health.* New Brunswick, NJ: Rutgers University Press.

Wang, V. L., Ephross, P., & Green, L. W. (1975). The point of diminishing returns in nutrition education through home visits by aides: An evaluation of EFNEP. *Health Education Monographs, 3,* 70–88. Also in J. Zapka (Ed.), *The SOPHE Heritage Collection of Health Education Monographs* (Vol. 3, pp. 155–173). Oakland, CA: Third Party.

Wang, V. L., Terry, P., Flynn, B. S., et al. (1979). Multiple indicators of continuing medical education priorities for chronic lung diseases in Appalachia. *Journal of Medical Education, 54,* 803–811.

Ward, W. B. (Ed.). (1987). *Advances in health education and promotion. Vol. 2.* Greenwich, CT: JAI Press.

Ward, W. B., Levine, D. M., Morisky, D., et al. (1982). Controlling high blood pressure in inner city Baltimore through community health education. In R. W. Carlaw (Ed.), *Perspectives on community health education: A series of case studies: Vol. 1. United States* (pp. 73–97). Oakland, CA: Third Party.

Ware, B. G. (1985). Occupational health education: A nontraditional role for a health educator. In H. P. Cleary, J. M. Kichen, & P. G. Ensor (Eds.), *Advancing health through education: A case study approach* (pp. 319–323). Palo Alto, CA: Mayfield.

Warner, K. E. (1977). The effects of the anti-smoking campaign on cigarette consumption. *American Journal of Public Health, 67,* 645–650.

Warner, K. E. (1981). Cigarette smoking in the 1970's: The impact of the anti-smoking campaign on consumption. *Science, 211*(13), 729–731.

Warner, K. E. (1986). *Selling smoke: Cigarette advertising and public health.* Washington, DC: American Public Health Association.

Warner, K. E. (1987). Selling health promotion to corporate America: Uses and abuses of the economic argument. *Health Education Quarterly, 14,* 39–55.

Warner, K. E. (1989). Effects of the antismoking campaign: An update. *American Journal of Public Health, 79,* 144–151.

Warner, K. E. (1992). Effects of workplace health promotion not demonstrated. *American Journal of Public Health, 82,* 126.

Warner, K. E., & Murt, H. A. (1983). Premature deaths avoided by the antismoking campaign. *American Journal of Public Health, 73,* 672–677.

Warner, K. E., Smith, R. J., Smith, D. G., & Fries, B. E. (1996). Health and economic implications of a work-site smoking-cessation program: A simulation analysis. *Journal of Occupational and Environmental Medicine, 38,* 981–992.

Warner, K. E., Wickizer, T. M., Wolfe, R. A., et al. (1988). Economic implications of workplace health promotion programs: Review of the literature. *Journal of Occupational Medicine, 30,* 106–112.

The Washington Post/Kaiser Family Foundation/Harvard University Survey Project. (1996). *Why don't Americans trust the government?* Menlo Park, CA: Henry J. Kaiser Family Foundation.

Waterworth, J. (1992). *Multimedia interaction with computers: Human factors issues.* New York: Ellis Horwood.

Weare, K. (1992). The contribution of education to health promotion. In R. Bunton & G. Macdonald (Eds.), *Health promotion: Disciplines and diversity* (pp. 66–85). London: Routledge.

Webb, G. R., Sanson-Fisher, R. W., & Bowman, J. A. (1988). Psychosocial factors related to parental restraint of pre-school children in motor vehicles. *Accident Analysis and Prevention, 20,* 87–94.

Wechsler, H., Levine, S., Idelson, R. K., Rothman, M., & Taylor, J. O. (1983). The physician's role in health promotion: Survey of primary care practitioners. *New England Journal of Medicine, 308,* 97–100.

Weiler, R. M. (1997). Foreword: Twenty-year subject and author index, volume 1, 1977–Volume 21, 1997. *American Journal of Health Behavior, 21,* 403.

Weinberg, M., Mazzuca, S. A., Cohen, S. J., & McDonald, C. J. (1982). Physicians' ratings of information sources about their preventive medicine decisions. *Preventive Medicine, 11,* 717–723.

Weinberg, N., Schmale, J., Uken, J., & Wessel, K. (1996). Online help: Cancer patients participate in a computer-mediated support group. *Health and Social Work, 21*(1), 24–29.

Weinberger, M., Mazzuca, S. A., Cohen, S. J., & McDonald, C. J. (1982). Physicians' rating of information sources about their preventive medicine decisions. *Preventive Medicine, 11,* 717–723.

Weinberger, M., Saunders, A. F., Bearon, L. B., et al. (1992). Physician-related barriers to breast cancer screening in older women [Special issue]. *Journals of Gerontology, 47,* 111–117.

Weiss, C. H. (1973). Between the cup and the lip. *Evaluation, 1*(2), 54.

Weiss, C. H. (1998). *Evaluation: Methods for studying programs and policies* (2nd ed.). Upper Saddle River, NJ: Prentice Hall.

Weiss, J. R., Wallerstein, N., & MacLean, T. (1995). Organizational development of a university-based interdisciplinary health promotion project. *American Journal of Health Promotion, 10,* 37–48.

Weiss, S. M., Herd, J. A., & Fox, B. (Eds.). (1981). *Perspectives on behavioral medicine.* New York: Academic Press.

Weitzel, M. H., & Waller, P. R. (1990). Predictive factors for health-promotive behaviors in white, Hispanic, and black blue-collar workers. *Family and Community Health, 13,* 23–34.

Welles, K. B., Lewis, C. E., Leake, B., Schleiter, M. K., & Brook, R. H. (1986). The practices of general and subspecialty internists in counseling about smoking and exercise. *American Journal of Public Health, 76,* 1009–1013.

Welles, K. B., Ware, J. E., & Lewis, C. E. (1984). Physicians' attitudes in counseling patients about smoking. *Medical Care, 22,* 360–365.

Welles, K. B., Lewis, C. E., Leake, B., & Ware, J. E. (1984). Do physicians preach what they practice? *Journal of the American Medical Association, 252,* 2846–2848.

Wells, B. L., DePue, J. D., Lasater, T. M., & Carleton, R. A. (1988). A report on church site weight control. *Health Education Research, 3,* 305–316.

Werden, P. (1974) Health education for Indian students. *Journal of School Health, 44,* 319–323.

Westberg, J. (1986). Gaining physician support for effective patient education. *Patient Education and Counseling, 8,* 407–414.

Wewers, M. E., & Ahijevych, K. (1995). Low-intensity smoking cessation intervention among African-American women cigarette smokers: A pilot study. *American Journal of Health Promotion, 9,* 337–339.

Wharf Higgins, J., & Green, L. W. (1994). The APHA criteria for development of health promotion programs applied to four healthy community projects in British Columbia. *Health Promotion International, 9,* 311–320.

Wholey, J. S., Hatry, H. P., & Newcomer, K. E. (1994). *Handbook of practical program evaluation.* San Francisco: Jossey-Bass.

Whyte, N., & Berland, A. (1993). *The role of hospital nurses in health promotion: A collaborative survey of British Columbia hospital nurses.* Vancouver: Registered Nurses Association of British Columbia and Vancouver General Hospital, Pub. 28). [See summary: Health promotion in acute care settings: Redefining a nursing tradition. *Nursing BC,* March–April, 1994, pp. 21–22.]

Wickizer, T. M., Wagner, E., & Perrin, E. B. (1998). Implementation of the Henry J. Kaiser Family Foundation's Community Health Promotion Grant Program: A process evaluation. *Milbank Quarterly, 76,* 121–153.

Wikler, D. (1987). Who should be blamed for being sick? *Health Education Quarterly, 14,* 11–25.

Willemsen, M. C., deVries, H., van Breukelen, G., & Oldenburg, B. (1996). Determinants of intention to quit smoking among Dutch employees: The influence of the social environment. *Preventive Medicine, 25,* 195–202.

Williams, A. F., & Wechsler, H. (1972). Interrelationship of preventive actions in health and other areas. *Health Services Reports, 87,* 969–976.

Williams, G. A., Abbott, R. R., & Taylor, D. K. (1997). Using focus group methodology to develop breast cancer screening programs that recruit African American women. *Journal of Community Health, 22,* 2245–2256.

Williams, L. S. (1986). AIDS risk reduction: A community health education intervention for minority high risk group members. *Health Education Quarterly, 13,* 407–422.

Williams, M. D. (1993). *A comprehensive review of learner-control: The role of learner characteristics.* New Orleans, LA: Proceedings of Selected Research and Development Presentations at the Convention of the Association for Educational Communications and Technology. ERIC Document Reproduction Service No. 362 211.

Williams, R. M. (1990). Rx: Social reconnaissance. *Foundation News, 31*(4), 24–29.

Williamson, J. W., & Chapin, J. M. (1980). Adverse reactions to prescribed drugs in the elderly: A multicare investigation. *Age and Aging, 9,* 73–80.

Williamson, N. B., Burton, M. J., Brown, W. B., et al. (1988). Changes in mastitis management practices associated with client education and the effects of adopting recommended mastitis control procedures on herd production. *Preventive Veterinary Medicine, 5,* 213–223.

Williamson, P. S., Driscoll, C. E., Dvorak, L. D., Garber, K. A., & Shank, J. C., (1988). Health screening examinations: The patient's prespective. *Journal of Family Practice, 27,* 187–192.

Wilshire, B. L., Kreuter, M. W., Kunyosying, A., et al. (1997) *Development of the STARLITE personal interest scale: A preliminary validation study.* Paper presented at the 1997 American Public Health Association Annual Meeting, Indianapolis, IN.

Wilson, R. W. (1986). The PRECEDE model for mental health education. *Journal of Human Behavior and Learning, 3*(2), 34–41.

Wilson, R. W., & Elinson, J. (1981). National survey of personal health practices and consequences: Background, conceptual issues, and selected findings. *Public Health Reports, 96,* 218–225.

Wilson, R. W., & Iverson, D. C. (1982). Federal data bases for health education research. *Health Education, 13*(3), 30–34.

Wilson, W. J. (1987). *The truly disadvantaged: The inner city, the underclass, and public policy.* Chicago: University of Chicago Press.

Winder, A. E. (1985). The mouse that roared: A case history of community organization for health practice. *Health Education Quarterly, 12,* 353–363.

Windom, R., McGinnis, J. M., & Fielding, J. E. (1987). Examining worksite health promotion programs. *Business and Health, 4,* 26–37.

Windsor, R. A. (1984). Planning and evaluation of public health education programs in rural settings: Theory into practice. In H. P. Cleary, J. M. Kichen, & P. G. Ensor (Eds.), *Advancing health through education: A case study approach* (pp. 273–284). Palo Alto, CA: Mayfield.

Windsor, R. A. (1986). An application of the PRECEDE model for planning and evaluating education methods for pregnant smokers. *Hygie: International Journal of Health Education, 5,* 38–43.

Windsor, R. A., Baranowski, T., Clark, N., & Cutter, G. (1994). *Evaluation of health promotion, health education, and disease prevention programs* (2nd ed.). Mountain View, CA: Mayfield.

Windsor, R. A., & Bartlett, E. (1984). Employee self-help smoking cessation programs: A review of the literature. *Health Education Quarterly, 11,* 349–359.

Windsor, R. A., & Cutter, G. (1983, July 10–15). A randomized trial to evaluate the effectiveness of a smoking cessation program for pregnant women: Study intervention, methods, and design. In *Proceeedings of the Fifth World Conference on Smoking and Health,* Winnipeg, Manitoba.

Windsor, R. A., Cutter, G., Morris, J., et al. (1985). Effectiveness of self-help smoking cessation interventions for pregnant women in public health maternity clinics: A randomized trial. *American Journal of Public Health, 75,* 1389–1392.

Windsor, R. A., Felknor, S. A., Friel, J., et al. (Eds.). (1988). *Conference proceedings: XIII World Conference on Health Education: Participation for All in Health, 1988, Houston, Texas, USA* (2 vols.). Atlanta, GA: Centers for Disease Control, Public Health Service, U.S. Department of Health and Human Services.

Windsor, R. A., Green, L. W., & Roseman, J. M. (1980). Health promotion and maintenance for patients with chronic obstructive pulmonary disease: A review. *Journal of Chronic Disease, 33,* 5–12.

Windsor, R. A., & Orleans, C. T. (1986). Guidelines and methodological standards for smoking cessation intervention research among pregnant women: Improving the science and art. *Health Education Quarterly, 13*(2), 131–161.

Winett, R. A., Altman, D. G., & King, A. C. (1990). Conceptual and strategic foundations for effective media campaigns for preventing the spread of HIV infection. *Evaluation and Program Planning, 13,* 91–104.

Winett, R. A., King, A. C., & Altman, D. G. (1989). Health in the workplace. In R. A. Winett, A. C. King, & D. G. Altman (Eds.), *Health psychology and public health* (pp. 285–313). New York: Pergamon Press.

Winickoff, R. N., Coltin, K. L., Morgan, M. M., Busbaum, R. C., & Barnett, G. O. (1984). Improving physician performance through peer companions. *Medical Care, 22,* 527–534.

Winkleby, M. A., Fortmann, S. P., & Barrett, D. C. (1990). Social class disparities in risk factors for disease: Eight-year prevalence patterns by level of education. *Preventive Medicine, 19,* 1–12.

Winkleby, M. A., Kraemer, H. C., & Varady, A. N. (1998). Ethnic and socioeconomic differences in cardiovascular disease risk factors: Findings for women from the Third National Health and Nutrition Examination Survey, 1988–1994. *Journal of the American Medical Association, 280,* 356–362.

Winslow, C. E. A. (1920). The untilled fields of public health. *Science, 51,* 23.

Witherspoon, D. (1990). Making wellness an effective tool for cultural change. *Employee Health and Fitness, 12,* 153–168.

Witte, K. (1994). Fear control and danger control: A test of the Extended Parallel Process Model (EPPM). *Communication Monographs, 61,* 113–134.

Wojtowicz, G. G. (1990). A secondary analysis of the school health education evaluation data base. *Journal of School Health, 60,* 56–59.

Wong, M. L., Alsagoff, F., & Koh, D. (1992). Health promotion: A further field to conquer. *Singapore Medical Journal, 33,* 341–346.

Wong, M. L., Chan, R., Koh, D., & Wong, C. M. (1994–1995). Theory and action for effective condom promotion: Illustrations from a behavior intervention project for sex workers in Singapore. *International Quarterly of Community Health Education, 15,* 405–421.

Wong, M. L., Chan, R., Koh, D., & Wong, C. M. (1996). Controlled evaluation of a behavioural intervention programme on condom use and gonorrhoea incidence among sex workers in Singapore. *Health Education Research, 11,* 423–432.

Wong, T. Y., & Seet, B. (1998). A behavioral analysis of eye protection use by soldiers. *Military Medicine, 162,* 744–748.

Woo, B., Woo, B., Cook, F., Weisberg, M., & Goldman, L. (1985). Screening procedures in the asymptomatic adult: Comparison of physicians' recommendations, patients' desires, published guidelines, and actual practice. *Journal of the American Medical Association, 254,* 1480–1484.

Woodruff, K. (1996). Alcohol advertising and violence against women: A media advocacy case study. *Health Education Quarterly, 23,* 330–345.

Woodruff, S. I., Candelaria, J., & Zaslow, K. A. (1996). Implementation factors related to outcomes of a nutrition education program for Latinos with limited English proficiency. *Journal of Nutrition Education, 28,* 219–222.

Worden, J. K., Flynn, B. S., Geller, B. M., et al. (1988). Development of a smoking prevention mass-media program using diagnostic and formative research. *Preventive Medicine, 17,* 531–558.

Worden, J. K., Flynn, B. S., Solomon, L. J., et al. (1996). Using mass media to prevent cigarette smoking among adolescent girls. *Health Education Quarterly, 23,* 453–468.

Worden, J. K., Solomon, L. J., Flynn, B. S., et al. (1990). A community-wide program in breast self-examination training and maintenance. *Preventive Medicine, 19,* 254–269.

Workman, S. (1989). (1988). The PRECEDE model applied: A comparison of two communities. In *Proceedings of the XIII World Conference on Health Education, Houston* (Vol. 1, p. 131, Abstract No. 4208-1). Houston, TX: U.S. Host Committee for International Union for Health Education, P.O. Box 20186, W-902 RAS Bldg.

Workplace health: Discovering the needs. (1990). Ottawa: Health and Welfare Canada.

World Health Assembly. (1985). *New policies for health education in primary health care: Technical discussions of the 36th World Health Assembly.* Geneva: World Health Organization.

World Health Organization. (1978). *Alma-Ata 1978: Primary health care* (HFA Ser. No. 1). Geneva: World Health Organization.

World Health Organization. (1979a). *Health for all by the year 2000* (HFA Ser. No. 1). Geneva: World Health Organization.

World Health Organization. (1979b). *Report of the Task Force on Health Education in Family Health* (Tech. Rep. Ser. 45). Geneva: World Health Organization.

World Health Organization. (1980). *International classification of impairments, disabilities, and handicaps: A manual of classification relating to the consequences of disease.* Geneva: World Health Organization.

World Health Organization. (1981). *Health program evaluation: Guiding principles.* Geneva: World Health Organization.

World Health Organization. (1983). *Expert committee on new approaches to health education in primary health care.* (Tech. Rep. Ser. 690). Geneva: World Health Organization.

World Health Organization. (1984, September). *Health promotion: A discussion document on the concept and principles.* Copenhagen: World Health Organization, Regional Office for Europe, ICP/HSR 602. Reprinted in (1986). *Health Promotion, 1,* 73–76.

World Health Organization. (1986a). Ottawa charter for health promotion. *Health Promotion International, 1,* iii–iv.

World Health Organization. (1986b). *Targets for health for all.* Copenhagen: World Health Organization, Regional Office for Europe.

World Health Organization. (1996). *Promoting health through schools: The World Health Organization's global school health initiative.* Geneva: Author.

World Health Organization. (1997). *Promoting health through schools: Report of a WHO expert committee on comprehensive school health education and promotion.* Geneva: WHO Technical Report Series 870.

World Health Organization and United Nations Children's Fund. (1986). *Helping a billion children learn about health: Report of the WHO/UNICEF international consultation on health education for school-age children, 1985.* Geneva: World Health Organization.

World Health Organization Quality of Life Group. (1996). What quality of life? *World Health Forum, 17,* 354–356.

Worrall, L., Hickson, L., Barnett, H., & Yiu, E. (1998). An evaluation of the Keep on Talking program for maintaining communication skills into old age. *Educational Gerontology, 24,* 129–140.

Wortel, E., de Geus, G. H., Kok, G., & van Woerkum, C. (1994). Injury control in pre-school children: A review of parental safety measures and the behavioural determinants. *Health Education Research, 9,* 201–213.

Wortel, E., de Vries, H., & de Geus, G. H. (1995). Lessons learned from a community campaign on child safety in The Netherlands. *Family and Community Health, 18,* 60–77.

Wurtele, S., Roberts, M., & Leeper, J. (1982). Health beliefs and intentions: Predictors of return compliance in a tuberculosis detection drive. *Journal of Applied Social Psychology, 53,* 19–21.

Wyllie, A., & Casswell, S. (1989). The response of New Zealand boys to corporate and sponsorship alcohol advertising on television. *British Journal of Addiction, 84,* 639–646.

Xin-Zhi, W., Zhao-guang, H., & Dan-yang, C. (1987). Smoking prevalence in Chinese aged 15 and above. *Chinese Medical Journal, 100,* 686–692.

Yandrick, R. M. (1990, June). With the release of two hallmark documents, EAPA is helping position our young profession for growth and development in the 1990s. *EAPA Exchange,* pp. 14–21.

Yeo, M. V. (1998). *Drug-related illness in the elderly: Patients' perceptions of factors affecting medication self-management practices.* Unpublished doctoral dissertation. Calgary: Department of Educational Psychology, University of Calgary, Alberta.

Yingling, L., & Trocino, L. (1997). Strategies to integrate patient and family education into patient care redesign. *AACN Clinical Issues, 8,* 246–252.

Young, M. A. C. (1967). Review of research and studies related to health education communication: Methods and materials. *Health Education Monographs, 1*(25), 18–24.

Yukl, G. (1994). *Leadership in organizations* (3rd ed.). Englewood Cliffs, NJ: Prentice-Hall.

Zabora, J. R., Morrison, C., Olsen, S. J., & Ashley, B. (1997). Recruitment of underserved women for breast cancer detection programs. *Cancer Practice, 5*(5), 297–303.

Zapka, J. G. (1985). Management functions of the health education director: Examples of data management activities. In H. P. Cleary, J. Kitchen, & P. Ensor (Eds.), *Advancing health through education: A case study approach.* Palo Alto, CA: Mayfield.

Zapka, J. G., & Averill, B. W. (1979). Self care for colds: A cost-effective alternative to upper respiratory infection management. *American Journal of Public Health, 69,* 814–816.

Zapka, J. G., Chasan, L., Barth, R., Mas, E., & Costanza, M. E. (1992). Emphasizing screening activities in a community health center: A case study of a breast cancer screening project. *Journal of Ambulatory Care Management, 15,* 38–47.

Zapka, J. G., Costanza, M. E., Harris, D. R., et al. (1993). Impact of a breast cancer screening community intervention. *Preventive Medicine, 22,* 34–53.

Zapka, J. G., & Dorfman, S. (1982). Consumer participation: Case study of the college health setting. *Journal of American College Health, 30,* 197–203.

Zapka, J. G., Harris, D. R., Hosmer, D., et al. (1993). Effect of a community health center intervention on breast cancer screening among Hispanic American women. *Health Services Research, 28,* 223–335.

Zapka, J. G., & Mamon, J. A. (1982). Integration of theory, practitioner standards, literature findings and baseline data: A case study in planning breast self-examination education. *Health Education Quarterly, 9,* 330–356.

Zapka, J. G., & Mamon, J. A. (1986). Breast self-examination in young women: II. Characteristics associated with proficiency. *American Journal of Preventive Medicine, 2,* 70–78.

Zapka, J. G., & Mazur, R. M. (1977). Peer sex training and evaluation. *American Journal of Public Health, 67,* 450–454.

Zapka, J. G., Stoddard, A., & Barth, R., et al. (1989). Breast cancer screening utilization by Latina community health center clients. *Health Education Research, 4,* 461–468.

Zapka, J. G., Stoddard, A. M., Costanza, M. E., & Greene, H. L. (1989). Breast cancer screening by mammography: Utilization and associated factors. *American Journal of Public Health, 79,* 1499–1502.

Zeldman, M., & Myrom, S. (1983). *How to plan projects and keep them on schedule.* San Diego, CA: Integrated Software Systems.

Zelnik, M., & Kim, Y. J. (1982). Sex education and its association with teenage sexual activity. *Family Planning Perspectives, 14,* 117–126.

Zhang, D., & Z. Qiu (1993). "School-based tobacco-use prevention: People's Republic of China, May 1989–January 1990. *Morbidity and Mortality Weekly Report 42*(19), 370–377.

Ziff, M. A., Conrad, P., & Lachman, M. E. (1995). The relative effects of perceived personal control and responsibility on health and health-related behaviors in young and middle-aged adults. *Health Education Quarterly, 22,* 127–142.

Ziglio, E. (1997). How to move towards evidence-based health promotion interventions. *Promotion and Education, 4*(2), 29–33.

Zill, N., & Rogers, C. C. (1988). Recent trends in the well-being of children in the United States and their implications for public policy. In A. Cherlin (Ed.), *Family change and public policy.* Washington, DC: Urban Institute Press.

Zimmerman, M. (1998). Editorial. *Health Education and Behavior, 25*(1), 1–3.

Zuckerman, A. E., Olevsky-Peleg, E., Bush, P. J., et al. (1989). Cardiovascular risk factors among black schoolchildren: Comparisons among four Know Your Body studies. *Preventive Medicine, 18,* 113–132.

Zuckerman, M. J., Guerra, L. G., Drossman, D. A., Foland, J. A., & Gregory, G. G. (1996). Health-care-seeking behaviors related to bowel complaints: Hispanics versus non-Hispanic whites. *Digestive Diseases and Sciences, 41,* 77–82.

Index